DIAGNOSIS AND TREATMENT
OF
PAIN OF
VERTEBRAL ORIGIN

A Manual Medicine Approach

DIAGNOSIS AND TREATMENT OF
PAIN OF
VERTEBRAL ORIGIN

A Manual Medicine Approach

ROBERT MAIGNE

Former Chef du Service de Rééducation et de Médecine orthopédique de l'Hôtel-Dieu (Université Paris VI)
Professeur au Collège de Médecine des Hôpitaux de Paris
Past President, International Federation of Manual Medicine

Translated by Georgette Kamenetz
with the editorial assistance of Walter L. Nieves, M.D.,
and Hillel M. Sommer, M.D.

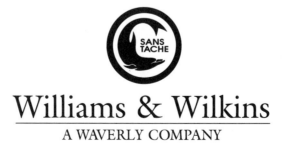

Williams & Wilkins
A WAVERLY COMPANY

BALTIMORE • PHILADELPHIA • LONDON • PARIS • BANGKOK
BUENOS AIRES • HONG KONG • MUNICH • SYDNEY • TOKYO • WROCLAW

Editor: John P. Butler
Managing Editor: Linda S. Napora
Production Coordinator: Carol Eckhart and Anne Stewart-Seitz
Copy Editor: Anne K. Schwartz
Designer: Norman W. Och
Illustration Planner: Lorraine Wrzosek
Cover Designer: Tom Scheureman
Typesetter: Maryland Composition, Inc.
Printer: Maple Press
Binder: Maple Press

351 West Camden Street
Baltimore, Maryland 21201-2436 USA

Rose Tree Corporate Center
1400 North Providence Road
Building II, Suite 5025
Media, Pennsylvania 19063-2043 USA

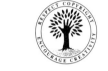

Accurate indications, adverse reactions and dosage schedules for drugs are provided in this book, but it is possible that they may change. The reader is urged to review the package information data of the manufacturers of the medications mentioned.

Printed in the United States of America

First Edition,

Library of Congress Cataloging-in-Publication Data

Maigne, Robert.
   [Diagnostic et traitement des douleurs commones d'origine
rachidienne. English]
   Diagnosis and treatment of pain of vertebral origin : a manual medicine
approach / Robert Maigne : translated and edited by Walter L.
Nieves.
      p.   cm.
   Includes bibliographical references and index.
   ISBN 0-683-05376-0
   1. Spine—Diseases—Treatment. 2. Manipulation (Therapeutics)
3. Pain—Treatment. I. Nieves, Walter L. II. Title.
   [DNLM: 1. Spine—anatomy & histology. 2. Spine—physiopathology.
3. Manipulation, Orthopedic. 4. Pain—therapy. 5. Spinal Diseases.
WE 725 M218d 1995a]
RD768.M28813 1995
617.3'75—dc20
DNLM/DLC
for Library of Congress   94-29321
                                              CIP

Translated by Georgette Kamenetz
with editorial assistance of
Walter L. Nieves, M.D., and Hillel Sommer, M.D.

The publishers have made every effort to trace the copyright holders for borrowed material. If they have inadvertently overlooked any, they will be pleased to make the necessary arrangements at the first opportunity.

95 96 97 98 99
1 2 3 4 5 6 7 8 9 10

FOREWORD

At a time in medicine when pain assumes a great proportion of disability and much is related to the neuromusculoskeletal system, all approaches merit exposition.

Dr. Maigne has been a strong proponent of diagnostic manual medicine and has offered a scientific basis for relief by manipulative techniques. He has written extensively in French, and his methods have been studied by physicians from many countries. Physicians and students, the world over, have been privileged to study his methods and techniques. His books have literally become tomes of valuable information and his concepts have become accepted in medical orthopedics.

Manipulative technique however is only a small, albeit prominent, aspect of this text. Dr. Maigne has scientifically verified and explained many peripheral impairments as being related to their origin at the vertebral level from the posterior radicular branches and minor articular or discal abnormalities. His neuoranatomical explanations are brilliantly illustrated and documented with a profound review of the literature. In today's epidemic disabilities resulting from neuromuscular etiologies, Maigne's concepts and clinical evaluation are welcomed.

The modality of vertebral manipulation has enjoyed advocacy for centuries, but the precise indications and the specific technique indicated for the pathology ascertained remain inaccurate. Dr. Maigne has developed diagnostic procedures that accurately ascertain the exact pathology and its vertebral site. Such accuracy has been deficient in most osteopathic and chiropractic specialties that advocate manipulation.

The concept of regaining lost joint range of motion, which is considered the basis of osteopathic and chiropractic techniques, by forcing that particular segment further is disputed by Maigne. He advocates manipulating in the direction that is free and contralateral to the direction that provokes pain. The direction, the precise vertebral segment, and its pathological significance are the basis of the Maigne techniques.

Manipulative technique also begs clarification and demands personal hands-on learning. This has been Dr. Maigne's success in personally training physicians from all over the world. The benefit he has given patients who have come from all over the world for his services affirms the benefit of his method.

In this text, his techniques are clearly and precisely demonstrated and allow the trainee to learn from reading. The illustrations for appropriate diagnosis and ultimate treatment are extremely well presented. To reiterate, however, the value of this text is to acquire the technique of manual evaluation of the mechanism of common pain of spinal origin that justifies manipulative intervention.

Many practitioners of medicine were denied this text because it was in French. Fortunately, it is now available for English-reading physicians and therapists and will become a mandatory text in all medical libraries and offices.

René Cailliet, M.D.
Professor Emeritus, Department of Physical Medicine
School of Medicine of the University of Southern California
Author of Neuromusculoskeletal Pain Series,
F.A. Davis Company, Philadelphia

PREFACE

The purpose of this book is to invite the reader to take a new look at common pains of spinal origin. My first book, *Les manipulations vertébrales*, published in 1960, aimed at recognition of this therapeutic method by the medical profession. At that time manipulation was widely criticized, rejected, and even considered a kind of charlatanism. It is true that manipulation was used as the only form of treatment by certain nonmedical schools who considered hypothetic vertebral microdisplacements the source of all disease. However, experience convinced me of their potential. Therefore, I attempted to present their indications and contraindictions precisely, to select the reliable techniques, describe them in an objective way, and assign a clear rule of application. I proposed the "rule of pain free and opposite motion." That is to say that the manipulation must be performed in a direction in which the range of *motion is free* and *opposite to the direction in which the motion is painful*, rather than simply attempting to restore a real or supposed limitation of the mobility of a vertebral segment.

This rationale for manipulation achieved recognition by the Faculty of Medicine, and in 1969, a diploma of "Orthopaedic Medicine and Manual Therapeutics" was created at the University of Paris VI (Broussals Faculty-Hotel-Dieu). I was offered the directorship of the program—a program that extended far beyond the simple teaching of these techniques and covered broadly common vertebral pathology. During the following 20 years, teaching founded on the same model was organized in other medical schools in France; Marseille being the first in 1975.

My second book, *Douleurs d'origine vertébrale et traitements par manipulations*, had the subtitle, *Les dérangements intervertébraux mineurs*.

The sometimes surprising results of these treatments compelled one to reflect. Often, in a very spectacular way, vertebral manipulation relieved a certain pain, whose spinal origin was evident (though the mechanism of action was not clear), and other pains, apparently unrelated to the spine, would disappear. However, when inappropriately executed, these techniques could provoke both types of pain.

Traditional practitioners of manipulation, coming for the most part from osteopathy, maintained that the loss of mobility of specific vertebral segments, which according to them was detectable by palpation, could explain and justify their maneuvers.

In fact, I noticed that the segments at the origin of a local or referred pain were themselves tender when certain maneuvers of direct pressure (segmental examination), were carried out. After a successful manipulation, these same segments became pain free on segmental examination. The key point, then, was the segmental tenderness and not the hypothetic loss of mobility; this finding corresponded perfectly with the application of manipulation according to the rule of "pain free and opposite motion."

I therefore proposed the term *painful minor intervertebral dysfunction* (DIM-French, PMID-English), for these painful, benign, self-sustained dysfunctions of the spinal segment. Frequently resulting from trauma, exertion, false movements, or secondary to static or postural problems, these painful minor intervertebral dysfunctions are usually reversible and have no radiologic findings. They can affect radiologically normal segments as well as segments with signs of degeneration.

While the PMID was first merely a hypothesis about the indications and actions of manipulation, it has now become an uncontested clinical reality extending far beyond the frame of manipulation even though the underlying pathophysiology has not yet been clearly established. Its everyday use shows us that it is at the origin of most common intervertebral pain syndrome.

Another element became apparent, both confirming and clarifying the role played by manipulation. With systematic palpation of the skinfolds, muscles, and tendons, I realized that the PMID frequently was associated with abnormal tissue reflexes in the homologous spinal segment. These changes became apparent through modifications in tissue consistency and sensitivity: painful thickening of the skinfolds to *pince-roule* (pinch-roll) throughout all or part of the dermatome, areas of focal muscular hypertonus among certain muscles of the myotome, and hypersensitivity to palpation of the tenoperiosteal insertion. Moreover, I also found these neurotrophic disturbances in the same distribution in other spinal segmental pain syndromes, for example, disc herniation or facet joint capsulitis or synovitis. These manifestations, which I group under the term *segmental celluloperiostiomyalgic syndrome*, can be the origin of certain misleading pains such as pseudoradicular, pseudoarticular, and pseudovisceral syndromes.

Furthermore, their topography is rather consistent for a given spinal segment, particularly in the case of cellulalgia, which allows one to demonstrate objectively the role played by the posterior rami in a number of painful syndromes of the back, such as cervicogenic dorsalgia and low back pain with an origin in the upper lumbar spine, as well as to describe some frequent but misunderstood syndromes such as that of the thoracolumbar junction or other junctional syndromes.

Radiographic imaging has made marked progress in recent years. It provides a nearly perfect means of detecting many of the serious spinal lesions, be they inflammatory, infectious, neoplastic, traumatic, or otherwise. However, it is not as useful in the domain of common pain syndromes. While these imaging techniques provide a sophisticated means of delineating degenerative lesions or other structural anomalies, the relationship between these images and the patient's pain complaint is often difficult to establish. While it has been known for quite some time that significant vertebral spondylosis as well as disk degeneration can be entirely painless, it is now readily apparent that there are also some cases of frank disk herniation, clearly visible on CT or MRI, that produces no discomfort whatsoever. Conversely, there are many patients who present with a significant degree of painful symptoms, who have normal imaging studies or studies that disclose lesions so benign that it is difficult to identify them as causative agents.

It is especially in these cases that the guidelines constituted by the painful minor intervertebral dysfunction and the segmental celluloperiostiomyalgic syndrome are of great value. These guidelines provide us with an understanding of many pains that are not well defined and, therefore, are not well treated; they furnish us with a kind of ''Ariane's thread'' to help us find our way in the maze of all these pains by which the physician is confronted on a daily basis; they broaden the semiology and restore to the clinical examination all its superiority.

Nevertheless, we shall neglect neither the traditional repertoire of the well-established semiologic, classic, and pathogenic notions nor the recent advances that facilitate diagnosis and treatment of common painful syndromes of the spine. Indeed, it is not sufficient merely to diagnosis; one must treat as well. For this reason, a significant segment of this book deals with treatment; particularly the manual therapies that when well executed are so often effective.

                                                                        R.M.

CONTENTS

SECTION I
ANATOMY

SECTION II
BIOMECHANICS

SECTION III
PAIN OF SPINAL ORIGIN

S E C T I O N   I V
EXAMINATION OF THE SPINE

S E C T I O N   V
TREATMENT

SECTION VI
CLINICAL ASPECTS OF PAIN OF SPINAL ORIGIN

xiv   CONTENTS

SECTION VII
MANUAL TECHNIQUES

I

ANATOMY

1

CURVATURES

The vertebral column, or spine, is the axis of the human body. Its functions are to protect the spinal cord and the nerve roots that emerge from it, to sustain the viscera that are fastened to it, and to provide support to the head and the shoulder girdle.

The spine is a flexible axis composed of articulated vertebrae that allow the column to readily deform its shape while still maintaining its rigidity. The vertebral column has been compared to a mast placed on a ship's hull (the pelvis), supporting a large transverse yard (the shoulder girdle). At all levels there is a musculoligamentous framework that braces the column. All of these structures, which are controlled by extrapyramidal pathways, readily adapt instantaneously and automatically to changes in posture, position, or physical exertion by a permanent adjustment in muscular tone.

The spinal column is composed of 24 articulated vertebrae (Fig. 1.1): 7 cervical, 12 thoracic, 5 lumbar, 5 sacral (fused into one), and 3 coccygeal (often fused into one). Fibrocartilaginous disks that act as shock absorbers are located between all articulated vertebrae with the exception of C1-C2.

TYPES

The spinal column is composed of three curves:

- A cervical lordosis
- A thoracic kyphosis
- A lumbar lordosis

These curves may vary in their degree of accentuation (Fig. 1.2). The degree of curvature in the sagittal plane can be measured using the "Delmas index," which compares the surface length of the entire column to its vertical height. The mean index is 95 (Fig. 1.3). A spine with an index lower than 94 is a spine with marked curvature, referred to as the "dynamic spine" of Delmas. A vertical axis passing through the body's center of gravity passes through the two extremities of the spine (Fig. 1.4):

- Superiorly, the craniocervical junction
- Inferiorly, the lumbosacral junction

This axis passes just posterior to the body of L3.

EMBRYOLOGY

At birth, the spinal column assumes the form of a C-shaped curve concave anteriorly; as the child progressively attains the ability to extend the neck, the *cervical lordosis* is formed. The *lumbar lordosis*, which develops as a result of the human's upright posture, begins at age 3 and becomes fully developed at around age 10 (Fig. 1.5).

The "keystone" vertebrae of these curves are the ones that are situated at the apex:

- C6 for the cervical curve
- T7 for the thoracic curve
- L3 for the lumbar curve

SPINAL CURVES AND RESISTANCE TO LOADING

The spinal curves increase the shock-absorbing capacity of the vertebral column and facilitate its stability and equilibrium. The ver-

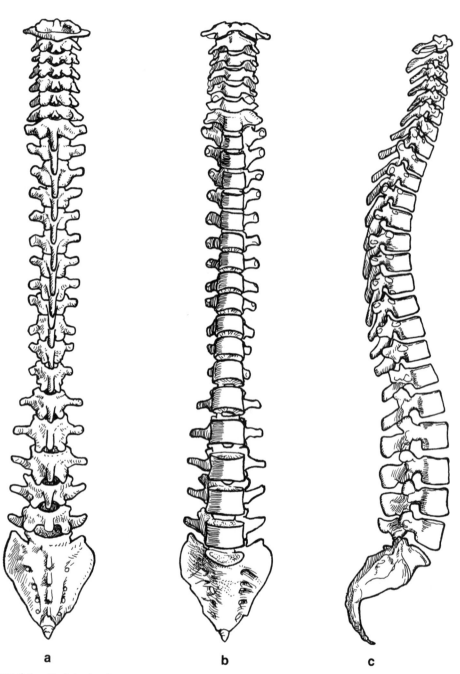

Figure 1.1. Vertebral column and sacrum. **a.** Posterior view. **b.** Anterior view. **c.** Lateral view.

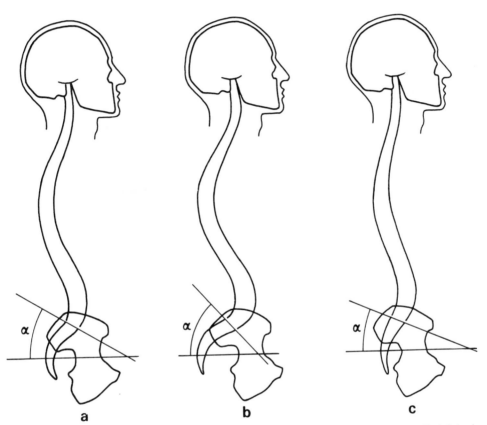

Figure 1.2.   Vertebral curves. **a.** Normal curve. **b.** Accentuated curvature. **c.** Attenuated or diminished curvature. There is a relationship between the degree of curvature and the inclination of the sacral promontory.

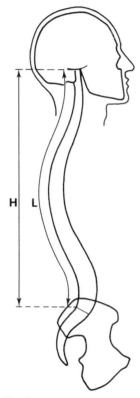

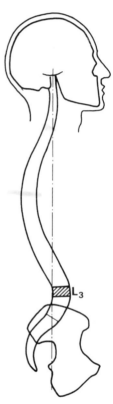

Figure 1.3.   The Delmas index: $H \times 100/L$, where L is the length of the entire vertebral column and H is the height of the vertebral column.

Figure 1.4.   The plumb line passes through the foramen magnum on a line tangent to the posterior aspect of $L3$ and through the middle of the sacral promontory.

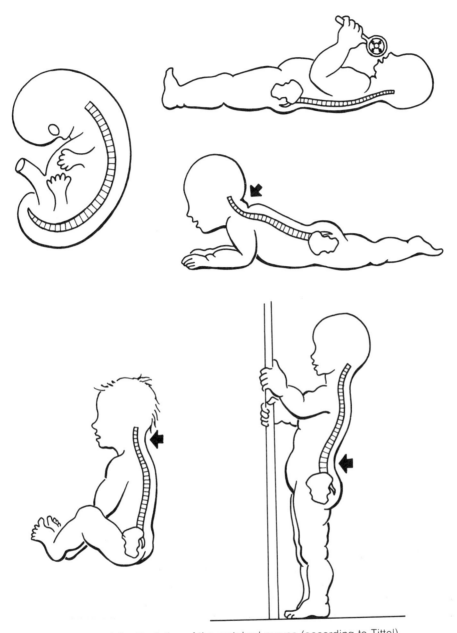

Figure 1.5. Evolution of the vertebral curves (according to Tittel).

tebral column acts like an elastic column with alternating curves. Because it has three curves, the spine is 10 times more resistant to loading than if there were no curves.

The law of physics that governs elastic columns with alternating curves is expressed as follows: if n is the number of curvatures and 1 is the resistance of a straight column system, the resistance of the system with alternating curves is equal to $n^2 + 1$, in this case $3^2 + 1 = 10$. Although this law cannot be strictly applied to the spine, it nevertheless gives us an appreciation of the effect of spinal curves on stability.

2

TYPICAL VERTEBRAE

DIFFERENT GROUPS OF VERTEBRAE

Each vertebra is unique and differs, sometimes very slightly, from its neighbor. There are three groups:

- Cervical vertebrae
- Thoracic vertebrae
- Lumbar vertebrae

The vertebrae in each group possess common characteristics, and each is a variant of the "typical vertebra" (Fig. 2.1) that serves as a prototype for description. The "typical vertebra" is composed of a posterior neural arch of a horseshoe shape that is attached to the posterior aspect of the vertebral body, thus forming the spinal canal. This arch gives rise to the zygapophyseal joints on either side, which are anchored to the vertebral body via the pedicles. Two laminae form the posterior aspect of the spinal canal and unite in the midline to form the spinous process. Two transverse processes are formed, one on each side of the body, at the posterior aspect of the arch near the articular pillars.

STRUCTURE OF THE VERTEBRAL BODY

Vertebral Endplate

The vertebral body is cylindrical. Its superior and inferior margins are referred to as endplates. These endplates are slightly concave in all directions. They are composed of two parts:

- A central part layered with cartilage and riddled with small apertures that play an essential role in the nutrition of the disk
- A peripheral part, white in color, that forms an annular pad into which the annulus fibrosus of the disk is inserted

This peripheral part is the ring epiphysis, which acts as the ossification center for the body; it fuses at about age 14.

Bony Framework

The vertebral body is composed of a trabecular system that projects in three directions: vertical, oblique, and horizontal. The function of the *vertical trabeculae* is to support the vertebral column. The oblique trabeculae are made up of two bundles (Figs. 2.2 and 2.3). One arises from the inferior aspect of the endplate and passes through the pedicles to form the superior articular facet and spinous process. The other arises from the superior endplate and passes through the pedicles to form the inferior articular process and spinous process. This creates a region of enhanced posterior resistance, the posterior column (described by G. Rieunau and P. Decoulx), which is composed of the posterior aspect of the vertebral body and the pedicles. Rieunau and Decoulx have therefore classified vertebral fractures as stable if they spare the posterior column and as unstable if they do not. The anterior surface of the vertebra, containing only vertical trabeculae, is a zone of least resistance and hence a frequent site of compression fracture. This region is triangular with a posterior apex and corresponds to the vascular equatorial zone. The *horizontal and radial trabeculae* join the lateral cortical trabeculae.

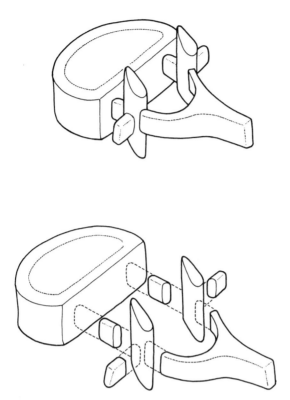

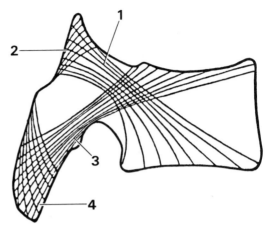

Figure 2.2.   The trabecular system: *1*, oblique superior trabecular bundle; *2* and *4*, supporting trabeculae of the facet joints; *3*, interior oblique bundle. Not shown in the diagram are the vertical system (the vertical trabeculae that aid in the essential function of weight bearing) and the horizontal radicular system of trabeculae (which radiate out from the axial line to the periphery).

Figure 2.1.   The typical vertebra.

Figure 2.3.   Osseous vertebral trabeculae: *1*, sheaf bundles; *2*, transverse bundles.

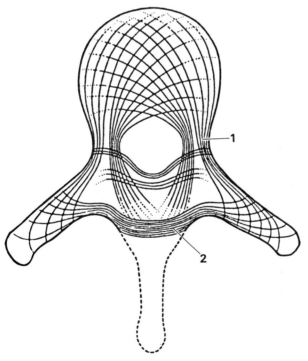

ARCHITECTURE OF THE POSTERIOR ARCH

The posterior arch is formed by (*a*) an inter-transverse trabecular system that extends from one transverse process to the other and passes through the laminae and (*b*) a U-shaped trabecular system bordering the superior part of the laminae between the two superior articular processes (Paturet). It is independent of the superior and inferior oblique trabeculae that open like a fan in the thickness of the superior and inferior articular processes.

CARTILAGINOUS ENDPLATES

Cartilaginous endplates are the reproductive zones that provide growth in height. They are thin in the adult and thick in the child in accordance with their respective degree of function.

Some pathologic processes can damage the endplates and impair bony growth, resulting in vertebral body malformations. The cartilaginous endplates detach more easily from the vertebral body than from the disk; in fact, they are considered part of the disk by H. Junghanns.

ZYGAPOPHYSEAL JOINTS

While the disk allows for vertebral mobility, the zygapophyseal joints (or facet joints) provide a restraint for vertebral motion.

Their orientation varies with the different vertebral levels. In the cervical spine, the superior articular processes face posteriorly and slightly laterally. In the thoracic spine, they face posteriorly; in the lumbar spine, they face medially. The angles of inclination of the facet joints in the horizontal plane are 45° for the cervical spine, 60° for the thoracic spine, and 90° for the lumbar spine (Figs. 2.4 and 2.5).

The superior articular process of the T12 vertebra is thoracic, while the inferior articular process is morphologically lumbar.

The articular surfaces of the facets are covered with cartilage. The facet joints are enveloped by a baggy capsule, which covers them

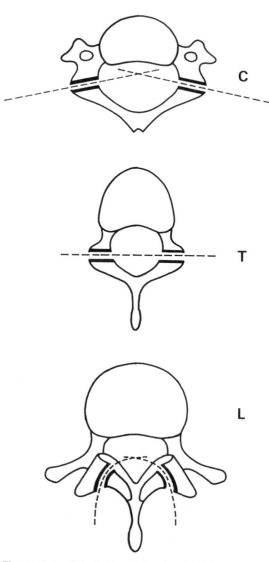

Figure 2.4. Orientation of the facet joints as seen from the frontal plane. *C*, cervical vertebrae; *T*, thoracic vertebrae; *L*, lumbar vertebrae.

like a hood and imparts to the joint a degree of elasticity. The degree of freedom of movement at each vertebral level is largely governed by the orientation of the facets.

Joint Capsule

The facet joint capsule is the most richly innervated part of the spine with respect to nociception as well as proprioception. This degree of innervation allows the proximal and distal supporting structures to adjust to the numerous combinations of tension and pressure imposed by various different postures or physical exertion. The elastic properties of the joint capsule provide for solid support at their superior and inferior poles and tend to maintain the articular surfaces in close contact with each other. Each movement must overcome the surface tension of the capsule, and as soon as the mobilizing force ceases, the articular processes recoil to their original positions. These elastic forces impart a stabilizing effect on the spine without augmentation of joint tension as is the case with the action of the musculoliga-

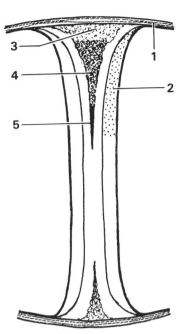

Figure 2.6.   Typical meniscoid formation (taken from a facet articulation) (according to Kos). *1*, capsule; *2*, cartilage; *3*, base of the meniscoid formation; *4*, medial aspect; *5*, terminal aspect.

mentous apparatus during exercise. The lateral aspects of the joint capsule are much more lax and contain fewer elastic fibers according to Töndury.

Meniscoids

Meniscoids were described by Schmincke and Santo and then later by Emminger and Zuckschwerdt and were studied in depth by Töndury and by Kos. They have incorrectly been referred to as "menisci." (Due to their potential role in certain vertebral pain syndromes, meniscoids are discussed in greater detail in Chapter 17.) They are composed of simple synovial folds, sometimes extremely thin, like cigarette paper.

According to Kos (1972), a "typical meniscoid formation" is made up of three parts: the capsular part, composed of loose connective tissue; the highly vascularized synovium; and a free terminal part, which is avascular and often contains chondrocytes (Fig. 2.6).

According to Töndury,

If the joint capsules are carefully removed from the nearby intervertebral foramina, careful dissection reveals small, shiny, semilunar-shaped wedges of a

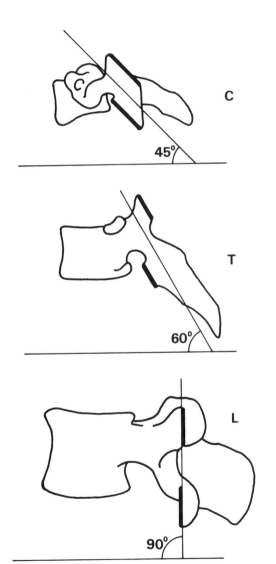

Figure 2.5.   Orientation of the facets in the sagittal plane. *C*, cervical vertebrae; *T*, thoracic vertebrae; *L*, lumbar vertebrae.

soft gelatinous consistency visible at the edge of the articular facet. In a fresh specimen, numerous small blood vessels are evident. According to their morphology, they are folds of synovial membrane connected to the periarticular filling and through to the intervertebral filling.

These inclusions exist in 84% of facet joints (Emminger). They form part of the usual structure of these joints and are maximally developed in the midlumbar region.

"Embryologically," according to Töndury, "their development is completely separate from that of a meniscus, even though in the adult, there is a certain structural similarity between these vertebral meniscoids and, for example, the meniscus of the knee."

When ossification of the vertebral arches begins in the embryo of 70 mm length, one can distinguish a clear articular split in the fold of synovial membrane at the medial aspect of the joint. These folds can either be composed of mesenchymal tissue (lumbar region) or result from a secondary invagination at the level of the intervertebral foramina (cervical region).

The regions of the capsule adjacent to the intervertebral foramina are well vascularized. They invaginate secondarily into the joint, forming small folds that, at their widened base, are connected to the tissue of the intervertebral foramina.

The definitive structure is formed at birth. In the adult they are of varying size, form, and thickness and are sometimes very thin. According to Engel and Bogduk, there are three types of intra-articular structures, each distinctive in its location within the joint and in its microscopic structure. The three types of structures are a connective tissue rim, an adipose tissue pad, and a fibro-adipose meniscoid. At least one type of structure was represented in every one of the joints examined, and 47 of 82 joints contained more than one type.

Giles and Taylor (1982) describe two types of formation located in the cervical spine and within the lumbosacral junction (L5–S1), in addition to adipose formations: (a) a thick inclusion projecting from the ligamentum flavum into the superior medial part of the joint, and (b) a wide synovial inclusion, well vascularized, projecting into the medial part of the joint.

Töndury suggests that these formations, unlike the disks and articular cartilage, do not degenerate with age due to their rich blood supply. When the cartilage degenerates, however, the meniscoid inclusions are exposed to abnormal biomechanical forces that may result in their "wearing out." It was his impression that the function of these meniscoids was to adapt to the incongruity of the articular surfaces. The meniscoids are readily able to adapt with the configuration of the joint surface, and their position within the joint varies dynamically with movement. Decreases in intra-articular pressure allow the meniscoid to penetrate more deeply into the joint; with increases in pressure, they are wedged toward the outside. Therefore, there is never any dead space within the joint (Töndury)[a].

---

[a] "Zygapophyseal Joints" was the theme of the Third Congress of the International Federation of Manual Medicine (1971), organized and presided upon by the author. The principal papers (H. Junghanns, G. Lazorthes, G. Töndury, J. Kos and J. Wolf, E. Emminger, A. Wackenheim, C. Gillot, R. Maigne) have been published in the *Annales de Medecine Physique* (1972), which has since become *Annales de Readaptation et de Medecine Physique* (see the remark in the bibliography under "Minor Intervertebral Dysfunction").

3

INTERVERTEBRAL DISK

The intervertebral disk is a fibrocartilaginous structure, biconcave in configuration, and situated between contiguous vertebral bodies. Although there are 24 vertebrae (26 if the sacrum and coccyx are included) and thus 25 intervertebral spaces, there are only 23 intervertebral disks. This discrepancy is due to the fact that there are no intervertebral disks between the occiput (C0) and the atlas (C1) or between the atlas (C1) and the axis (C2). The first disk is therefore located between C2 and C3. *The ratio of the disk to vertebral body height* determines the amplitude of segmental motion.

- In the cervical spine, the disks measure between 5 and 6 mm in height, with a disk to vertebral body height ratio of 1:3 (atlas and axis not included).
- In the thoracic spine, the disk height varies. The thoracic disks are smallest (3–4 mm) between T2 and T6, where the vertebral spinal index shows a functional reduction. Above T2, and especially below T6, the disk height becomes larger. On average, the disk to vertebral body height ratio is approximately 1:5 to 1:6 in the thoracic spine.
- The lumbar spine contains the largest disks in the spine (10 mm on average). However, the disk to vertebral body height ratio is only 1:3, as the vertebral bodies of the lumbar spine are also high and massive.

Of all the spinal segments, the least mobile are those in the thoracic spine because of the relatively smaller size of the intervertebral disks (i.e., one-sixth vertebral height) compared with the cervical (one-third vertebral height) and the lumbar (one-third vertebral height) disks (Fig. 3.1). The larger intervertebral disks in the cervical and lumbar spines allow for more segmental motion.

The shape of the disk determines the curvature of the vertebral column. When the anterior disk height is noticeably greater than the posterior height, the vertebral bodies within that segment will be slightly extended. The opposite is true for intervertebral disks with a higher posterior border. The cervical and lumbar disks are both thicker anteriorly than posteriorly (especially at the lumbosacral junction). The thoracic disks, on the other hand, are thicker posteriorly than anteriorly.

The disk is composed of a central part, the nucleus pulposus, and a peripheral part, the annulus fibrosus (Figs. 3.2 and 3.3). The nucleus pulposus, or central core, is gelatinous in substance and situated slightly posterior to the center of the disk. It has characteristic noncompressibility and plasticity that one associates with fluids and is basically a ground substance in which are embedded collagen fibers and isolated chondrocytes. It is encapsulated in a kind of "box" between the vertebral endplates by the annulus fibrosus. If there is a distinct difference between the annulus and nucleus macroscopically, the passage from one to the other is actually gradual, and microscopically, no sudden transition actually exists (Fig. 3.3).

The image of the nucleus as a "round marble within a fibrous ring" must be abandoned. The nucleus acts as a hydraulic chamber without clear boundaries (Rabischong et al.).

The annulus fibrosus, or "fibrous ring," is composed of thin layers of fibrocartilage in which are embedded flattened chondrocytes, creating a very firm consistency and thick texture. The fibers in each layer are oriented obliquely, with each layer running in the direc-

Figure 3.1. Relative height of the intervertebral disks and the body of the spinal vertebrae. **a.** At the cervical level, approximately one-third. **b.** At the thoracic level, approximately one-sixth. **c.** At the lumbar level, approximately one-third.

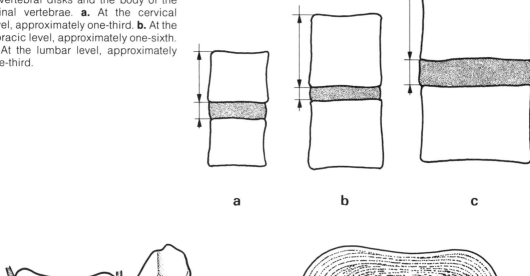

a   b   c

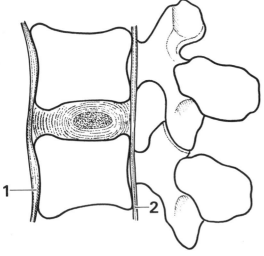

Figure 3.2. Sagittal section of an intervertebral disk. *1,* Anterior longitudinal ligament seen in the front; *2,* posterior longitudinal ligament seen in the rear.

Figure 3.3. Transverse section of an intervertebral disk. At the *center* is the nucleus pulposus. *Peripherally* is the annulus fibrosus.

tion opposite to the adjacent layer (Fig. 3.4). The degree of obliquity increases from the periphery of the disk to the center. Thus, the central layer of fibers are directed more in the horizontal plane. These fibers blend into the cartilaginous surface of the vertebral endplate. The annulus fibrosus is thus firmly adherent to the margin of the endplate, providing the disk with a structure that is highly resistant to tensile loads. The anterior border of the annulus fibrosus is the most resilient, since these fibers blend and penetrate deeply into the anterior vertebral rim via Sharpey's fibers; the pos-

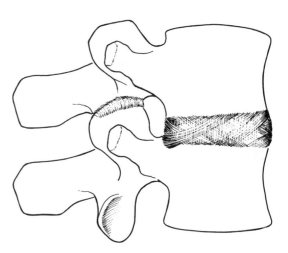

Figure 3.4. Lateral external view of an intervertebral disk. Note the oblique orientation and the crisscrossing of the fibers of the annulus.

terior portion of the annulus fibrosus is its weakest point.

The water content of the annulus fibrosus varies with age, but to a lesser degree than at the nucleus. At birth the annulus is 79% water, and this decreases to approximately 70% by age 70. The annulus is able to absorb pressure generated by the nucleus pulposus in an elastic manner; this is done, however, with the relatively little real elasticity of 15%. This unique characteristic, in addition to the alternating obliquity of the annular fibers, helps the healthy disk to maintain its shape under normal pressures.

Hydrophilic Properties

The intervertebral disk is well suited to absorb pressure by both dissipating it and redirecting it. This is achieved by means of its structure. The central aspect of the intervertebral disk or the nucleus pulposus is composed of a hydrophilic center that is high in water content and is therefore essentially noncompressible but deformable in shape. Pressure on this fluid center is dissipated radially to the annulus fibrosus, which, due to its toughness and relative elasticity, is able to absorb the pressure without a significant alteration in size or shape.

If the disk is sectioned in the transverse or sagittal plane, the gelatinous material inside spurts out as if it were jelly. The ability of the disk to dissipate pressure and tension is directly linked to its hydrophilic properties and high water content. It is noteworthy that the water content is not constant for all ages, being approximately 88% in a newborn and showing progressive dehydration with time so that by age 14 it is 80% and by age 70 it is approximately 70% (Keyes and Compere).

The disk is avascular in the adult. It relies on osmosis to meet its nutritional needs. Numerous microscopic pores allow nutrients to flow from the nucleus to the vertebral body via the cartilaginous endplate. When the disk is exposed to prolonged pressure (such as in the standing position), some of its water content diffuses into the vertebral body. As a result, one's disks are thinner in the evening and the person is actually somewhat shorter. This decrease in height can reach up to 2 cm in some people, with restoration after resting. With age, the hydrophilic properties of the disk are less pronounced, with a corresponding decrease in the shock-absorbing capacity of the disk. In conjunction with the increased incidence of vertebral body compression fractures and accentuation of the spinal curves that occur with aging, the loss in hydrophilic properties contributes to the gradual decrease in height seen among older people.

The mechanism of this hydration is not yet fully understood. The contents of the nucleus are governed by the laws of osmosis. The nucleus behaves like a solution bound by a semipermeable membrane (the cartilaginous endplate). Depolymerization of the polysaccharides augments the osmotic pressure and thus the force drawing water from the vertebral bodies through the multiple pores of the endplate. With age, the passage of water becomes increasingly difficult, and the nucleus loses its hydration capacity: this is called the "imbibition factor." The force one must apply to a colloidal jelly to separate the dispersed phase from the dispersing phase is called the "imbibition pressure." Within the disk, these two phases refer to the proteoglycan matrix and the interstitial fluid, respectively. The imbibition pressure is significant in young people, reaching approximately 250 mm Hg (Charnley). This pressure varies both with age and from day to day, along with the pressure transmitted to it by the nucleus.

In an attempt to study the hydrational characteristics of the intervertebral disk, Nachemson, Lewis, Maroudas, and Freeman (1970) utilized radiographic contrast materials and radioisotopes to study the permeability of liquids through the cartilaginous endplate to the disk and the lacunae of the subchondral bone. They concluded that only the central part of the disk was permeable.

LIGAMENTOUS SYSTEM

ANTERIOR LONGITUDINAL LIGAMENT

The anterior longitudinal ligament forms a long fibrous network from the anterior tubercle of the atlas to the sacrum. It is essentially attached to the anterior and anterolateral part of each vertebral body. It is not attached to the margin of the vertebral body and adheres only slightly to the disk, from which it can be easily detached. It has a high degree of tensile strength and in general maintains its integrity in vertebral compression fractures (Figs. 4.1 and 4.2).

POSTERIOR LONGITUDINAL LIGAMENT

Unlike the anterior longitudinal ligament, the posterior longitudinal ligament is firmly adherent to the disk. It is widest at its point of attachment to the disk and narrows as it borders the vertebral body (Fig. 4.3). The paraspinal venous plexus is situated posterior to the vertebral bodies, thus separating the ligament from attaching to the vertebrae. Pathophysiologically, the posterior longitudinal ligament plays an important role, since it reinforces the disk posteriorly where the annulus is at its weakest point, and thus provides a barrier to disk extrusion.

The posterior longitudinal ligament is composed of (*a*) long, superficial, ribbonlike, median fibers that extend over four or five contiguous vertebrae and (*b*) a deep layer of short arciform fibers that skip alternate vertebrae and attach on the side opposite to their origin. This ligament is strongest in the thoracic spine and weakest at the lumbar levels.

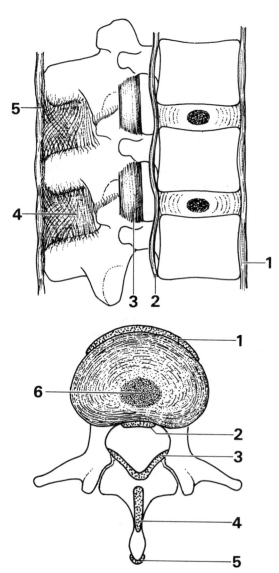

Figure 4.1. Sagittal section (**top**) and transverse section (**bottom**) showing the different ligaments of the spinal vertebrae. *1*, Anterior longitudinal ligament; *2*, posterior longitudinal ligament; *3*, ligamentum flavum; *4*, interspinous ligament; *5*, supraspinous ligament; *6*, nucleus pulposus.

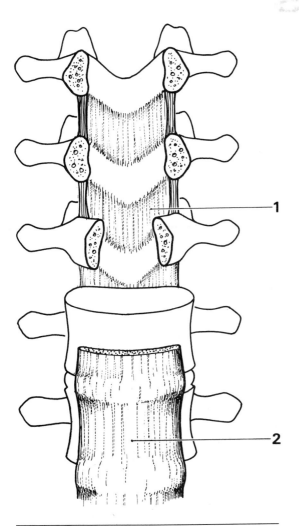

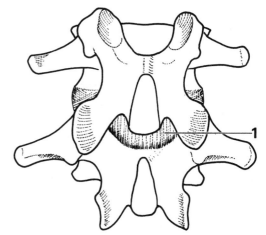

Figure 4.2. Vertebral sections at the level of the pedicles to demonstrate the superior dorsal aspect of the vertebrae. **Left,** Anterior view. **Right,** Posterior view. *1,* Ligamentum flavum; *2,* anterior longitudinal ligament.

INTERSPINOUS LIGAMENT

The interspinous ligament connects the contiguous spinous processes and is reinforced by the supraspinous ligament. It plays a major role in limiting spinal flexion.

LIGAMENTUM FLAVUM

The ligamentum flavum is composed of two halves that meet in the midline, adjoining the vertebral laminae and thus closing the vertebral canal. This ligament's high content of elastin affords it a high degree of resilience and also accounts for the yellow color (*flavos* is the Greek word for yellow). The ligamentum flavum is also attached to the medial aspect of the facet joints and thus restricts their range of motion.

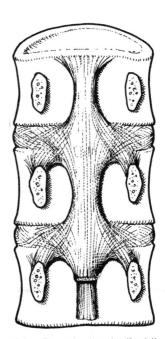

Figure 4.3. Posterior longitudinal ligament.

5

SPINAL CHARACTERISTICS BY REGION

CERVICAL SPINE

The cervical spine is composed of seven vertebrae, forming a curve that is convex anteriorly. The apex of the curve is situated at C4, and its convexity continues distally until T2 (Figs. 5.1 and 5.2).

The two most proximal cervical vertebrae, the atlas and the axis, are distinguished from the other typical cervical vertebrae as there is no intervertebral disk between them (Fig. 5.3). The first intervertebral disk is located between C2 and C3. There are several characteristics that distinguish the cervical spine from other regions of the vertebral column that are necessary to note here.

Facet Joints

The cervical facet joints are obliquely oriented, with a gradual increase in obliquity from the horizontal as one descends from top to bottom. Beginning with the facets of the axis, which are quasi-horizontal, there is a progressive increase in inclination, reaching a maximum of approximately 45° in the distalmost cervical vertebrae. In the sagittal plane, the articular surfaces of the facets face dorsally and slightly medially. This alignment facilitates gliding of contiguous surfaces in all directions, especially in flexion and extension (Figs. 2.4 and 2.5).

Spinous Processes

The atlas has no spinous process. The size of the spinous process increases gradually from C3 to C7. The orientation of the spinous processes is nearly horizontal, and in hyperextension they come into contact with each other. On palpation, C7 is the first spinous process that differs from the other cervical segments; it is the only one that is not bifid, and it is the most prominent of the neck (Figs. 5.1 and 5.2).

Supraspinous Ligament

In both the thoracic and the lumbar spines, the supraspinous ligament is a flattened tissue layer closely adherent to the posterior aspect of the interspinous ligament. In the cervical spine, it is much more developed and forms the ligamentum nuchae, attached proximally to the occiput and distally to the spinous process of all the cervical vertebrae with the exception of C1 and C7.

In certain animals, such as the horse, this ligament is highly developed. Its strength and resiliency assist the cervical extensors by passively supporting the weight of the head.

Uncinate Processes

The uncinate processes are unique to the cervical vertebrae from C3 to C7. These processes are situated laterally and give a saddle-shaped appearance to the vertebral body (Fig. 5.4a). The inferior aspect of the vertebral body has a reverse shape with a notch on each side that is complementary to the uncinate processes.

The significance of these "articulations" lies chiefly in their proximity to the vertebral artery and the sympathetic chain in close juxtaposition to it.

These processes can be the source of spondylosis with formation of osteophytes that may extend posteriorly toward the vertebral canal, encroaching on the nerve root or the vertebral

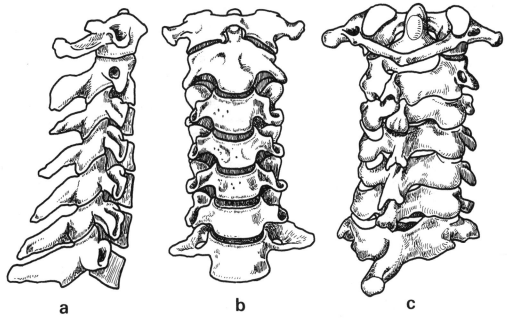

Figure 5.1.   Cervical spine. **a,** Lateral view. **b,** Anterior view. **c,** Oblique view.

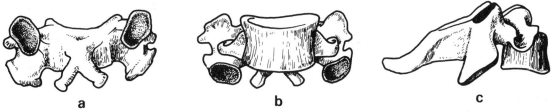

Figure 5.2.   Cervical vertebrae. **a,** Posterior view. **b,** Anterior view. **c,** Lateral view.

artery. Luschka was the first to point out this peculiarity.

Since Luschka, the fissures between the uncovertebral joints and the disk have been considered true articulations with a joint cavity, articular cartilage, and a joint capsule. The anterior part of the joint capsule blends with the annulus fibrosus of the disk (Fig. 5.4b).

In a degenerating disk, the nucleus pulposus can impinge upon the arthritic uncovertebral joint. Contact made by nuclear material with osteophytes originating from the uncinate process forms a nodule that may bulge into the intervertebral foramina. This nodule was named the "disco-osteophytic nodule" by de Seze. Cervicobrachial neuralgia is often the result of nerve root impingement by this nodule. These nodules are often referred to by a sur-

geon as "hard herniations," as opposed to "soft herniations" that are formed when the nucleus herniates through an annular tear.

According to Töndury (Fig. 5.4c), there is no formal "uncovertebral joint." He states that "lateral disk fissures" appear at approximately age 10 and progressively widen medially with age, eventually communicating with the nucleus pulposus, allowing it to reach the periphery and form the disco-osteophytic nodule.

Töndury bases his opinion on study of the uncus in relation to age. The uncinate processes belong to the neural arches of the cervical vertebrae. In the fetus, collagen fibers join the processes of contiguous vertebrae, and no fissure is evident. The disks extend only to the epiphyseal cartilage. In the newborn, the collagen fibers of the uncinate processes become adherent to the peripheral laminae of the disks. Even in children of ages 6–7, there is no evidence of a true uncovertebral "articulation." These fissures, still very narrow, first begin to

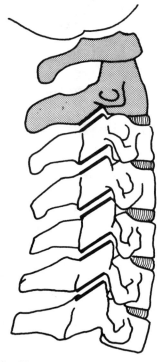

Figure 5.3. There are no intervertebral disks between the occiput and the atlas and between the atlas and the axis. The first intervertebral disk is seen between C2 and C3.

appear in the disks of the inferior cervical spine in children of approximately 9–10 years of age. Töndury showed, with the aid of microscopic sections, that these fissures are not articular splits but ruptures in the collagen fibers that are initially limited to the lateral aspects of the disk. Examination of disks in adults of various ages demonstrates that fissures extend progressively toward the center of the disk, eventually communicating with the gelatinous nucleus; in extreme cases, the fissure may extend from one end of the disk to the other. When this occurs, a lateral disk extrusion can result, narrowing the intervertebral foramina; this extrusion is the "disco-osteophytic nodule."

Transverse Processes and the Vertebral Artery

The cervical transverse processes arise from the midpoint of the lateral masses by two roots. These roots form the transverse foramen (Fig. 5.5).

Foramina are located on all the cervical vertebrae. However, at C7, the opening is much smaller, allowing passage of the vertebral vein only. The foramina of the first six vertebrae form a discontinuous canal through which the vertebral artery (a branch of the subclavian artery), its sympathetic plexus, the vertebral vein, and the spinal nerve pass (Fig. 5.6).

In the superior cervical spine, the artery takes a complex route, as the transverse fo-

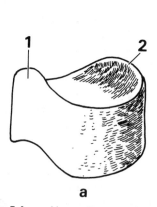

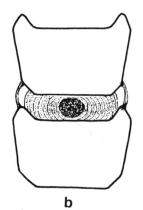

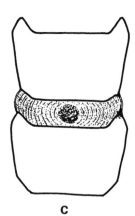

Figure 5.4.   **a,** Uncus. It causes the superior cervical endplate of the cervical vertebrae to take the form of a stirrup (*1* and *2*). **b,** The classic interpretation is that there exists an articular cavity (Luschka). **c,** Töndury's interpretation is that there is no uncovertebral articulation, but after 10 years of age there is formation of lateral fissures in the annulus. These fissures progressively make their way to the central disk.

ramina of the atlas are situated much more laterally than those of the axis; the artery thus has to pass laterally and then medially, thus making a double bend before reaching the foramen magnum (Fig. 5.7). Jung notes that the artery, whose dimensions are the same as those of the transverse foramen, often appears cramped in this passage. One can easily envision the stretch to which the artery is subjected with extreme movements of the head. Arteriography has shown that when a subject posi-

tions the neck in extension and external rotation, the circulation is compromised on the side contralateral to the rotation (Fig. 5.8).

The close proximity of the vertebral artery to the cervico-occipital junction explains the possibility of injury to the arterial wall that may occur with inappropriate maneuvers of the cervical spine. Serious accidents have been described after certain "manipulations," or even after some prolonged abnormal postures of the cervical spine that can result in vertebral artery compression and thus restrict blood flow between the atlas and the occiput. In normal patients, the transient interruption of the vertebral artery circulation is normally com-

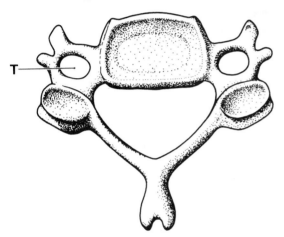

Figure 5.5.   Neural foramen (*T*).

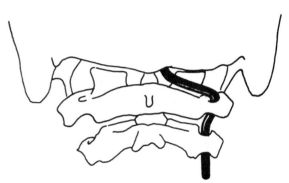

Figure 5.7.   Intervertebral canal.

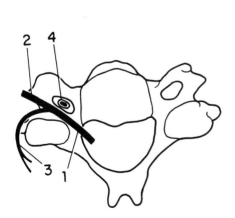

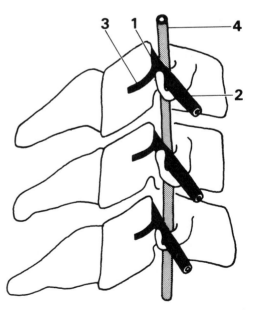

Figure 5.6.   Spinal nerve (*1*), with the anterior primary ramus (*2*), posterior primary ramus (*3*), and vertebral artery (*4*).

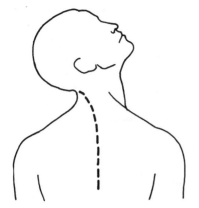

Figure 5.8.   Rotation with hyperextension of the head impairs blood flow in the vertebral arteries on the side contralateral to the rotation.

pensated by the blood supply of the contralateral vertebral artery. This is not the case if the latter is narrowed by atheroma or is hypoplastic. Anatomic variations and anomalies are indeed very frequent at this level.

Uncinate spondylosis and, less frequently, facet arthrosis can create bends or segmental narrowings of the vertebral artery.

Anomalies of the Cervico-occipital Junction

Anomalies of the occipitocervical junction are not uncommon. Many are subclinical and can go on to produce serious neurologic sequelae that are often discovered or aggravated by trauma.

Cranial Settling

The most common anomalies of the cervico-occipital junction may result in cranial settling. This is characterized radiologically as a rise in the odontoid process above Chamberlain's line (which, in a lateral radiograph of the cervical spine, connects the posterior edge of the bony palate and the posterior edge of the foramen magnum) (Figs. 5.9 and 5.10).

Another landmark is Fischgold's line (Figs. 5.11 and 5.12). This line is seen on a standard anteroposterior radiograph of the cervical spine (forehead and nose on plate) as a line joining the two mastoid processes, which normally passes through the atlanto-occipital ar-

ticulation. With cranial settling, the odontoid process ascends above this line.

Other Anomalies

Cranial settling can be accompanied by other anomalies such as occipitalization of the atlas, spina bifida occulta of the atlas, stenosis or deformation of the foramen magnum, subluxation or dislocation of the atlas on the axis, cervical block vertebrae, spina bifida, or platybasia.

These bony anomalies are often associated with neurovascular anomalies. Often, patients with such anomalies have a short neck, a low hairline, and restricted neck range of motion.

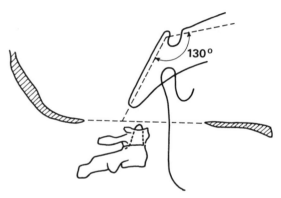

Figure 5.9.   Chamberlain's line. This line connects the posterior border of the bony palate to the posterior border of the foramen magnum. In normal individuals, the odontoid process is found below this line. The basal angle is normally 130°. It can be greater in persons with conditions such as platybasia.

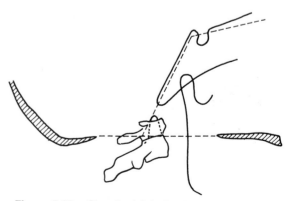

Figure 5.10.   Chamberlain's line in cases of cranial settling. The odontoid process is noted to be above this line.

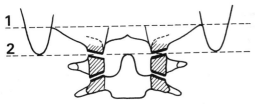

Figure 5.11. Fischgold's line (frontal tomography passing through the mastoid processes). In the normal individual, the bimastoid line (*2*) passes through the occiput-atlas articulations and is tangential to the upper pole of the odontoid process. The digastric line (*1*) passes above the base of the cranium and 1 cm above the level of the atlanto-occipital articulations.

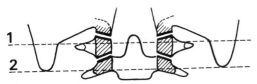

Figure 5.12. In cases of cranial settling, the odontoid process is seen to be significantly above the bimastoid line (*2*). This is also noted for the atlanto-occipital articulation. *1*, digastric line.

Sudden maneuvers should be avoided in these susceptible spines.

THORACIC SPINE

The thoracic spine is composed of 12 vertebrae. The vertebral bodies are taller than the disks. The articular surfaces of the facets are oriented in close approximation to the frontal plane and are inclined 60° from the horizontal. The superior articular processes face posteriorly, slightly superiorly, and laterally (Rouvière). The spinous processes are long and directed obliquely and inferiorly. The ribs articulate with the thoracic vertebrae (Figs. 5.13 to 5.17).

The vertebral body is semicylindrical in shape, hence the semicircular appearance of the vertebral endplates. The intervertebral foramen is circular. Two costal demifacets (superior and inferior) are situated on each side of the posterolateral aspect of the vertebral body with the exception of T1, T11, and T12. Each of the latter three vertebrae has a complete articular facet for the homologous rib (Fig. 5.14).

The transverse processes are massive and extend posterolaterally. With the exception of T11 and T12, they have an articular facet on their anterior surface for the homologous rib (costotransverse articulation) (Figs. 5.14 and 5.16). The spinous processes are directed obliquely in such a manner that the tip of the

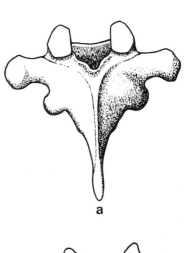

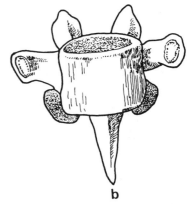

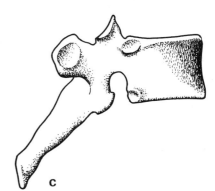

Figure 5.13. Thoracic vertebra seen posteriorly (**a**), anteriorly (**b**), and in lateral view (**c**).

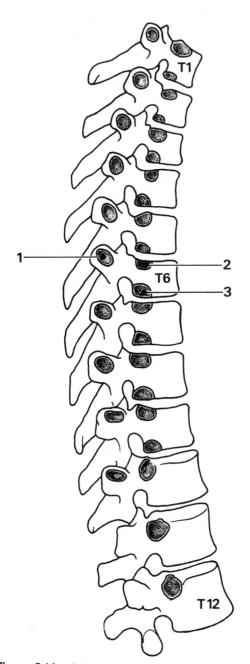

Figure 5.14. Articular facets of the thoracic vertebrae associated with the ribs, consisting of two semi-facet articulations, one superior and one inferior at the head of the rib (*2* and *3*), and one articular facet for the tuberosity of the ribs (*1*). This last one does not exist for the last two vertebrae, which articulate with a facet that is between T11 and T12.

process of T6 lies at the level of the superior part of the body of T8 (Fig. 5.15). This degree of obliquity increases progressively downward to T8 and then gradually decreases for the final four thoracic vertebrae, whose spinous processes are somewhat shorter. The spinous processes of the last two vertebrae more closely approximate those of the lumbar spine.

The facets are oriented 60° from the horizontal plane and lie in the frontal plane. This facilitates mobility in all directions (Figs. 2.4 and 2.5).

LUMBAR SPINE

The lumbar spine is composed of five vertebrae arranged in a lordotic curve that is convex anteriorly (Fig. 5.18). The disks are thick and measure approximately one-third the height of the corresponding vertebral body. The facets are oriented in such a way as to considerably limit lateral flexion (Figs. 5.19 and 5.20). Rotation would thus be impossible were it not for some laxity between them. Indeed, the superior articular process is flattened transversely; its medial aspect has an articular surface in the shape of a vertical sulcus whose concavity faces medially and slightly posteriorly. The inferior articular processes, in contrast, have a convex articular surface shaped like a cylindrical segment facing laterally and slightly anteriorly, which permits the disk to glide into the concavity of the superior articular process of the vertebra beneath it. Anomalies of the facets are frequent.

T12 is a transitional vertebra with superior articular processes that are typically thoracic in morphology and inferior articular processes that are typically lumbar. On occasion, T11 plays the role of a transitional vertebra.

Spinous Processes

The spinous processes are massive. They are directed horizontally and are shaped like a knife blade ending in a vertically lengthened tuberosity.

Transverse Processes

In the lumbar spine these processes are called "costiform." They are long and serve as the insertion site of powerful muscles.

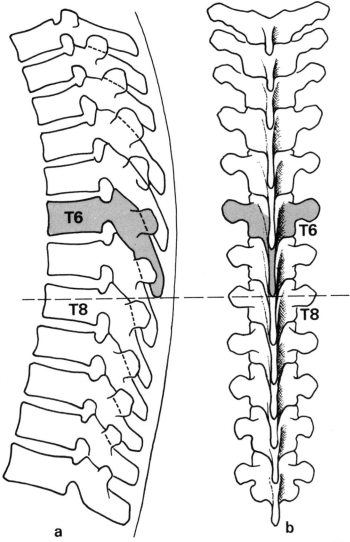

a   b

Figure 5.15.   The tip of the T6 spinous process is found to reach approximately one-third of the way down the vertebral body of T8.

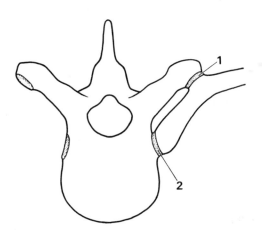

Figure 5.16.   Costotransverse articulation (*1*) and costovertebral articulation (*2*). At T11 and T12, the ribs are noted not to be true ribs, as they do not have costotransverse articulations.

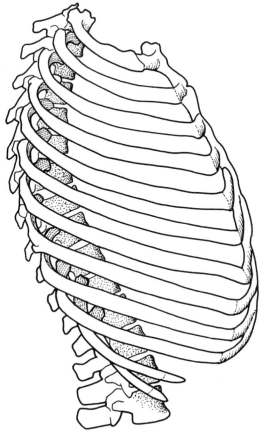

Figure 5.17.   Rib cage.

Figure 5.18. Lumbar vertebrae and sacrum seen posteriorly (**a**) and in lateral view (**b**).

SACROILIAC JOINT

The pelvic girdle represents the junction between the spine, which rests on top, and the lower limbs below. It is formed by two symmetric iliac bones, the right and the left, and by the sacrum, a median triangular segment composed of five fused vertebrae. Thus, the sacrum articulates on each side with an iliac bone (Fig. 5.21).

The symphysis pubis joins the iliac bones anteriorly. The pelvic girdle is in the shape of a funnel with the opening facing superiorly: the pelvic inlet. The pelvis is wider, broader, and shorter in women than in men.

The sacrum is triangular with its apex inferior and its base superior; thus it acts like a keystone between the two iliac bones. The sacrum articulates with the two ilia via the sacroiliac joints:

1. The lateral aspect of the sacrum is shaped like a circular arc (articular surface). The center of that circle is situated at the level of the tubercle of S1, which represents the point of insertion of the powerful supporting ligaments.
2. The coccyx, located at the posteroinferior

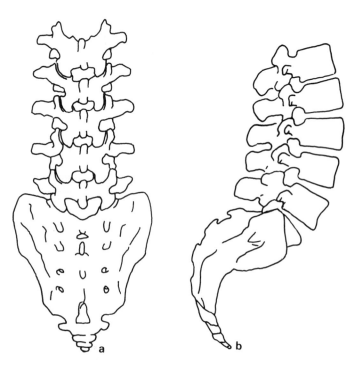

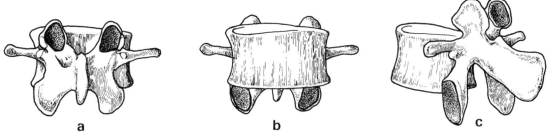

Figure 5.19.   Lumbar vertebrae seen posteriorly (**a**), anteriorly (**b**), and in oblique view (**c**).

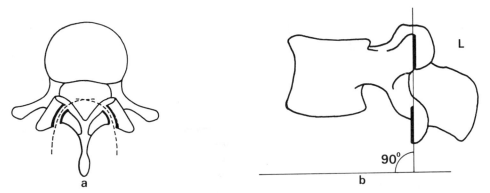

Figure 5.20.   Facet joint orientation at the lumbar level. This orientation does not allow for rotation.

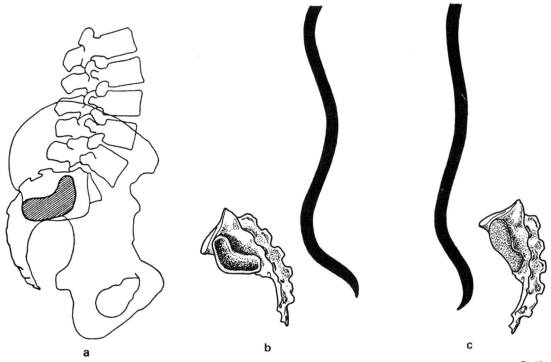

Figure 5.21.   **a,** Sacroiliac articulation. **b,** Dynamic-type sacroiliac articulation according to Delmas. **c,** Static-type sacroiliac articulation according to Delmas.

aspect of the sacrum, has an articular surface identical in contour to that of the sacrum. Its shape is also like an arc of a circle or a crescent. The midpoint of the circle corresponds to the level of the iliac tuberosity, on which are inserted supportive ligaments.

These surfaces have highly irregular contours; they are neither flat nor symmetrically curved. The coccygeal surface has been compared to a rail (Farabeuf), because its longitudinal axis has a bulge separating two depressions. The inferior sacral surface is rather convex, while the superior and middle portions are rather flat.

Delmas has described two types of sacroiliac joints:

• The first, which he refers to as "dynamic" (Fig. 5.21), is typical among those who must stand for prolonged periods and whose spinal curvatures are thus accentuated.
• The second, which he refers to as "static"

(Fig. 5.21), is common among individuals whose spinal curves are attenuated.

The "dynamic" type of sacrum, which is seen in 25% of the population, tends to be oriented horizontally, and the concavity of the articular facets are more pronounced. This type of sacroiliac joint is capable of greater mobility and is more prevalent in females.

The "static" type, which can be found in 25% of the population, tends to be oriented vertically with the articular facets very elongated, vertical, and almost flat. This type is most characteristic of primates. It is an articulation that has more limited mobility and a greater capacity for weight bearing and effort and is a characteristically masculine feature.

Between these two schematic types, there are intermediary forms (50%). The articular surfaces are lined with cartilage.

The sacroiliac joint and its ligaments are innervated by the dorsal rami of L5 and S1, as well as by branches originating from a posterior plexus formed by the dorsal rami of the inferior lumbar roots and the roots of S1 to S3.

6

THE MUSCLES

The muscles are the power source of the spine. They can be categorized as intrinsic, such as the paravertebral muscles, which are made up of short bundles that act directly on individual spinal segments with a short lever arm, and extrinsic, which act via a long lever arm and play a role in stabilizing spinal movement.

Figures 6.1 to 6.4 depict the superficial and deep muscles of the back.

PARASPINAL MUSCLES

The paraspinal muscles have been categorized by C. Gillot according to their position relative to the plane of the transverse processes. He describes them as follows:

Muscles Located Anterior to the Plane of the Transverse Process

Muscles located anterior to the plane of the transverse process are situated along the lateral surface of the vertebral body and the anterior surface of the transverse processes. They are well developed in the lumbar and cervical levels and are absent from T4 to T11.

a. At the cervicothoracic level are the longus colli and the rectus capitis anterior muscles. These muscles are flexors and accessory rotators. They are completed by the rectus capitis lateralis, a flexor and lateral flexor of the occiput.
b. In the lumbar spine, the psoas muscle acts as a flexor of the hip (or of the trunk, depending on whether it acts in an open or closed kinetic chain) as well as an external rotator of the hip.

Muscles Located between the Transverse Processes

These muscles are situated in the frontal plane as follows:

a. In the cervical spine, the scalenus anterior, medius, and posterior. These muscles are ipsilateral lateroflexors and assist in contralateral rotation.
b. In the lumbar spine, the quadratus lumborum is a lateral flexor of the trunk, or, when the spine is fixed, it elevates the ipsilateral hemipelvis toward the spine.
c. At both the lumbar and cervical spine are small intertransverse (intertransversaria) muscles, which are replaced by ligaments in the thoracic spine. These muscles assist in lateral flexion (Gillot).
d. In the thorax, Delmas and Gillot consider the intercostal muscles as paravertebral muscles.

All of the above muscles, with the exception of the intertransverse muscles, are innervated by branches of the anterior primary rami.

Muscles Located Posterior to the Plane of the Transverse Processes

These are the muscles of the paravertebral sulcus. According to Gillot, they can be categorized as (a) the small deep muscles situated at the craniocervical junction and (b) the erector spinae muscles within the vertebral sulcus.

Small Deep Muscles of the Neck Situated at the Craniocervical Junction

There are four small deep muscles situated at the craniocervical junction (Fig. 6.7):

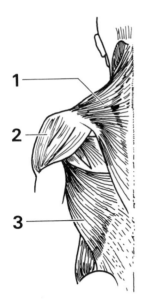

Figure 6.1. Superficial muscles of the trunk. *1*, Trapezius; *2*, deltoid; *3*, latissimus dorsi.

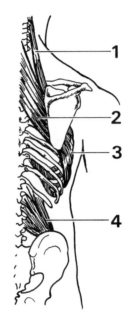

Figure 6.3. Deep muscles of the trunk. *1*, Levator scapulae; *2*, rhomboideus; *3*, serratus anterior; *4*, quadratus lumborum.

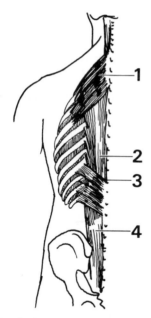

Figure 6.2. Deep muscles of the trunk. *1*, Serratus posterior superior; *2*, iliocostalis; *3*, serratus posterior inferior; *4*, sacrospinalis.

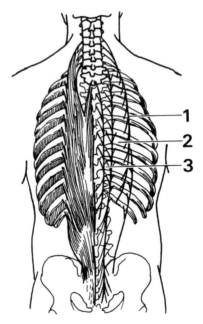

Figure 6.4. Deep muscles of the trunk. *1*, Iliocostalis; *2*, longissimus thoracis; *3*, multifidus.

- Rectus capitis posterior
- Rectus capitis anterior
- Obliquus capitis superior
- Obliquus capitis inferior

These are the "vernier muscles" of Kapandji that offer fine tuning to the movements of the upper cervical spine. The obliquus capitis superior is a rotator; the rectus capitis posterior is an extensor and assists in rotation; the rectus capitis major acts as a rotator; the obliquus capitis inferior acts as an extensor and an accessory rotator. These muscles are innervated by the posterior ramus of C1. The obliquus superior also receives some fibers from C2.

Erector Spinae Muscles within the Vertebral Sulcus

These muscles extend from C3 to the sacrum, and their description is very complex. They are

- Multifidus, the deepest layer
- Iliocostalis, located most laterally

Along with the longissimus thoraces they form a group of spinal muscles whose inferior insertion on the sacrum constitutes a common mass.

In the cervical spine are the splenius and semispinalis muscles: the semispinalis capitis maintains the cervical lordosis and is essential in maintaining the head in the upright position. The splenius, which lies more superficial, is a rotator and acts as an antagonist to the sternocleidomastoid.

The right sternocleidomastoid rotates the head to the left, whereas the right splenius rotates it to the right. Both muscles, however, are synergists in lateral flexion to the ipsi-

lateral side. All these muscles are innervated by branches of the dorsal primary rami.

ABDOMINAL MUSCLES

The abdominal muscles play a very important role as flexors of the thoracic and lumbar spine, in maintaining vertebral balance, and in reducing strain on the lumbosacral spine. They are, laterally, the obliquus externus abdominis, the obliquus internus abdominis, and transversus abdominis, all located on both sides of the midline.

The rectus abdominis is located on either side of the *linea alba*. Unilateral contraction of the abdominal muscles results in rotation and lateral flexion of the trunk; rotation is contralateral for the external oblique and ipsilateral for the internal oblique.

MUSCLES OF THE NECK AND BACK

The trapezius muscle acts as an extensor of the head (Fig. 6.1).

The sternocleidomastoid muscle, when contracted unilaterally, acts as a powerful lateral

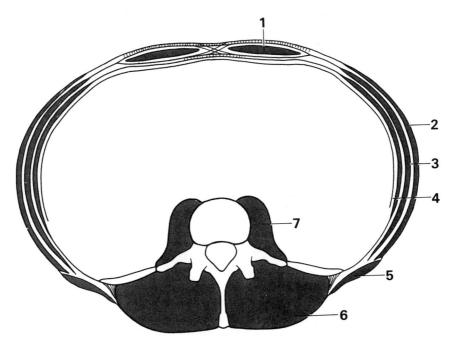

Figure 6.5. Muscles of the abdominal wall (seen in section). *1*, Rectus abdominis; *2*, obliquus externus; *3*, obliquus internus; *4*, transversus abdominis; *5*, latissimus dorsi; *6*, erector spinae; *7*, psoas.

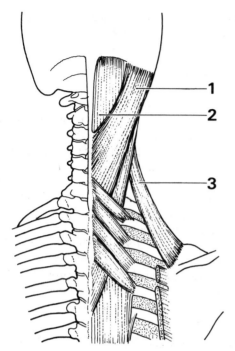

Figure 6.6. Posterior muscles of the neck. *1*, Splenius; *2*, semispinalis capitis; *3*, levator scapulae.

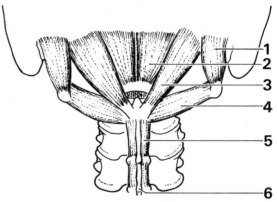

Figure 6.7. Muscles of the occipital region. *1*, Obliquus capitis superior; *2*, rectus capitis posterior minor; *3*, rectus capitis posterior major; *4*, obliquus capitis inferior; *5*, interspinal ligament; *6*, supraspinal ligament.

flexor of the cervical spine with contralateral rotation. When both sternocleidomastoid muscles contract simultaneously, they act as flexors of the inferior cervical spine.

During cervical rotation, the sternocleidomastoid acts synergistically with the contralateral splenius capitis muscle. In the upper cervical spine, the obliquus is the principal rotator.

MUSCLES OF THE LUMBAR REGION

The lumbar spine is supported by powerful muscles. It looks like a central column surrounded by four thick muscular pillars: the two psoas muscles anteriorly and the erector spinae masses posteriorly, forming a "composite beam" composed of bone and muscle (Rabischong, Dolto) (Fig. 6.5).

VASCULAR SUPPLY OF THE SPINE

ARTERIAL SUPPLY

Each radicular artery gives rise to an intercostal or a lumbar artery. Prior to entering the intervertebral foramen, each artery subdivides into three tributaries:

- One supplying the spinal nerve accompanied by the radicular artery;
- One that courses along the midline of the posterior aspect of the vertebral body and subdivides into two branches: one that penetrates the corresponding vertebral body and a second that descends one level and penetrates the vertebral body below;
- One that courses along the inferior aspect of the pedicle and gives rise to a few branches that supply the posterior arch and the most-medial paravertebral muscles. The most-lateral muscles are supplied by a posterior collateral branch of the intercostal or lumbar artery.

VENOUS SUPPLY

The venous system is composed of two parts, the intraspinal venous plexus and the extraspinal venous plexus (Fig. 7.1).

Intraspinal Venous Plexus

The veins of the intraspinal venous plexus are located within the epidural space, and on each side they consist of two ascending plexiform cords (plexus venosi vertebrales externi and interni). They course away from the disk and converge in the interpedicular space. They

are united by a transverse anastomotic vein (plexus transversale) that receives the basivertebral vein, which also drains the vertebral body. This vein also forms an anastomosis with the paraspinal plexus.

Perispinal Venous Plexus

The veins of the perispinal venous plexus are located along the anterior and lateral aspect of the vertebral body (anterior vertebral plexus) and on the posterior aspect of the posterior neural arch (posterior vertebral plexus). They communicate with the intraspinal plexus via the veins of the intervertebral foramina.

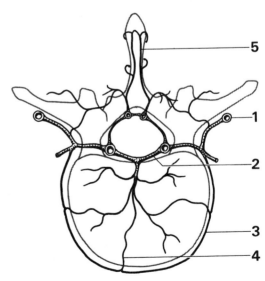

Figure 7.1. Vertebral basilar veins. *1*, Azygos; *2*, intervertebral venous plexus; *3* and *5*, perispinal venous plexus; *4*, vertebral draining veins.

Depending on the level, the vertebral blood supply may drain via any of the ascending lumbar veins (lumbalis ascendens), the azygos veins, the hemiazygos veins, or the posterior intercostal veins (venae intercostales posteriores).

Venous pressure is very low in the spinal veins. Therefore, even the slightest degree of venous compression anywhere along their course in the intervertebral foramen can result in venous congestion in the territory drained by these vessels.

INNERVATION OF THE VERTEBRAL STRUCTURES

The vertebral structures are innervated by the posterior primary rami as well as the sinovertebral nerves.

POSTERIOR PRIMARY RAMI

The spinal nerve is formed by the union of the ventral motor root and the dorsal sensory root. As it exits the intervertebral canal, it subdivides into a large anterior primary ramus and a much smaller posterior primary ramus. C1 and C2 represent exceptions to this rule. The posterior ramus courses around the facet joints, giving rise to branches supplying the joints, ligaments, and all the segmental spinal muscles as well as providing for the cutaneous supply over the back from the vertex to the coccyx. In their anatomic studies, Lazorthes and Gaubert (1956) demonstrated the intimate relationship between these nerves and the zygapophyseal articulations that they surround and innervate (Figs. 8.1 to 8.3).

Each posterior ramus divides into a lateral branch and a medial branch. The first is a muscular branch, and the second has both muscular and cutaneous supply. Distal to T8, the first is muscular and cutaneous, while the second is muscular.

In the lumbar spine the medial branch passes within 1 cm of its origin, through a 6-mm-long fibro-osseous tunnel, where it is flattened against the root of the transverse process (Bradley). It then passes between the intermamillary and mamillostyloid fascicles of the intertransverse muscle and travels inferiorly and medially, skipping one or two vertebrae (Fig. 8.4).

The medial branch innervates the structures that lie between the two facet joints: interspinal muscles (interspinalis), the transverse spinal muscles (multifidus), the innermost portion of the erector spinae (sacrospinalis), the joint capsule, the ligamentum flavum, and the supraspinous and interspinous ligaments.

The lateral branch innervates the intertransverse (intertransversarii) muscles, the iliocostalis and longissimus muscles, and the dorsal lumbar fascia.

Not all posterior rami have a cutaneous branch. For example, C1, L4, and L5 are exclusively motor nerves. While most authors agree on these exceptions, there is some disagreement as to whether a cutaneous branch exists for C6-C7 and C8. Certain authors (such as Grant, Lazorthes, and Töndury) deny the existence of cutaneous branches for these lower cervical segments. Our clinical findings support those of the above authors and suggest

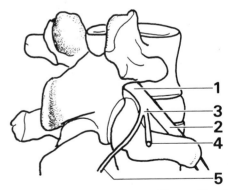

Figure 8.1. The spinal nerve root (*1*) on exiting from the intervertebral canal branches into an anterior primary ramus (*2*) and a posterior primary ramus (*3*). The latter further divides into a lateral (*4*) and a medial (*5*) branch.

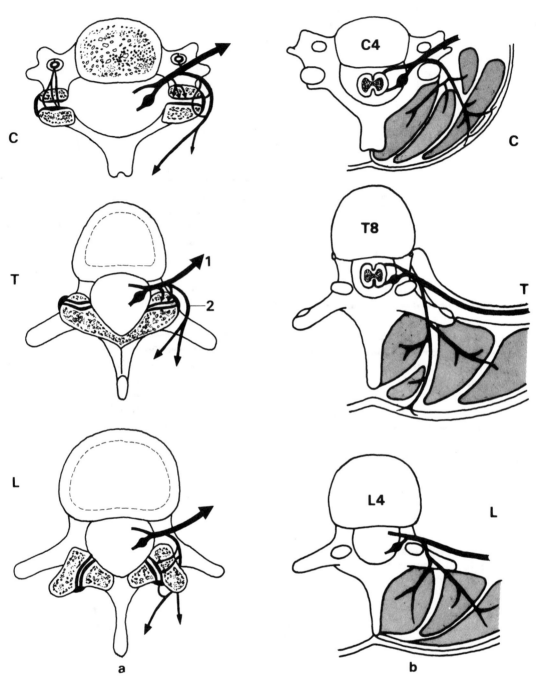

Figure 8.2. a, Posterior primary rami of the spinal nerve and the facet joint (according to G. Lazorthes). **b,** The posterior primary rami of the spinal nerves innervate the intrinsic muscles of the spinal column and the skin overlying the trunk (according to G. Lazorthes). *C*, at the cervical level; *T*, at the thoracic level; *L*, at the lumbar level.

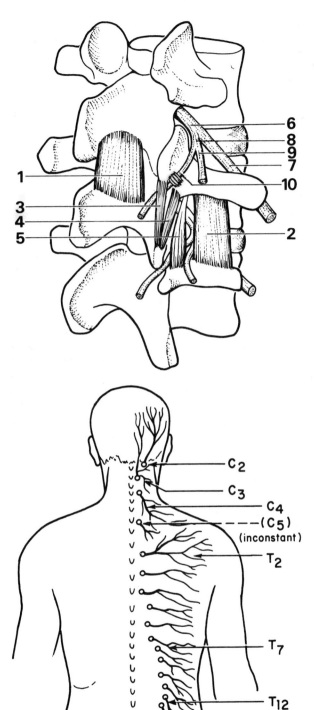

Figure 8.3. At the lumbar level, the branches of the posterior primary rami of the spinal nerve follow the contours of the facet joints and pass through a fibro-osseous tunnel (Bradley). Then they enter the intermamillary fascia and mamillostyloid and transverse spinal muscle. *1*, Interspinous muscle; *2*, intertransverse process muscle; *3*, intermamillary fascicles; *4*, mamillary styloid fascicles; *5*, interstyloid fascicles; *6*, spinal nerve root; *7*, anterior primary ramus of the spinal nerve root; *8*, posterior primary ramus of the spinal nerve root; *9*, external branches of the posterior primary ramus; *10*, internal branches of the posterior primary ramus and the osteofibrous canal.

Figure 8.4. Cutaneous branches of the posterior primary ramus. Individual variations are frequent. The cutaneous branches of C5 are not constant. This diagram is a summary of clinical investigations performed by the author.

that the cutaneous branches of C5 and T1 are also inconsistent.

The cutaneous territory of the posterior rami is always located distal to the level of the corresponding vertebra, with the exception of C2 and C3. The displacement increases progressively from superior to inferior. For example, the skin overlying the posterior aspect of the buttocks is innervated by the posterior rami of the thoracolumbar junction.

Most dermatome charts do not appear to correspond with these clinical findings, especially the depiction of the cutaneous supply of the upper and midthoracic regions. Keegan and Garett's chart, probably the most well known, shows the dermatomes of C5, C6, C7, and T1 as small strips distributed in a fishbone-like manner overlying the superior thoracic region. In fact, we have noticed, in a series of dissections, that the cutaneous branch of T2 is often much larger than its neighbors and supplies a much larger cutaneous territory. The cutaneous branch of T2 becomes superficial at the T5 level before ascending toward the acromion. The neighboring territory of cutaneous supply is that of C4 superiorly and T3 inferiorly (Fig. 8.5) (see Chapter 36).

We have also studied the innervation of the skin overlying the upper buttocks. This region is supplied by the cutaneous branches of the posterior rami of T12, L1, and L2. Occasionally there is a contribution from L3 to this region, but this branch is inconsistent (J.Y. Maigne). Again, the classic dermatome charts do not appear to correspond with these clinical findings (see Chapter 41).

A Chinese team at Ninghsia College studied the lumbar region and noted the frequency of anastomoses between the medial and lateral branches at the various levels near their origin. At the sacral level, the branch of S2 is the largest. In conjunction with branches from S1, S3, and S4, it forms a true plexus innervating the lumbosacral muscles and the periosteal and peri-ligamentous surfaces. The terminal branch in this plexus is the *posterior gluteal nerve* (Trolard), which in fact does not have a cutaneous branch. This nerve, approximately 10 cm in length, courses along the inferior aspect of the sacrum, giving rise to a few branches to the sacrococcygeal articulation before terminating in two branches. The first ascends to the second sacral foramen and in-nervates the overlying skin; the second terminates in the coccygeal region (Lazorthes).

SINOVERTEBRAL NERVE

The sinovertebral nerve (Fig. 8.6), which is the size of a thick thread (Hovelacque), is formed by the junction of a spinal nerve with a sympathetic nerve root. The branch from the spinal nerve originates immediately after its exit from the intervertebral foramen. Occasionally it arises from either the posterior or the anterior primary ramus. The branch from the sympathetic chain arises from the adjacent white communicating ramus; most often subjacent. Once formed, the sinovertebral nerve courses posteriorly and enters the intervertebral foramen following a *recurrent* course anterior to the spinal nerve. Lazorthes, Poulhis, and Espagno (1948) have described the distribution of its terminal branch as purely segmental. The branches are distributed to the vertebral body, the laminae, the posterior longitudinal ligament, the epidural tissues, the dura mater (G. Lazorthes), the anterior longitudinal ligament, the annulus fibrosus (Jung and Brunschwig), and the disk above the corresponding vertebral body via numerous fibers and occasionally to a disk below. Hovelacque writes, "We have never seen the nerve divide into two terminal branches: one ascends and one descends with reciprocal anastomosis between the branches of the nerves above and below." Lazorthes confirms Hovelacque's opinion concerning the lumbar region. Luschka, however, has described such anastomoses.

INNERVATION OF THE DISK

The disk is not innervated except at the superficial layers of the posterior and posterolateral regions of the annulus. Hirsch et al. discovered some free nerve endings of small-caliber myelinated fibers in the superficial layer of the annulus adjacent to the posterior longitudinal ligament.

Cloward noted that the superficial anterior layers are also innervated, at least in the cervical region. This innervation depends on the sinovertebral nerve, but this is debatable.

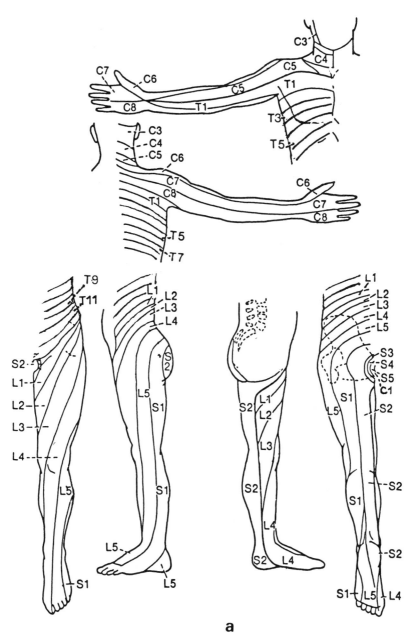

a

Figure 8.5. **a,** Dermatomes according to Keegan and Garrett. This is the most frequently reproduced diagram of the dermatomes. We do not believe that this diagram is consistent with clinical findings, particularly with regard to the dermatomes of the posterior half of the body, including the trunk. **b,** Dermatomes consistent with results of our research. This diagram represents generally accepted territories that involve the upper and lower limbs, including the anterior part of the trunk. This diagram is consistent with our findings, particularly with regard to the dermatomes of the posterior half of the limbs and trunk. (*Figure continues*)

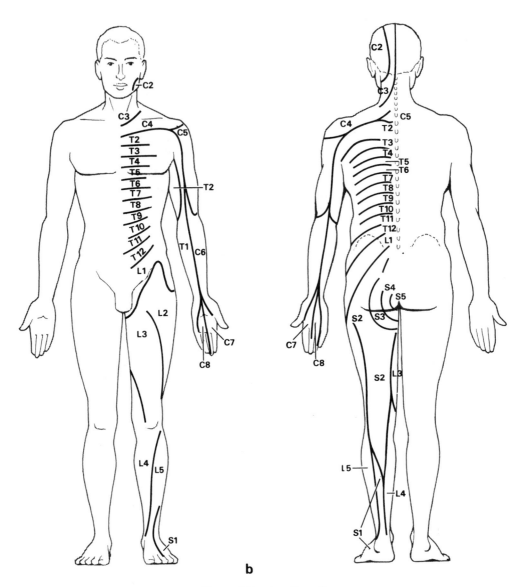

b

Figure 8.5. *(continued)*

Rabischong and Serrano-Vella have noticed numerous nerve fibers in the anterior and posterior longitudinal ligaments, in the region separating them from the annulus, and even 1–2 mm inside the annulus. They add that this innervation does not come exclusively from the sinovertebral nerve, but also from some "nerve fibers that are most likely unmyelinated."

INNERVATION OF THE FACET JOINTS

The facet joints are innervated by the posterior primary rami, with the exception of the occipito-atlanto-axial articulations, which are innervated by branches of the anterior ramus.

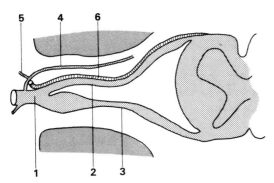

Figure 8.6. Spinal nerve in the intervertebral foramen. *1*, Spinal nerve root; *2*, anterior primary ramus; *3*, posterior primary ramus; *4*, sinovertebral nerve formed by a single nerve root coming from the spinal nerve and a sympathetic root from the gray ramus communicantes (*5*); *6*, artery.

The joints are supplied by a branch from the homologous level as well as one from the subjacent level. Moreover, Paris et al. (1980), in their study of the lumbar spine, were able to show the existence of an ascending branch arising from the medial division of the posterior ramus. This branch courses laterally through the space bounded by the intertransverse ligament and ascends to the facet joint above it. The facet capsules are richly innervated, as are the joint surfaces themselves. Hirsch et al. noted

1. Free endings of myelinated fibers of small diameter (3 μm)
2. Nonencapsulated endings of medium diameter (5–12 μm) typical of Golgi tendon organs or Ruffini's corpuscles
3. Encapsulated endings typical of Golgi-Mazzoni and pacchionian corpuscles

The articular cartilage is not innervated.

INNERVATION OF THE LIGAMENTS

The supraspinous and interspinous ligaments are innervated by the posterior primary ramus.

The anterior longitudinal ligament, the posterior longitudinal ligament, and the ligamentum flavum are innervated by the sinovertebral nerve. Both free and encapsulated endings can be found in these ligaments. The posterior longitudinal ligament is richly innervated. Hirsch et al. discovered some free nerve endings in the superficial and posterior layers of the ligamentum flavum. However, Jackson et al. have found none.

INNERVATION OF THE VERTEBRAL PERIOSTEUM

The vertebral periosteum is innervated by the sinovertebral nerve. Hirsch et al. discovered free nerve endings, as well as nonencapsulated endings of medium-diameter myelinated fibers.

INNERVATION OF THE SPINAL MUSCULATURE

The spinal muscles are innervated by motor branches arising from the posterior primary rami. Electromyographic studies performed by Gough et al. on subjects with paraplegia or quadriplegia demonstrated that motor innervation of muscles supplied by the posterior primary rami originate below the level of the nerve of origin, sometimes as far away as six vertebral segments for nerves that originate in the inferior cervical spine. This is much lower, according to these authors, than is cutaneous innervation.

Walts, Koepe, and Sweet, in a similar study, demonstrated the existence of anastomoses among branches of the cervical posterior rami in monkeys.

MUSCLE AND TENDON RECEPTORS

According to Sherrington, 40% of the nerve fibers assigned to muscle are sensory. They are fibers that end on neuromuscular spindles, Golgi tendon organs, and free nerve endings.

Motor outputs originate in the medulla and descend via the corticospinal tract, terminating on the anterior horn cells. The axial musculature is controlled by the medial part of the anterior horn, while the limbs are controlled by the lateral part.

Neuromuscular Spindles

Neuromuscular spindles (Figs. 8.7 and 8.8) are long formations distributed within the muscle according to the degree of complexity of that muscle's function. They measure only a few millimeters (3 mm on average). A spindle is composed of two components in parallel alignment with the extrafusal muscle fibers. The two ends of the spindle are formed by very fine intrafusal muscle fibers that contain numerous motor endplates. The central part (equatorial zone) has no muscle fibers and is purely sensory.

Efferent Fibers

The intrafusal fibers are innervated by small-diameter gamma motor neurons originating from the gamma cell of the anterior horn.

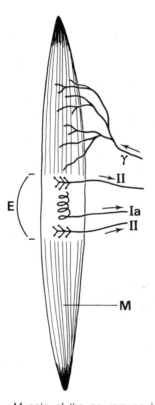

Figure 8.7. Muscle of the neuromuscular muscle spindle complex. *M*, Intrafusal fibers; *E*, midregion of the fiber bundle; γ, gamma fibers; *Ia*, sensory fibers carrying afferent input from the terminations of the spiral center situated in the muscle bed; *II*, sensory fibers carrying afferent information from the terminal ends of the muscle spindle.

The extrafusal fibers are innervated by alpha motor neurons. Gamma motor neurons, although very fine individually, constitute a relatively important mass, since their volume represents approximately one-third of the total mass of the efferent nerves located in the anterior root.

Afferent Fibers

The afferent fibers innervate the equatorial region of the spindle. The annulospiral, or type 1A fibers, surround the equatorial zone of the spindle in a *spiral fashion*. They are of large diameter and conduct rapidly. They are particularly sensitive to the rate of change in length. A few scattered type II fibers are also found in the primary ending. These fibers are of smaller diameter and are more sensitive to the absolute change in length. Any type of stretching action, be it passive (caused by the muscle itself) or active (caused by contraction of the intrafusal fibers under gamma control), will cause these fibers to increase their firing rate. The intrafusal fibers are maintained under some degree of tension (gamma tone) in a muscle at rest, thus allowing for the maintenance of resting muscle tone. This gamma tone is capable of modifying the muscle's reaction to stretching.

When a muscle is lengthened, the spindle is stimulated, resulting in reflex extrafusal contraction. Conversely, if the muscle is shortened, the activity of the spindle decreases. This characteristic of the muscle spindle causes the muscle to resist changes in length. This role is essential for the maintenance of posture.

Gamma Loop

The gamma loop is the name given to a reflex circuit. It consists of the gamma motor neuron of the anterior horn, whose axon ends on intrafusal muscle fibers and in the afferent Ia and type II fibers that leave the equatorial zone of the spindle and enter the spine through the dorsal root. It is this circuit that produces the myotatic reflex, which is most often monosynaptic.

The Myotatic Reflex. Liddell and Sherrington have shown that passive stretching of a muscle provokes a reflex contraction of this muscle that is often accompanied by relaxation

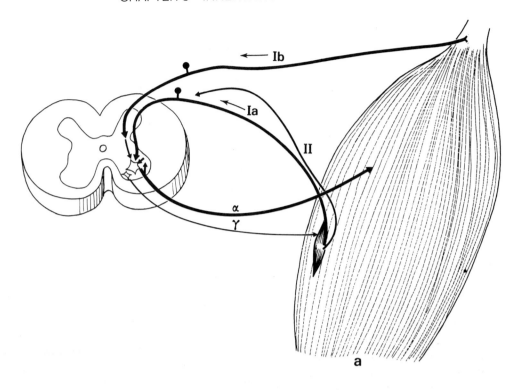

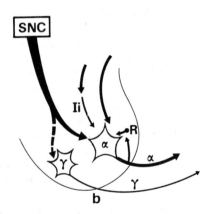

Figure 8.8.   Spinal reflexes. **a,** General scheme. **b,** Detailed scheme. α, Motor neuron to the muscle; γ, motor neuron to the muscle spindle; *R*, inhibitory Renshaw cell; *Ii*, inhibitory interneurons; *SNC*, corticospinal tract; *Ia*, primary afferent fiber; *II*, secondary afferent fiber; *Ib*, afferents from the organ of Golgi. The myotactic (monosynaptic) reflex circuit can be described as $\gamma\rightarrow$la$\rightarrow\alpha$. The inverse myotactic reflex (bisynaptic) can be described as Ib$\rightarrow$li$\rightarrow\alpha$. The Renshaw inhibitory circuit can be described as R$\rightarrow\alpha$. The cortical spinal modulation of the system is performed by two means: (*a*) direct, through the modulation of the activity of the alpha motor neuron, and (*b*) indirect means on the activity of the gamma motor neurons.

of the antagonist muscle (law of reciprocal innervation). It is the myotatic reflex that occurs when a neuromuscular spindle is activated by muscle stretch. This reflex helps maintain a constant tone in the antigravity muscles. Clinically, this reflex is applied when one taps the tenoperiosteal junction with a reflex hammer.

The Inverse Myotatic Reflex.   This reflex causes relaxation of the agonist that occurs suddenly in a muscle initially subjected to a strong and prolonged stretch. This reflex is activated by the Golgi tendon organ.

Renshaw Loop

Renshaw demonstrated the existence of a small cell located in the anterior horn of the spinal cord near the anterior horn cell. The alpha motor neuron, prior to exiting the anterior horn, gives rise to a collateral branch with a recurrent course that terminates on the Renshaw cell. From there an interneuron arises, terminating on the motor neuron from which the original collateral branch originated.

This Renshaw loop has an inhibitory effect,

in contrast to the excitatory gamma loop. Its purpose is to facilitate fine movement control.

The gamma cell is under the control of the central nervous system, which may have an inhibitory or an excitatory action. The degree of sensitivity of the gamma system can be modulated by descending tracts from the central nervous system and allow fine adjustments in the gamma sensitivity to movement. Emotional states also have an important influence on the gamma system and, in certain cases, can adversely affect muscle coordination, which can produce excessive strain on a joint that is under too much tension.

Golgi Tendon Organs

Golgi tendon organs are located within the tendon at the musculotendinous junction, as well as in the intramuscular aponeurotic wall. They are sensitive to tension placed on the tendon, either through muscular contraction or passive stretching of the muscle. Because these receptors are aligned in series with the muscle, rather than in parallel as is the case with the neuromuscular spindle, these receptors are sensitive to stretching at the musculotendinous junction rather than to stretching of the entire musculotendinous unit. These receptors have a quasi-permanent baseline activity whose firing rate is increased with significant increases in muscle tension that stretch the musculotendinous junction. Thus there is a threshold that must be exceeded by a sufficient increase in tension to increase the firing rate proportional to the amount of tension produced.

Afferent impulses are transmitted via type IB sensory fibers that enter the dorsal root and terminate on inhibitory interneurons (Renshaw cells). Their activity thus results in a inhibition of the agonist muscle, resulting in a decrease in muscle tension if the firing threshold is exceeded. They thus facilitate the action of the antagonist muscle.

Free Nerve Endings

Free nerve endings are found in muscles and tendons in the vicinity of blood vessels. They relay nociceptive impulses that may be produced when the muscles or tendons are pinched.

ARTICULAR RECEPTORS

The articular and periarticular structures have receptors that relay messages to the central nervous system about position, tension applied to them by the tendons, and muscle length.

The facet joints are innervated by the posterior primary ramus. They receive the majority of their innervation from a branch of the posterior ramus from the homologous vertebral level, which courses close to the joint surface. However, each facet joint also receives input from branches from the posterior ramus above as well as from the one below. Several types of different nerve endings have been described.

Because of certain similarities, these nerve endings were given the name of Ruffini, or Pacchioni by analogy. This terminology is now avoided (Brodal), and a neutral terminology has been proposed (Freeman, Wyke). These authors identify four categories, each having distinct characteristics but all having in common sensitivity to tension.

In articular and periarticular structures are located type I, type II, type III, and type IV receptors. Types I, II, and III are mechanoreceptors. The type IV receptors are nociceptors.

Type I receptors are found mainly in the joint capsules and are analogous to the Ruffini corpuscles. They are sensitive to changes in joint position as well as to the velocity of their movement. They have a baseline firing rate and are sensitive to stimuli that exceed this threshold. They are innervated by thin myelinated fibers of 5–8 μm in length.

Type II receptors are approximately twice as large as the type I receptors. Their axons are composed of thicker myelinated fibers of approximately 8–12 μm. These receptors resemble the pacchionian corpuscles and react rapidly to changes in joint position. These receptors are located within the capsule.

Type III receptors are the largest of this group. Their axons are composed of thick, myelinated fibers. They are extracapsular and are located within the ligaments resembling Golgi tendon organs. They react slowly and have a high excitation threshold. The function of these receptors has not yet been well defined.

Type IV receptors are composed of a plexus of fine unmyelinated nerve fibers located within the joint capsule, ligaments, and fat pads. They have never been found in the synovial membrane (Wyke). These receptors are nociceptors. A stimulus of sufficient strength to activate the type IV receptors results in contraction of the periarticular muscles, resulting in immobilization of the joint.

9

AUTONOMIC NERVOUS SYSTEM

The autonomic nervous system regulates the function of the various organ systems. It not only involves visceral innervation but also acts on vasomotoricity, glandular secretion, smooth muscle, joint capsules, connective tissue, and the central nervous system (CNS) itself. Sympathetic efferent fibers have been found among numerous nociceptors and mechanoreceptors.

Although the autonomic nervous system is not under voluntary control, it is integrated into the function of the CNS. That is, it is not a separate system but rather a subsystem that can be thought of as having characteristics that are particular to it.

The autonomic nervous system is made up of CNS nuclei that extend down and into the spinal cord. The outflow information of this system is provided via hormonal and neural output. The neural output or efferent activity is conducted by two types of fibers in the autonomic system, the sympathetic and parasympathetic. Although there is no histologic difference between these two fiber types, each is an anatomically discrete system with separate functions and neurotransmitters.

SYMPATHETIC SYSTEM

The sympathetic system (Figs. 9.1 and 9.2) is composed of two types of neuron:

- *Preganglionic fibers* situated in the lateral column of the spinal cord (located between T1 and L2 only)
- *Postganglionic fibers* situated in the ganglionic chain

The axons of the sympathetic preganglionic fibers are myelinated. They exit via the ventral root and then, as the white rami communicantes, enter the ganglionic sympathetic paravertebral chain.

The sympathetic paravertebral chain is segmented. At certain stages the ganglia may fuse, however, and thus in the cervical spine one finds three cervical ganglia known as the superior, the medial, and the inferior ganglion. (Occasionally, the medial ganglion is absent.) Otherwise, these are named the stellate ganglia, which are traversed by the vertebral artery. Approximately 12 thoracic ganglia, 3–5 lumbar ganglia, and 3–5 sacral ganglia exist. Thus there are approximately 22 ganglia for 30 spinal nerves.

Some fibers synapse in the paravertebral ganglion. The unmyelinated postganglionic fibers reenter the spinal nerve (forming the grey rami communicantes) to form the sympathetic component of the peripheral nerves. The distribution of these fibers does not strictly correspond to their radicular level, since the lateral column does not extend throughout the entire spinal cord.

The superior preganglionic thoracic fibers ascend to the cervical ganglia. The lower thoracic and lumbar fibers can, in a similar fashion, descend to the lumbosacral ganglia. These fibers are destined to reach the muscles, organs, and cutaneous tissues; the efferent effect of the sympathetic systems affects numerous receptors of various types, including nociceptors and mechanoreceptors. The organs are predominantly innervated by the sympathetic system (G. Lazorthes).

Other fibers traverse the ganglia without synapsing there, but rather in the perivisceral (prevertebral) ganglia. These form the prevertebral plexus, cardiac plexus, solar plexus, and hypogastric plexus. These plexuses are also involved in the innervation of glandular secretion and various other organ functions.

The existence of afferent sympathetic fibers is controversial. English and American authors do not believe that the few afferent fibers that accompany this system are actually part of the sympathetic system. French authors, however, accept their existence (Delmas, Lazorthes).

PARASYMPATHETIC SYSTEM

The parasympathetic system is also composed of two fiber types:

• Preganglionic fibers
• Postganglionic fibers

Preganglionic fibers have myelinated axons that arise from cell bodies in the gray matter of the brainstem and the middle three segments of the sacral cord. In the brainstem, these fibers are incorporated as part of cranial nerves III, VII, IX, and X.

The postganglionic fibers have unmyelinated axons and are found in association with ganglia, annexed to the cranial nerves (ophthalmic, sphenopalatine, optic, and submaxillary ganglia) and in prevertebral and perivisceral ganglia for the pneumogastric and erectile nerves (Lazorthes).

In contrast to the sympathetic postganglionic fibers, the postganglionic fibers are quite short. Similar to the sympathetic fibers, however, there probably exists an afferent component.

The sympathetic system functions through the use of intermediary neurotransmitters:

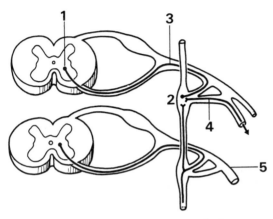

Figure 9.1. Organization of the sympathetic nervous system. *1*, Spinal center (spinal cord gray matter); *2*, sympathetic trunk ganglion; *3*, preganglionic fibers; *4*, postganglionic fibers; *5*, spinal nerve.

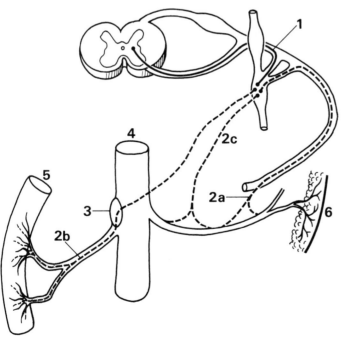

Figure 9.2. Generalized distribution of the sympathetic system (according to G. Lazorthes). *1*, preganglionic fiber; *2*, postganglionic fiber: *2a*, sympathetic collaterals to the spinal nerve; *2b*, periarterial visceral plexus; *2c*, periarterial somatic plexus; *3*, perivisceral ganglion; *4*, artery; *5*, visceral organ; *6*, skin.

- Acetylcholine is the neurotransmitter for both sympathetic and parasympathetic pre-ganglionic fibers, as well as for parasympathetic postganglionic fibers. These fibers are referred to as cholinergic.
- Adrenalin (epinephrine) is the neurotransmitter for sympathetic postganglionic fibers (adrenergic), with the exception of the sympathetic postganglionic fibers that innervate the sweat glands. These latter fibers exert their effect through acetylcholine (sympathetic cholinergic).

Most organs are under the dual influence of both sympathetic and parasympathetic systems. In most cases, these two systems have antagonistic effects on their end organs, including increasing/decreasing the heart rate or dilating/constricting the bronchial airways.

The autonomic nervous system (ANS) is under reflex control at the level of the spinal cord (e.g., micturition). In addition, modulation occurs through relays in the brainstem, which are under supranuclear influence. The extent of all the anastomoses between the CNS and the ANS is not fully known.

The sympathetic system is also involved in the modulation of pain pathways. This is frequently manifested in referred pain phenomena, such as the arm referral that occurs with cardiac ischemia. This may occur as nociceptive afferent input is relayed to the stellate ganglion via sympathetic afferents. From there, they enter the spinal cord to synapse on efferent fibers destined for the upper limb. As a result, the cortex interprets the origin of the pain to be in the arm. There is concordance between the spinal (radicular) level of the viscera and the dermatomal level where pain is referred. Pain, however, can be referred in a more diffuse fashion, as is the case with referral to the jaw with cardiac ischemia. Bourreau noted that sometimes the zone to which pain is referred is a function of a patient's prior painful experiences. He also noted that acute pain might be referred to a previously injured scar zone or chronic lesion.

The sympathetic system is also implicated in reflex sympathetic dystrophies (causalgia), as well as in any pain syndrome characterized by cutaneous hypersensitivity. These conditions cannot simply be explained on the basis of nociceptive relays (as in referred pain); instead, there seems to exist a dysregulation of the system—more precisely, a hyperactivity—that appears to be the source of the pain. Because of this, sympathetic neural blockade is often beneficial in the treatment of certain pain syndromes.

It is important to keep in mind that the hypothalamus is under the control of higher cortical centers, and thus both consciousness and autonomic functions are highly coordinated (Gouaze).

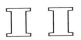

BIOMECHANICS

10

SPINAL KINEMATICS

The vertebral column is a flexible structure that readily adapts to a variety of different positions while still maintaining the ability to withstand compressive loads at each segmental level. The delicate precision by which it continuously adapts to changes in posture ensures the protection and mobility of the fragile neurovascular structures contained within the bony framework.

With the exception of the first two cervical segments (which lack an intervertebral disk), segmental motion is a function of the disk. Posteriorly, the facet joints limit and direct segmental motion.

During flexion, the nucleus pulposus migrates posteriorly, and the articular processes diverge slightly (Fig. 10.1).

During extension, the nucleus migrates anteriorly while the articular processes converge toward each other (Fig. 10.2).

Lateroflexion results in nuclear migration toward the contralateral side, with ipsilateral convergence and contralateral divergence of the articular processes (Fig. 10.2). Rotation results in displacement of the ipsilateral transverse process posteriorly and the contralateral transverse process anteriorly (Fig. 10.3).

THE MOBILE SEGMENT

H. Junghanns, known for his work on the spine in collaboration with Schmorl, considered all the elements that adjoin or separate two adjacent vertebrae as a functional unit. He coined the term "the mobile segment" referring to the intervertebral disk, facet joints, and the adjoining ligamentous system that form the unit (Figs. 10.4 to 10.6).

The vertebral column consists of 23 "mobile segments," with each one representing a unit of spinal mobility. There is a very close relationship among the elements of the mobile segment and the intervertebral foramina (Fig. 10.7).

The mobile segment, or intervertebral joint, is an integrated unit. Any mechanical perturbation affecting any one of its elements affects the others; just as any movement of a large segment of the column, even if only to maintain balance, affects all the other segments. The spinal curves are also interdependent: a lumbar lordosis results in a thoracic kyphosis and a cervical lordosis.

Automaticity of Spinal Function

The concept of the mobile segment as a mechanical unit of the spinal column helps to explain the mechanical relationships among the different elements of the spine during movement and of the consequences of lesions to these elements.

This concept is not enough, however, to explain the automatic functions of the vertebral column. Proprioceptive input, indispensable to maintenance of posture and motion, is received from all elements of the motion segment, including the facet joints, muscles, and tendons.

Through the action of proprioceptors, any change in position, whatever its origin, alters the distribution of force on the elements of the motion segment, resulting in a redistribution of muscular contraction. In addition, the mobile segment also receives input from Golgi tendon organs (type Ib afferents) and muscle spindles (type Ia and II afferents). All of these inputs are ultimately under the kinesthetic monitoring of the cerebral cortex. Thus the complexity of this *autoregulation*, which results from the

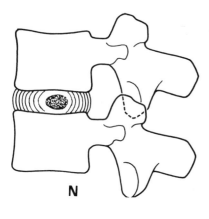

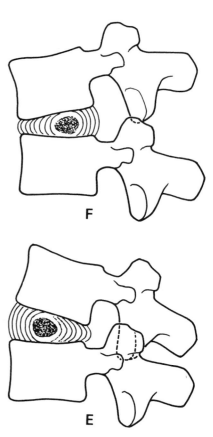

Figure 10.1. Spinal segmental motion. *N*, Neutral position; *F*, flexion; *E*, extension.

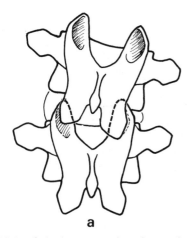

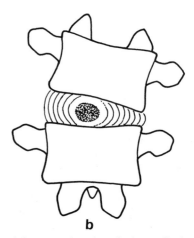

Figure 10.2. Spinal segmental motion. **a,** Lateroflexion to the right; posterior view. **b,** Lateroflexion seen in section through the nucleus pulposus.

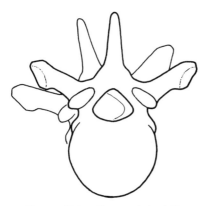

Figure 10.3. Segmental rotation.

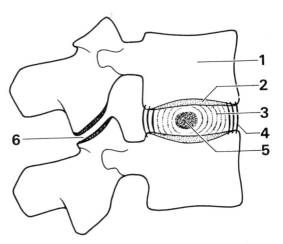

Figure 10.6. Elements of the mobile segment: *1*, vertebral body; *2*, cartilaginous end plates; *3*, annulus fibrosus of the disk; *4*, Sharpey's fibers; *5*, nucleus pulposus; *6*, facet joints.

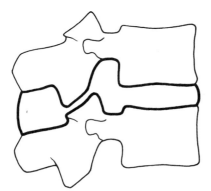

Figure 10.4. The mobile segment of Junghanns, lateral view.

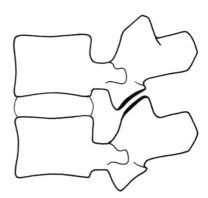

Figure 10.7. Intervertebral foramen.

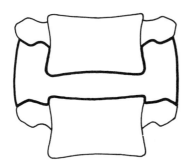

Figure 10.5. Mobile segment of Junghanns, anterior view.

continuous relaying of afferent and efferent input from each motion segment, is infinite.

Therefore, it would be an oversimplification to consider vertebral lesions only in regard to mechanical implications, especially since the spine is subject to neural regulation, allowing it to function with a high degree of automaticity. Any richly innervated element, if affected, will produce a "wrong note" in the harmonious function of the spine by stimulating protective muscle guarding (spasm) as a local protective measure. The role of "spasm" is essential, therefore, to the concept of "painful minor intervertebral dysfunction." Since muscles are not unisegmental in innervation, however, a mechanical displacement that affects only one vertebral segment (most often) may result in multisegmental sequelae. Thus, the spine is a biomechanical structure of extraordinary complexity, and segmental motion is far from simple.

REGIONAL SPINAL MOTION

At each spinal region, global movement is a product of motion at each of its mobile segments. At each spinal segment, the segmental physiodynamics change, resulting in marked regional differences. For example, the kinematics of cervical segments differ significantly from those of lumbar segments. The disk to vertebral body height ratio, the vertebra's width to height ratio, and the orientation of the articular processes determine the motion available to each spinal segment and, to a large extent, the mechanical displacements that can occur. The functional features of the mobile segments also help to determine and explain which types of therapeutic modalities are efficacious. We shall study spinal motion, which varies with age, at the cervical, thoracic, and lumbar levels.

Cervical Motion

The cervical spine is extremely mobile, and yet remarkably resistant to loading. It supports the head, which weighs 4–5 kg, in a variety of different positions and is able to withstand great stress.

Cervical segments are the most mobile of all the spinal motion segments. This is due to

- The disk to vertebral body height ratio (1:3 for the cervical spine, 1:6 for the thoracic spine, and 1:3 for the lumbar spine)
- The relatively small anteroposterior and transverse diameters in relation to the body height
- The presence of the uncinate processes
- The anatomy of the first two cervical segments, the atlas and the axis, which form the cervico-occipital junction

The cervical spine can be divided into two functional units (Fig. 10.8):

- The superior cervical spine, formed by the first two vertebrae
- The inferior cervical spine, formed by the remaining five

These two units complement each other functionally and allow precisely coordinated movement in every plane. The inferior cervical

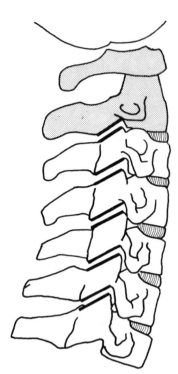

Figure 10.8. Cervical spine. Physiologically, one should distinguish between the upper cervical spine and the rest of the cervical spine (see the text).

spine is capable of two degrees of freedom: flexion/extension and coupled side bending with rotation. The superior cervical spine, on the other hand, has three degrees of freedom, allowing precise adjustments in positioning the head in space.

Superior Cervical Segments

The superior cervical spine is composed of the atlanto-axial articulation and the atlanto-occipital articulation. The movement at these two joints can be analyzed separately. In reality, however, these two articulations form a functional unit that must be considered as a whole.

Atlanto-Occipital Articulation

Flexion/Extension. Flexion/extension is the primary articular motion. In our civilization, it represents the "yes" movement that is accomplished by anteroposterior translation of the occipital condyles on the facets of the atlas for flexion, and posteroanterior for extension. The amplitude of this movement varies with the individual. Figures given for normal range of motion at this articulation vary according to the method of examination and the population examined; an average of 30–60° for the complete range of motion has been established; Fielding assigns 25° for extension and 10° for flexion (Fig. 10.9).

Lateroflexion.   Lateroflexion is possible in the range of 5–8°.

Rotation.   Rotation is not possible at this articulation.

Atlanto-Axial Articulation.   The atlanto-axial articulation, which is the most mobile segment of the spine, allows mostly rotational movement, though small degrees of flexion/extension and lateroflexion are possible.

Flexion/Extension.   Flexion/extension is possible because of the relative laxity of the transverse alar ligament in the atlanto-odontoid articulations as well as a certain degree of translation in the atlanto-axial articulation. This movement is in the range of 2° in extension and 9° in flexion (Kottke and Mundale) to 10° in extension and 5° in flexion (Fielding).

Lateral Inclination.   Lateral inclination is in the range of 5°.

Rotation.   Rotation is the ''no'' movement. This movement, which is not a pure rotation, is important, since it represents a range of motion of 30–35° in each direction (approximately half of available cervical rotation). Rotation about the longitudinal axis results in translation of the two lateral masses of the atlas in an anteroposterior plane, but in opposite directions on the lower adjacent facets. Rotation of the head results in anteroposterior translation of the ipsilateral lateral mass and posteroanterior translation for the contralateral lateral mass. The marked convexity of the facets in the anteroposterior direction makes this motion like that of a screw, with the atlas descending 2–3 mm during rotation. This simultaneous axial depression that occurs with rotation compensates for the twisting action on the spinal nerve roots and the vertebral artery (G. and C. Oliver).

Inferior Cervical Segments

The inferior cervical spine is composed of the inferior five cervical vertebrae. Not withstanding some slight variations from one vertebra to another, the movements are the same at each segmental level. The inferior cervical spine functions as a distinct biomechanical unit.

Movements that are possible are flexion/extension, lateral flexion, and rotation. Physiologically, the latter two are coupled and therefore inseparable.

Flexion/Extension.   During flexion/extension (Fig. 10.10), there is a true migratory movement on the ball bearing formed by the nucleus pulposus on the subjacent vertebra (Fig. 10.11). During flexion, the nucleus is compressed toward the rear of the disk, placing pressure on the posterior annular fibers and gapping the articular processes of the facet joints; the superior articular process glides anteriorly on the inferior process.

The absence of nuclear migration and a marked anterior pinching during flexion are the first signs of disk degeneration; this has been documented on 50 slow-motion cineradiograhic examinations (Figs. 10.12 and 10.13). Flexion is limited by ligamentous tension in the posterior longitudinal ligament, the liga-

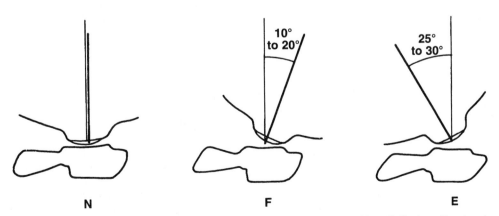

Figure 10.9.   Movement of the atlanto-occipital articulation. *N*, Neutral position; *F*, flexion; *E*, extension.

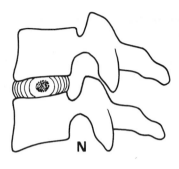

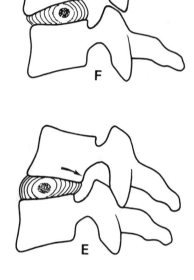

Figure 10.10. Movement at the mid or lower cervical spine level. *N*, Neutral position; *F*, flexion; *E*, extension.

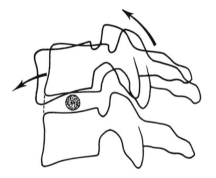

Figure 10.11. Flexion produces a "translation" of the lower adjacent vertebra, as though it were sliding on "ball-bearing" disks.

mentum flavum, the interspinous and supraspinous ligaments, and the facet joint capsule. For this reason, anterior subluxations can occur in sudden flexion injuries such as "whiplash," in which the constraints of these ligamentous structures are overcome. An example of this occurs with "jumped" cervical facets where the inferior articular process slips out from underneath the superior process. This condition is often associated with spinal cord injury, and the reduction of the facet dislocation is very difficult. This is the only example

of a dislocation without fracture at this level of the spine.

In extension, the nucleus is compressed toward the front, while the articular processes converge on each other; nuclear migration, however, prevents the articular processes from closing completely, and there is a slight gap anteriorly that remains at end range. Extension is limited by abutment of the neural arches, by contact made between the superior articular process of the subjacent vertebra and the transverse process of the upper adjacent vertebra, as well as by tension in the anterior longitudinal ligament. Several authors have studied extension. Raou studied movement in cadavers, while de Sèze, Djian, and Abdelmoula studied radiographs of live subjects. Their results are presented in Table 10.1. Kottke and Mundale's results, obtained from subjects of 15–30 years of age, are shown in Table 10.2. By analyzing lateral flexion/extension views, Kapandji determined a total amplitude of 100–110° for flexion/extension of the inferior cervical spine.

Rotation and Lateral Flexion. Rotation and lateral flexion are large-amplitude movements in the inferior cervical spine. Fick and Lovett demonstrated these two movements to be coupled at this level; during rotation, the vertebra

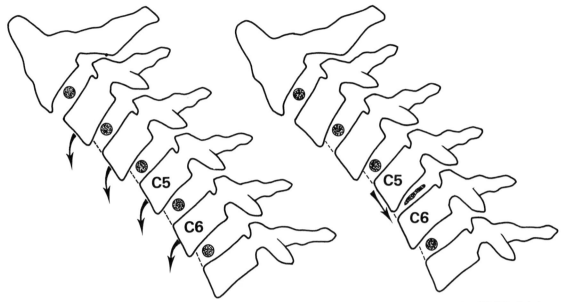

Figure 10.12. Normal cervical spine in flexion. Note that each vertebra slides on top of the subjacent vertebra in a gliding movement.

Figure 10.13. In this example, the C5-C6 disk has degenerated, and translation of C5 is not possible. In flexion, therefore, an anterior impingement is produced between C5 and C6.

Table 10.1

	Flexion	Extension	Total
C2–C3	5°	8°	13°
C3–C4	5.5°	10°	15.5°
C4–C5	7°	12°	19°
C5–C6	9°	18.5°	27.5°
C6–C7	6.5°	11°	17.5°
Total	33°	59.5°	92.5°

Table 10.2

	Flexion	Extension	Total
C2–C3	8°	3°	11°
C3–C4	7°	9°	16°
C4–C5	10°	8°	18°
C5–C6	10°	11°	21°
C6–C7	15°	5°	18°
Total	50°	36°	84°

undergoes simultaneous ipsilateral side flexion (Fig. 10.14).

The amplitude of these movements is difficult to evaluate. Kapandji has estimated lateral flexion to be 37° and rotation to be 66–76° in the inferior cervical spine.

Global Cervical Motion

Global cervical motion is a synthesis of the motions of the two functional units: the inferior and superior cervical spine. The base is formed by the inferior unit, while the superior segments adapt to perform precise movements.

Thus, in complete right lateral flexion or right rotation of the cervical spine, the movement of the inferior cervical segments is similar; it is the superior cervical spine that determines the final outcome of this triplanar motion by positioning the head in the desired position. In lateral flexion, the superior cervical segments rotate contralateral to the inferior segments to maintain the face in the frontal plane, while in rotation, the superior segments are ipsilateral to the inferior segments.

Numerous combinations are thus possible. The small, phasic muscles that govern superior cervical segmental motion are

• Rectus capitis major

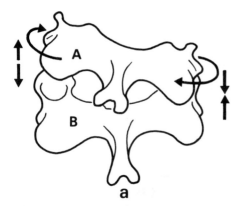

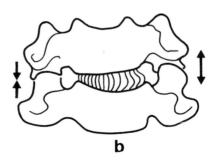

Figure 10.14.   Intervertebral movement is complex. The motions of lateral flexion and rotation are coupled. Thus, a right lateral flexion of vertebra *A* on *B* is ac-companied by a posterior right rotation on *B*. **a,** Posterior view. **b,** Anterior view.

• Rectus capitis minor
• Obliquus capitis superior
• Obliquus capitis inferior

Range of Motion.   The variability of the values assigned by different authors to motion that a priori seems relatively simple is noteworthy. The results are dependent on the author and on the method employed: whether studying live or cadaveric subjects, and whether performing radiographic studies or goniometric measurements.

Total Cervical Flexion/Extension.   Using goniometry on young students, Buck et al. obtained the following average results:

Young Men
• Total flexion 66°
• Total extension 73°

Young Women
• Total flexion 69°
• Total extension 81°

Complete Cervical Lateral Rotation.   Raou measured the maximum range of motion on cadavers and obtained 30–50° for the entire cervical spine bilaterally. Kottke assigns 45° ± 10°.

Complete Cervical Rotation.   For total cervical rotation, Buck et al. assign 146° for young men and 147° for young women. Kottke gives 75° ± 10° for rotation to either side.

Thoracic Motion

In the thoracic spine, the disk to vertebral body height ratio does not allow much mobility. On the other hand, the orientation of the facet joints would otherwise allow rotation and lateroflexion were it not for the ribs restricting their mobility (Fig. 10.15).

The plane of the facets faces posteriorly and slightly superolateraly. Moreover, the articulations form concentric circles with the center of the corresponding vertebral body (Fig. 10.16). The movement of rotation of the upper thoracic spine would theoretically be great were it not for the rib cage. At this level also, rotation is coupled with lateral flexion and is similarly restricted. In the lower thoracic spine, these movements can be produced with greater ease, as there are only a few false ribs to restrict movement.

When the thorax is flexible, as in young people, thoracic rotation is easy. It becomes more difficult with age, when the thorax becomes a semirigid cylinder.

Flexion is limited by the tension in the interspinous ligaments, the ligamentum flavum, the posterior longitudinal ligament, and the facet joint capsule. Thoracic extension is limited by the abutment of the articular and spinal processes.

Range of Movement
Rotation.   In cadaveric studies, Raou found a range of 35° available bilaterally for each thoracic vertebra, with the T8-T9 zone being (without ribs) the most mobile. Kapandji, citing the works of Gregersen and Lucas, measured 35° bilaterally at each thoracic level.

Lateroflexion.   Lateroflexion   was   measured as being up to 3–5° for each vertebra.

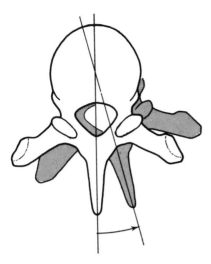

Figure 10.15.   Thoracic rotation.

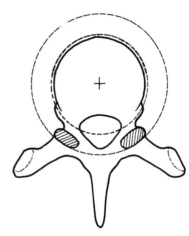

Figure 10.16.   Rotation is facilitated by the fact that the facet joints and the axis of the thoracic vertebral body show a common point from which one can inscribe concentric circles.

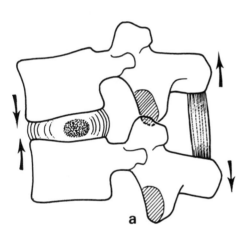
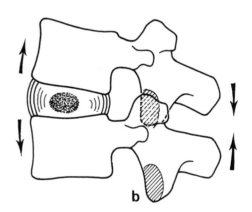

Figure 10.17.   Lumbar vertebrae. **a,** Flexion. **b,** Extension.

When it is slight, it produces an ipsilateral rotation (Rouvière, Lovett). Gonon et al. have shown the range to be greater at the inferior thoracic vertebrae: 6° for T10-T11, 10° for T11-T12, and 8° for T12-L1. Kapandji cites 20° of total thoracic lateroflexion bilaterally.

Flexion-Extension.   There are about 5° for flexion and 5° for extension at each level (Raou). Kapandji assigns 45°, totally, for flexion and 25° for extension, but he emphasizes the great variability with age and the individual. Gonon et al. give 6° for T10-T11, 9° for T11-T12, and 10° for T12-L1.

Lumbar Motion

Flexion-extension is the cardinal movement of the lumbar spine. All elements of the vertebrae at this level contribute to this type of movement (Fig. 10.17): the disk to vertebral body height (one-third) and the orientation of the articular facet joints. The alignment of the articular processes limits rotation at L1 and L2, and it is only the elasticity of the disks and the ligaments that permits rotation below L1 and L2 (Figs. 10.18 and 10.19).

On the other hand, lateral flexion is facili-

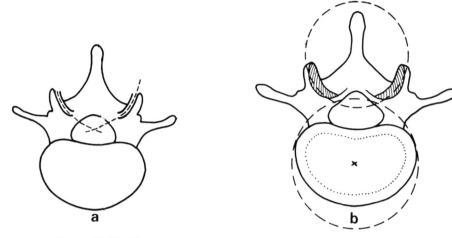

Figure 10.18. The orientation of the facet joint blocks lumbar rotation.

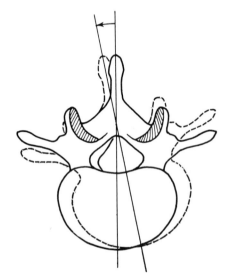

Figure 10.19. A slight amount of rotation is possible at the lumbar level and is primarily performed by a lateral translation of the body of the vertebrae aided by the elasticity of the intervertebral disk.

tated by contralateral divergence and by ipsilateral convergence of the articular processes.

Flexion-Extension. Extension is limited by the spinous processes, which are large at this level, while flexion is limited by the tension in the interspinous and supraspinous ligaments, the posterior longitudinal ligament, and the ligamentum flavum.

Raou, in cadaveric studies, found 20–36° of total flexion and 16–21° of total extension. In radiographic study, Kapandji measured 60° for total flexion and 35° for total extension. Cho-

pin determined an average range of extension to be 70–80°, while flexion was found to be 40° with respect to neutral.

Farfan cited flexion-extension as representing 80–90° for the entire vertebral column. Allbrook found an average of 62° in young men and a much greater mobility in young women.

Farfan found the following figures: 7.5° (flexion plus extension) for L1-L2 and L2-L3, 18° for L3-L4, 22° for L4-L5 (these figures are half for extension and half for flexion), and 18° for L5-S1, i.e., 6° for extension and 12° for flexion.

Gonon et al. give the following figures for each segment:

L5-S1 20°
L4-L5 15°
L3-L4 12°
L2-L3 12°
L1-L2 10°
T12-L1 10°

Lateral Flexion. According to Raou, lateral flexion was found to be in the range of 20–30°. According to Kapandji, it was found to be 10° to each side. According to Chopin, it was in the 20–30° range. The iliolumbar ligament limits movement at the level of L5-S1.

Rotation. Rotation is very limited at this level and, in general, is considered to be 1° per level, except for some authors who believe it to be in the range of 5–6° at L5-S1. This rotation is not pure, and there is an associated coupling with ipsilateral lateroflexion. In cadaveric studies, Raou noted 7–14° on each side. On fresh cadavers we have been able to observe that this rotation increased when the spine is slightly flexed and becomes virtually impossible with the spine in hyperextension. Gonon et al. give the following figures for each segment:

L5-S1 4°
L4-L5 7°
L3-L4 10°
L2-L3 8°
L1-L2 6°
T12-L1 18°

11

BIOMECHANICS OF THE SACROILIAC JOINT

Since Hippocrates, who was the first to note it, it has been universally accepted that the sacroiliac joints play an important role in childbirth. In contradistinction to prior authors (Vésale included), Ambroise Paré confirmed that a certain mobility also existed outside the state of pregnancy and also in men. The works of Delmas and Weisl uncovered facts that led to an understanding of the anatomy and physiology of this articulation that differed greatly from the classic concept of Farabeuf.

TYPES OF ARTICULATIONS

Delmas studied the anatomy of the sacroiliac joint in bipedal primates (gorilla, chimpanzee, orangutan, and gibbon, proceeding from the lesser to the more highly evolved species). Indeed, the gorilla is quadrupedal, the orangutan is exceptionally bipedal, and the gibbon is bipedal on the ground. The changes that occurred in the articular surfaces were significant and directly paralleled the stages of evolution leading to the erect position and walking. In the gorilla the articular surfaces are interlocked, in the gibbon they are flattened (planes), and in the human they are concave on the sacral side.

In humans, the final stage of the evolution, Delmas finds three types of articulations, which he refers to as dynamic, static, and intermediary.

- *Dynamic type*. The dynamic articulation occurs in 25% of humans. It is freely mobile, highly evolved, and "overadapted," corresponding to optimal adaptation for bipedal locomotion. The sacral auricle is concave, and the areas of ligamentous attachment are taut. These subjects have accentuation of their spinal curvatures (Fig. 11.1).
- *Static type*. The static articulation occurs in 25% of humans. In this type of articulation, the articular surfaces are flat, and the areas of ligamentous attachments are more lax. These subjects have moderate spinal curvatures and resemble the primates more closely (Fig. 11.2).
- *Intermediary type*. The intermediary is the most widespread type and occurs in 50% of humans. The sacroiliac articulations are firmly maintained by very strong ligaments. Weisl describes the ligamentous system in a very original and schematic manner. He divides the fibers of the posterior ligaments into two groups: caudal with cranial direction and cranial with lateral direction, which is distended in the nutation movement, i.e., the act of nodding, especially involuntary nodding. These two ligamentous systems balance the weight of the trunk.

JOINT MOTION

Nutation results in rotation of the sacrum on an imaginary "axis of nutation" formed by the iliac bones. Movements about this axis are classically described as follows: forward inclination of the anterior surface of the sacrum is termed nutation, while backward inclination is called counternutation (Figs. 11.3 and 11.4).

Interpretations of the Axis of Movement

Numerous studies and discussions, especially among obstetricians, have focused on determining the exact location of the axis.

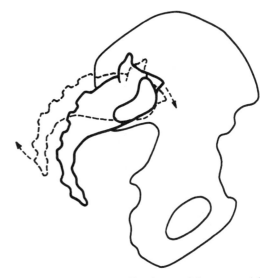

Figure 11.3. Nutation. The base of the sacrum is antetilted, and the coccyx moves posteriorly.

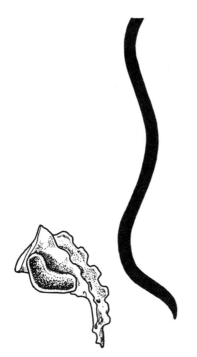

Figure 11.1. "Dynamic" spine of Delmas in a subject with pronounced vertebral curves. The sacral auricle is indented.

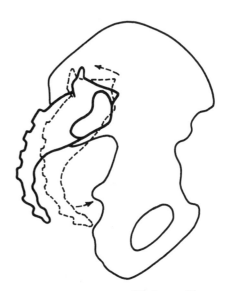

Figure 11.4. Conternutation. The base of the sacrum is retrotilted, and the coccyx is displaced anteriorly.

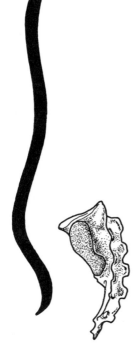

Figure 11.2. "Static" type of curvature of Delmas in which there is a reduction in the vertebral curvature. The auricle is flat.

Bonnaire defended the theory of an axis passing through a point of the articular surface (auricular axis) (Figs. 11.5 and 11.7). Others, especially Farabeuf, maintained that the axis passes to the rear of the auricle through the axial ligament (retroauricular axis) (Figs. 11.5 and 11.8). This concept was highly criticized, and modifications of it were offered, especially by Delmas and Weisl.

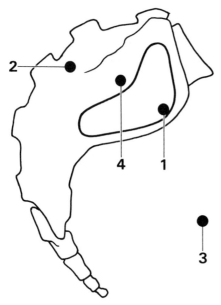

Figure 11.5. Different axes of movement of the sacroiliac articulations according to Bonnaire (*1*), Farabeuf (*2*), Weisl (*3*), and J. B. Mennell and, later, Bakland and Hansen (*4*).

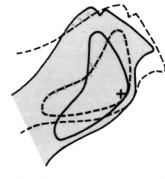

Figure 11.7. Movement according to Bonnaire.

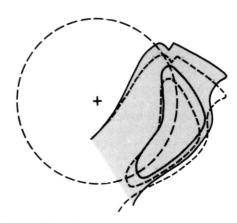

Figure 11.8. Movement according to Farabeuf.

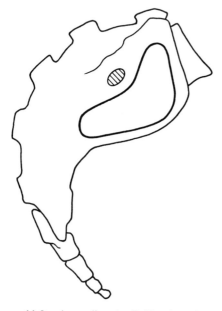

Figure 11.6. According to Bakland and Hansen, there exists an axial articulation.

Weisl's Concept

Weisl, after conducting extensive radiographic studies, formulated a new concept:

- There is no rotational movement at the sacroiliac articulations (Figs. 11.4 and 11.10, 11.5 and 11.9).
- Movements of the sacroiliac articulation are posterior-anterior movements, but the rostral segment of the articular surface is submitted to a more severe displacement than is the caudal segment (Fig. 11.9).
- This displacement, which is almost a transference, is around a virtual axis located about 5–10 cm below the promontory (preauricular axis). The seat of that axis varies from one individual to another and in the same individual by the movement performed (the displacement of that axis could then exceed 5 cm). In 12–14% of subjects, this is a simple

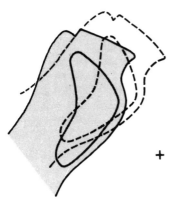

Figure 11.9. First type of movement according to Weisl (86–88% of individuals).

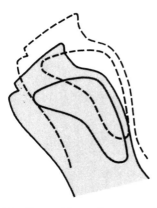

Figure 11.10. Second type of movement according to Weisl (12–14% of individuals). It represents a translation.

movement of transference from front to back; therefore, there is no axis of nutation in these individuals.

Wilder et al. have studied sacroiliac joint motion and have made the following remarks:

- Given the prominence of the articular surfaces (in the sagittal and frontal planes), rotation could not be accomplished about the proposed axes.
- If rotation occurred according to the described axes, a notable separation of the auricular surfaces would be necessary, but this is impossible because of the ligamentous restraint.
- A certain transference can be performed, provided there exists a sufficient amount of

spacing for the articular surfaces. This spacing is necessary because the surfaces are not planes. The most favorable axis for this translation is called by the authors the "rough axis."

Axial Sacroiliac Articulation

Accessory sacroiliac articulations have been described that are inconstant and located in the rear of the principal articulation (Fig. 11.6). Hadley describes a superficial articulation at the level of the second sacral foramen as well as a deep one at the level of the first sacral foramen. What is curious is that the incidence of these articulations increases with age, which may be explained by the mechanical work of these formations.

Bakland and Hansen, restudying sacroiliac articulations, described an axial sacroiliac articulation located 15 mm in the rear of the sacroiliac articulation (very much at the level of the deep accessory articulation of Hadley). It is, according to these authors, constant in the adult. It is formed by an iliac protuberance and a sacral cavity opposing each other very narrowly. These surfaces are slightly incongruous, but this incongruity is decreased by the juxtaposition of a loose conjunctive tissue rich in adipocytes. The iliac protuberance is often lined with articular cartilage. These authors think that the axis of rotation of the sacroiliac articulation goes through this axial sacroiliac articulation. It is noteworthy that this corresponds to the opinion of J. B. Mennell, who described an axis of rotation going through an "iliac protuberance and a deep sacral depression," which corresponds perfectly with the axial articulation as described by Bakland and Hansen.

Motion Evaluation

A certain degree of sacroiliac joint motion is available. Proof of this is the existence of a layer of articular cartilage covering the articular surfaces; but its appearance, grayish red with shaggy extensions, shows that it is very mobile (Olivier).

Pregnancy accentuates the normal mobility of this articulation but does not create any particular movement at that level (Sureau).

Displacements of the Sacrum According to Positions

These displacements have been studied, especially by obstetricians. They are caused by movements of the trunk and lower limbs. Crouzat in 1881 and Walcher in 1889 tried to use this concept to widen the superior aperture during delivery (Sureau). Weisl showed these relations radiographically:

- The promontory is displaced posteriorly during trunk or hip extension. Forward displacement occurs with flexion.
- Moving from supine to standing, which corresponds to the maximum range of motion of the sacroiliac articulation, results in an anterior displacement of the promontory in 90% of the cases.

In standing, the sacrum is close to the anterior limit of its course. In the supine position, it is close to the posterior limit of its course.

Sureau remarked that in a subject in the upright position where the sacrum is already in maximum anterior tilt, trunk or hip flexion cannot add to the existing nutation. Trunk extension in standing more or less displaces the promontory posteriorly. In the supine position, however, flexion of the thighs can displace the promontory anteriorly, but further extension does not lead to further displacement of the promontory posteriorly.

According to Testut, displacing the base of the sacrum by 2 mm results in a movement of 5–6 mm at the top of the coccyx. This motion is, of course, accentuated during delivery.

Nutation is maximal when one is standing and carrying a heavy load on the shoulders. The movement of counternutation is maximal in acrobats doing the "bridge."

Asymmetry of the Movement

Stracha et al. (cited by Piedallu) have studied the pelvis and vertebral column in a cadaveric study. They immobilized one of the iliac bones in a vise, leaving the pubic symphysis free to move. The displacements were recorded by the movements of rods and sliders fixed to the sacrum and to the free iliac bone. The lumbar spine was then flexed, extended, rotated, laterally flexed, distracted, and compressed axially. The authors concluded that the movements of the sacroiliac articulation are complex, combining translation with rotation. This is similar to Weisl's concept and shows the asymmetry of function of the two sacroiliac articulations. In 1949, Ingelrans and Oberthur noted that outside of pregnancy the movements were reduced, but they drew attention to the movements of torsion and lateroflexion that occur simultaneously and in opposite directions in each sacroiliac joint: "during ambulation, i.e., during the stance phase, the ipsilateral iliac wing tilts posteriorly, while the sacrum antetilts slightly." This is what is described as the position of "anterior sacrum" by osteopaths. In France, it is referred to as the position of the forward step (Piedallu).

Studies of Living Anatomical Relationships

Colachis et al. studied the problem of sacroiliac mobility in vivo. To study the live anatomic relationships, they drove Kirschner's wires into the posterior superior iliac spine of 12 medical student volunteers. Two pins were placed in one side of the spine and one in the other side. This was done to avoid any error that could occur if there was only one pin on each side; i.e., rotation of the sacroiliac joint could occur without any modification of the distance between the two pins, while with two pins on one side, there is a fixed plane of reference.

The authors avoided subjects who were obese, and they inserted the pins at the most superficial part of the bone, so that the traction of the soft tissues on the pin during movements would not be a source of error. Movements executed by the volunteers included sitting, standing, forward trunk flexion, and maximal flexion of a thigh on the trunk with the contralateral thigh in maximal extension. The authors came to the following conclusions:

- Sacroiliac joint motion did in fact occur in the examined subjects (young men).
- This motion was very small and varied very much from subject to subject.
- The greatest motion was seen during anterior trunk flexion, when a 5-mm separation of the iliac spines was noted in the most marked case.

This study was not an attempt to measure the articulation between the iliac and sacrum but was an attempt to measure the relative movements between the two iliac bones.

Using the photogrammetric technique of Suh, Lavignolle et al. (1983) studied the displacement of the iliac bones on the body in relation to the sacrum and the amplitudes of these displacements in precise movements. There were only five cases in this study, but the findings are interesting:

- The position of the axes was variable from subject to subject; nevertheless, the axes were in a rather consistent position in front of and below the sacroiliac articulations.
- The types of displacements of the iliac bones were identical in all subjects, uniting rotation and translation on these axes with a phenomenon of anterior "unlocking" of the articulations.
- Joint range of motion was reduced and variable, depending on the individual, but was on average 10–12° of rotation and at 6 mm of translation (they were young subjects, less than 25 years of age).

The range of the motion is greater here than in the movements measured by Egund et al. (1977), who used a stereophotogrammetric method and noted a range of motion of about 2°.

CONCLUSION

Wilder considered the functional role of the sacroiliac joint to remain an enigma. Given the results of most studies, however, he believed it would be safe to say that the joint played a role in acting as a shock absorber, absorbing the energy imparted by its powerful ligamentous system.

We are in agreement with this broad conclusion. These articulations have a very variable morphology, depending on the individual. But it is evident that regardless of their differences of mobility, they all still have, with more or less efficiency, the same functions:

- In women, the sacroiliac joint plays a role in labor and delivery.
- In all individuals, this articulation is like a shock absorber, absorbing the enormous pressures transmitted by the spine through ligamentous tension and joint microdisplacements.

12

FORCES ACTING ON THE VERTEBRAL COLUMN

THE DISK: SHOCK ABSORBER AND PRESSURE DIFFUSER

The disk absorbs shock and diffuses pressure on the spine. The farther down the spinal column toward the lumbar region one goes, the more the pressure loading of the column increases.

The superior cervical spine is, nevertheless, capable of supporting the head and performing precise movements without the aid of intervertebral disks. Thus, in spite of its apparent fragility and thin articular surface, it is submitted to considerable loads.

In the normal vertebral spine, the healthy disk is perfectly homogeneous and very hydrophilic. When it is loaded axially, its height decreases (Fig. 12.1), and the annulus bulges at the periphery like a tire under an excessive load. The decrease in the height of the disk space can be 1.5 mm for the lumbar disk of an individual carrying 100 kg on the shoulders. In fact, one must first add to this 100-kg weight the weight of the trunk and of the head, which is about 40 kg for a man weighing 80 kg, and then the intrinsic compressive force produced by muscular contraction that increases compression on the disk. This means that the disk will have to support a load of more than 150 kg when the individual is upright and the disk is in normal position. If the individual bends forward, the pressure on the nucleus pulposus will be transmitted most forcefully to the posterior annular fibers, which are the weakest of the fibers that make up the annulus fibrosus.

PRESSURE

Some authors have calculated the approximate compressive and distractive forces on the mobile segment in different anatomic positions, both with and without extrinsic loads. Here are a few examples taken from the studies of Herbert:

- *Subject standing, without overload:* the lumbar disk is submitted to a pressure of 15 kg/cm^2 in the nucleus, taken in tension by the annulus, and to a strain of shearing of 13 kg in the corresponding facet joints.
- *Subject in forward flexion:* the disk is submitted to a pressure of 58 kg/cm^2 in the nucleus, taken in tension by the annulus, and to a shearing of 47 kg in a plane perpendicular to the axis of the column, absorbed in compression of the facet joints.
- *Subject in full flexion, lifting up a bar of 100 kg:* the disk is submitted to a compression of 144 kg/cm^2 in the nucleus, taken in tension by the annulus, and to a shearing of 126 kg supported by the facet joints, absorbed in compression.

In this case, theoretically, there is a total pressure of 1000 kg on the nucleus. This demonstrates the enormous pressures brought on the intervertebral segments.

By measuring the intradiscal pressure, Nachemson introduced some new notions: (*a*) load on the nucleus is greater when sitting than when standing (measured on the L3 disk); (*b*) pressure is maximal during sitting, with the subject bent forward and lifting a load, arms

68

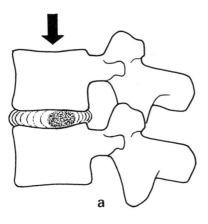

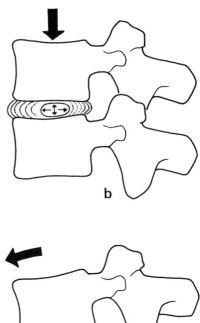

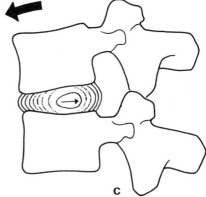

Figure 12.1. **a** and **b**, The axial pressure dissipated by the disk is transmitted to the annulus fibrosus and to the vertebral endplates. **c**, During anterior flexion, the nucleus pulposus moves posteriorly.

hanging; (c) the lowest pressure is measured with the subject supine; and (d) intradiscal pressure increases 45% with coughing and 45% with trunk rotation. For a 70-kg man in the upright position (Fig. 12.2), for example, the pressure on the L3 disk is 70 kg. It is about 120 kg if he bends forward 20°, and it is 340 kg if he lifts a load of 20 kg with his legs extended.

In a preliminary study, Drevet, using a material capable of taking both static and dynamic measures (a miniaturized piezo-resistive capacitor), noted the following:

- Important variations in the basal pressures in subjects of the same age and of identical morphotype
- Extremely rapid variations according to exogenous factors (suspension, carrying loads, etc.)
- Piezo-resistive measurements ranging from 1 to 3, depending on contraction of the muscles.

The lumbar spine is not alone in being subjected to such stresses. There is, for example, the cervico-occipital junction, with its narrow bony structures and slender articular surfaces that support and allow for the mobility of the large 5-kg ball that is the head. The latter rests in equilibrium on two small facets the size of nails, and it can be mobilized in all directions. Some persons carry on their heads loads of over 50 kg, which are transmitted in their entirety to the articulations of the first two vertebrae, since at that level there is no disk to dissipate compressive loads (Fig. 12.3).

ROLE OF THE ABDOMINAL WALL

Intra-abdominal pressure generated by the contraction of the abdominal musculature has to be taken into account (Bartelink) when evaluating the effective load that the lumbar spine

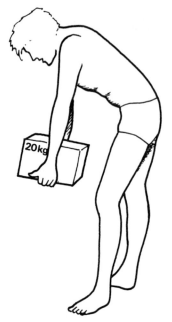

Figure 12.2. For a 70-kg standing man, the pressure on the L3 disk is on the order of 70 kg. It changes during forward flexion, when the angle reaches 20° from the vertical, to a pressure on the order of 120 kg. When a weight of 20 kg is lifted with the legs extended, the pressure reaches 340 kg (numbers according to Nachemson). Intradiscal pressure, however, depends not only on the weight lifted but also on the intensity of the contraction of the muscles involved.

must support. Any lumbar effort in effect "leans" on contracted abdominal muscles. The intra-abdominal pressure absorbs part of the load: 30%, according to Morris et al. The contraction of the abdominal muscles can be replaced or supplemented by the resistance that a corset or belt provides (as in a weight lifter's belt). The way that a corset or belt helps is that it provides an inelastic resistance against which an elastic, contracted, or lax abdominal wall cannot expand, thus increasing the intra-abdominal pressure. Thus, good abdominal muscle tone and a strong diaphragm and pelvic floor aid in reducing the load on the lumbar spine by reducing the pressures that it must support. Furthermore, because of their attachment to the thoracolumbar fascia, the abdominal muscles create an extensor moment upon the spine when they contract, imparting further stability.

ROLE OF THE VERTEBRAL BODY AS A SHOCK ABSORBER

The disk may not be the only shock-absorbing element of the spine. In light of the studies of Lamy and Farfan, it appears that the verte-

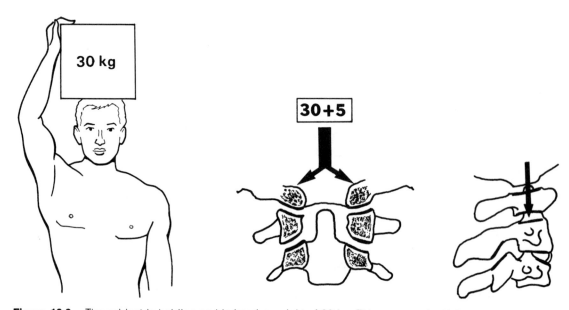

Figure 12.3. The subject is holding on his head a weight of 30 kg. This mass and weight are transmitted to the atlanto-occipital and the atlantoaxial articulations. The first disk to encounter this pressure is between C2 and C3.

bral body itself functions as a shock absorber with variable resistance. First, the authors expressed the liquid contained in a vertebral body, approximately 0.8–1 mL for each vertebral body. Then they studied 60 cadavers. From 30 of them they squeezed out half of the vertebral liquid, using pipettes placed in the vascular holes, which amounted to 0.5 mL per vertebra. The other 30 cadavers remained untouched and formed the second group. To each of the columns they applied increased axial loads. Under weak loading, the two groups behaved similarly. When the load was increased gradually, the normal vertebrae of the second group demonstrated increased resistance in contrast to the vertebrae of the first group. The authors concluded that the vertebral body has an automatic hydraulic system that modifies its resistance according to the load received. They also believed that when the lumbar spine is in a flexed position, the posterior ligaments act like a valve, blocking venous circulation on its return course, while intra-abdominal pressure is sufficient to block the external venous system. These two mechanisms that block intervertebral venous circulation act synergistically to increase the elastic resistance of the vertebral body during effort.

ROLE OF THE SACROILIAC JOINTS

It seems clear that the essential role of the sacroiliac joints is that of being a very powerful shock absorber (see Chapter 11).

13

THE AGING SPINE

EFFECTS ON THE VERTEBRAL BODY

Aging results in progressive bone loss, which begins at 30–40 years of age and continues for the remainder of the person's life. This process accelerates considerably in women for 8–10 years following menopause. It mainly affects trabecular bones, especially the vertebral bodies. Bone loss is from 1–2% per year and can reach 12% 2 years following oophorectomy (Genant, Riggs). This loss of bone mass, or osteopenia, results in compression fractures, often spontaneous or following trivial trauma.

EFFECTS ON THE INTERVERTEBRAL DISK

With age, the intervertebral disk dehydrates, and the physicochemical state of the ground substance is altered. The result is that the collagen fibers, which are few and slender at the beginning of life, become tight, thicken, and tend to group together with age, in almost parallel direction, and form fibrous bundles. This can be seen on macroscopic sections of the aged disk. It is called the "maturation of collagen," and its quantity increases notably in the second part of life, after about age 40; the rate of mucopolysaccharide production increases briefly, and then progressively diminishes for the duration of life.

Nucleus Pulposus

Little by little, the nucleus pulposus loses its gelatinous homogeneous character, the very qualities that make it a remarkable shock absorber. While this is occurring, the biaxial alignment of the fibers of the annulus fibrosus changes; they become unidirectional bundles, resulting in a significant loss of elasticity. They become less hydrophilic as the years go by, with water occupying a smaller proportion of the disk (79% in young children to 70% at 70 years of age). As we have previously remarked, this process of aging also affects the cartilaginous endplates, reducing possible sources of nutrition for the nucleus, which gets its nutrition from the apertures of the endplates. The more this osmotic exchange decreases, the more rapidly the disk deteriorates. Fortunately, this process occurs without clinical manifestations. At the same time that the disk ages, the ligaments stiffen and progressively limit spinal motion. As humans age, however, they progressively reduce their activities, and therefore, usually, between a fragile disk and reduced disk mobility, an equilibrium can most often be established (de Sèze) (Fig. 13.1).

For various reasons (e.g., trauma), some disks degenerate earlier than others. A disk can be old in a young subject. When a disk becomes vulnerable, it is generally the posterior annulus fibrosus that is most affected. This is the part that is subject to most of the compressive loading and thus fails; it is either compressed, forced back, or torn, resulting in a posterior or posterolateral disk herniation.

Formation of Osteophytes

De Sèze states,

In other cases, under the isolated or combined influence of aging, professional activities, and constitutional weakness, while the central nucleus pulposus

72

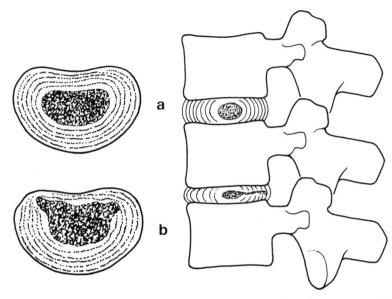

Figure 13.1. **a**, Normal intervertebral disk. **b**, Degenerative disk, including deterioration of the annulus fibrosus and nucleus pulposus.

degenerates, the annulus fibrosus is progressively driven anteriorly toward the periphery, where it comes in contact with the anterior longitudinal ligament. At this point a process of subligamentous ossification will occur, resulting in the formation of an osteophytic ring around the degenerated disk [Figs. 13.2 and 13.3].

This osteophyte originates at the vertebral body in the subligamentous zone that is found between the anterior longitudinal ligament (which, as we noted previously, adheres loosely to the disk but firmly to the vertebral body on the side of the endplate) and the attachment of the annulus fibrosus. It is molded on that ligament, which, due to disk degeneration, will bulge more and more. This explains the tendency for osteophytes to form horizontally when a very deteriorated disk is flattened; their orientation is more vertical when the disk is less flattened (Fig. 13.3).

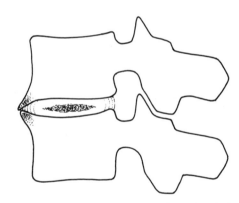

Figure 13.2. Formation of an anterior osteophyte (in section).

EFFECTS ON THE FACET JOINTS

Prior to stiffening of the ligamentous system, loss of disk height creates instability of the intervertebral joint and, in some cases, joint hypermobility (Junghanns). The degenerating disk will also affect other elements of a mobile segment: facet joints (Figs. 13.4 and 13.5), which become arthrotic, and the interspinous ligament. In hyperlordosis, two spinal segments can come into contact in the lumbar region. This is known as the "kissing spine" or, if it has progressed by one more degree, is a true arthrosis with molding of the spine at contact (syndrome of Baastrup) (see L2, L3, and L4 on Fig. 13.6).

In a study of 30 postmortem examinations of subjects 30–70 years of age, Rissanen showed that there were an equal percentage and parallelism between the degeneration of

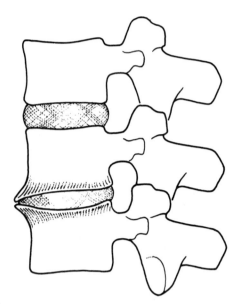

Figure 13.3. Lateral view. The osteophyte has formed a ring.

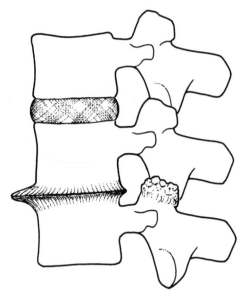

Figure 13.5. Lateral view of a segment with complete disk degeneration and arthrosis of the facet joint.

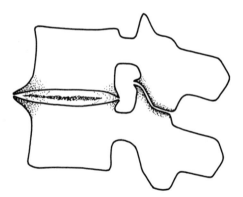

Figure 13.4. With further disk deterioration there is increased stress on the facet joints, resulting in posterior element arthrosis.

the disk and the degeneration of the interspinous ligament.

Trophostatic Syndrome of Menopause

All the consequences of intervertebral disk degeneration of maximum intensity can be seen in what de Sèze and Caroit have called the "trophostatic syndrome of the menopausal woman." Heaviness and loosening of the abdomen, together with postural collapse and compression of the vertebral column, produce

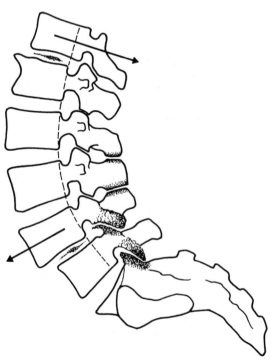

Figure 13.6. Postmenopausal trophostatic syndrome of de Sèze and Caroit.

the following deformations. Hyperlordosis occurs, which results in increased stress on the lower lumbar facet joints. This increased stress results in increased shearing and a tendency toward anterolisthesis. As a consequence of the same stress, retrolisthesis of the vertebrae of the superior lumbar region can occur, which results in the vertebrae resting, in a posterior position, on the subjacent vertebra, producing shearing of the facet joints. As a result of the deformation, the spinous processes come into contact with each other to produce an arthrosis of the spinous processes.

Intervertebral Foramen

The intervertebral foramen also undergoes changes as a result of the proliferation of osteophytes and disk degeneration. This occurs particularly at the level of the cervical spine because of the existence of the uncinate process and the formation of disco-osteophytic nodules (Fig. 13.7) and because of the frequency of spondylosis of the facet joints. The latter causes a narrowing of the posterior neuroforamina and is most commonly seen at its superior aspect. The inferior aspect is affected only in the advanced stage of the spondylosis. At the cervical level, posterior spondylosis can exist without a concomitant discal lesion (Hirsch, Payne et al., Friedenberg et al.).

The evolutionary formation of the disco-osteophytic nodule is debated. For some, there is an uncovertebral articulation with an articular cavity and a synovial membrane. This articulation could become arthrotic. When a fragment of the nucleus of the degenerated disk bulges into the articulations, it creates a "hard her-

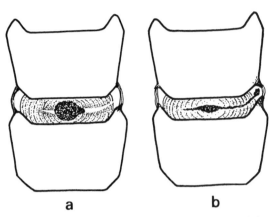

a   **b**

Figure 13.8. Formation of the osteophytic nodule: classic theory. **a**, There is an uncovertebral articulation with an articular cavity and synovial tissue. This articulation can thus undergo arthritic degeneration. **b**, The disk degeneration produces fissures in the annulus in the region of the nucleus pulposus. This can cause enlargement and reach the periphery. As a result, a fragment of the nucleus pulposus can then slip out into the arthrotic articulation and create a hard discal herniation known as a discal osteophyte.

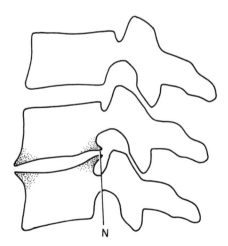

Figure 13.7. Osteophytic nodule (*N*) at the cervical level.

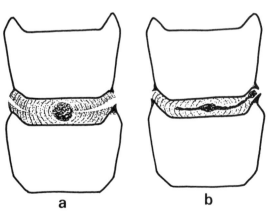

a   **b**

Figure 13.9. Formation of the osteophytic nodules: Töndury's theory. **a**, There is no uncovertebral articulation. **b**, After the age of 10, there is fissuring of the annulus fibrosus, which allows a progressive movement of the nucleus pulposus outward. As this happens, the material of the nucleus pulposus hardens in the fissures and, on gaining entry into the periphery, forms the osteophytic nodules.

niated disk." This is called the disco-osteo-phytic nodule (Fig. 13.8).

According to Töndury, there is no uncovertebral articulation (Fig. 13.9). He believed that from age 10, fibrous fissures form in the annulus at the periphery, gradually extending toward the center. When they reach the annulus, the discal jelly reaches the periphery, forming a hard herniated disk (Figs. 13.8 and 5.4).

At the level of the cervical spine, these formations affect not only the elements going through the foramen intervertebrale but also the vertebral artery that extends into the transverse openings. This was demonstrated on arteriograms, but it could not be definitely affirmed that these formations, as those seen in spondylosis, have a direct pathologic role, since images of sinus arteries are seen in asymptomatic patients. In spite of this, the success of uncinate processectomies has been demonstrated in some cases (Jung).

III

PAIN OF SPINAL ORIGIN

14

EXPERIMENTALLY PROVOKED PAIN

Pain is one of the most frequent presenting complaints among patients with vertebral pathology leading to medical consultation. It may be felt and described in many diverse ways, varying from patient to patient. It is the major symptom in those conditions where the prognosis is rarely in question and where the functional prognosis is only rarely so.

It results from a complex process combining central sensory phenomena with affective and emotional processes. Its repercussion depends on the personality of the subject. Acute pain is an alarm symptom, while chronic pain can become an illness by itself, without any relation to the initial lesion. A modern understanding of the anatomic structures and the neuromediators involved in the transmission of nociceptive impulses has led to a better understanding of some pain phenomena.

The nociceptive impulses coming from the peripheral receptors reach the central nervous system via several routes, with synaptic relays in the posterior horn of the spinal cord gray matter, the nuclei of the thalamus, and the cerebral cortex.

These impulses are regulated by a negative feedback loop. One theory of how inhibitory controls work is called the gate control theory (Melzack and Wall). According to this theory, nociceptive impulses are modulated at the segmental level in the spinal cord; stimulation of large-diameter proprioceptive fibers can inhibit the activity of the smaller-diameter nociceptive fibers.

Another inhibitory system at work is the system of suprasegmental verification that, via a descending serotonergic pathway, is capable of blocking the transmission of nociceptive impulses at the spinal cord level. It has been shown that electrical stimulation of certain cerebral regions, notably the periaqueductal gray matter, can bring on analgesia (Reynolds). This control can be inactivated, however, by the morphine antagonists, naloxone and nalorphine. The endorphins (β-endorphins and enkephalins) intervene at several levels in this verification, playing a role in the modulation of pain.

On a practical level and in the framework of common vertebral pain syndromes, it is important is to try to understand what creates pain at the vertebral level, in order to best be able to determine the involved segments (to know the relays and referral patterns in relation to its origin). We know that clinically pain can be local, regional, or radicular in distribution, but it can also be referred at a distance and be difficult to diagnose.

In this section, we look at experimentally provoked pains arising from different spinal structures and their resemblance to those seen clinically. We then consider the different vertebral lesions, be they degenerative, mechanical, or static, seen in current pathology. We then consider that the lesions in the classical repertoire do not correspond to or explain the nature of these painful disorders or the often rapid and favorable responses that carefully performed spinal manipulation can provide.

In most pathology, the lesions detected radiographically are in many cases irrelevant and not responsible for the pain complaint; in many cases, even the most sophisticated examinations leave us without diagnostic answers. Often, however, an attentive clinical examination including segmental palpation techniques, which are normally painless, reveals a specific painful vertebral segment. The "lesion" detected is an example of a "painful minor intervertebral dysfunction" (PMID) (Maigne), consisting of painful segmental vertebral dysfunctions that are often associated with skin hypersensitivity and altered tissue texture in a metameric distribution: cellulalgic, myalgic, and tenoperiosteal. They constitute the "segmental vertebral celluloperiosteomyalgic syndrome" of the author, of which the PMID is often the source.

Pain can only arise from the irritation of an innervated structure or from the nerve itself. The anatomy shows us, for example, that the nucleus pulposus is not innervated. It cannot, therefore, be a source of pain. However, it can precipitate pain if it irritates an innervated element or the nerve root itself. This occurs when the nucleus bulges and imparts tension to the superficial and posterior annular fibers, the posterior longitudinal ligament, or the nerve root.

Experiments confirm these facts. They have delineated the sensitivity of different spinal structures and revealed the local and referred pain patterns of experimentally provoked pains. The comparisons that can be made between experimentally provoked pains and the ones seen daily at clinic are highly useful in telling us something about the origins of these pains.

In this chapter, we look first at pain resulting from the irritation of the spinal nerve roots, then at pains provoked by the irritation of each of the components of the mobile segments (annulus fibrosus, facet joints, anterior and posterior longitudinal ligaments, interspinous ligament), and finally at pains that originate in muscles and tendons.

THE SPINAL NERVE ROOT

Sensory Root

Experimental stimulation of the sensory root provokes sharp pain in the area of the corresponding dermatome. It is demonstrated easily by irritative infiltrations of the nerve. Pricking the nerve provokes a sharp and sudden flash of pain all along its pathway. During interventions on the cervical spine, Cloward directly excited the sensory root and obtained the same result.

If a nerve root is subjected to sustained pressure, however, pain is not elicited; numbness occurs instead (Inman and Saunders, Burke). According to Inman and Saunders, "the usual concept that sciatic pain is only due to pressure on the nerve root is not supported by experimental evidence."

Neither does nerve root traction appear to be the cause of root pain. Falconer performed animal experiments in which small pieces of wax were placed under the nerve roots, at the level of the lumbar intervertebral disks. When the animals woke up, a paralysis in the corresponding area was seen, with the animal returning to its normal behavior in 48 hours without paralysis. A reintervention showed that the wax did not move, the nerve had adjusted. Such a stretching, therefore, is not sufficient to cause pain. Admittedly, in cases of radicular pain of mechanical origin, such as sciatica, reactive inflammation of the nerve root is often implicated in pain production, making the nervous fibers hyperexcitable.

Another notion, held by Frykholm, is of great interest in understanding the radicular pains of mechanical vertebral origin. Frykholm noticed that the compression of a cervical root by a hard hernia (disco-osteophyte nodule) can be tolerated a long time. To cause pain, another mechanical element must intervene, suddenly provoking a forceful or strenuous variation of pressure, or a fibrosis of the cul-de-sac of the dura mater must occur, or a reactive inflammation must start.

This notion that a forceful or strenuous variation of pressure is necessary to cause pain is interesting. It helps to understand why a patient with a herniated disk can have violent pain after a sudden movement, and why pain can, in many cases, with or without treatment, decrease or disappear while the herniated disk remains unchanged.

Motor Root

It is not usual to consider that irritation of the motor root can provoke pain. However, Frykholm, then Cloward, excited the motor root of the cervical nerves and provoked pains in patients that reproduced the "typical pain" that they had experienced during cervical radicular irritation as a result of a herniated disk. This provoked pain was described as being "deep, exasperating," very different from the one brought by excitation of the sensory root.

For these two authors, the common radicular pain is made up of two pains: one is due to the irritation of the sensory root, while the other is myalgic, i.e., due to the irritation of the motor root. This is consistent with the sensation felt by patients with sciatica or cervicobrachial neuralgia. Remember that cramps are frequent sequelae in the patient with sciatica; they are very painful and often associated with fasciculations. Electromyographic examinations often reveal fibrillation potentials, which are spontaneous single muscular fiber discharges seen in association with nerve root pathology. In some cases of sciatica or femoral neuralgia, this myalgic element is characteristic (see Chapter 43, "Sciatica," and Chapter 44, "Femoral Neuralgia").

THE DISK

All authors agree that the nucleus pulposus is not innervated while the superficial annular fibers are. Wiberg studied the sensitivity of different vertebral structures at the lumbar and cervical levels in patients under local anesthesia. He concluded that in the lumbar spine pressure on the posterior surface of the disk and posterior longitudinal ligament resulted in lumbosacral pain in every case. It is a deep pain ipsilateral to the side of excitation. Anesthesia of the corresponding spinal nerve does not modify the result.

At the lumbar level, Cloward arrived at the same conclusions as Wiberg. By irritation of the superficial fibers of the lumbar hemidisk, Cloward provoked pains radiating to the sacroiliac region, the hip, and the buttock of the same side. He concluded that these pains are related to an irritation of the sinovertebral nerve that innervates the peripheral fibers of the disk and the ligaments that surround it. He drew a distinction between this "discogenic" pain and the "neurogenic" pain arising from irritation of the spinal root:

An intradiscal injection of 0.2–0.3 mL of opaque radiologic liquid does not cause any pain if the disc is normal. However, if the fibers of the annulus are torn and if the solution injected under pressure reaches the periphery of the disc, pain is felt. Its localization, its character [,] and its intensity will depend on the site and the extent of the discal tear.

This point is debatable. Holt made 148 discograms on 50 young volunteers without any vertebral pains. He noted that the intradiscal injection of the contrast liquid can be painful without the presence of a tear in the annulus. However, in patients with discal pathology, it is the exact reproduction of their typical pain during discography that is felt to be significant in addition to the morphologic features seen radiographically.

The results obtained by these authors are very much the same at the cervical level as at the lumbar level where irritation of the posterior surface of the annulus and posterior longitudinal ligament is concerned. When the inferior cervical spine is involved, pain is referred to the shoulder and the upper arm (Falconer et al., Wiberg, Cloward). Cloward also noted the possibility of provoking referred pain by pinching or pressing the anterolateral part of the last cervical disks. He thus produced a dorsal periscapular pain aften associated with cervical herniated disks. There, too, he found that the sinuvertebral nerve of Luschka played an important role.

Cloward's observation is consistent with our own studies of periscapular pain of low cervical origin. But we believe that the source of this pain referral can arise from certain cervical spinal structures other than the disk. Our clinical observations do not allow us to share Cloward's opinion on this point or on the mechanism of that referred pain (see Chapter 36, "Chronic Thoracic Pain").

Rabischong and Serrano-Vela have found many small nerve endings in the anterior longitudinal ligament, in the feltwork separating this ligament from the disk, and in the superficial laminae of the annulus. They do not believe that this innervation is exclusive of the sinuvertebral nerve.

THE FACET JOINTS

By injecting 11% hypertonic saline into the lumbar facet joints, L4-L5 or L5-S1, Hirsch et al. noticed the appearance of a sharp lumbar pain after a few seconds. A few moments later, the pain radiated to the sacroiliac and gluteal regions and to the great trochanter, and then in a few minutes disappeared.

Taillard's findings were a little different. After irritating the capsules of the lumbar facet joints under local anesthesia in patients with spondylolisthesis, he provoked referred pains producing a sciatic, pseudoradicular referral pattern:

[I]nteresting observations have been made in patients operated under local anesthesia. It is easy to obtain a good Novocaine infiltration in the subcutaneous tissues, the lumbar fascia, the paravertebral muscles, the periosteum of the laminae. But in general[,] this anesthesia is not strong enough to make the capsules of the facet joints insensitive. It is almost always possible to reproduce the patient's typical pain complaint by pinching or rubbing the capsule close to the joint. Not only the lumbar pain, but also the sciatic pain radiating into the thigh, the calf[,] and sometimes even the foot, are produced.

Since the publications of Rees (1971) and Shealy (1975), the lumbar facets have been in the forefront of work evaluating the patterns of lumbar pain. By various means, such as injection of hypertonic saline solution (Mooney and Robertson, 1976) and electrical stimulation (Bogduk and Don Long, 1980), lumbar pains have been provoked that are referred to the inferior limbs in a diffuse, vague, and generalized fashion, often suggestively reproducing a more or less radicular topography; i.e., the pain is referred in a sclerotomal pattern.

Such pain referral patterns are frequently seen in clinic. They are often relieved by infiltration of the corresponding facet joint if the latter was found painful on examination (see Segmental Examination in Chapter 20, "General Principles"). During the injection, it is not rare to momentarily exacerbate the referred pain. These pains have an apparently radicular distribution.

Sometimes, facet injection provokes, transitorily, referred pains that do not apparently correspond to any diagram of anatomic or embryologic distribution. Thus we have noticed that infiltration of the thoracolumbar junction facets occasionally reproduces a transitory pain in the posterior aspect of the leg ipsilaterally, a sciatic distribution, although it usually does not extend below the superior gluteal region.

THE INTERSPINOUS LIGAMENTS

Kellgren injected a few drops of 5% hypertonic saline in the interspinous ligaments after anesthesia of the skin and provoked local and distant pain. According to Kellgren, the topography of this pain corresponded to the referral pattern expected for the innervating spinal roots, with some differences at the level of the limbs. This pain was characterized as a profound deep pain. Still according to him (1948), the infiltration of the interspinous ligaments L1-L2 provoked pain in an area that was noticeably the area of the L1 root. But this pain seemed more like the pain of renal colic than the pain of a radiculitis, and it was accompanied by retraction of the testicle (Fig. 14.1).

Feinstein (1954) used the method of Kellgren and obtained similar results. Studying five subjects, he made up a map of the pain provoked by injection in each of the interspinous ligaments from the occiput to S3. Pain had a constant recurrent characteristic topography that could be demonstrated in subjects when reexamined after an interval of several days. It lasted for about 10 minutes after the injection, but in some cases, it persisted for several days. It radiated locally and at a distance. The extent of the zone of diffusion varied according to the quantity of the liquid injected (0.2–1 mL); tolerance varied from one subject to another. Some did not tolerate the maximal dose.

Feinstein insisted that this distribution did not correspond to the dermatome; it was, as he says, "segmental." It corresponded to the whole of the tissues innervated by the corresponding sensory nerve root (muscle, bone, ligaments, skin), not just to the cutaneous area (dermatome).

We are concerned here with where the pain was "felt." Each of the five subjects gave the precise area where it was felt. The *dark areas* indicated in Figure 14.2 are where all subjects felt pain and where it was strongest. Feinstein remarks that when examining the objective sensitivity, there is often a slight hypoesthesia, more rarely a hyperesthesia, in these areas.

Glover (1960), using a pin, regularly found zones of hypersensitivity in patients with back pain; he looked for them in the paravertebral

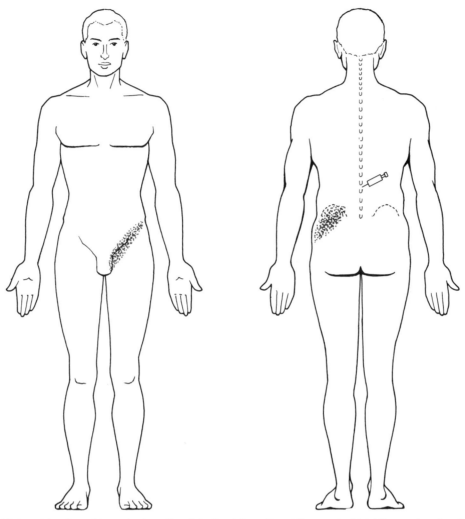

Figure 14.1.   Injection of hypertonic saline into the interspinous ligament of L1-L2 provokes low back pain and a pain in the inferior abdominal region radiating toward the testicle (according to Kellgren).

region. To elicit pain, the pin must be inclined to 40° and lightly pressed against the skin. The sensations reported by the patients are included in remarks such as "you press too much," "it is scratching," and "it tickles." Sometimes, the patients reported an electric feeling. A spot was often found to be particularly sensitive, most often 4–5 cm lateral to the midline, in the middle of a region that was less sensitive.

Glover also remarks that 90% of these spots disappeared after manipulation, at the same time that the pain disappeared. He did not notice any difference in temperature between these zones and the painless symmetric zones. In one of two cases, however, he found that the electric impedance of the skin was lowered, probably related to the start of perspiration, which was not observable on other objective tests.

The zones of hyperesthesia of the back described by Glover correspond well to the ones described by Kellgren (1939) and by Inman and Saunders (1944). As is shown later, these zones coincide, for the most part, with the zones where we find cellulalgic hypersensitivity during the "pinch-roll" test; hypersensitivity that was not looked for by the preceding

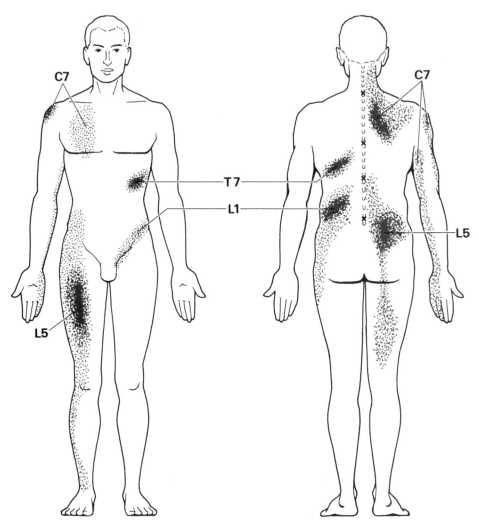

Figure 14.2. Pain obtained after the injection of different interspinal ligaments of different intervertebral segments with hypertonic saline (according to Feinstein).

authors (see Chapter 18, "Segmental Vertebral Celluloperiosteomyalgic Syndrome").

THE POSTERIOR AND ANTERIOR LONGITUDINAL LIGAMENTS

It is difficult to differentiate, experimentally, the irritation of the superficial fibers of the disk from the irritation of the posterior longitudinal ligament closely joined to it.

All authors recognize that the posterior longitudinal ligament has a very rich innervation. According to Hirsch, it was the irritation of

this ligament that was believed to give rise to the particular type of pain associated with the herniated lumbar disk. Its role in painful vertebral pathology is very important, especially at the lumbar level.

Remember the experiments made by Smyth and Wright during interventions for sciatica. They attached fine nylon threads to the sacrolumbar fascia and to the facet joints, to the ligamentum flavum and to the posterior part of the annulus fibrosus, to the posterior longitudinal ligament and to the nerve root. Three to 4 weeks later, when the threads were pulled, these formations were irritated. The patients reexperienced their former pain, which had been lumbosciatic in nature, when a traction was performed on the threads of the annulus fibrosus, the posterior longitudinal ligament, and the nerve itself. Rabischong and Serrano-Vela found nerve endings in the anterior longitudinal ligament. They thought that pressure on this ligament could be responsible for some pains.

THE LIGAMENTUM FLAVUM

Pressure on the ligamentum flavum is not painful (Wiberg). Stretching of this ligament, as in the experiment of Smyth and Wright, is not painful either.

THE VERTEBRAL BODY

Pressure on the posterior side of the vertebral bodies provokes no pain (Wiberg).

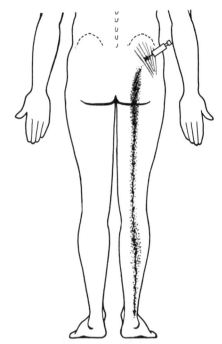

Figure 14.3.   Injection of an irritating substance into the gluteus minimus provokes pain that radiates into the lower leg in a pseudosciatic distribution.

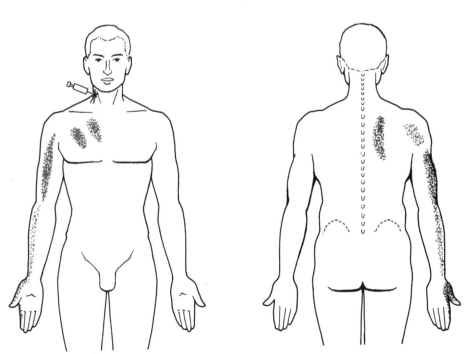

Figure 14.4.   Injection of several drops of hypertonic saline into the scalene muscle provokes pain that radiates diffusely to the upper arm and the anterior chest.

THE MUSCLES

It has often been observed that the intramuscular injection of an irritating liquid in the gluteal region causes a pseudosciatic pain along the thigh, even if this injection is performed at the external iliac fossa, which is distant from the sciatic trunk (Fig. 14.3).

Kellgren and Lewis studied these pain referral patterns. After anesthesia of the skin, they injected a solution of 5% hypertonic saline in different muscles and tendons. While the pain provoked in the tendons remained local, the one provoked by the injection in the muscle was distant. An injection in the distal triceps resulted, for example, in a pain extending from the medial side of the forearm to the fifth finger. An injection in the trapezius caused pain that radiated to the occiput. An injection in the scalene muscle caused pain that radiated in a diffuse manner to the arm and chest (Fig. 14.4). If performed on the infraspinatus muscle, it produced pain referred to the anterior side of the shoulder, radiating into the arm (Fig. 14.5).

Kellgren established precise diagrams of these referral patterns and came to the following conclusions:

- The distribution of pain for a given muscle is the same for all subjects. There might be some intrasubject variations, with some having a dorsal predominance, while others have a ventral one, and the pattern is more or less distal, depending on the part of the muscle that has been injected.
- The referral pattern is related to the nerve root innervating the muscle under consideration, so that the muscles innervated by this same root have a common pain diagram.
- The topography of the referral pattern coincides with the spinal root that innervates the muscle in question.
- Pain is independent of the mode of stimulation. The same experimental pain can be provoked by the injection of hypertonic saline or by electric stimulation performed during some surgical interventions.

According to Travell and Simons, the pain referral of certain trigger points, by pressure or by pin, does not correspond to any radicular

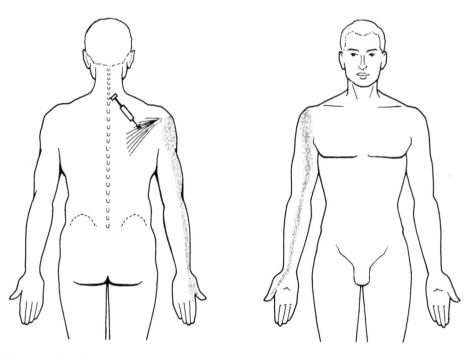

Figure 14.5.   Injection of several drops of hypertonic saline into the infraspinatus muscle provokes pain in the anterior shoulder and radiates into the arm.

or segmental distribution. Daily experience confirms their remarks. Some muscles (e.g., glutei medius and minimus), however, have a pain referral pattern starting in the area corresponding to the nerve that innervates them. As for the paravertebral muscles, injection in the trigger points of the low thoracic region causes pain toward the ischium, while injection in spots of the high lumbar region causes pain higher in the lumbar fossa, toward the iliac crest.

15

VERTEBRAL LESIONS AND COMMON PAIN SYNDROMES

Back pain is often attributed to lesions of the intervertebral disk or facet joints or to static disorders. But many of these lesions, visible on x-rays, are painless, and many patients with painful backs have normal x-rays.

INTERVERTEBRAL DISK LESIONS

Besides the lesions brought on by normal aging, which are generally well tolerated, the disk can demonstrate apparently similar degenerative changes at an earlier than expected age, which, because of their premature character and location, can be pathologic.

There are strong analogies, but not complete similarities, between the aberrations of the aged disk and those of a degenerated disk in the young patient. In the aging process, the rate of mucopolysaccharide production increases for a short time around age 40 and then returns to a rate equal or slightly inferior to that at its starting point. On the other hand, in cases of herniated disks, the decline in mucopolysaccharide production is rapid, significant, and progressive. In patients 20 years of age, one can already notice slight localized degeneration of fibers in the deep layers of the annulus, most often posteriorly. Gradually, their number and size increase and form (about at age 40) small fissures in the laminae. By age 30, these areas become susceptible to injury by tearing or enlarged by pressure on the nucleus. There are two types of rupture of the annulus: radial tears and concentric splits or tears. The latter form cracks in the shape of an arch, parallel to the laminae localized usually to the lateral and anterior parts of the disk.

The radial tears start at the contact region between the nucleus pulposus and the annulus fibrosus and extend to the periphery. They are predominant in the posterior or posterolateral aspect of the disk. They are of variable size, narrow or wide, and generally unique; there may be two or three (de Sèze).

When they are wide, a segment of the nucleus pulposus can protrude into it. If the fragment goes toward the front or the sides, there will be no pain, but it will lead to the formation of osteophytes. On the other hand, fragments extending posteriorly will bulge and contact the superficial annular fibers. The distention of these fibers and the forceful or strenuous pressure put simultaneously on the posterior longitudinal ligament will cause pain of the acute lumbar disk type. Finally, frank rupture of the superficial annular fibers many occur, resulting in extrusion of the nucleus pulposus. This is known as a noncontained herniated disk (Fig. 15.1).

The substance of the nucleus pulposus can also infiltrate through a tear in the annulus fibrosus. This is the mechanism of painful internal disk disruption. Finally, the posterior superficial laminae distended under the influence of postural forces or exertion effort can be a source of chronic lumbar disk pain.

The production of pain need not be solely a mechanical phenomenon. Soft tissue injury can produce many types of substances with algogenic potential. Thus, for example, the rupture of a herniated disk has been shown to provoke the liberation of a primary mediator of the inflammatory cascade, phospholipase A_2, which acts as the rate-limiting step in the production of prostaglandins and leukotrienes (J. S. Saal, R. C. Franson, R. Dobrow, J. A. Saal, A. H. White, and N. Goldthwaite).

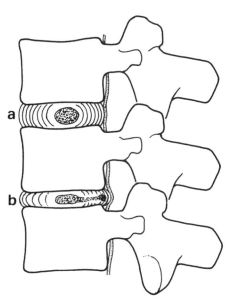

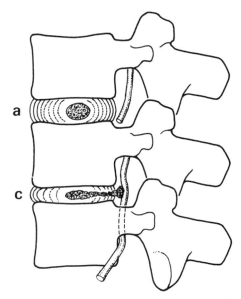

Figure 15.1. Horizontal flexion. **Left.** Posterolateral herniated disk with compression of the nerve root. **Right.** Median disk herniation compromising the dural sac and cauda equina. *a,* Normal disk; *b,* bulging disk due to merely an outward bulging of the superficial fibers of the annulus fibrosus, which are not broken; and *c,* herniated disk with the superficial fibers of the annulus fibrosus ruptured and the nucleus pulposus able to gain exit and compromise the spinal nerve.

Herniated Disks

The posteriorly herniated disk can come into contact with the nerve root, compress it, irritate it, and cause inflammation, which is the primary source of pain. This is the usual mechanism of the common femoral neuralgia and sciatica.

At the cervical level, foraminal stenosis due to osteophyte formation (de Sèze) is most often the cause for the cervicobrachial neuralgia. The protrusion of a fragment of the nucleus, generally after excessive activities, is very rarely the cause.

Herniated disks are most frequent at the lumbar level. In statistics given by the Clinique Universitaire de Neurochirurgie de Zurich on 2941 cases, there were

- 1098 herniations of the L5-S1 disk
- 1667 herniations of the L4-L5 disk
- 135 herniations of the L3-L4 disk
- 14 herniations of the L2-L3 disk
- 7 at the level of the inferior dorsal spine
- 20 at the level of the last cervical disks

At the Lumbar Level. The herniations are most often posterolateral, as the posterior longitudinal ligament reinforces the intervertebral disk posteriorly. Some herniations remain subligamentous, but others break through this ligament (Fig. 15.3).

Posterolateral Herniation. Posterolateral herniations are the most frequent type of herniated disk often leading to compression or irritation of the corresponding spinal root (Figs. 15.1 and 15.2). It can compress the nerve root from either lateral or medial side. It can also compress the root of the subjacent level superiorly, or extend inferiorly via a sequestered fragment. It is then said to be in superior or inferior sublaminar position.

Posterior Herniation. The posterior herniation can deform the posterior longitudinal ligament and compress the dural sac without irritating the nerve roots. It can be responsible for chronic lumbar pain with acute exacerbations or for subacute lumbar pain with lumbar stiffness (Fig. 15.2).

Transligamentous Herniation. Among the herniations (sometimes small) that have broken the posterior longitudinal ligament, some remain in continuity with the disk while others are separated into multiple sequestered fragments that pose difficulty for surgical dissection. These free fragments can be visualized on magnetic resonance imaging (MRI) and in certain cases, with sacroradiculography.

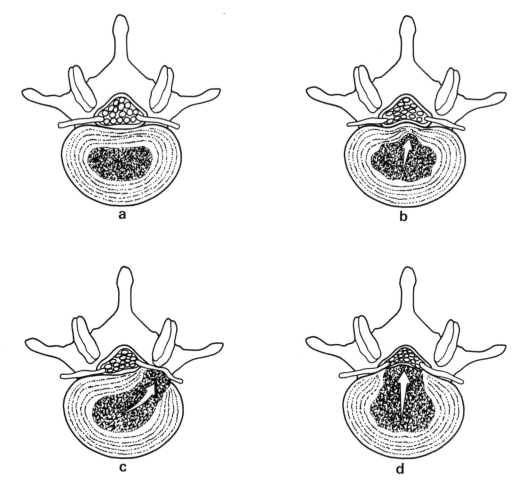

Figure 15.2. Transverse section showing different modes of compression by a herniated disk. **a,** Normal state. **b,** Simple protrusion. **c,** Posterolateral disk herniation. **d,** Posterior disk herniation.

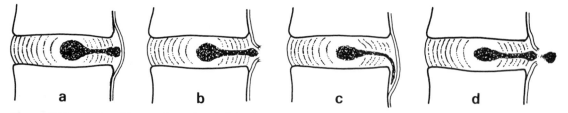

Figure 15.3. Different types of herniated disks (according to Junghanns). **a,** Without rupture of the posterior longitudinal ligament. **b,** With rupture of the posterior longitudinal ligament. **c,** Disk extrusion beneath the posterior longitudinal ligament. **d,** Sequestered fragment.

Discography may also be useful in demonstrating the existence of an anterior or lateral herniation. Classically, these types of herniations are asymptomatic. Schmorl's nodules are also a form of herniation into the vertebral body. These lesions can contribute to some instability of the segment (see Chapter 17,

"Painful Minor Intervertebral Dysfunctions").

At the Thoracic Level. Disk herniations are rare in this region. They produce thoracic pain or pain referred to the pelvic region and the legs. Often, they are accompanied by nocturnal paresthesias (hyperesthesia, burning pains, stiffness). The motor deficit can range from a simple impression of weakness in one leg to total paraplegia. MRI is the imaging study of choice to detect them.

At the Cervical Level. At the cervical spine level, there are hard herniations formed by the disco-osteophytic nodule, a spondylotic reaction at the level of an uncinate process, and the true herniated disks, called soft herniations, which are much rarer. These can be

- Posterolateral, compromising the spinal nerve (Fig. 15.4, *1*)
- Intraforamenal, threatening the spinal nerve also (Fig. 15.4, *3*)
- Much more rarely, posterior and median, threatening the dura mater, spinal cord, and anterior spinal artery (Fig. 15.4, *2*)

MRI or computed tomography (CT) scanning after injection of myelographic contrast can be of help in identifying them.

LESIONS OF THE FACET JOINTS

The facet joints can be associated with acquired or congenital anomalies, degenerative lesions, and lesions due to mechanical pain. Thanks to various scanning devices and arthrography, they have been studied completely and thoroughly.

Anomalies

Congenital Anomalies. Congenital anomalies have been chiefly noted in the lower lum-

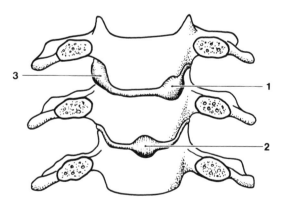

Figure 15.4. Different varieties of herniated cervical disks: *1*, posterolateral protrusion; *2*, posteromedial protrusion; and *3*, intraforaminal protrusion (as per Frykholm). In this scheme, the posterior arch is resected for better viewing.

bar areas. Anomalies involving the position of the facet joints and asymmetry of the articular facet joints have been well studied.

The facet asymmetries have been verified and evaluated by using CT scanning. They have not only been seen at the lumbosacral junction but have also been found at the level of the thoracolumbar junction (Malmivaara et al., Maigne et al.).

It is possible that such anomalies can induce an instability at a segment and cause articular spondylosis. When there is a significant asymmetry in the inclination of the posterior articular spaces, a CT scan demonstrates a strongly condensed aspect of the articular edges or subcortical gaps expressing the articular hypertension.

Acquired Anomalies. Gillot, working on cadavers, noted the prevalence of small and transverse bony crests on the inferior lumbar articular surfaces in old patients. This was believed to be due to the reduction of articular play during flexion and extension associated with the aging process. The crests were thought to be evidence of the successive loss of range of motion.

Degenerative Lesions

Facet Arthrosis

Facet joint arthrosis is located at the level of the lordotic regions of the spine, the neck and lumbar region. It is, indeed, the result of excessive pressure caused by hyperlordosis or discal deterioration. Arthrosis is, in fact, very rare at the levels of the articulations without a disk, such as at the occiput and atlas and at the atlas-axis, which are extremely mobile and sustain significant pressure. Arthrosis can, however, affect the atlas-odontoid articulation.

Arthrosis can also be found on segments with apparently intact disks. Most often, however, they are segments adjacent to segments presenting very severe disk lesions.

At the cervical level, posterior articular arthrosis is especially located between C2-C3 and C3-C4, but it can affect the inferior levels. At the lumbar spine level, arthrosis is frequently seen in patients over age 50. Most often, it is localized to only one level; it is seen in 45% of cases according to Louyot, i.e., 1% in L2-L3, 8% in L3-L4, 17% in L4-L5, and 19% in L5-S1. It affects several articulations in 17%

of the cases and is generalized in 38% of cases.

The mechanical factors that foster it are found together in the "trophostatic syndrome of the postmenopause," which affects women past 60 years of age who are hyperlordosed, often obese, and have a slackening of the abdominal wall. The L4-L5 level is most often affected. The L4-L5 and L5-S1 levels can be affected simultaneously. Sometimes, the lesions extend to L2-L3.

Pathologic Role.   Arthrotic lesions, when significant, can modify the morphology of the vertebral canal, lead into acquired stenosis that can be superimposed on a congenital stenosis, resulting in a myeloradiculopathy at the cervical level and the lumbar stenosis syndrome at the lumbar level. At the lumbar level also, facet hypertrophy can narrow the lateral recess and facilitate a radicular pain syndrome. At the cervical level, osteophytes can compress the vertebral artery in the transverse canal.

In the above cases, facet arthrosis plays a direct and mechanical role. These represent, however, just a small percentage of the cases of vertebral arthrosis usually seen.

Vertebral arthrosis is painful during inflammatory attacks. Some people experience them often, episodically, and some rarely or never.

It can be uncomfortable because of the numbness it produces; if it is not painful, however, the patient may not complain. Finally, acting like rust on a hinge, it can promote painful minor intervertebral dysfunction, which generally improves after mobilization and sometimes improves after manipulations if the state of the spine allows it.

Facet Joint Periarthritis

CT scans allow the detection of calcification of the capsules and ligaments of the facet joints. Calcification is common at the thoracolumbar junction, localized to the facet joint capsule and/or the ligamentum flavum (Maigne et al.). Para-articular reactions without any radiologic evidence are probably much more frequent at all levels.

Other Lesions

Facet joint arthrography has shown the existence of lesions not revealed by conventional radiography: hydrarthrotic manifestations, di-

verticular formations, and, more rarely, synovial cysts or communication between the adjacent articulations.

Synovial cysts can compress the root in the neuroforamen. The communication between adjacent articular cavities corresponds to the junction of several cystic cavities (Chevrot et al.). Thanks to CT scanning, hypodense images of the joint of gaseous type have been shown, revealing an articular void. This void is usually associated with a posterior articular arthrosis.

Meniscoid Formations

The lesions of the synovial fold are discussed in Chapter 17, "Painful Minor Intervertebral Dysfunctions."

OBJECTIVE MUSCULAR LESIONS

In popular language, acute lumbar pain occurring after lifting is most often attributed to a "muscular tear." This type of lesion is not rare in athletes, but it is uncommon in the thoracic or lumbar muscles.

Apart from the usual reflex protective guarding, the role of the muscle in vertebral pain syndromes is rarely raised. However, a careful examination of the paravertebral muscles can help to identify, in some cases, small firm cords the size of a match that are very painful to palpation. They can be the source of severe pain distally. These "trigger points" found on palpation do not correspond to any objectively demonstrable lesion. They seem to be due to a functional perturbation that tends to become permanent. They can be relieved, sometimes permanently, by injection of local anesthetic.

Nevertheless, Drevet (1983) has shown that some myalgic points, which are localized to the lumbar muscular and are responsible for unilateral lumbar pain, correspond to abnormal zones that are often hypoechogenic on ultrasonographic examination. His morphologic and structural studies of the samples have shown an intensive perimysial and endomysial fatty infiltration massively invading the muscular bundles. This could explain the building of the hypoechogenic image and of the pain-associated phenomena (see Chapter 39, "Chronic Lumbar Pain").

16

POSTURAL DISORDERS AND PAIN

When a patient with vertebral pain presents with a postural disorder, one is tempted to accept it as the cause of the pain. Such static disorders can consist of scoliosis, dorsal hyperkyphosis, lumbar hyperlordosis, or flat lumbar curve. It can also take the form of a spondylolisthesis that is not really a static disorder but is a malformation.

SCOLIOSIS

Scoliosis is usually a painless disorder in the adolescent. In the adult, however, many vertebral pains are usually attributed to scoliosis, although many patients with scoliosis do not experience pain. According to Stagnara, a scoliotic adolescent has a 50% chance of having spinal pain when an adult, but the percentage of scoliotic patients with pain is similar to that of patients without scoliosis. Stagnara studied 100 cases of adult scoliosis with spinal pain and concluded that neither the patient's sex, nor the patient's profession, nor the angle of the scoliosis played a determinant role in who would have pain. Jackson et al. arrived at the same conclusion after studying pain in 197 scoliotic adults (more than 18 years of age) with a median age of 31 and comparing them to 180 nonscoliotic patients. The frequency of pain was the same in both groups (51%).

However, it is clear from the study by Jackson et al. that when pain was present, scoliotics had more severe pain than nonscoliotics, and the progression of the pain was different. Spontaneous resolution occurred in 64% in the scoliotic group and in 83% in the nonscoliotic group. The pain and severity of the scoliosis were noted to worsen with age; the pain's ori-

gin was essentially related to the concavity of the spine but could also be of discal, articular, or radicular origin. Nevertheless, there is general agreement among those who work with lumbar scoliotics that they suffer severe social and professional handicaps as a result of their condition.

According to Stagnara, physical rehabilitation alone was able to ameliorate pain in 40%. Orthotic devices including the use of corsets for limited periods of time helped in 60% of cases. Surgery was reserved for the most severe cases and was able to help reduce pain in 65% of the cases.

Minor Scoliosis

Physicians not specialized in the treatment of scoliosis rarely see severe cases. Most of the cases they treat are of the minor scoliotic variety, i.e., scoliosis of less than 30°. These patients present with thoracic and lumbar spine pain of mild to severe intensity. Almost all of these individuals are diagnosed as having pain due to their scoliosis. Most of the patients have the same clinical picture as can be noted in nonscoliotics, in that they also present with interscapular thoracic pains of cervical origin (see Chapters 36 and 37 on thoracic pain) or lumbar pain of thoracolumbar junctional origin. Treatment is similar for those with scoliosis as for those without scoliosis, and similar results are obtained. In the absence of precise statistics, it is difficult to say whether recurrence is more common for scoliotics than for nonscoliotics; this tendency, however, is not evident to us. Mild to moderate scoliosis should not, therefore, be automatically diagnosed as the cause for all pain of vertebral origin.

THORACIC HYPERKYPHOSIS

Exaggeration of the thoracic kyphosis is most often due to Scheuermann's disease. It is usually the sequela in the adult with spondylosis. In the adolescent, a kyphotic posture should be distinguished from true kyphosis.

Kyphotic Posture in the Adolescent

In the kyphotic posture seen in preadolescents and adolescents, shoulders coil forward, and the lumbar region appears hollow. It is important to note that there is no radiologic lesion and that the kyphosis is reducible.

Conversely, true kyphosis is not reducible, and there are radiologic lesions. In the beginning, however, the diagnosis is not always easy to make; therefore, regular supervision is necessary.

Hyperkyphosis Due to Dystrophic Spinal Growth

Scheuermann described a developmental abnormality of the thoracic spine, which is named after him. It is due to an impairment of the fibrillar system of the cartilage of the vertebral endplates during growth. These impairments are benign and precocious. They can be seen in the very young about age 4 but are generally seen after age 8; they are numerous and extensive in some patients. They then form zones of least resistance to pressure, making the vertebral body vulnerable to compression, especially in its anterior part. Increased anterior loading squeezes this fragile zone, which increases the kyphosis, further increasing the pressure anteriorly, leading to more damage, and a vicious circle is started.

In the adolescent, pain is rare and generally moderate (20% of cases). It appears on waking up, disappears during the day, and reappears in the evening. Severe cases are treated by rest and, when it is not possible, by immobilization in a plaster cast to reduce pain. The midthoracic region is most often affected.

In the adult, dystrophic growth produces spondylosis, which is rarely painful. When these patients have interscapular thoracic pain, the origin is very often the inferior cervical spine (Maigne) (see Chapters 36 and 37 on thoracic pain).

When the thoracolumbar junction is affected, low lumbar pain is frequent, especially in the adult. In the adolescent, according to Fauchet, 90% of lumbar conditions are painful, presenting as posturally exacerbated low back pain. This condition can result in the reduction or disappearance of the normal lumbar lordosis. In the early stages of the condition, the kyphosis is evident only in the sitting position; it appears in the standing position only when the vertebra has become wedge shaped. An early sign is the pigmentation of the skin at the level of the spinous processes of the affected vertebral segments.

The lumbar pain of youth, if left untreated, can continue and become serious in the adult. If treatment such as plaster cast, corset, and physical therapy is applied before bony vertebral maturity occurs, the dystrophic vertebrae will be able to remodel themselves and reduce or eradicate the development of future lumbar pain.

TRANSITIONAL ZONE ABNORMALITIES

Lumbosacral transitional zone abnormalities are frequent. Their frequency is estimated at 20% by all authors, be it the lumbarization or hemilumbarization of S1 or the sacralization or hemisacralization of L5. Although they do not play any direct role in lumbar pain, it is often admitted that they can play a fostering role.

In a study by Schiano et al., a comparison was made between 200 patients with lumbar pain and 200 patients of the same median age without lumbar pain. In both groups, the frequency of transitional zone abnormalities was the same. Castellini studied 200 cases of herniated disks and found a transitional zone abnormality in 60 patients. He classified these malformations and studied their influence on the incidence of herniated disks. He was able to classify them into four groups (Fig. 16.1):

- Group I had one or two big transverse processes of more than 19 mm in height. There was no pathologic incidence of a herniated disk noted in this group.

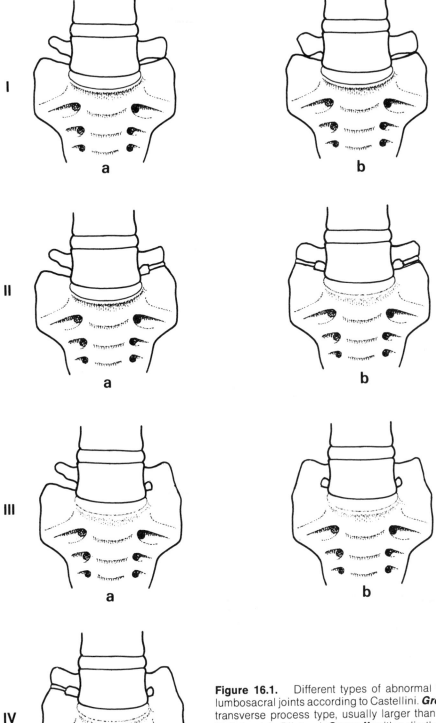

Figure 16.1.   Different types of abnormal transitional lumbosacral joints according to Castellini. **Group I:** large transverse process type, usually larger than 19 mm. **a,** Unilateral. **b,** Bilateral. **Group II:** with a diarthrodial articulation between the transverse spine and the sacrum. **a,** Unilateral. **b,** Bilateral. **Group III:** osseous union between the transverse process and the sacrum. **a,** Unilateral. **b,** Bilateral. **Group IV:** mixed type, with the osseous union on one side and a diarthrodial articulation on the other.

- Group II had an incomplete unilateral or bilateral sacralization. There was a diarthrodial articulation between the transversarium and sacrum. This group had the highest incidence of herniated disks at the level subjacent to the abnormality, but also at the level of the transition, contrary to generally accepted opinion.
- Group III represented a unilateral or bilateral fusion of the transverse process to the sacrum. No pathologic incidence of herniated disks was noted. No increase in the frequency of herniated disks at the subjacent level in relation to normality was noted either.
- Group IV represented a unilateral fusion with arthrodial articulation of the transverse process with the sacrum on the other side. The same conclusions as for group III were noted in this group, except that there was no increase in the frequency of herniated disks.

SPONDYLOLISTHESIS

Spondylolisthesis is relatively frequent. Most authors agree that about 5–7% of the total population is affected. It seems that there are some variations according to race. Stewart found the condition in 27.4% of Eskimos, 6.3% of American Indians, and 2.8% of African Americans.

In European countries, the frequency is from 1.5 to 3%, depending on the author. Spondylolisthesis can be classified according to a system of stages that depends on the degree of displacement between the vertebrae, with stage I having a displacement of less than 30% and stage II having a displacement of 30–40%. Stage III demonstrates spondylolisthesis with a major displacement or sliding of more than 40%. In stage I, the L5-S1 disk is normal. In stage II, it is slightly degenerated. In stage III, it is completely destroyed where there is also a major dysplasia of L5 (Roy-Camille).

The evolution of spondylolisthesis over time is most often asymptomatic if the displacement is under 40%, as is seen in groups I and II. The prognosis is much worse for patients in stage III. Nevertheless, spondylolisthesis with significant displacement can long remain asymptomatic in people who perform heavy work or other activities but can manifest itself by lumbar pain or by benign episodic sciatic pain.

The disk subjacent to the listhetic vertebra is most often asymptomatic, whether it is normal or demonstrates a benign degeneration on discography. In cases of severe sciatica, it is usually the listhetic disk that is usually responsible, rarely the subjacent disk (Roy-Camille).

The facet joints of the listhetic vertebra when submitted to excessive pressure can be the origin of sciatic pain (Taillard). Frequently, there is an involvement of the thoracolumbar junction (Maigne), which can be responsible for low lumbar pain falsely attributed to the listhetic segment.

Spondylolisthesis is frequent in athletes who start when they are very young and whose sport demands hyperextension of the lumbosacral spine or repeated falls (judo, gymnastics). Coned lumbosacral radiographic studies of young athletes with lumbar pain can show a fissure of the internal edge of the isthmus, which can be strengthened by rest. This constitutes the early stage of a spondylolisthesis.

ASYMMETRY OF THE LUMBAR TRANSVERSE PROCESS ORIENTATION AND FACET JOINT DEVELOPMENT

Asymmetric development of the lumbar facet joint spaces, pedicles, and transverse processes is frequent, particularly in the lower lumbar vertebrae. In studying 550 subjects who were without pain, Southworth and Bersack found 26% to have asymmetric spaces at the L4-L5 level and 17.4% to have asymmetric spaces at the L5-S1 level. Putti (1930) thought that this asymmetry was a source of facet pain, lumbar pain, and sciatica.

Asymmetry modifies the distribution of the mechanical pressure. It seems reasonable to assume that it could have some pathologic consequences. Farfan noted that of 52 patients who had an operation for herniated disk, 38 showed a posterior articular asymmetry at the concerned level. The herniated disk in 94.7% of cases was localized contralateral to the side of the sacralized facet joint.

The unilateral sacralization of an articular space can provoke a mechanical overloading of the contralateral posterior hemiarch and cause an isthmic lysis (Maldague and Malghem). Then the isthmus and the pedicle on the sagittal side endure increased mechanical forces, causing a condensation of the isthmus and of the pedicle (anisocoria). The evolution can remain stable or continue toward a bilateral isthmic lysis.

SHORT LEG

The "short leg" syndrome is often held indiscriminately responsible for all types of spinal pain. Here we are not referring to significant shortening of 3 cm or more, which is part of the orthopedic domain and which deserves to be recognized and treated. Instead, we are concerned with small inequalities of leg length on the order of 1 cm.

Statistical studies have shown that 2 out of 5 persons have one leg shorter than the other, in the 0.5- to 1.5-cm range. What is the real influence of these inequalities on the spine? What is their role in the painful pathology of the spine? Should the condition be corrected and, if possible, how? Opinions on these points vary.

Evidence

Clinical Evaluation

An inequality in the length of the inferior limbs is suspected when there is a slight lumbar scoliosis with convexity on the side of the suspected short leg. To verify the presence or absence of the short leg, the patient is examined in the following manner. First, the patient is examined in the standing position, with the legs in a symmetric stance; the height of the iliac crests and of the posterior and superior iliac spines is then inspected. This same examination is performed with the patient in a sitting position on a hard and horizontal plane, and verification is made to see if the scoliosis persists in this position. It disappears if it is the result of a short leg. It disappears also if the patient is made to stand on an inclined plane that compensates for the difference in the length of the limbs. Finally, with the patient lying down, a comparison of the medial malleolus is performed. This gives an approximation, which can be fairly exact with practice.

But it is not enough. This examination has no value in an acute lumbar pain, where there is lumbar contracture.

Radiologic Evaluation

Radiologic studies are the only way to prove the existence of a short leg. The technique is properly performed with the patient in the standing position. The x-rays must pass horizontally at the level of the femoral heads. Teleradiography can show the entire spine and allows a better assessment of the effect of the shorter leg on the vertebral alignment. The important point to evaluate is the horizontal plane of the sacral endplate.

False and True Short Leg

Radiologic examination will show (*a*) either the true shortening of one leg, with its repercussion on the sacral endplate and the spine, inclination of the sacral endplate on the short side, flexion of the lumbar spine (with convexity on the short side), and compensation at the level of the dorsal and/or cervical spine, or (*b*) equality of the two legs with the horizontal plane of the sacral endplates. Clinical examination may demonstrate a difference in length; it is a false short leg.

False Short Leg

Piedallu and classic osteopaths consider the false short leg to be one of the signs of blocking in malposition of the sacroiliac joint in "anterior sacrum," i.e., in position of nutation. To correct for this malposition, the iliac ala is rotated anteriorly in relation to the sacrum. This technique is described under "in lordosis" (see "Manual Techniques"). After performing this maneuver, the clinical examination may immediately show a return to equal length of the legs and the disappearance of the other signs. The resulting return of symmetric leg length is, for supporters of the concept of sacroiliac blocking, the evident proof of the existence of "sacroiliac blocking." The return of symmetric leg length is also used to justify the value of the signs of the examination they perform and of the corrective techniques they use.

This interpretation is controversial and highly debatable. Given what is known about such cases, it would seem more reasonable to ascribe false short legs to postural changes resulting from pain caused by deep lumbosacral muscular contractures or painful lumbar dysfunctions.

True Short Leg

The true short leg is confirmed by radiologic examination. It is used to confirm the clinical impression. These studies are used to confirm the presence of a difference of at least 1 cm in the height of the femoral heads. The position of the sacral endplate is verified by this technique:

- If it is level, asymmetry of the sacrum or of the iliac ala compensates the shortening of the leg; then there is nothing to correct.
- If it is not level, then the possible use of compensatory techniques such as the use of the footpad can be considered.

Determining what therapeutic route will be taken depends on factors such as spinal flexibility and patient age.

Procedural Considerations.

Young Subject with a Flexible Spine. In the young with a flexible spine, the condition should be corrected, and the sacral endplate should be brought to a horizontal plane. It is safe to start with half of the correction; the other half can be performed a month later. Periodic controls are to be made during the growth period.

Subjects with an Inflexible or Stiff Spine. In older subjects, one would think that the spine became adapted and that the use of a heel lift would perturb the acquired functional balance. Nevertheless, there are cases where trying a foot pad is reasonable. This is particularly true in patients presenting with lumbar or thoracolumbar pain, especially in the standing position, which is temporarily relieved by vertebral treatments.

During the first month, a heel pad corrects half of the true shortening. If the result is favorable and sufficient, the correction is maintained. If it is insufficient, the correction is set at three-fourths of the measured leg length discrepancy. In all cases, the patient is seen again 3 months later.

It is surprising to note sometimes the positive effect of a heel lift of 5–6 mm on lumbar thoracic or cervical pain, even in cases where the spine is arthrotic and stiffened. One can think of it as a favorable modification of pressure placed on the concerned vertebral segment. It is noteworthy that there are some patients who feel very relieved by a heel lift they have mistakenly placed on the side of the long leg. Does this mean that there is a favorable mechanical effect regardless of the logic used to determine which side should be treated, or is this a signal that we are dealing here with a placebo or purely psychologic effect?

17

PAINFUL MINOR INTERVERTEBRAL DYSFUNCTIONS

Many common pain syndromes of spinal origin do not correspond to lesions that are radiographically visible. Our hypothesis, consistent with clinical reality, is that these pains often have their origin in the painful dysfunction of one or more vertebral segments, which we call "painful minor intervertebral dysfunction" (PMID). These PMIDs are often the result of trauma, forced movements, or postural or static disturbances.

Spinal manipulation often relieves these benign segmental pains, which have a reversible character. Although spinal manipulation may be of help, it is not the only technique available to manage this condition and may be insufficient by itself or even contraindicated.

DEFINITION

Painful minor intervertebral dysfunction, or PMID, is generally a reversible benign, painful, segmental vertebral dysfunction of mechanical and reflex origin (Maigne). This term (1964) is purposely vague, since we are not certain as to the mechanism that generates the benign painful dysfunction. These dysfunctions appear to be the common denominator of common local or regional vertebral pain and can also act as the origin of referred pain:

- Pain associated with the region served by a spinal nerve, most often of its dorsal ramus
- Referred pain due to irritation of some constituents of the spinal segment (facet joints, ligaments)
- Pain for which a common denominator is the PMID, including also cellulalgic reactions and tenoperiosteal or myalgic reflexes (seg-mental vertebral celluloperiosteomyalgic syndrome of Maigne)

DIAGNOSIS

The diagnosis of PMID is based on finding a painful spinal segment on segmental examination and on the absence of any clinical or radiologic features revealing a significant pathologic process. The absence of these features allows one to conclude that a benign mechanical process is the cause of the pain.

In Chapter 20, in the section entitled "Clinical Examination of the Spine," we discuss the segmental examination in detail. For now, in brief, the examination consists of examining each spinal segment (Fig. 17.1) by selected palpation maneuvers. These maneuvers do not provoke pain in normal segments but are painful in the symptomatically involved segment. These maneuvers are always painful in cases of a PMID (Fig. 17.2).

The segmental examination consists of the following:

- Axial pressure on the spinous process.
- Transvese pressure against the spinous process. In PMID, pain is most often elicited by pressure applied in one direction (from right to left or from left to right), but in some patients, it may be present in both directions. This maneuver provokes vertebral rotation about an oblique axis.
- Friction overlying the facet joints. Facet joint pain to palpation is a constant sign in PMID. It is usually painful on one side only.
- Transverse pressure on the interspinous ligament of the concerned segment, performed with the tip of the finger or, better yet, with a key ring, is often painful (inconstant sign).

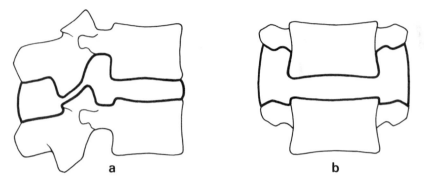

Figure 17.1. Mobile segment of Junghanns. **a,** Lateral view. **b,** Frontal view.

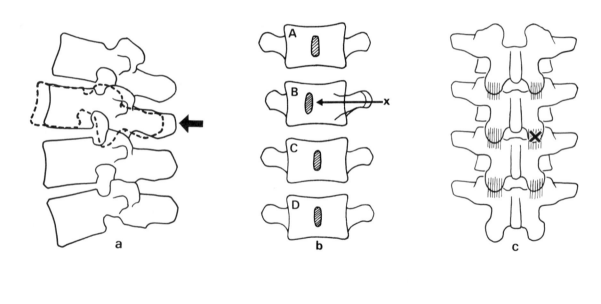

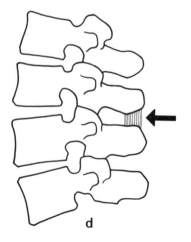

Figure 17.2. A segmental examination uses maneuvers that allow one to study the different segmental vertebrae. The examination is usually nonpainful in normal segments. If pain is provoked, it suggests the existence of underlying pathology of the segment. This pathology may be benign or malignant. This determination can only be made in the context of further clinical and radiologic evaluations. **a,** Axial pressure. **b,** Transverse pressure on the spinous process. **c,** Friction- pressure over the facet joint. **d.** Transverse pressure on the interspinous ligament.

DIFFERENTIAL DIAGNOSIS

Segmental pain uncovered by segmental examination does not necessarily point to or indicate a diagnosis of PMID (Fig. 17.3). The segmental examination helps to focus our attention on a segment that needs to be explored. Among the common causes of segmental pain, besides PMID, are inflammatory conditions, spondylosis, and disk herniations.

Acute Synovitis

It is not necessary for the spondylosis to be radiologically severe to present as an episode of acute synovitis. Usually, the cervical spine is involved. It can be difficult to differentiate between mechanical causes of pain and acute synovitis, particularly when the examination reveals severe painful sensitivity of several of the facet joints and when mobilization is painful in all directions. It is even more difficult when only one facet is affected. The tests of repeated mobilization centered on the concerned spinal segment can aid in the diagnosis. The spinal segment is usually painful in one direction, right or left, if it is due to a PMID; the spinal segment is always painful in both directions if it is due to an acute synovitis.

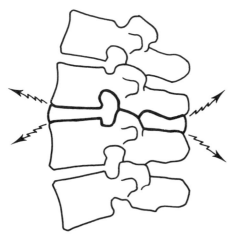

Figure 17.3.   PMID due to a benign painful dysfunction of the spinal segment, which is mechanical in nature and reflex in origin. The segmental examination (Maigne) allows one to demonstrate the painful dysfunction of the spinal segment.

Confusion in determining the suitability of manipulative therapy for this type of condition is rare, though certainly the use of manipulation in the case of synovitis could aggravate the condition. The reason that there is little confusion is that when the rule of manipulation only in the painless range of motion—the rule of no pain—is used, the lack of any range of movement that is nontender would dictate that no manipulation be performed.

PMID and the Herniated Disk

With regard to herniated disks, the situation is somewhat different. Manipulation can be of utility in some cases of disk degeneration characterized by disk bulge or a true hernia, as can, at times, be seen in sciatica. A herniated disk is not a "minor dysfunction." There is no problem in terminology where there is a herniated disk irritating a nerve root.

But there are some situations that are less clear; e.g., on examination a painful segment demonstrates a discopathy with a disk bulge but without a radicular pain syndrome. Is the discopathy directly responsible for the segmental pain, or has a PMID been fostered by this discopathy?

If manipulation is possible and produces a lasting relief, does this mean that we are dealing with a case of PMID? But if the clinical findings and the development of the condition demonstrate that the symptoms are due to the disk lesion itself, then support for the diagnosis of PMID would not be as clear. This situation is seen often in daily practice. In fact, the issue is more one of semantics, which has little bearing on the actual outcome of these cases.

DIFFERENT TYPES OF PMIDs

PMIDs can be acute or chronic, "active" (responsible for pain) or "latent" (not responsible for pain).

Acute PMIDs

PMIDs can present acutely. It occurs most often as a result of a sudden movement or strenuous effort and is accompanied by strong muscular spasms.

Chronic PMIDs

Chronic PMIDs are the commonest form of PMID. It usually develops without an initial acute phase. When it is responsible for chronic episodic pain, the findings on examination are constant, though attenuated, and present even during the nontender phase of the condition. This should be emphasized, as it is very important for making the diagnosis. The same is true for the cellulalgic tenoperiosteomyalgic chronic PMID.

"Active" PMIDs

Active PMIDs are responsible for pain, either directly or through celluloperiosteomyalgic and neurotrophic manifestations.

"Latent" PMIDs

Sometimes, the segmental vertebral examination demonstrates subclinical PMIDs not associated with episodes of spontaneous or ongoing pain. In fact, these segments are rarely totally "inactive" but cause only very slight discomfort or occasional mild pain that is quickly forgotten and is usually ascribed to other causes such as stiffness or fatigue.

LOCALIZATION AND NUMBER

PMIDs can be found at all levels of the spine. However, it is in the segments of the transitional zones of the spine that it is especially frequent.

For a given region, there is usually only one segment involved with PMID. Rarely, two adjacent segments may be involved. Involvement of three segments is very rare. In the same patient, however, it is not rare to find several nonadjacent segments involved with PMID, some asymptomatic, some not, localized to different spinal regions, such as the cervical and thoracic regions.

ASSOCIATION OF PMID AT DIFFERENT LEVELS

Finding PMID at different spinal levels is rather frequent in chronic cases. In a patient with a chronic lumbar pain coming from L4-L5, the examination will often show some PMID localized to T12-L1, C6-C7, and C2-C3 or to a nearby segment; they can simply be examination discoveries or can be responsible for the production of pain. These PMIDs practically always present with a painful facet joint on the same side, right or left, at all levels. They are generally at the level of the transitional zones of the vertebral column. Thus, a "syndrome of the transitional zones" can be defined (Maigne) by the association and grouping of these painful segments (see Chapter 29, "Syndrome of the Transitional Zones").

PMID AND THE PAIN THRESHOLD

Certain PMIDs can remain asymptomatic (inactive MIDs) or disappear spontaneously without having produced discomfort. Others manifest themselves by episodic pain, while the examination demonstrates findings that point to the involved segment and can persist during nonpainful periods.

Thus there is a threshold of tolerance at which the PMID provokes pain and below which it may not provoke any. This threshold varies from one patient to another and can vary over time in the same individual. There are patients with a "low threshold" and others with a "high threshold." Psychologic factors may play a role, especially in cases where depression or anxiety exists.

Spasmophilia (with all the reservations this term can arouse) is a frequent factor capable of potentiating PMID by lowering the tolerance threshold and by neuromuscular hyperexcitability.

But the threshold of pain can also be altered by

- Mechanical factors aggravating PMID, such as strenuous effort, poor posture or position at work or during sleep, or forced movements.
- Internal, digestive, gynecologic causes or other organic causes, or a state of fatigue due to overwork or lack of sleep, which decreases the tolerance of the subject.
- External causes, such as exposure to irritations such as cold or air drafts, which will

increase the sensitivity of the tissues. It seems also that the PMID can be "reactivated" or become symptomatic by irritation of one of the cellulalgic, tenoperiosteal, or myalgic manifestations that it provokes, as we shall see in Chapter 18, "Segmental Vertebral Celluloperiosteomyalgic Syndrome" (of Maigne).

TREATMENT

There is no standard treatment for PMID. The treatment must be tailored according to the underlying cause, the general state, the vertebral state, and the state of the area and associated neurotrophic manifestations.

Acute Cases

Treatment often consists of immobilization, but facet joint injection or manipulation can be used in many cases.

Chronic Cases

Manipulation is often the treatment of choice. For various reasons, it can be contraindicated in some cases. Articular injection is useful if there is a strong para-articular reaction; injection of the interspinous ligament is sometimes necessary. When manipulation and infiltration are contraindicated, electrotherapy in association with modalities such as diathermy and ultrasound is the best treatment. Local treatment of the associated celluloperiosteomyalgic manifestations is often indispensable.

Treating the whole patient is important. Many PMIDs start only if the tolerance of the patient decreases, as is seen in fatigue, depressive states, spasmophilia decompensation, and concurrent illnesses. Postural disorders should get attention, and the patient should be made aware of incorrect postural habits and be reeducated.

Recurrent PMID

Patients are often seen who present with a painful syndrome whose connection with PMID has been well established. They are typically relieved by the treatment, but the condition recurs 3 or 4 months later. Usually, examinations of these patients reveal the same PMID, and the same maneuver produces relief in one or two sessions. Between two painful episodes, the segmental examination often demonstrates a progressive reappearance of the PMID. The PMID in these cases often remains latent for long periods of time before again becoming symptomatic.

The causes of these recurrences are multiple. Poor postural habits are most often the cause. The cervical spine can be affected by sleep positions, especially sleeping on the abdomen, which results in excessive rotation of the neck, made possible by the increased laxity of the muscles during sleep. It can also be due to repetitive occupational maneuvers such as turning the head to look at something behind or making numerous movements in parking a car.

Seats or work stations can be also the cause. All these recurrent factors should be looked for attentively during the interview. A "short leg" or postural disorders of the feet can sometimes be found on examination, but their correction rarely produces the solution.

The syndrome of the transitional zones (Maigne) (see Chapter 18) can be a cause of these chronic and recurrent pains and should be looked for. As we have seen, it is characterized by the existence of a PMID on several spinal segments belonging to transitional vertebral zones. Even when "latent," they can facilitate the recurrence of the PMID. In these cases, all the presenting PMIDs should be treated.

Finally, the persistence of neurotrophic manifestations (see page 109) depending on the PMID, such as cellulalgia infiltrates and trigger points from which arise nociceptive impulses and which contribute to the maintenance of a vicious circle, should be treated. Physical therapy is essential.

Should "Latent" PMIDs Be Treated?

Latent PMIDs should be treated if they seem to contribute to the maintenance of other PMIDs that are "active" (see Chapter 18), provided they are isolated and their treatment is easy. Otherwise, they should be watched regularly, and the patient should be aware of the positions or movements to be avoided.

DO PAINFUL MINOR INTERVERTEBRAL DYSFUNCTIONS HAVE VISCERAL REPERCUSSIONS?

The segmental dysfunction that produces somatic neurotrophic manifestations probably has repercussions on the sympathetic visceral system. However, if it does exist, as has been the hypothesis of osteopaths, no objective clinical demonstration of this yet exists.

In the practice of manipulative therapies, clinical observations are sometimes made suggesting that some minor visceral functional disorders may be related to PMIDs, especially those arising from the thoracolumbar region, which can be accompanied by flatulence or constipation, which disappears after vertebral treatment. Flatulence can be exaggerated in the hours following manipulation. But given these few facts, we are unable to leap to the conclusion that the spine is at the origin of most functional disorders or organic visceral disorders.

HYPOTHESES ON THE MECHANISM OF THE PMID

The notion of PMID is perfectly consistent with the findings of the clinical examination. But the mechanism provoking this dysfunction is not evident.

It is logical to look first for a mechanical element, not visible on the radiographs, which is capable of explaining the segmental dysfunction. If such a reversible lesion were to exist, it would most likely have to involve the disk or facet joints.

Possible Role of the Discal or Facet Joint Pathology

Discal Pathology

Discal pathology modifies the function of the mobile segment often resulting in stress on the facet joints. Some authors (Copeman, Taillard, Brugger, etc.) consider (and rightly so) facet joint dysfunction to be an additional source of pain in the herniated disk.

One can imagine that some intradiscal lesions, though unrevealing by themselves, could cause a painful dysfunction of the facet joints or of the interspinous ligament. This could be a mechanism of PMID that could possibly explain the beneficial effects of manipulation that would unlock the incarcerated disk fragment.

If there are cases where this mechanism could occur, the PMID is most often localized to segments where the disk appears normal on the radiographs and remains so for some years. Moreover, some MIDs are seen at superior cervical levels where there is no disk. The role of the disk lesions cannot, therefore, be rejected but does not provide a sufficient explanation for the vast majority of cases seen.

Facet Joint Pathology

The common lesions of these articulations capable of giving rise to mechanical dysfunction are essentially arthrosis and malformations. Some authors have also considered the role of meniscoid formations in the cause of these lesions.

Spondylosis. The segmental examination of a patient with a facet spondylosis is usually painless. It becomes painful only in the case of an acute synovitis.

Can it favor PMID? It may be possible, though most of the arthrotic segments are painless on segmental examination. When there is PMID on these arthrotic spines, it is also found frequently on the segment that is apparently the least affected. In some cases, the arthrotic state of the segment seems to complicate the PMID, make the treatment more difficult, and foster recurrences. Most often, the spondylosis seems to foster segmental stiffness, more than does the PMID.

Articular Malformations. Articular malformations were previously described. Remember that Putti (1927) gave to the facet joints the usual responsibility for lumbar pain and sciatica. Besides the arthrotic lesions, he gave some importance to their asymmetry of surface and orientation. These lesions can now be uncovered on computed tomography sections, but nothing has been found that would convincingly prove the causal connection between these facet tropisms and painful states.

Gillot and Freudenberg have noticed the frequency of such abnormalities at the level of the lumbosacral spine. The other vertebral regions have not been studied as far as we know. Gillot has also emphasized the frequency of transverse crests on the surfaces of the lumbosacral articulations and thought that they could be responsible for ''joint blockage.'' Farfan noted that these crests are frequent in old people or in people with significantly developed discopathy at the same level, but they do not play any role in possible ''blockage.''

Though these lesions may explain certain cases of segmental dysfunction, they do not explain all cases.

Meniscoid Formations.   Some authors have thought that they could explain the favorable action of the manipulations by the release that they would cause to intra-articular blockage of the meniscoid formation (see ''Mode of Action of Spinal Manipulation'' in Chapter 22).

Entrapment of a meniscoid formation would result in alteration in tension of the richly innervated facet joint capsule to which it is attached, resulting in reflex muscle guarding. The latter then further increases capsular tension and thus propagates a vicious circle.

This fascinating mechanism evoked by Kos (1972) was refuted by many. Taking up their anatomic study, Bogduk (1984) noticed that most of these ''meniscoid'' formations have a form that could not permit such a blockage, and even if this blockage could be possible, the laxity of its base would preclude any increased tension on the facet joint capsule.

According to Giles (1986), this is incorrect as far as the lumbosacral articulations are concerned. He criticized Bogduk's study, which concerned only the lumbar articulations and not the lumbosacral articulations. At that level, as at the cervical level, Giles noted two types of ''synovial inclusions'' that were susceptible to entrapment between the articular surfaces during some movements and thus resulted in increased tension on the facet joint capsule, with associated reflex muscle guarding. They are a large, fatty vascular inclusion localized at the inferomedial aspect of the joint and a dense and fibrous inclusion arising from the ligamentum flavum and localized to the medial aspect of the joint. This discussion is very interesting, but the PMIDs are found not only at the cervical level but also at the level of L5-S1.

The problem is to know if these synovial folds are innervated or not. According to Moo-

ney and Robertson (1976), the synovial membrane is richly innervated, but they did not produce any histologic proof. According to Wyke (1981), there are no nerve endings of any kind in synovial joints or in the pseudomeniscus of these articulations. But Giles and Taylor (1982) showed, by the silver impregnation method, the existence of nerve endings in the synovial folds of the inferior lumbar facets, ''which seem to be some afferent nerves having probably a nociceptive function.''

If these studies are confirmed, it will remain to be shown that these endings exist at all levels of the spine.

Reflex Mechanism

Most of the PMIDs seen in daily practice are localized at vertebral segments that seem devoid of disk or facet pathology, in the present state of possible investigations. We must remark, however, that in the particular system that is the spine, with a strictly automatic functioning, it does not seem necessary to think of the existence of a permanent mechanical element to explain a lasting segmental dysfunction.

Both a single macrotrauma as well as repetitive microtrauma can lead to dysfunction of the facets or interspinous ligament and lead to reflex muscle guarding to protect the segment. This muscle guarding can only partially protect the involved segment, given the enormous lever arms playing on the sensitive elements during rapid forceful movements or during some positions. They are perpetual opportunities to reactivate the vicious circle and maintain it. This characteristic of vertebral functioning can be illustrated as follows. If one suffers a slight ankle sprain, one limps, if one walks without thinking (automatic walk), because the painful stimuli coming from the affected ligament creates a functional blockage that tends to maximally immobilize the joint. But if one does not want to limp and if the pain can be mastered, it may be possible to impose normal movement on the muscles and the joint and use the foot normally. This is not possible at the vertebral level. The most courageous person can neither normally straighten out with an acute lumbar pain nor oblige the neck to be flexible with torticollis (wryneck). Any attempt to overcome the blockage will only exaggerate the reflex muscle action. Because of the automatic functioning of the axial spinal muscles, volitional control over these muscular groups or on such vertebral segments is lost. Spinal motion is a global movement. It brings into play a significant number of muscles with complex insertions that must function in perfect synergy to perfectly distribute the loads imparted on the mobile segment during movements or efforts. The proprioceptive impulses relayed to the spinal cord come from the richly innervated spinal ligaments, muscles, and facet joints.

If a spinal segment becomes painful, there is an immediate response from the muscles that tend (without really succeeding because the pressures are powerful) to functionally block or splint segmental motion. These pressures will self-reactivate perpetually unless there is complete rest of the region and this parasite circuit. The persistent reflex produces a functional surcharge at the level of the concerned muscles, which becomes a source of pain, while with time, periarticular reactions settle in. The out-of-control mechanism has a progressively reduced tendency to spontaneous normalization. Everything tends to maintain it, at least while the pressure weighing on the concerned segment from weight persists. Often, temporarily resting the affected segment (bed, collar, etc.) will break the self-maintained mechanism.

It is not always easy or possible to rest a reflex already put into action. The dorsal ramus of the spinal nerve is also concerned; it innervates these joints and muscles. It is wrapped against the articular pillar, as Lazorthes has shown, and its medial branch passes through a narrow muscular passage composed of the mamillomamillary and mamillostyloid bundles (Winckler), both of which are affected by reflex muscle guarding.

In this mechanism of maintained pain, the role of algogenic substances, resulting from the irritation of the nerve, is also to be considered.

The reflex that maintains the PMID is probably not just local. As seen in Chapter 18, the PMID is often accompanied by reflex modifications of the sensitivity of the tissues (skin, muscles, tendon, periosteum) and even of their texture (cellulalgic thickening, indurated myalgic cords) in a metameric distribution. This is why a thickening of the cutaneous fold, painful under the "pinch-roll" maneuver, is practically constant in the cutaneous area of the dorsal ramus of the spinal nerve corresponding to the PMID. The nociceptive influx coming from these "cellulalgic conditions" and from these myalgic cords "maintain the vicious circle which contributes to the maintenance of the segmental dysfunction."

The PMID appears as the common denominator of a great number of common vertebral pains, either directly or through the reflex manifestations that they determine, which can be responsible for or may misleadingly produce pseudoradicular, pseudovisceral, or pseudopara-articular pain syndromes.

PMID AND THE FACET SYNDROME

The term "facet syndrome" is, at present, very much in use. Ghormley was the first to use it in 1933. This term implied that facet joint arthrosis was responsible for the origin of sciatica. He was not the first to suggest a role for these joints in sciatic pain. Others pointed it out before him: Goldthwait in 1911, Danforth in 1925, Putti in 1927, and Ayers in 1927. But he was the first to give it a name that was going to be used. He was also the first to demonstrate radiographic evidence of the narrowing of the intervertebral foramen. This was considered to be the cause of sciatica and felt to be due to facet joint arthrosis or to an excessive encasing of these articulations. He emphasized that he could cure sciatica with a facetectomy, but he advised fusing it to a lumbosacral and sacroiliac graft. At that time, the sacroiliac articulation was thought to be a common source of lumbosacral pain and, according to Ghormley, was part of the "facet syndrome," since it was a synovial articulation.

Shortly thereafter, Mixter and Barr, with their publication in 1934, began the period of the disk that overshadowed the "facet syndrome" until the publication by Rees in 1971 of "Bilateral Percutaneous Rhizolysis of the Segmental Nerves in the Treatment of the Intervertebral Disc Syndrome," with which he had 99.8% success (i.e., denervation of the posterior articulations of the last three lumbar levels, which he did with a scalpel, using the percutaneous approach). His work was taken up by Shealy (1974), who proposed denervation of the facets by "percutaneous radiofrequency rhizotomy" under fluoroscopic guidance; a technique used since by numerous authors.

The term "facet syndrome" was taken up again by Mooney and Robertson (1975), who proposed to extend it to the pain referred into the inferior limb from the facets of the last lumbar segments. They also proposed the use of the "facet block" for diagnosis of this condition, i.e., anesthetic injection performed under fluoroscopic control in the three contiguous articulations from which the pain was supposed to come. In case of success, percutaneous rhizotomy was performed on these three articulations, i.e., the last three lumbar segments. In the English literature, the term "facet syndrome" is usually used to designate the pains coming from articulations that are arthrotic or unstable due to discal pathology and concerns only the inferior lumbar articulations.

Facet joint tenderness is a consistent finding in what we have defined as a PMID. One could, seeing things superficially, consider this facet tenderness of a PMID as being a "facet syndrome," since in some cases, facet joint

injection can effectively relieve the patient. But this does not explain the usual pain of the other constituents of the mobile segment. If the facet tenderness is often dominant in the PMID, it is sometimes secondary to the pain of the interspinous ligaments or of a muscle directly affecting the segment in question. Moreover, these MIDs are seen at all levels of the spine, not just at the inferior lumbar region, and most often, no lesion is seen on radiography.

Since 1960 we have used facet blocks at all levels of the spine to determine the role of the facet joint in referred pain when the segmental examination as described in this book demonstrates a precise pain of that articulation. It has provided us with a means of studying the role played by facet joint dysfunction of the inferior cervical spine in the generation of interscapular mediodorsal thoracic pain (1964), in some pain syndromes of the shoulders and epicondyles and of the superior cervical spine in numerous headache syndromes, and, a little later (1970), the role played by the thoracolumbar junction in some low back pain syndromes.

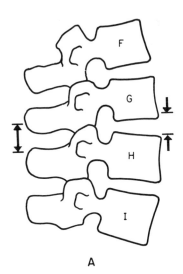

A

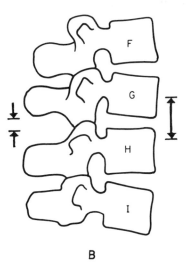

B

Figure 17.4. "Osteopathic lesion" with regard to somatic vertebral dysfunction. This is, above all, defined by osteopaths as a modification of the vertebral segment mobility. It is believed to consist most often of hypomobility; sometimes, however, hypermobility is cited. The diagnosis of hypomobility or hypermobility is made by palpation of the spinous processes and by movement of the transverse processes. **A,** An osteopathic lesion (in segment *GH*) indicated by "segmental movement restriction." The spinous processes of vertebrae *G* and *H* separate poorly during the flexion movement. This is described as a lesion in "extension." The inverse of this is noted in **B**, where the spinous processes of vertebrae *G* and *H* come together poorly in the movement of extension. This is called a lesion in "flexion." One could create similar schemes for rotation and lateroflexion.

PMID AND THE "OSTEOPATHIC LESION"

Osteopaths and chiropractors, convinced of the efficacy of their manipulations, have tried to justify their use with concepts such as "osteopathic lesion" (osteopaths) and "subluxation" (chiropractors). A "subluxation" would show itself by a deviation of the vertebra, found by palpation. Radiographs could show it objectively. It is treated by manipulation, which is supposed to "readjust" the subluxation.

The "osteopathic lesion" (now referred to as "somatic dysfunction") is defined as a dysfunction of the vertebral segment characterized by a modification of its mobility: "hypomobility" most of the time, "hypermobility" sometimes. Osteopaths state that the aim of mobilization is to "restore the normal joint play" of the concerned segments (Fig. 17.4) (see also Chapter 22, "Vertebral Manipulation"). In osteopathic medicine, there is not a reference to pain provoked by these maneuvers in the vertebral segment. (The notion of hypomobility and hypersegmental mobility is fundamentally different from that of a concept entertained in "minor intervertebral derangements" of Dr. Maigne, which are defined as painful dysfunction.) This essential point is found in the osteopathic literature and has been confirmed to us by some American osteopathic authorities. This concept of "segmental dysfunction," founded only on the loss of segmental mobility, has been adopted by most schools of manual medicine in the world.

The concept of "painful minor intervertebral dysfunction" or PMID (Maigne), on the contrary, defines a minor dysfunction whose characteristic feature is pain. The concerned segment is painful when it is called into play by maneuvers exaggerating its movements. In our definition, we do not take into account the mobility of the segment, in as much as it can be noted. Besides, it is reasonable to suppose that only a segment whose functioning is painful can be at the origin of nociceptive influxes sufficient to result in or produce local referred pains.

CONCLUSION

The concept of PMID gives a medically acceptable and clinically logical substratum to the use of manipulations. It also widely extends beyond the frame of this therapeutic means, since it explains a great number of common vertebral pain syndromes for which manipulation is not always indicated.

18

SEGMENTAL VERTEBRAL CELLULOTENOPERIOSTEOMYALGIC SYNDROME[1]

Under the title of "segmental vertebral cellulotenoperiosteomyalgic syndrome" (SVCPMS), we describe a group of palpable modifications of the texture and sensitivity of the soft tissues—cutaneous (cellulalgia), muscular (trigger points), and tenoperiosteal (in relation to a segmental spinal dysfunction). These manifestations are localized to a constant territory for a given spinal segment. Clinically, this territory correlates well with that of the corresponding nerve root, but at some levels, the cellulalgia extends beyond this area, and a cellulalgic zone can be common to two or three adjacent spinal segments.

The manifestations of this syndrome can be "active" and responsible for pains that are often misleading: pseudoradicular, pseudopara-articular, or pseudovisceral. They can also be "latent," simply discoveries on the examination.

In the framework of common pain syndromes, the most frequent cause of segmental dysfunction responsible for these manifestations is the "painful minor intervertebral dysfunction" (PMID). Segmental dysfunction can also be due to a herniated disk or an acute synovitis or spondylosis.

By systematically palpating the muscles and cutaneous tissues in common radicular sciatica and in femoral neuralgia, we have noticed the existence of trigger points whose mechanism of appearance seemed different to us, since it was tied to the spinal segmental dysfunction. These trigger points were always localized to the same muscles and often to the same part of these muscles for the same root. Another remarkable fact is that they were often associated with a localized zone of cellulalgia specific for L5, S1, L3, and L4 and demonstrated similar findings with the pinch-roll maneuver (Fig. 18.1). These manifestations could disappear with the termination of the episode or could persist partially and sometimes be responsible for chronic pain (Maigne, 1961).

Given their distribution, these manifestations seemed to be tied to the irritation of the dorsal primary ramus of the spinal nerve, especially since they did not refer to the lower limbs as in the case of pure lumbar pain (without sciatica) coming from L4-L5 or L5-S1. Later, we were able to note the existence of such manifestations in cases of segmental dysfunction without radicular pain syndrome, in the trunk and upper limbs (Fig. 18.2).

It is from these remarks that the "cellulo-periosteomyalgic syndrome of the segmental vertebral dysfunction" was described (Maigne 1968).

"Vertebrospinal" syndromes fostering some pain with nonradicular topography have been described. They are essentially referred pains provoked by experimental irritation of different vertebral structures (Kellgren, Feinstein), as discussed above (see "The Intraspinous Ligaments," in Chapter 14). They are pains felt by the patient in a given area and not modifications of texture or sensitivity of the tissues found on the palpation examination.

Later in this chapter, we discuss the studies that have pointed out, in the past and under different names (myogelosis, hartspann, trigger points), in the center of some muscles, the presence of indurated cords responsible for local or radiating pains. These cords can be thought of as an explanation for the surcharge

[1] In this book, we use the terms "segmental vertebral cellulotenoperiosteomyalgic syndrome" (SVCPMS), "segmental vertebral neurotrophic syndrome" (SVNS), or, more briefly, "segmental vertebral syndrome" (SVS) interchangeably to designate this syndrome and its manifestations.

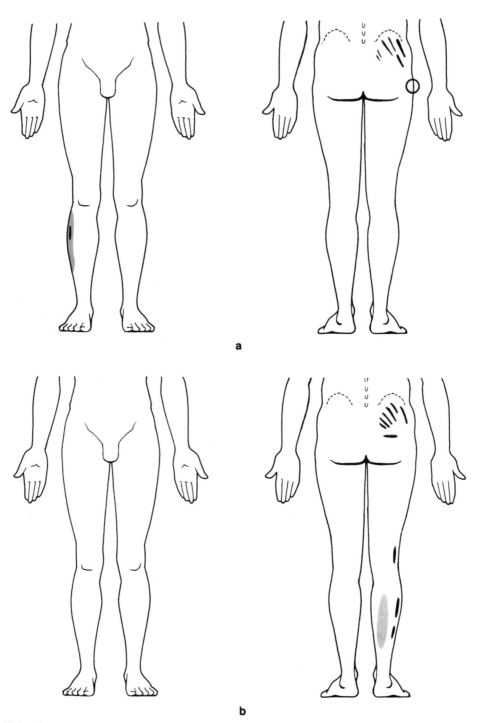

Figure 18.1. Cellulalgic, myalgic, and tenoperiosteal manifestations that one can find by palpation of the sciatic nerves L5 (**a**) and S1 (**b**). *Dark zones* represent trigger points, *gray zones* represent cellulalgic zones, and *circles* represent painful tenoperiosteal sites.

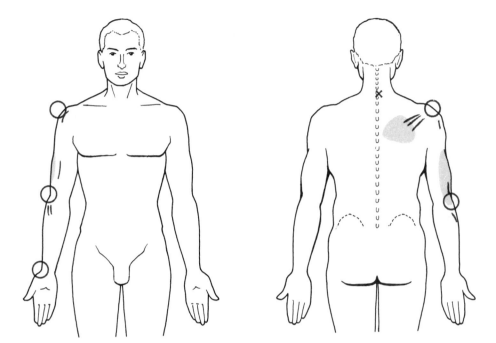

Figure 18.2. Cellulalgic, myalgic, and tenoperiosteal manifestations that can be found on palpation in cases of C5-C6 segmental dysfunction (see the explanations for the various zones in Fig. 18.1). Areas shown here are only those most commonly found.

of activity due to forceful movement, static problems, or fatigue.

Some authors, in a few isolated cases, have thought of a possible vertebral origin for a cellulalgia responsible for a pseudovisceral or referred pain (May et al., Judovich and Bates). Others have described some modifications of texture and sensitivity of muscles and of paravertebral tendons ("systematic tendinomyositis") in the neighborhood of the involved segment, by vertebral or sacroiliac dysfunction (*Ecole ostéopathique*). Brugger also described some "tendinomyose" tied to the distress of the joints of the limbs and of the facet joints, provoked by postural disorders. For example, he mentions the reflex tendomyosis of the musculature of the cervical or thoracic spine, tied to a facet joint dysfunction, and the reflex tendomyosis of the paraspinal and gluteal muscles, tied to dysfunction of the lumbar facet joints.

As far as we know, however, no one described, prior to us, the neurotrophic changes systematically uncovered by palpation in the presence of segmental spinal dysfunction localized to a constant area for a particular segment, essentially that of the dermatome, which involved simultaneously the skin and subcutaneous tissues (cellulalgia), the muscles (trigger points), and the tenoperiosteal insertions

CLINICAL MANIFESTATIONS OF THE SEGMENTAL VERTEBRAL SYNDROME

Segmental dysfunction usually alters the sensitivity and texture of the soft tissues detected by careful palpation of the cutaneous, muscular, and tenoperiosteal tissues. These soft tissue findings are consistently found in the same location in the involved tissues in a manner unique to each segmental level and in the territory of the corresponding spinal nerve root.

These cellulalgic, tenoperiosteal, and myalgic manifestations always affect the same muscles, the same cutaneous zones, and the same tenoperiosteal insertions for a given spinal segment. This altered soft tissue sensitivity and texture, associated with segmental spinal dysfunction, constitute the SVCPMS (Maigne).

For a given spinal segment, this syndrome groups

- Skin and subcutaneous swelling and induration in all or part of the dermatome
- Indurated myalgic cords (trigger points) localized in some muscles of the myotome
- Hypersensitivity of the tenoperiosteal insertions (entheses) of the sclerotome on palpation

Recall that embryologically, sclerotome refers to that part of the somite that will develop into the axial skeleton (spine). In the English literature, however, this term is currently used to indicate also the bones of the limbs developing from the same somite. This is the meaning we use in this book.

These manifestations are reversible and disappear when the segmental spinal dysfunction resolves. In chronic cases, however, they can become organized and persist autonomously. They are usually unilateral, and all are localized to the same side, the side of the dysfunctional facet joint uncovered by the segmental examination. They can be bilateral if the dysfunction is also bilateral, but this is rare.

All the elements of this syndrome need not necessarily always present together. Especially in the trunk, cellulalgia is generally an isolated manifestation. To find these manifestations, the palpation examination should be thorough, with side-to-side comparison as well as any adjacent zones.

Segmental spinal dysfunction can lead to perturbations that are more extensive than the ones perceived only by clinical examination. In practice, however, we can rely only on the clinical examination and note the radicular topography of their distribution.

Some overflow is possible; there are some areas where cellulalgia has a topography common to two or three adjacent spinal segments. This is the case in the cervical spine and, to a lesser degree, at the thoracolumbar junction. The same trigger points of a given muscle can also be facilitated by dysfunction of two adjacent spinal segments, which is normal, since all muscles (with the exception of the rhomboids) are innervated by more than one spinal nerve root.

These manifestations, generally improved by spinal treatment, can sometimes be responsible for local, regional, or referred pains that are often misleading. They also constitute a source of nociceptive influx maintaining a vicious circle.

This SVCPMS gives a better understanding of the persistence of some pains and explains why some purely spinal treatments often instantly relieve the tendinous, muscular, or pseudovisceral signs and symptoms that otherwise do not appear to have a spinal source.

Cellulalgia

Cellulalgia, or skin and subcutaneous tissue irritability, is the most frequently seen manifestation and the only one easily detectable in the trunk. It is characterized by increased texture thickness with acute tenderness to pinch-rolling, the key maneuver of this examination.

Examination: The "Pinch-Roll" Test

To perform the pinch-roll examination, a fold of the skin is pinched firmly between the thumb and index finger. Tension is applied to the skinfold as it is rolled between the fingers in one direction and then in the other—as if rolling a cigarette—maintaining a firm pinch throughout. The pinch should never be released during the maneuver (Fig. 18.3). It is better to use both hands for this maneuver.

The examination should be performed bilaterally and symmetrically throughout all cutaneous surfaces. Consistent pressure is necessary. The examination is generally performed over the trunk from inferior to superior and transversely for the limbs. All the tender cutaneous areas covering a wide zone should be explored. This maneuver, apparently simple, requires a certain practice to be performed appropriately. It should be measured by performing the same examination on a nontender or normal cutaneous zone. In practice, several trials with different degrees of pressure should be made, comparing both sides.

Of the involved zones, two observations can be made:

- The skinfold is thickened.
- The maneuver is very painful.

The thickening of the fold is more or less significant, depending on the region of the body and on the subject. Sometimes, it is very thick and firm, giving the impression of a sau-

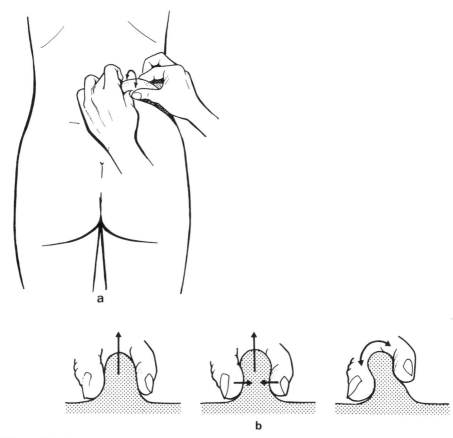

Figure 18.3. **a,** Pinch-roll maneuver at the lumbar level. **b,** Different phases of the pinch-roll maneuver. Using both hands, grasp the skin between the thumb and index finger, firmly pulling it away from the under-lying tissue, continually maintaining traction as it is rolled upward. In the course of this, a pinch-roll motion is carried out.

sage between the fingers; at other times it is so edematous that it is impossible to grasp between the thumb and index finger. In some subjects the thickening is hardly noticeable; only pain is present. Often, these persons have thin skin. Pain on the pinch-roll examination is constant and sometimes intolerable if the pinch is a little firm in the involved zone. As for the thickening of the fold, comparison should be made between the symmetric zone and the adjacent zones while maintaining an equal pressure.

In some subjects, especially obese women with significant diffuse global thickening of the soft tissues and regions of subcutaneous fat deposition (nape, shoulders, arms, loins, buttocks, hips, internal side of the knee, etc.), examination may be difficult because of unilateral, cellulalgic, and limited zones tied to a segmental vertebral syndrome (SVS). Nevertheless, in these subjects, it is generally possible to find a true hypersensitivity in a small zone of involvement in relation to the contiguous zones in the same nerve root distribution.

Topography

The affected zone is more or less extensive. It coincides with all or part of the dermatome and is usually unilateral. In the trunk, especially over the dorsal aspect, its topography coincides reliably with the cutaneous area of the dorsal primary ramus of the corresponding spinal nerve. It gives the only semiologic sign that is convenient (Maigne).

Careful study of the dorsal cellulalgic zones at our clinic in relation to the involved spinal segments has caused us to reconsider the cutaneous path and distribution of these posterior rami. We noted that they did not always correspond to the generally accepted sensory distributions (C4, T2, T12, L1, L2) as depicted in classical dermatomal maps. Verifications by dissection have confirmed our clinical findings.

Over the ventral aspect of the trunk, the cellulalgic zones are found in the areas corresponding to the usually accepted areas of the dermatome. They are less constant than are those over the dorsal region (Fig. 18.4).

In the lower limbs, the cellulalgic areas of L2, L3, and L4 also correspond to the classical dermatomes, while the areas of L5 and S1 are reduced to a very limited zone. What is noticeable for these last two segments is that the cellulalgia exists only when the segmental dysfunction at L4-L5 or L5-S1 is accompanied or was accompanied by a sciatica.

In the upper limbs, the topography is less clear. The cellulalgic zones of spinal origin are seen only in the upper arm and the superolateral forearm.

The presence of a localized cellulalgic zone, especially if it is unilateral, requires a careful examination of the corresponding spinal segments and a search for other neurotrophic manifestations (trigger points, tenoperiosteal hypersensitivity). It is often the only objective sign found in cases of neuralgia in which there is no hypoesthesia or hyperesthesia to touch or pinprick. These cellulalgic zones can be responsible for misleading pains, which can be felt superficially or as a burning pain but are more usually felt as a deep pain mimicking visceral pain of abdominal or thoracic origin (Fig. 18.3). In the back, these zones result in regional pain (thoracic pain, lumbar pain) clearly localized below the involved spinal segment, since they noticeably cover the cutaneous territory of the dorsal rami whose territory lies somewhat inferiorly to the corresponding vertebra (Fig. 18.3). Thus, pain arising from the segments of the thoracolumbar junction, T11-T12-L1, is often felt by the patient over the buttocks and can simulate a low abdominal pain or a gynecologic pain anteriorly.

In the limbs, it is possible to have a limited cellulalgic zone, found only after a detailed ex-

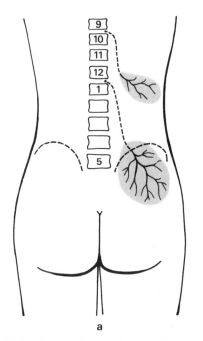

a

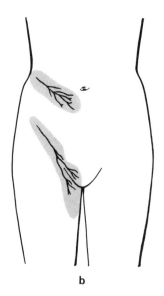

b

Figure 18.4.   Cellulalgic zone involved in segmental dysfunction of T9-T10 and T12-L1. These zones are situated in the territory of cutaneous branches of the corresponding posterior primary rami overlying the torso. **a,** Constant findings of the anterior branches overlying the abdomen. **b,** Findings not constant.

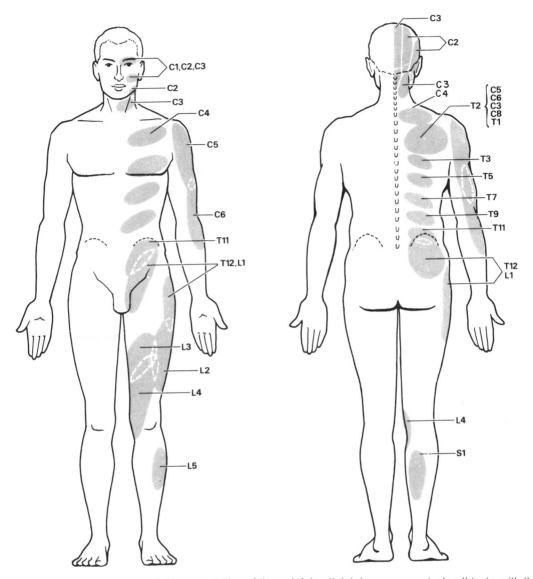

Figure 18.5. SVCPMS (Maigne). Representation of the painful cellulalgic zones on pinch-roll tests, with their usual associated segmental dysfunctional level. At the hairline level, the pinch-roll test is replaced by the "friction sign."

amination, which can be responsible for the persistence of regional or pseudoradicular pain.

Injection of local anesthetic into the cellulalgic zone can momentarily suppress the refractory pain. These zones are usually ignored by the patient, who is surprised when they are revealed.

These cellulalgic zones disappear when the segmental dysfunction that precipitated them resolves. In chronic cases, they can persist partially, being less painful and less thick on pinch-rolling and, moreover, not responsible for pain (Fig. 18.5).

Myalgic Indurated Cords (Trigger Points)

Myalgic indurated cords present as one or several taut bands that (when found) are very tender to palpation. They vary in diameter (from the size of a needle to the size of a cigar, depending on the involved muscles) and are usually a few centimeters long (Fig. 18.2).

Palpation of the muscle should be performed with the palm of the hand with fingers slightly flexed, rubbing the relaxed muscle fibers perpendicular to their orientation, as if one were strumming the strings of a guitar (Fig. 18.6). The pressure applied with the pad of the finger on the most sensitive point of the taut band often reproduces the pain felt by the patient and its referral pattern. Injection of this point with a few drops of local anesthetic often reproduces, at the start of the injection, the acute local and referred pain. This pain disappears rapidly with the effect of the anesthetic. The same injection performed in an adjacent part of the muscle a few millimeters away from it may not reproduce any reaction. Injection at the most sensitive point often produces a sudden muscle twitch, which is palpable and visible, and thus this point is called a "trigger point."

Target Muscles

Remarkably, these trigger points are most often localized to the same part of the same muscles for the same spinal segment. They are "target muscles." Some seem to be specific to a segment. The short head of the biceps femoris, for example, is practically always involved in sciatica (S1) as are the fibers of the lateral head of the gastrocnemius. As mentioned above, however, these muscles are in-

nervated by two or more spinal segments, therefore, the gluteus maximus, medius, and minimus muscles are always involved when there is a segmental dysfunction of either one of the last two lumbar segments. Piriformis muscle involvement helps distinguish L5 from S1 dysfunction, as it is involved only when S1 is affected. Similarly in the upper limbs, the "target muscles" are the supraspinatus, infraspinatus, teres minor (C5, C6), supinator (C5, C6), extensor carpi radialis longus and brevis (C6, C7), triceps, common extensor (C7), subscapularis (C6), etc.

Trigger Points and Referred Pain

These trigger points may become chronic sources of refractory pain. They can be responsible for the persistence of pseudoradicular pains in femoral neuralgia, sciatica, or cervicobrachial neuralgia. Only one taut band of the inferior aspect of the biceps femoris, for example, can produce a persistent sciatica increased in the sitting position, since in that position the muscle fibers in question are compressed against the seat. A trigger point of the gluteus medius or minimus can be a perpetuating factor in an L5 sciatica, while a trigger point in the infraspinatus can mimic shoulder pain, etc. Although not all taut bands result in painful syndromes, they surely play a role when the pressure performed on a particular point of the cord reproduces the pain at a distance ("trigger point"), known by the patient.

Regional pain or referred pain, for which they are responsible, is very misleading. The painful projection is the same as that resulting from injection of a few drops of hypertonic saline in the same normal muscle.

The painful muscular points attributed to local muscular fatigue by most authors seem often to have a spinal origin.

If local treatment of the trigger point momentarily relieves the local or referred pain, then a spinal treatment alone may have a long-lasting effect when the trigger point is affected by a SVS and is due to segmental dysfunction. However, it is not uncommon for some trigger points of a SVS to be aggravated and be made more sensitive if the involved muscle is over-worked because of direct activity or poorly maintained posture.

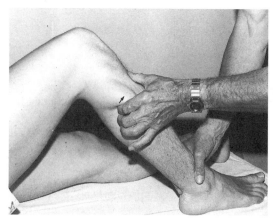

Figure 18.6.   Palpation of a taut band involving the triceps surae.

Tenoperiosteal Hypersensitivity

Tenoperiosteal hypersensitivity is seen frequently. Sometimes, it presents as a spontaneous pain; most often, however, it simply is discovered on examination. The sensitivity of the tendon can be discovered by the contraction of the muscle against resistance or, better, by comparative palpation. It can disappear or decrease considerably as soon as the segmental spinal dysfunction responsible for it resolves or decreases. This is why the effect of manipulation or facet joint injection on this sign can be quasi-instantaneous. This tendinous sensitivity of spinal origin is particularly frequent in the shoulder (supraspinatus, infraspinatus, biceps). Many apparent cases of "tendinitis" disappear immediately after spinal treatment. In these cases, there are always one or more trigger points in the involved muscle.

Epicondylar palpation will be tender in a patient with a segmental dysfunction of C5-C6 or C6-C7 due to a PMID or synovitis, in 70% of the cases ipsilateral to the facet joint tenderness. This epicondylar hypersensitivity is usually ignored by the patient. If, however, these patients take up activities to which they are not accustomed (using a screwdriver, using pruning shears to trim a tree, playing tennis excessively, or playing tennis with a different racket, i.e., one that modifies the patient's musculoarticular habits), epicondylar pain often results, which will respond quickly, sometimes immediately, to cervical treatment. In cases where the irritation is light, local treatment of the epicondyle (injection) can be sufficient. If the cervical factor is more pronounced, however, this treatment may be ineffective or have only a temporary effect, or the epicondylar pain will recur at the first opportunity (see Chapter 53). It is the same for other tenoperiosteal insertions such as certain types of pubalgia, which are often of spinal origin or have a spinal component (T12, L1) (Fig. 20.19) (see Chapter 56, "Pubic Pain and Spinal Factors") or of pseudotendinitis of the "crossroads" (L3, L4) or of the trochanter (L5) (Figs. 18.7 and 20.12) (Maigne).

It appears that tenoperiosteal hypersensitivity of spinal origin sometimes provokes and often facilitates "enthesites" or "pseudotendinitis." The significance of the role played by local stress and its ability to provoke spontaneous pain are inversely proportional to the degree of spinal facilitation. General factors such as an individual's characteristics can also play a role.

Cellulotenoperiosteomyalgic Manifestations, Active and Latent

Many cellulotenoperiosteomyalgic (CTPM) manifestations of the SVS that are asymptomatic on systematic examination can be found in the area corresponding to a segmental spinal dysfunction. They are "silent" or "latent"; the ones responsible for spontaneous pain can be called "active."

When there are several CTPM manifestations tied to segmental dysfunction, frequently only one of them is found to be active; it can be a cellulalgic zone, a trigger point, or a tenoperiosteal insertion. The others are inactive, but they can, at any moment, become "active" as a result of (a) accentuation of the segmental spinal dysfunction, (b) a local irritation, or (c) a decrease in the pain tolerance threshold.

Even when latent, they sometimes seem to be able to maintain this vicious circle of pain. Thus in some cases, when they do not yield to spinal treatment, it becomes necessary to institute a local treatment to make these "latent" manifestations disappear, to obtain the complete disappearance of the "active" CTPM manifestations that are affecting the same segment and are responsible for the complaint of pain. These CTPM manifestations, themselves, are the source of nociceptive impulses capable of maintaining reflex reactions, periphery-center-periphery, perpetuating and reactivating the segmental spinal irritation.

Hypotheses on the Pathophysiology of These Manifestations

Only hypotheses are available to explain the pathophysiologic basis for these manifestations, i.e., cellulalgic, tenoperiosteal, and myalgic pain of spinal origin. This mechanism is probably related to spinal cord function; however, the topography and the clinical characteristics of these tissue perturbations suggest a "focusing" factor, probably the irritation of the corresponding spinal nerve or of one of its branches.

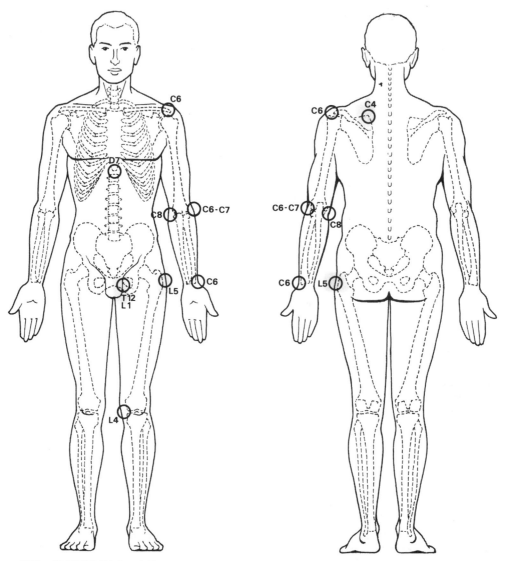

Figure 18.7. SVCPMS (Maigne). This diagram represents tenoperiosteal zones that are often hypersensitive to palpation in cases of segmental spinal dysfunction. Often, these points are apt to present as tenoperiosteal insertional tenderness in situations in which the attached muscles are overworked.

If a nociceptive impulse bombards the spinal cord almost constantly, it can bring about a state of facilitation of the neurons whose cellular body is localized to the same spinal cord segment and provoke motor (anterior horn) and autonomic (intermediolateral horn) responses (Korr, Perl). Sato and Schmidt have shown that sympathetic response to nociceptive stimuli, measured on the white rami communicantes, takes place in a very segmental way. But from there, this modality can be upset, since the efferent impulses are going to reach the periphery in a much more diffuse way, either because of the distribution of the preganglionic fibers to several ganglions of the paravertebral chain or the ratio of preganglionic fibers to postganglionic fibers, which can reach 1:80 (Astegiano). This diffusion effect is restricted to the sympathetic system. In some regions (lower limbs and trunk), however, the CTPM manifestations are often clinically very localized (localized cellulalgia, "target muscles") and, as we have remarked in our earlier publications, are in an area corresponding to all or part of the area of the spinal nerve or one of its branches. Here we should suspect the existence of some superimposed local factors.

Indeed, another element must be taken into consideration: we have regularly noticed that discopathy of L4-L5 or L5-S1 may not provoke the same manifestations if it is responsible for a pure lumbar pain or a sciatic neuralgia. It is, however, the same segmental dysfunction.

- In the case of lumbar pain, there are always some taut bands in the glutei and, often for L5, tenoperiosteal tenderness of the trochanter.
- In the case of sciatic pain, the same elements can be found. In 90% of cases, however, there are also taut bands in the lateral gastrocnemius and biceps femoris (at its inferior aspect) if it is sciatica (S1); and in 60% of cases, there is also a small cellulalgic zone localized to the posterior surface of the calf for S1 and at the anterolateral surface of the leg for L5. These neurotrophic manifestations of the lower limb exist only when there is or was a sciatic neuralgia. The irritation of the nerve thus also plays a role.

The irritation of the nerve is probably the case for the dorsal primary ramus of the spinal nerve. If the cellulalgia is more constant in its area than in the area of the anterior ramus, it appears likely that the posterior ramus is victim to a constant irritation in its difficult course after its emergence from the spine between muscular bundles that are tight and contractured.

Upton and McComas (1973) have shown that pressure in series on the course of a nerve facilitates the creation of a distal pathology: this is what is called the "double crush syndrome." For example, in carpal tunnel syndrome, compression of the distal part of the nerve can readily provoke pain when the axons constituting the median nerve have been irritated or compressed in their proximal course at the level of the root or plexus. Both authors evoke the possibility of a perturbation in the axonal flux, resulting in trophic neural dysfunction. A fundamental part of their hypothesis is that the nerve fibers normally have a "safety factor" that can be reduced by numerous mechanical factors (stretch or chronic pressure on the nerve) or general factors. Such a mechanism could then play a role in the formation of the CTPM manifestations of the SVS.

Cellulalgia

It is surprising how quickly the neurotrophic disorder of cellulalgia can disappear when it is recent, especially when it is in a zone of the back corresponding to the area of a dorsal primary ramus of the spinal nerve. It is sufficient to inject a few drops of 0.5% lidocaine into the painful facet of the segment affected by the PMID, an injection that also involves the posterior ramus attached to it, and in a few minutes one notices that the fold of the skin that was thick, lumpy, and painful to pinch-rolling becomes supple and painless. The same result can be obtained by manipulation if the maneuver makes the segmental pain disappear. When the cellulalgia is more chronic, the effect is less complete, but the skin becomes less thick and less painful.

An axon reflex may be at the origin of cellulalgia. It could start the local liberation of algogenic substances, creating a local vasodilation with extravasation and local edema. These local reactions perpetuate the quantity and intensity of painful impulses reflexively.

Trigger Points

The trigger points that are part of an SVS are found in the same part of the same muscles for the same segment. But similar taut bands can also be seen under other circumstances. They have been described by many authors under varied names ("myogelosis," "hartspann," "taut bands," "muscular trigger points," etc.). They are attributed to a functional adaptation of the muscle, resulting from static and postural disorders or muscle fatigue due to overwork or impairment of the articulation they move (e.g., coxarthrosis). Thus they are theoretically different from the ones we classify in the SVS. But the usual descriptions include all the taut bands, the ones of local origin and the ones we consider part of an SVS from which they are not differentiated.

This relationship is confirmed by the coexistence of a localized cellulalgic zone located in the same nerve root distribution, by the discovery of the tenderness of the corresponding spinal segment, and especially by their lessening or disappearance after spinal treatment. Several studies have been done on the mechanism or nature of these localized muscular indurations attributed to a local origin, but none has resulted in a totally satisfactory explanation (see Chapter 19).

19

MYOFASCIAL PAIN OF NONVERTEBRAL ORIGIN (PANNICULALGIA, MYOGELOSIS, TENDOMYOSIS, TRIGGER POINTS)

The origin of local or referred soft tissue pain, presenting as alterations in tissue consistency and sensitivity, has long been recognized by numerous authors. Various names have been used for this condition: "cellulitis" and "panniculalgia," for the skin and subcutaneous edema; "fibrositis," "myogelosis," "tendomyosis," "myofascial pain," "hartspann," "trigger points," etc., for the taut muscular bands. The distribution and mechanism for soft tissue pain reproduction is different from those of the segmental vertebral celluloperiosteomyalgic syndrome of Maigne that is described in the preceding chapter. But there is no doubt that much of the pain of myalgic cords resulting in this syndrome disappears with vertebral treatment has been attributed by other authors to different causes.

CELLULALGIA OR PANNICULALGIA

Cellulalgia or panniculalgia was first described by Balfour in 1816 and has been studied by numerous authors, especially Wetterwald, since then. It is a painful sensitivity of the subcutaneous adipose tissue localized preferentially and symmetrically in some regions, most often in the nape of the neck, the supraspinous fossa, the lateral shoulder, the periphery of the hips, and the medial fat pad of the knees. It affects women primarily. It can be responsible for diffuse, generalized, or localized pains and is aggravated by heat. The skin is thickened and adheres to the deeper tissue planes; pinching a fold of skin demonstrates the phenomenon of "orange peeling,"

revealing the dilation of the pores. Pinching and kneading the skin is very painful and feared by the patient.

There seems to be a genetic factor. Cellulalgia is often familial, tied to general and neurohormonal factors. Pain is attributed to compression of free nerve endings by internal pressure. It is increased by external pressure. Numerous painful symptoms have been attributed to it. In France, Laroche and Meurs-Blatter and May et al., among others, have published observations of misleading abdominal pain due to the cellulalgia. In the English literature, the term "fibromyalgia" includes altered sensitivity of the skin and subcutaneous tissues—muscles and tenoperiosteal insertions—which include the cellulalgia as just described and the musculotendinous pain described below.

Remarks
The localized cellulalgic edema that we describe in the framework of the segmental spinal cellulotenoperiosteomyalgic syndrome is different. It can be seen in any subject and can be located in any region of the body. It is generally unilateral and occupies only a small surface. It can be more marked in some patients than in others. It can be superimposed upon a regional cellulalgic condition, making the diagnosis more difficult to establish. The topography is, of course, directly linked to the corresponding spinal segment.

TENDOMYOSIS

Under the name "tendomyosis" or other names (myogelosis, hartspann), are pain syndromes of muscle and tendon that are not normally included in the category of classic pathology (tendinitis, tenosynovitis, bursitis).

The English word "fibrositis" includes, in a rather vague way, all pains of the soft tissues. Some authors have divided it into muscular fibrositis, subcutaneous fibrositis, or tendinous fibrositis or enthesitis, etc. The word "tendomyosis" underlined the usual concomitant sensitivity of muscle and tendon. According to Brugger, "tendomyosis is a painful functional disorder, acute or chronic, without a humoral or anatomic pathologic substratum that is known at present. It is a syndrome characterized by precise muscular characteristics, provoked by different pathogenic factors." Tendomyosis links pain with movement—making it and limiting it. The affected muscle is indurated or nodular. In these painful reflex states, Brugger sees four groups of etiologic factors:

1. Muscular strain due to excess activity or poor posture.
2. Painful projection in some muscles. For example, after a severe attack of migraine, there are often pains in the musculi cutanei of the face, especially the frontalis muscle; and in a patient with angina pectoris, tendomyosis of the deltoid and the supraspinatus can exist, since cardiac pains are referred to these zones.
3. Local trauma. Muscular pain can persist after trauma. There can be pain not only at the level of the contusion but also at the level of the corresponding tendon.
4. Reflex of articular origin. This is the case for the painful tendinous and muscular states found, for example, in osteoarthritis of the hip and knee. The clinical aspect is sometimes less clear. This is the case for tendomyosis of the shoulder girdle, provoked by the dysfunction of the acromioclavicular joint; musculotendinous pain here is most significant. The articular dysfunction is not always clear and should be looked for. Injection of the joint immediately suppresses the spontaneous pain and the reflex tendomyosis. These types of tendomyosis can then be responsible for local pain that occasionally has a periarticular or pseudoradicular component. The role of the facet joints is the same as that of the other synovial articulations, i.e., a possible source of a tendomyosis of the paraspinal muscles.

The pathogenic mechanism of these types of tendomyosis is not clear. According to Brugger, it is "an alteration in muscle function, mediated by neural reflex mechanisms and presenting with symptoms that inhibit function." This "starts by pain with contraction and leads to alterations in motor unit recruitment (fasciculations) until the appearance of muscular blocking (fascicular muscle spasm, rigidity)." Tendomyosis is, therefore "the expression of an effect of neuroautonomic blocking" and is among the most important autonomic reflexes. These types of "tendomyosis" or "myogelosis" can precipitate and perpetuate regional pain, especially some with a pseudoradicular component.

MUSCULAR TRIGGER POINTS

The term trigger points is used to convey the fact that they can "release" regional or referred pain. They are located in taut bands of muscle whose center is particularly painful; palpation performed on this point or contact with a needle often reproduces the pain referral pattern for which it is responsible. Anesthetic injection reduces the pain immediately.

Travell made these "trigger points" known and, along with Simons, studied them and mapped out their pain referral patterns. Their topography is rather constant for a given part of the muscle, as the same muscle can present several trigger points whose referral patterns are different. These authors attribute the taut bands to a fatigue of the concerned muscle due to overuse or static or postural problems (e.g., short leg). Thus, they are manifestations analogous to the ones described under the name of myogelosis or tendomyosis in the Germanic countries. But the research there to find the smallest taut band capable of presenting a "trigger point" whose treatment would relieve a given referred pain seems finer and has been done more carefully.

In our experience, though some of these taut bands may have a local source, many belong with their trigger points to a "segmental vertebral syndrome" and respond to spinal treatment. When they have become chronic or when a local factor (of mixed origin) increases them, however, local treatment is also necessary. Several studies have been done on these "trigger points."

Electromyographic examinations do not reveal anything in particular when the needle penetrates in the indurated bundle. But if the needle is put into a "trigger point" of the cord, it provokes a brief visible twitch of the muscular bundle. At that moment, some repetitive high-frequency brief-duration discharges have been recorded, while the rest of the muscle behaves normally (Travell and Simons). A thermoelectric couple introduced into a "muscular trigger point" demonstrates first a temperature higher than that of the surrounding tissues, then rapidly (15–60 seconds) the temperature falls to the level of the nearby tissues.

Numerous explanations have been proposed for the characteristically firm consistency of these taut bands—fibrous conjunctive tissue, local edema, myogelosis (modification of the colloids of the muscle)—but these explanations have never been confirmed. Palpation of the muscle gives the impression of a localized "contraction" of this muscle. However, the electromyograph may not reveal any motor unit activity; besides, how can the nervous system order the isolated contraction of some muscle bundles while others are left relaxed?

This is why Simons thinks that there is a localized "muscle contracture" (contraction without action potentials). As a result of effort that exceeds the capacity of the contractile elements, this muscle contracture could lead to microlesions responsible for local metabolic disturbances from repetitive muscle pressure, resulting in an identical process on a vulnerable part of the muscle. The injured region would then become incapable of getting rid of the excess of liberated calcium ions, which would provoke this permanent local muscle spasm with strong vasoconstriction. The circulatory disturbance seems well established with the study of the temperature, and many authors have admitted that trigger points are a region of local ischemia. The common characteristic of all these trigger points of local or vertebral origin is their hyperirritability, as if the afferent neurons of the muscle were sensitized.

The role of agents such as serotonin, histamine, bradykinin, or prostaglandin is often raised. The biopsies by Awad, which at the electron microscopic level show numerous plaques (which free the serotonin) and mast cells (which free histamine), are not contrary to that hypothesis. The hypersensitivity of the cords and particularly of their central point could be due to mechanoreceptors or sensitized nociceptors. As in the case of cellulalgia, there seems to be both a peripheral factor and a spinal reflex that facilitates this state. We should think here also of the studies of Drevet (see "Objective Muscular Lesions" in Chapter 15).

FIBROMYALGIA

Since the beginning of the 20th century, the word "fibrositis" has been used in some English-speaking countries for some imprecise cervical, thoracic, or lumbar pain syndromes or limb pain, when palpation detected soft tissue pain in the region. This idea was taken up by Yunus (1981) who, under the name of "fibromyalgia syndrome," described pain involving muscle, joint, and tenoperiosteal insertions.

This fibromyalgic syndrome is usually found in women of about 50 years of age who are fatigued and complain of diffuse pain, early morning stiffness, emotional hypersensitivity, and excessive reactivity to physical stress, headaches, irritable bowel symptoms, etc. On examination, they have an essential sign: multiple "tender points." Smythe could find 12 or 14 sites of such pain. The number of points and sites has varied according to the authors. These sites are generally symmetric (trochanters, supraspinous fossae, epicondyles, etc.).

Nonrestorative sleep is frequent in these patients, and there is a significant amount of interrupted deep sleep that needs to be explained (Moldofsky). Personality and psychologic disorders are frequent. Generally, the tricyclic antidepressants (Hérisson et al.) are very useful in the management of this condition.

The bilaterality of the pain and the multiple painful zones make this "polyenthesopathy," also called "diffuse idiopathic polyalgic syndrome," a condition still vague but very different from the cellulotenoperiosteomyalgic syndrome or from the types of postural myalgia with trigger points.

IV

EXAMINATION OF THE SPINE

20

GENERAL PRINCIPLES

The spinal examination should always be preceded by a clinical history in order to become better acquainted with the patient's presenting complaint and past medical history. It is essential to know the precise location of the pain, its character, its evolution, and its possible impact on the patient's activities of daily living and daily work, while trying at the same time to develop an appreciation of the patient's psychologic behavior.

In many cases of so-called typical back pain, the physical examination alone can uncover the source of the patient's complaint and identify the responsible spinal segment. It is important to inspect for any postural asymmetries, assess the range of motion for limitation, and examine the soft tissues for any signs of increased muscle tone or contracture. The spinal examination should be performed scrupulously according to the techniques indicated below, including a segmental examination to elicit the signs of the cellulotenoperiosteomyalgic syndrome that corresponds to the painful spinal segment.

The neurologic examination follows the spinal examination. It's purpose is to find all objective signs of nerve involvement as manifested by motor, sensory, or reflex dysfunction. Sometimes signs of upper motor neuron involvement can be detected indicating a possible spinal cord or cortical lesion.

Certain isolated trigger points or segmental spinal dysfunctions may be the source of pain referred distally, occasionally of a nonradicular pattern. Depending on the results of the clinical examination, ancillary testing, including imaging and electrodiagnostic assessments, may be performed. In most cases, the benign nature of the spinal disorder is confirmed, but occasionally a more ominous diagnosis of a spinal disorder is uncovered including inflammatory, metabolic, metastatic, or infectious conditions.

The psychologic component of painful spinal disorders should not be overlooked. Furthermore, referred pain of visceral origin can occasionally be mistaken for spinal pain, especially when the clinical features are nonspecific. Finally, in the presence of subclinical spinal pain, one must consider the possibility of an intraspinal disorder, as some evolve very slowly and can be clinically misleading for a long time.

CLINICAL HISTORY

The clinical history should elicit the following information:

- The precise location of the pain, its referral pattern, aggravating and relieving factors, consistency of referral pattern, the change in pain with respect to rest, exertion, and work, and the extent to which the patient has modified behavior in response to the pain.
- The mode of onset, whether acute (as in trauma, overexertion, or a sudden movement) or insidious, without any apparent cause.
- A history of any previous episodes and their similarity to the current presentation.
- The evolution: whether static, progressively worsening, or with a consistent baseline but with acute flares (whose frequency and duration should be given precisely). Certain patients may complain of isolated attacks occurring during overexertion or sudden movement or occasionally, spontaneously. Therefore, the effect of various positions in-

cluding standing, sitting, and lying should be given precisely—standing (stamping, walking), lying down (hard, firm, or soft bed), sitting (firm, soft, high, or low seat), stooping, positions of effort (carrying, lifting) and time the pain appears.

These latter points may help to distinguish pain of inflammatory origin, which is usually associated with morning stiffness and improves with activity. Conversely, pain of mechanical origin is usually improved by rest, while the pain of neoplastic conditions is frequently worse at night and subsides in the morning.

In addition, one should keep in mind that a soft bed that offers poor support can be an underlying cause of severe nocturnal pain, as is the case with ordinary lumbar pain; cervical pain is usually aggravated in the recumbent position when the neck is unsupported and cannot find a comfortable position.

It is essential to know

- The nature of the patient's work, including degree of effort, work place ergonomics, and whether there is a need to drive a long distance to and from the work place.
- The patient's leisure activities: tinkering, gardening, sports, etc.
- Past medical history, including an inquiry into the patient's review of systems and any ongoing treatments. A previous history of a peptic ulcer, diabetes, or hypertension will help clarify which treatment strategies may or may not be used.
- The manner in which a patient describes the problem and responds to questions often helps in interpreting whether any psychologic component is modifying the patient's pain complaint. The detection of significant inorganic features, including pain behavior, can play an essential role in the diagnosis and management of the patient. An organic cause for the patient's pain complaint should be ruled out prior to attributing the patient's presentation to psychologic factors.

PHYSICAL EXAMINATION

Physical examination of the spine includes
- A general inspection, static and dynamic, in the standing position

- Range of motion assessment in flexion, extension, rotation, and side bending of the cervical, thoracic, and lumbar regions
- The segmental examination (Maigne) to assess for any specific painful segments.

General Inspection: Static

The patient should be standing comfortably with the legs extended. Curvature abnormalities in both the frontal and sagittal planes should be looked for. The patient is examined

- From the rear: both shoulders, the top of the scapulae, and the iliac crest should be on the same horizontal plane with respect to the sagittal bisector formed by the spinous processes (Fig. 20.1).
- From the front: the anterior superior iliac spines should both be on the same horizontal plane (Fig. 20.1).
- From the side: the sagittal curvatures are examined with a plumb line held tangentially at the top of the thoracic kyphosis to determine the size of the curvatures. The static examination is completed with a study of the lower limbs, including thighs, legs, and feet.

This examination can reveal abnormalities of the curvatures in the frontal or sagittal plane.

Frontal Plane Anomalies

Frontal plane anomalies are due to (a) scoliosis or pseudoscoliosis and (b) antalgic posturing.

Antalgic Posturing. During an acute episode of low back pain, with or without sciatica, the patient may manifest a lateral lumbar shift either ipsilateral or contralateral to the painful side. Often, there is a loss of lumbar lordosis and, occasionally, a lumbar kyphosis. This posturing is involuntary and nonreducible, either actively or passively. This posturing can be distinguished from true scoliosis by the lack of a rotatory component to the involved vertebrae. The lumbar shift is thought to arise from positioning the spine in a manner that decreases the pain, and it is maintained by involuntary muscle guarding. These findings resolve spontaneously with resolution of the factors that led to the acute attack (Fig. 20.2).

Scoliosis and Pseudoscoliosis. In pseudoscoliosis, there is no rotoscoliosis. The curve

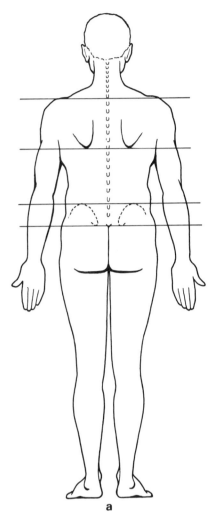 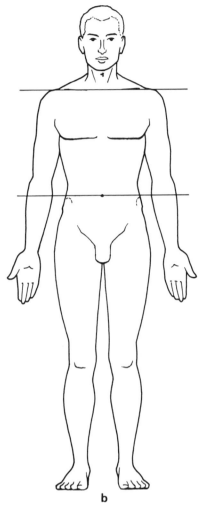

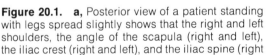

a   b

Figure 20.1. **a,** Posterior view of a patient standing with legs spread slightly shows that the right and left shoulders, the angle of the scapula (right and left), the iliac crest (right and left), and the iliac spine (right and left) are all level. **b,** Anterior view showing the biclavicular line of the shoulders and the horizontal line of the iliac spine anteriorly and superiorly.

asymmetry corrects when the patient bends forward at the waist while keeping the knees extended (Fig. 20.3). A leg length discrepancy can produce static postural asymmetry resulting in obliquity of the sacral base and a convexity in the frontal plane. A wedge placed under the short limb levels the pelvis, and the pseudoscoliosis resolves (Figs. 20.4 and 20.5).

In true scoliosis, there is a rotatory component to the involved segments that produces the characteristic gibbous deformity. Furthermore, the scoliotic curve does not resolve in forward bending (Fig. 20.6). Radiographs performed in the prone or supine position can dis-

tinguish between scoliosis and pseudoscoliosis, as the latter condition corrects in nonweight-bearing positions, while the former does not. The major curve and the minor (compensatory) curve are clearly delineated radiographically.

The scoliotic deformity may be either balanced or unbalanced. In a balanced scoliosis, a plumb line propped from the spinous process of C7 falls in the midline between the two gluteal folds; in an unbalanced scoliosis, the same plumb line falls to one side of the midline (Fig. 20.7).

The degree of scoliosis may be assessed

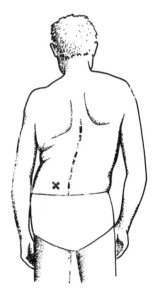

Figure 20.2. Antalgic posture or painful scoliosis. A lateral lumbar shift can be due to protective muscle guarding as is seen in sciatica resulting from disk disease or acute low back pain.

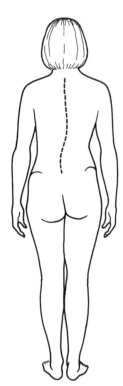

Figure 20.4. Short leg can be responsible for scoliotic posture.

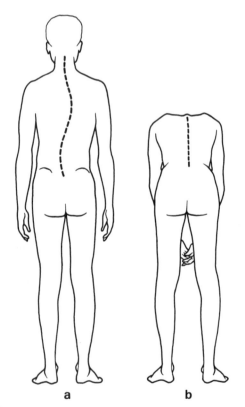

a   b

Figure 20.3. **a,** Scoliotic posture. **b,** It disappears with forward flexion. There is no rotation of the vertebrae.

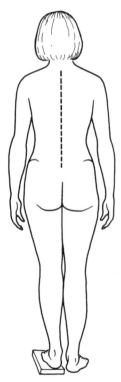

Figure 20.5. A wedge under the foot can reequilibrate the vertebral spine.

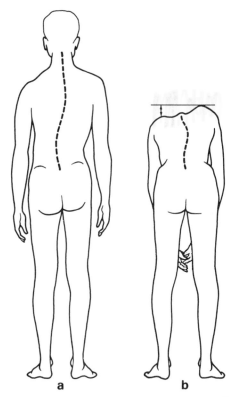

Figure 20.6.   a, True scoliosis is due to a rotation of the vertebrae. **b,** In true scoliosis, forward flexion results in a gibbous deformity that can be measured as the difference between the high and the low point of the back.

clinically in terms of the gibbous deformity that manifests in forward flexion. This can best be appreciated when the examiner stands behind the patient and inspects tangent to the spinous processes (Fig. 20.6). This angle can be measured radiologically by the Cobb method. In this method, lines are extended tangent to the superior or inferior endplate of the most inclined superior and inferior vertebrae, respectively. The angle formed by the intersection of perpendiculars dropped from each of these two lines is the Cobb angle, which represents the angle of curvature of the scoliosis (Fig 20.8).

Most cases of scoliosis may be classified as idiopathic (80%). The curve may be thoracic, lumbar, thoracolumbar, or in two of the above regions.

Sagittal Plane Anomalies

The sagittal plane curves may be

- Exaggerated, resulting in lumbar hyperlordosis or thoracic hyperkyphosis
- Attenuated, producing a "flat back"
- Reversed, resulting in lumbar kyphosis and thoracic lordosis

The thoracic kyphosis is considered to be excessive when the angle of curvature exceeds 50°. The measurement is made from a lateral upright radiograph of the thoracic spine. Kyphotic curves can be separated into those curves with a smooth gradual angular deformity as well as those with acute angulation (Stagnara).

The apex of the thoracic kyphosis usually is situated at T7-8 where the plumb line rests tangent to the spine (Fig. 20.9). The perpendicular distance from the plumb line to the C7 and L3 spinous processes can be measured readily,

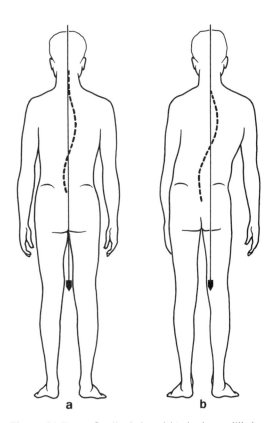

Figure 20.7.   a, Scoliosis is said to be in equilibrium when a plumb line is able to pass through the middle of the occiput and the natal cleft (intergluteal groove). **b,** Scoliosis is said to be in disequilibrium when a plumb line does not pass through the middle of the occiput and the natal cleft.

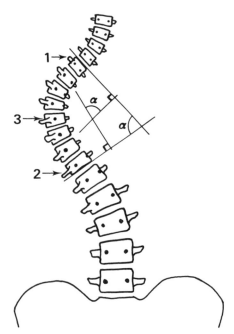

Figure 20.8. Measurement of the angle of the scoliotic curves. *1*, vertebral upper limit; *2*, vertebral lower limit; and *3*, vertebral apex. Tangential lines are extended through the endplates of the vertebrae at the superior and inferior limit of the scoliotic curve, which is usually the vertebrae most inclined from the horizontal plane. The angle formed by these two tangential lines is described as the angle of scoliosis (α). It is easy to obtain this angle by dropping perpendiculars from these tangents, as is demonstrated in the drawing.

and in the adult, usually equals 60 and 90 mm, respectively. The angle of curvature of the kyphosis can be derived radiographically at the intersection of tangential lines extending from the superior and inferior endplates of the upper- and lowermost vertebrae of the curve, respectively. Photographic techniques are also used to assess the degree of kyphosis. The subject is upright and photographed in side view against a background grid of 5-cm squares.

Kyphosis is of clinical significance in the adolescent population, with the most common presentation being that of Scheuermann's apophysitis. The thoracic spine is most frequently involved, but occasionally the lumbar region is affected. The latter case is most evident with the patient in the seated position, as the lumbar lordosis is replaced by a kyphotic curve.

General Inspection: Dynamic

Assessment of Forward Flexion

The patient is asked to bend forward at the waist from the upright position while keeping the legs adducted and the knees extended (Fig. 20.11). One should note

- A normal lumbopelvic rhythm with smooth reversal of the lumbar lordosis.
- The persistence (as in scoliosis) or the reversal (as in pseudoscoliosis) of any frontal plane anomalies.
- Pain limiting flexion (measured as the distance from fingertips to floor (Fig. 20.12).
- The presence of paraspinal muscle fullness (spasm) or a lumbar shift, which may only

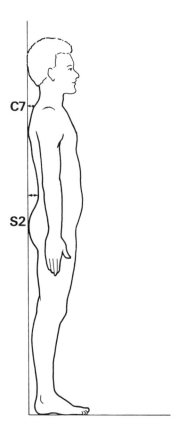

Figure 20.9. Posture in the sagittal plane is measured by dropping a plumb line tangent to the most posterior part of the spinal column. This apex is usually at approximately T7-T8. From this line one can then measure the distance between C7 and that line, which in the normal individual is in the range of 30 mm and demonstrates a similar distance at the L3 level.

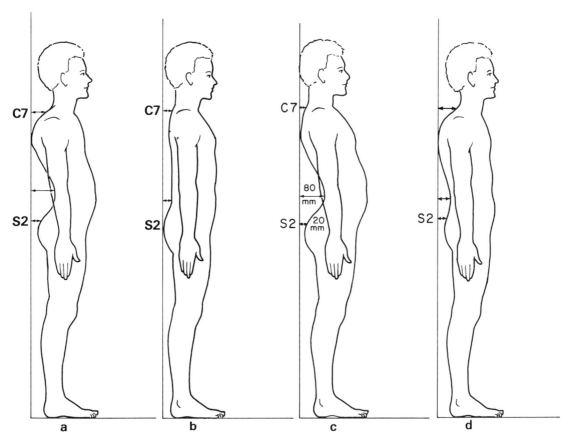

a   b   c   d

Figure 20.10. Subjects with abnormal curves. **a,** Accentuated curves. **b,** Attenuated curves. **c,** Lumbar hyperlordosis. **d,** Thoracic hyperkyphosis. (The *arrow* that measures the lordosis does not measure the lordosis itself. One must deduct the sacral distance to obtain this measure. In case **c,** for example, the L4 *arrow* measures 80 mm, and the S2 *arrow* measures 20 mm. 80 mm − 20 mm = 60 mm. Thus the subject is said to have a measured lordosis of 60 mm.)

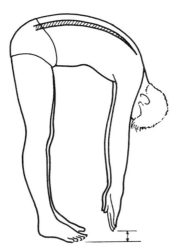

Figure 20.11. Forward flexion with the legs extended. This motion requires a flexible spine or flexible hamstrings.

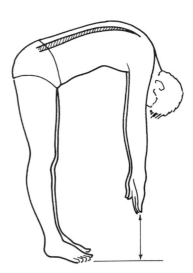

Figure 20.12. If the spine is rigid, the lumbar lordosis does not reverse on forward flexion.

be present during a small arc of flexion, then resolve with further flexion.

- Whether the limitation in flexion (fingertips to floor) is due to painless stiffness of the spinal extensors or hamstring muscles. This is frequently the case in those subjects with otherwise normal lumbopelvic rhythm. This lack of resiliency can increase the stress on the lumbosacral junction. Conversely, some patients can occasionally touch their fingers to the floor, despite a stiff spine, if the hamstrings are loose enough (Figs. 20.13 and 20.14). Schober's test measures the degree of lumbar excursion (see "Examination of the Lumbar Spine" in Chapter 21). Badelon's *rachimeter* can precisely measure the excursion of the spine and the hamstrings (supra- and infrapelvic excursion).

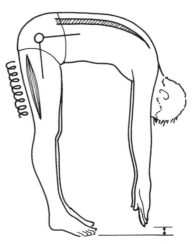

Figure 20.14. Conversely, an individual who has a stiff low back but can stretch the hamstring may be able to easily touch the floor.

Assessment of Side Bending

In the upright position, with the legs slightly abducted and knees extended, the patient is asked to bend laterally to the right and then to the left, sliding the hand down the leg.

One should note whether the spinal curves are smooth and symmetric side to side or if there appears to be any segmental stiffness that may be more pronounced in one direction, and whether or not this is associated with pain. The fingertip-to-floor measurement may be used to quantify the amount of lateroflexion (Fig. 20.15). Alternatively, the position where the fingertip overlies the thigh can be compared on both sides.

Assessment of Extension

This aspect of the examination is more specifically addressed in the regional spinal assessment. However, a global sense of the degree of extension, and whether or not there is pain or stiffness, can be inferred by asking the patient to bend backward with the hips and neck in extension and the shoulders retracted.

Assessment of Rotation

This examination is performed as part of the regional assessment.

Assessment of Regional Mobility

This portion of the examination assesses the components of triplanar motion made up of flexion/extension, right and left rotation, and right and left lateroflexion. Each spinal region—cervical, thoracic and lumbar—is assessed.

First, the subject is requested to perform the active range of motion, followed by passive range assessment by the examiner. Attention is given to whether there is any specific segmental stiffness and which degrees of freedom are restricted or painful.

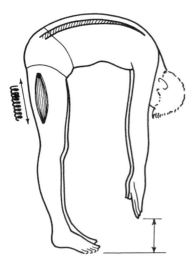

Figure 20.13. Patients who lack hamstring flexibility may have limited forward flexion, as measured by the distance between the fingers and the floor, despite normal vertebral flexibility.

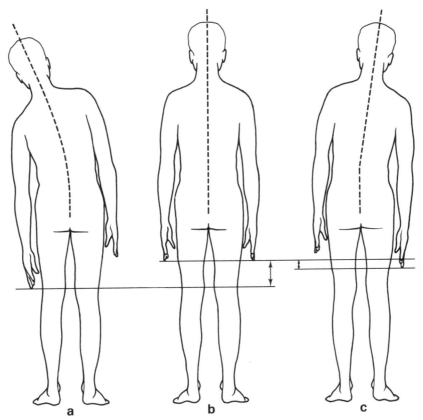

Figure 20.15.   a, Trunk side-bending produces a smooth C curve of the spinal vertebrae. **c,** Loss of lumbar mobility translates to an abnormality called the sign of Cassure.

The degree of discomfort is noted as well as where in the arc of motion it is produced. A "star diagram" (Maigne and Lesage), in which each of the six primary movements is represented by an arrow, is a convenient way to record this information (Fig. 20.16).

Previously, the degree of pain or motion restriction was indicated by hatches (from 1 to 3, according to degree) assigned to the branch of the involved plane of motion. This diagram can be improved upon by distinguishing painless restriction (-) from painful restrictions (X). The position of the markings on the branch (i.e., the distance from the center) indicates where in the arc of motion the restriction occurs. The intensity of the pain or limitation is indicated by the number of X's or strokes, respectively. A painful but unlimited arc is marked with a circle (Fig. 20.17). Thus, all possible combinations can be readily visualized, and a markedly restricted but painless arc of

motion can be distinguished from a marked restriction that is mildly painful (Fig. 20.18–20.20).

Segmental Examination

The segmental examination assesses each spinal segment individually. Its purpose is to elicit tenderness in a spinal segment by one or more specific maneuvers. Segmental tenderness may be indicative of many different pathologies; mild, severe, benign, or malignant.

Basic Maneuvers (Fig. 20.21)

The four basic maneuvers of the segmental examination are as follows:

1. Posteroanterior pressure over the spinous process
2. Transverse pressure against the lateral aspect of the spinous process

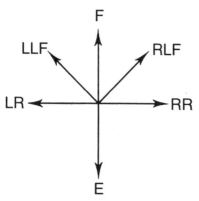

Figure 20.16. Star diagram of Drs. Maigne and Lesage. *E,* Extension; *F,* flexion; *LLF,* left lateral flexion; *RLF,* right lateral flexion; *LR,* left rotation; and *RR,* right rotation.

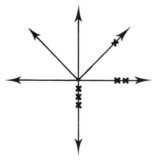

Figure 20.18. If one wishes to be more precise in terms of documenting the results of the examination, one can place the *bars* or *X*s closer or farther from the center according to the level of severity obtained or the movement limitation. In this case, one would place the *X*s closer to the center if they appear early in the movement, or farther out along the *branch* if they occur late in the movement. One would translate this diagram as follows: severe pain on extension at the onset of movement, severe pain on right rotation, and mild pain at the end of right lateral flexion.

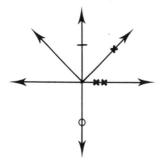

Figure 20.17. A *bar* placed on one of the *branches* of the star is used to mark a limited but nonpainful range of motion. Depending on the severity of this limitation, one can note one, two, or three *bars*. *X* indicates a painful limitation in range of motion. One can note one, two, or three *X*s, indicating increasing severity. A *circle* indicates a normal range of motion with a painful arc.

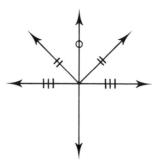

Figure 20.19. This diagram represents a region of the spine where the flexion-extension is free, with pain on flexion; right and left lateral flexion and right and left rotation are very limited though not painful.

3. Longitudinal friction overlying the facet joints
4. Pressure against the interspinous ligament

PA Pressure over the Spinous Process (Fig 20.22). This is best performed with the pad of the thumb. Firm, gradual anteriorly directed pressure should be applied to the spinous process and held for a few seconds. It may be preferable to interpose the other thumb between the spinous process and examining thumb.

Transverse Pressure against the Spinous Process. This maneuver can be used for all spinal

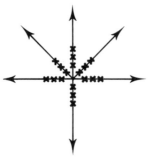

Figure 20.20. This diagram represents pain without any free movement.

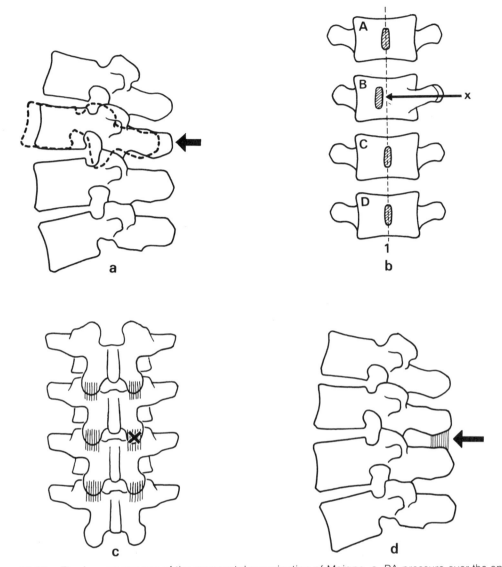

Figure 20.21.   The four maneuvers of the segmental examination of Maigne. **a,** PA pressure over the spinous process. **b,** Transverse pressure against the spinous process. **c,** Longitudinal friction overlying the facet joints. **d,** Pressure against the interspinous ligament.

segments except the cervical segments above C7 and in some cases C2. Slow gradual pressure is applied to both sides of the spinous process, right and left alternately, in the plane of the skin (Fig. 20.23). This maneuver imparts rotation about an oblique axis on the involved vertebral segment. The example in Figure 20.23 depicts vertebra *B*, which is tender with transverse pressure from right to left, or right rotation. Contralateral pressure to either vertebra *A* above or *C* below helps distinguish which of the two motion segments, *AB* or *BC*, is involved.

Remarks

   It is essential that pressure truly be applied transversely to the spinous process rather than obliquely to the junction of the spinous and transverse processes. The latter maneuver can produce false-positive results through irritation of the underlying branches of the posterior rami.

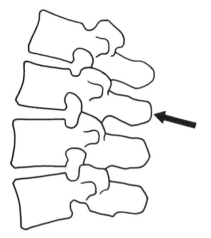

Figure 20.22.   PA pressure over the spinous process. This procedure is performed with the thumb or both thumbs superimposed over the top of the spinous process. This imparts a posteroanterior motion to the spinal vertebrae.

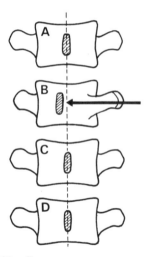

Figure 20.23.   Transverse pressure against the spinous process. This is performed from right to left and then from left to right on each vertebra. It imparts a movement of rotation about an oblique axis to the vertebrae.

Contralateral Pressure (Maigne).   While applying transverse pressure to a vertebra in the painful direction, the opposite thumb may apply a contralateral transverse pressure to the spinous process of the vertebra above or below. Usually, one of these two maneuvers will increase the tenderness provoked with unilateral transverse pressure, allowing for

precise localization of the segmental dysfunction. In the example in Figure 20.24, vertebra *B* is painful to transverse pressure applied from right to left. This pressure on *B* is maintained while a simultaneous contralateral transverse pressure is applied from left to right. When this counterpressure is applied to vertebra *A*, the pain is not modified. However, when the same counterpressure is applied to vertebra *C*, the pain is notably increased. One can conclude that the origin of the provoked pain is segment *BC*. The most effective position for the thumbs is shown in Figure 20.25.

Longitudinal Friction Overlying the Facet Joints.   Facet joint tenderness is elicited by longitudinal friction (Fig. 20.26). This maneuver does not provoke pain in the absence of dysfunction involving one (rarely, both) of the facet joints. The friction is applied to the subcutaneous tissues and paraspinal musculature that is superficial to the facets. In the cervical assessment, the paracervical muscles readily relax in the supine position. This facilitates this maneuver, allowing nearly direct palpation of the articular pillars. This direct palpation is not present in the thoracic or lumbar regions. Nevertheless, when longitudinal friction is applied and produces tenderness one fingerbreadth lateral to the midline, the location of the tender point practically always corresponds (except in the midthoracic segments, T4-7) to the facet joint, as has been verified fluoroscopically. This is seen in the context of other signs of segmental dysfunction.

Pressure against the Interspinous Ligament (Fig. 20.27).   Interspinous ligament sensitivity is often seen in spinal segmental dysfunctions. Ligamentous tenderness is elicited by transverse friction over the ligament, applied by the pad of the index finger or, preferably, with a key ring.

Sources of Error and Precautions in the Segmental Examination

Faulty examination technique can lead to spurious conclusions. Excessive and improperly applied pressure can provoke tenderness in normal segments, leading to false positives. More importantly, false negatives occur when insufficient pressure is applied to involved spinal segments.

All of the maneuvers of the segmental examination should be applied gradually, progressively, and firmly. The examination should be

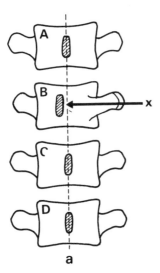

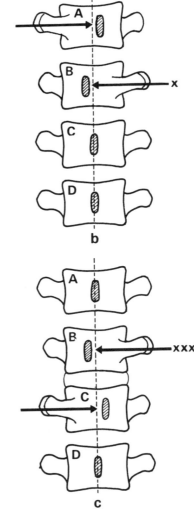

Figure 20.24. Restricted transverse pressure. To make the prior examination more sensitive, one can use lateral counterpressure simultaneously (Maigne). **a,** For example, one can produce tenderness to pressure from right to left on *B,* indicated by *X.* One would like to know if this pain is due to involvement of segment *AB* or segment *BC.* **b,** While maintaining pressure on *B* from right to left, one simultaneously applies a counterpressure on *A.* This maneuver did not increase the provoked pain. **c,** By contrast, the same maneuver executed on *C* notably increased the pain provoked by the isolated pressure on *B* (indicated by *XXX*). Thus segment *BC* is identified as the cause of the pain.

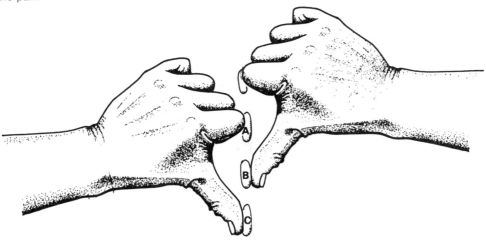

Figure 20.25. Lateral counterpressure method applied to the spinous process.

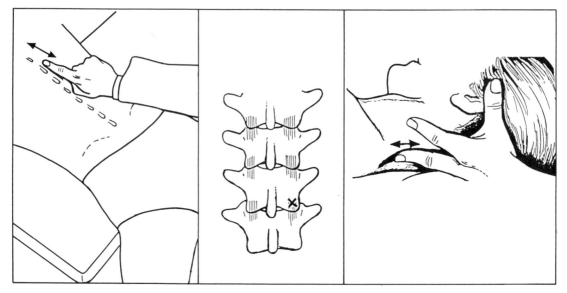

Figure 20.26. Longitudinal friction maneuver over the facet. Facet joint tenderness is consistently found in many common vertebral pain disorders. In this case, there is thoracolumbar pain (*left*) and cervical spine pain (*right*).

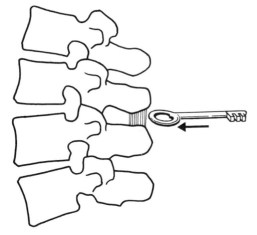

Figure 20.27. Pressure can be applied against the interspinous ligament with the fingertips or, more easily, with the head of a key.

unhurried, repeated, and compared with that of adjacent spinal segments. The pressure applied to each side should be equivalent. Proficiency in these techniques requires a degree of practice. Practitioners skilled in these methods consistently concur on the level of segmental findings in a given patient.

Errors to avoid:

- Pain with PA pressure on the spinous process may, in some cases, be due to periosteal sensitivity (apophysitis) rather than to painful segmental motion. Pain with friction over the spinous process that is of the same intensity as pain with PA pressure is most suggestive of apophysitis. A few milliliters of local anesthetic, applied subcutaneously over the spinous process, usually eliminates this apparent segmental tenderness (Fig. 20.28).
- Entrapment of a skinfold against the spinous process with PA or transverse pressure (Fig. 20.29) is often a source of false positives. This is most commonly seen in the midthoracic level (see Chapter 36). It is therefore important to be certain that the portion of skin receiving the pressure with these maneuvers is not overly sensitive to pinch-rolling (Fig. 20.30).
- In the midthoracic spine, particularly at the level of T5-6, sensitivity one fingerbreadth from the midline can result from an irritable facet joint or irritation of the cutaneous branch of the dorsal ramus of T2 as it runs superficially at this level (see Chapter 36). This is the only site where the superficial emergence of the cutaneous branch of the

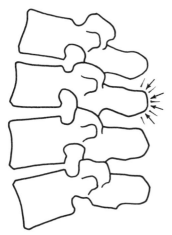

Figure 20.28. Source of error in the segmental examination: pain is produced by friction over a tender spinous process. This type of pain tends to be superficial and usually disappears after injection of local anesthetic.

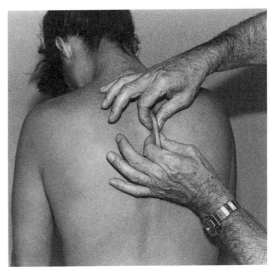

Figure 20.30. To avoid error when performing the segmental examination, one should always start by examining the skin with the pinch-roll technique.

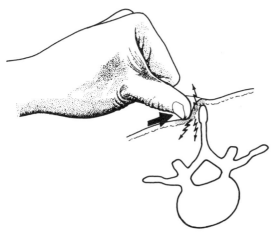

Figure 20.29. Another source of error in the segmental examination: if one pinches the soft tissues against the spinous process, a region of skin that is unusually sensitive or cellulalgic may falsely reproduce tenderness. The same error may occur when looking for painful facets or ligaments.

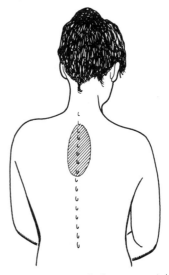

Figure 20.31. Most errors in the segmental examination are made in the interscapular region, since these areas are often cellulalgic.

dorsal ramus overlies a facet joint. Below T6, the emergence of this branch is more lateral. When this tender point is detected, the adjacent skinfolds should be examined by pinch-rolling. Sensitivity to pinch-rolling indicates irritation of the dorsal ramus of T2, and the tender point corresponds to the site of its superficial emergence. Confusion with a T5-6 segmental dysfunction can be eliminated by finding tenderness to pinch-rolling in the territory of the dorsal ramus of T5, which corresponds to the level of T9 (Fig. 20.31).

21

REGIONAL APPLICATIONS

EXAMINATION OF THE CERVICAL SPINE

Range of Motion Assessment

Patient Seated

With the patient seated, the global range of flexion/extension, rotation, and side bending can be assessed. The active range of motion is assessed first by asking the patient to initiate the movements. This is followed by passive range of motion performed by the examiner with the patient maximally relaxed. The movements that are painful or restricted are carefully noted.

When assessing *flexion and extension*, the examiner grasps the patient's chin with one hand, while stabilizing the base of the neck with the other. A normal range of motion allows the patient to flex the chin to the chest and extend so that the eyes are oriented vertically. In practice, it is difficult to measure this range goniometrically; it can, however, be measured radiographically with flexion/extension lateral views depicting a normal range in flexion as 80° and extension as 70° (Figs. 21.1 and 21.2).

Rotation is assessed by grasping the patient's chin and guiding the head to the right and then the left while the opposite hand stabilizes the shoulder girdle (Fig. 21.3).

Lateroflexion is assessed by guiding the head to the right and then the left, using one hand as a guiding hand and the other as a stabilizing counterforce on the contralateral side (Fig. 21.4).

Finally, the *compound triplanar movements* such as rotation with flexion or extension are assessed (Figs. 21.5 and 21.6).

It is evident that the range of all of these movements diminishes with age.

Patient Supine

The examination of cervical segmental mobility is facilitated by patient relaxation. This is best achieved with the patient supine and the head supported by the examiner. The passive range of cervical rotation and lateroflexion increases in supine. First the global range is assessed, followed by a more precise localization of the site of restriction, whether at the upper, mid, or lower cervical level (Figs. 21.7–21.15).

In cases of mild restrictions, each vertebral segment is examined using the techniques of mobilization and manipulation described below. These are performed bilaterally at each segmental level, taking up the slack passively and without excessive force. The maneuver is applied with the fingertips and repeated by oscillating the segment at end range. This is most important in assessing rotation and lateroflexion.

Axial Traction and Compression

Axial pressure may be applied to the vertex with the patient seated or supine. This maneuver may temporarily exacerbate pain of cervical origin (Fig. 21.16). Of greater importance is the test of manual traction (Fig. 21.17), which is indispensable in relaxing the patient prior to treatment, when it results in pain relief. Occasionally, traction can exacerbate the pain and should therefore be avoided.

Segmental Examination

After assessing the active and passive cervical range of motion in sitting and supine, the cervical spine can be examined segmentally.

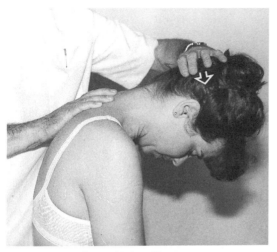

Figure 21.1.   Flexion.

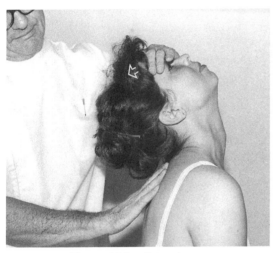

Figure 21.2.   Extension.

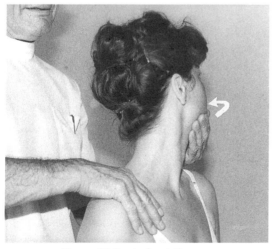

Figure 21.3.   Left rotation.

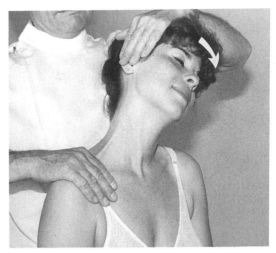

Figure 21.4.   Left lateral flexion.

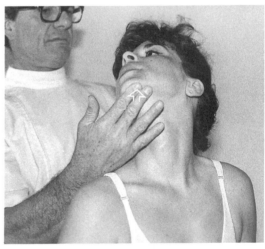

Figure 21.5.   Right rotation with an associated extension.

It is not unusual in cases of pain syndromes associated with chronic segmental dysfunctions to have the global active or passive range of motion be full and painless, while the segmental examination reveals abnormal hypersensitivity of the involved segment. This segmental dysfunction can be due to a painful minor intervertebral dysfunction (PMID), an inflamed facet or uncovertebral joint, or occasionally a more ominous pathology. The diagnosis is reached in the context of the clinical and radiologic examinations.

In the cervical spine, segmental dysfunction

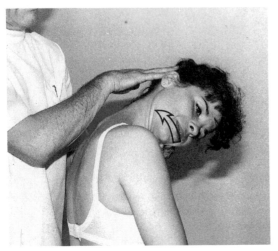

Figure 21.6. Left rotation in full flexion.

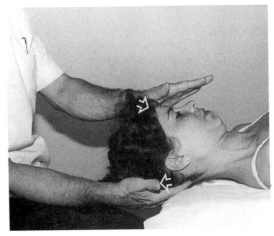

Figure 21.8. Flexion limited to the upper cervical spine.

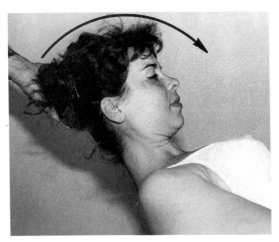

Figure 21.7. Total flexion of the neck.

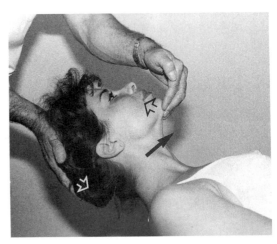

Figure 21.9. Flexion of the midcervical spine and lower cervical spine. The upper cervical spine is maintained in a neutral position.

is essentially detected by finding tenderness to palpation over the articular pillars (sometimes two) with the patient in supine. In the sitting position, the involved segment may be painful to PA pressure over the spinous process. Transverse pressure to the spinous process can be applied at C7 only. The segmental examination is completed by looking for signs of the cellulotenoperiosteomyalgic syndrome in the distribution of the anterior or posterior ramus of the involved nerve root.

Examination of Facet Joint Irritability

This step is the most important part of the segmental assessment of the neck (Fig. 21.18). With the patient in the supine position, the examiner, seated at the patient's head, cradles the occiput with the palms of the hands, extending the fingers over the cervical paraspinals. The middle or index fingers, placed symmetrically on each side of the neck, are utilized for palpation.

To best achieve the desired muscular relaxation, it may be necessary to gently rotate the head from right to left several times. Once relaxed, the paraspinal muscles are easily displaced for deep palpation, allowing the pad of the examiner's finger to contact the posterior aspect of the articular pillars at each segmental level. It is most efficacious to begin palpation at the cervicothoracic level and proceed superiorly to the suboccipital region to C2-3, which is the most rostral level palpable.

The palpation technique involves slow longitudinal strokes with the fingerpad creating friction against the articular pillar. With a consistent pressure, palpation progresses centimeter by centimeter to adjacent segmental levels, allowing comparisons between ipsilateral and contralateral vertebrae. In cases of zygapophyseal spondylosis, a bony prominence can often be discerned beneath the palpating finger. Often, this is painless and without a doubt not the cause of the painful symptoms; on other occasions, this palpation can be very painful.

Occasionally, the articular pillar may feel boggy and tender as can be seen in traumatic

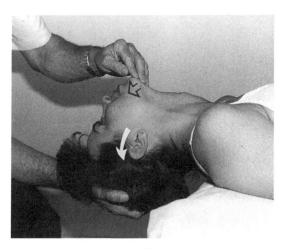

Figure 21.10.   Total extension.

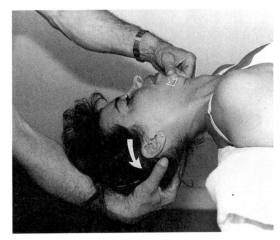

Figure 21.12.   Extension limited to the midcervical and lower cervical spine. The upper cervical spine is maintained in flexion.

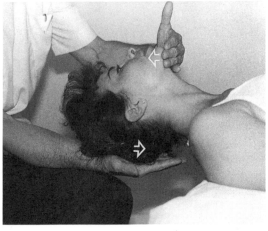

Figure 21.11.   Extension limited to the upper cervical spine.

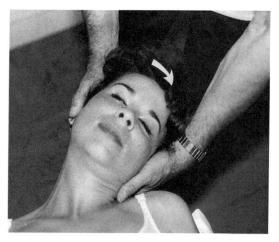

Figure 21.13.   Total left lateral flexion.

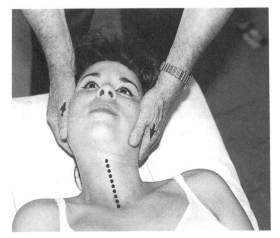

Figure 21.14.   Left lateral flexion of the upper cervical spine.

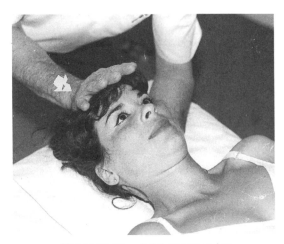

Figure 21.16.   Axial compression.

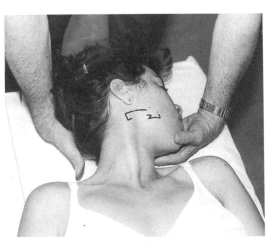

Figure 21.15.   Full rotation.

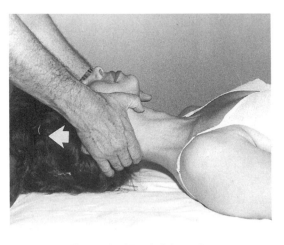

Figure 21.17.   Axial traction.

sprains or inflammatory synovitis. Most often, only the involved segment is tender to palpation, while adjacent and contralateral levels, examined in a similar fashion, are asymptomatic. With practice, one can detect focal muscular hypertonus restricted to the involved level. In these instances, a minor intervertebral dysfunction (MID) may be present and must be distinguished from more ominous pathology.

PA Pressure on the Spinous Process

After having established that superficial tenderness of the spinous process is not pres-

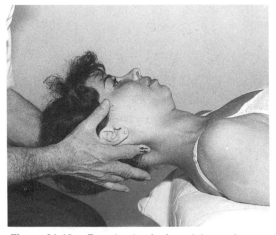

Figure 21.18.   Examination for facet joint tenderness.

ent to light superficial rubbing, a firm poster-oanteriorly directed pressure is applied (Fig. 21.19). This maneuver should be repeated with the spine in neutral position, flexion, and extension.

Transverse Pressure against the Spinous Process

This maneuver can be performed only at C7. The right thumb applies pressure from right to

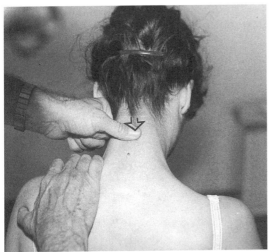

Figure 21.19. Pressure applied to the spinous process.

left, followed by opposite pressure directed by the left thumb (Fig. 21.20).

Pressure against the Interspinous Ligament

Interspinous ligamentous tenderness can be elicited with pressure applied by a key ring. This sensitivity is occasionally the only source of refractory posttraumatic cervical pain (Fig. 21.21).

The Anterior Cervical "Door Bell" Sign (Maigne)

This maneuver is sometimes quite useful in assessing segmental dysfunctions of the cervical region. With the pad of the thumb (the right for the patient's left side and vice versa), the examiner applies firm transverse pressure to the anterolateral aspect of the cervical vertebrae one segment at a time. This pressure should be held for a few seconds (Fig. 21.22).

It is evident that pressure applied in this fashion is distributed over many anatomic structures. Nevertheless, the soft tissues are readily retracted, allowing the thumb to contact the vertebra's transverse process.

A positive sign consists of the reproduction of arm pain or, in some instances, periscapular pain, confirming the cervical origin. Used systematically, this maneuver has allowed us to

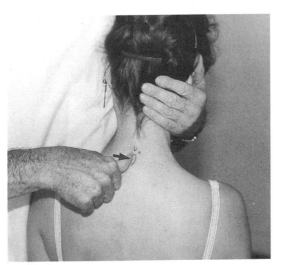

Figure 21.20. Lateral pressure against the spinous process (this examination is variable only for C7 at the cervical level).

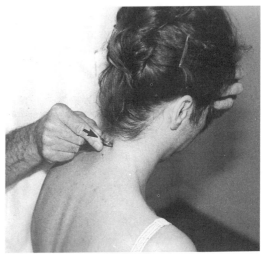

Figure 21.21. Evaluation of the interspinous ligament for pain.

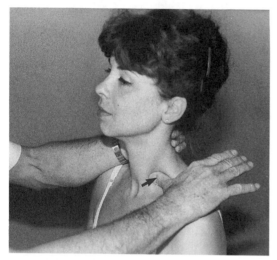

Figure 21.22. Doorbell point. Horizontal pressure is applied with the pad of the thumb to the involved segment, which can reproduce pain of cervical origin in the arms and periscapular region.

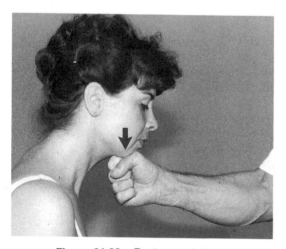

Figure 21.23. Testing neck flexors.

show a cervical origin for dorsal or periscapular pain. It is also useful in the assessment of acroparasthesiae, when one considers the possibility of a cervical source. Finally, it is important to assess resisted motion of the cervical spine in flexion (Fig. 21.23), extension (Fig. 21.24), and rotation (Fig. 21.25).

Examination of the Cervical Spinal Nerve Roots

Cervical spinal nerve root examination is performed by assessing the integrity of sensa-

tion, motor power, and stretch reflexes within their distribution. Following this evaluation, the patient should be examined for cellulotenoperiosteomyalgic manifestations of the "segmental vertebral syndrome."

Anterior Rami

Cutaneous Topography. The cutaneous territory of the anterior rami is shown in Figure 21.26. Depending on the author, there are a few variations. The dermatomal maps usually depicted are those of the anterior rami, which usually do not take into consideration the territorial differences for the dermatomes of the posterior rami.

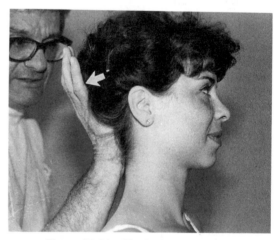

Figure 21.24. Testing neck extensors.

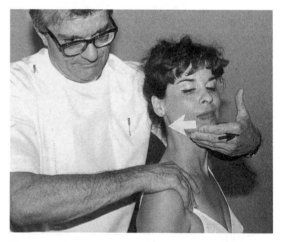

Figure 21.25. Testing rotator muscles with the patient seated.

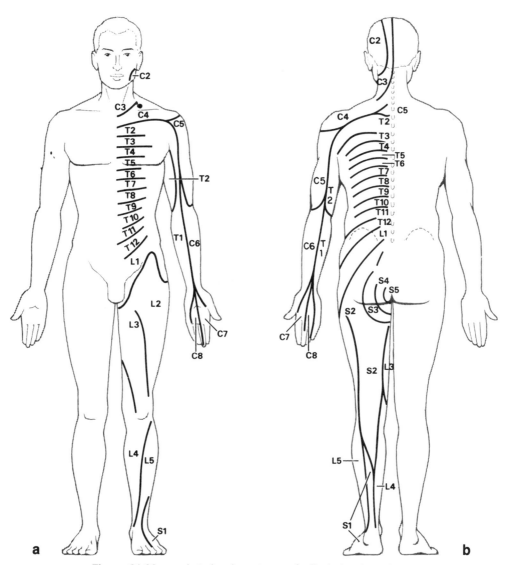

Figure 21.26. **a,** Anterior dermatomes. **b,** Posterior dermatomes.

Muscles. Table 21.1, as adapted from Grossiord, depicts the myotomal distribution of the anterior rami. Schematically, the C5 root governs abduction of the arm; C6, flexion at the elbow; C7, extension at the elbow, wrist, and fingers; and C8-T1, the intrinsic muscles of the hand, especially those innervated by the median for C8 and by the ulnar for T1. Muscular strength is evaluated by classical manual muscle testing.

Reflexes. Testing of reflexes of the anterior rami is performed as follows.

C5: BICEPS REFLEX. Tapping the biceps ten-don at the elbow crease produces flexion of the forearm upon the arm.

C5-6: BRACHIORADIALIS REFLEX. The brachioradialis tendon is tapped at the radial styloid, resulting in flexion and supination of the forearm.

C7: TRICEPS REFLEX. The triceps tendon is tapped just proximal to the olecranon, producing extension of the forearm.

C6-7: PRONATOR REFLEX. The ventral surface of the radial styloid is tapped with the forearm in supination, resulting in pronation of the wrist.

Table 21.1.
Muscular Innervation of C4–T1

	C4	C5	C6	C7	C8	T1
Rhomboids		■				
Deltoid		■	░			
Biceps		■	░			
Brachialis		■	■			
Coracobrachialis		■	■			
Supinator		■	■			
Extensor carpi radialis longus and brevis			■	░		
Triceps				■	░	
Extensor indicis proprius				■	░	
Extensor digitorum longus				■	░	
Flexor carpi ulnaris					■	░
Anconeus				■	■	
Pronator teres			■	░		
Palmaris longus				■	░	
Flexor digitorum sublimis				░	■	░
Flexor digitorum profundus				░	■	■
Flexor policis longus				░	■	░
Extensor carpi ulnaris					■	░
Intrinsic muscles of the hand					░	■
Infraspinatus		░	■			
Supraspinatus	░	■				
Teres minor		■	░			
Teres major		■	■			
Pectoralis major			■	■	░	░
Latissimus dorsi			■			

C8: FINGER FLEXOR REFLEX. The long flexors are tapped over the carpal tunnel or the pads of the fingers, resulting in finger flexion.

Posterior Rami

The posterior ramus of C4 innervates the entire superior surface of the shoulders and back. The dermatome immediately adjacent to C4 is T2, as the cutaneous branches of the posterior rami of C5, C6, C7, C8, and T1 are either vestigial or nonexistent. This is due to their embryogenesis. The inferior cervical dermatomes are distributed throughout the upper limb. Clinically, however, the cutaneous branch of the T2 dorsal ramus, which is physically quite large and covers a vast cutaneous territory, encompasses the cutaneous contributions of the dorsal rami of C5, C6, C7, and C8 (Maigne) that are nonexistent (C6, C7, C8) (Lazorthes, Töndury) or inconsistent (C5). The T2 posterior ramus becomes superficial at the level of T5 and supplies an area extending superiorly toward the acromion (Hovelacque) (Fig. 21.26) (see Chapter 36, "Chronic Thoracic Pain"). The ramus of T3 sometimes seems affected. The only way to explore the dysfunction of these nerves is examination of the skinfolds by the pinch-roll test as we have proposed (see "Examination: The 'Pinch-Roll' Test" in Chapter 18).

Muscles.   The posterior rami innervate the axial spinal muscles. This area of innervation extends down very low, as it has been noted in some tetraplegics or some paraplegics. Cough noted some muscle innervations extending down 5–6 levels below their anatomic level of origin. There is no easy exploration of these muscles.

Examination for Manifestations of the "Segmental Vertebral Neurotrophic Syndrome" of Maigne

The search for the cellulalgic tenoperiosteomyalgic manifestations resulting from painful dysfunction of a spinal segment should be an integral part of the spinal examination. Below, we give their most usual topography.

Cellulalgia

Posteriorly.   A disorder of the inferior segments (C5–T1) presents as a cellulalgia affecting a large dorsal and common zone extending from T5 to the acromion. This large cellulalgic area is present in all the inferior cervical spinal (C5–T1) irritations and is common to all these segments. It depends, in fact, on the posterior ramus of T2. The cutaneous branch of T2 seems to represent all of the posterior cutaneous contingent of the last cervical segments (Maigne) (Figs. 21.27 and 21.28) (see Chapter 36, "Chronic Thoracic Pain").

Just above the T2 dermatomal territory lies

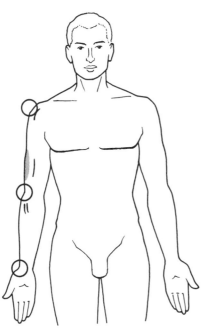
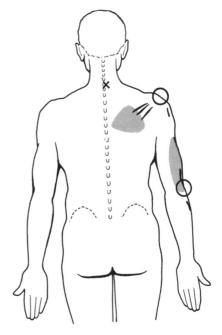

Figure 21.27.   Segmental vertebral syndrome of C6. *Cellulalgia:* lateral aspect of the arm and the superior lateral forearm. Cellulalgia is noted in the interscapular region and is common with inferior cervical segment involvement. *Trigger points:* the muscles most often involved are the infraspinatus, biceps, supinator, and the pectoralis. *Tenoperiosteal insertion:* the lateral epicondyle and the radial styloid.

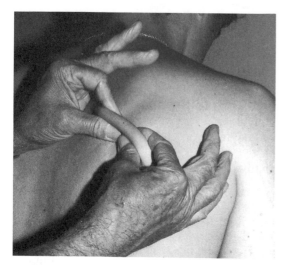

Figure 21.28. Pinch-roll test in the interscapular region (the segmental vertebral syndrome of C5, C6 or C7, C8).

a zone corresponding to the C4 segment, which includes the skin overlying the supraspinous fossa. The C3 segment corresponds to the nape of the neck (with C2 for the superior part and C4 for the inferior part) (Fig. 21.32).

The pinch-roll maneuver is not used for examination of the scalp. It is replaced by the "friction maneuver" (Maigne). Firm pressure is applied to the scalp against the skull as if shampooing. This maneuver, usually painless, becomes painful if the nerve root innervating the concerned zone is irritated (see Chapter 48, "Headaches of Cervical Origin" and Fig. 21.38). If one considers the area of scalp situated posterior to a line passing through the vertex and joining the two ears, one finds

- Near the midline, the zone corresponding to the posterior branch of C3
- More laterally, the middle zone corresponding to the posterior branch of C2
- Supra-auricular and retroauricular regions innervated by branches arising from the anterior rami of C2 and C3

Anteriorly. The clavicular region corresponds to C4. The anterolateral surface of the neck corresponds to C3 (Figs. 21.32–21.35). For C1 and C2 (and sometimes C3) we have described an astonishing sign situated in the area of the ophthalmic division of the trigeminal nerve, the "eyebrow sign" (Maigne) (Figs. 21.37 and 21.39). It consists in a thickening of the skin of the superciliary region, with pain on the pinch-roll test. It can sometimes be associated with the "cheek sign" on the same side (Maigne); i.e., pinch-roll testing of the skin of the submandibular region produces pain. These signs are described in detail and their mechanism is discussed in Chapter 48, "Headaches of Cervical Origin." Cellulalgic edema of the region of the angle of the jaw corresponds to C2 (Fig. 21.39).

The zone corresponding to C5 is at the lateral aspect of the shoulder. The zone corresponding to C6 is at the middle portion of the lateral aspect of the arm and the superior lateral forearm.

Trigger Points

C1 trigger points are located in the suboccipital muscles.

The trigger points of C3-4 involve the scapular rotators (levator scapulae). For C2, they also sometimes involve the sternocleidomastoid muscle, and for C3, they involve the trapezius muscle.

For C5, C6, and C7, they involve the muscles of the shoulder girdle and upper limb, including some "target muscles": supraspinatus, deltoid, infraspinatus (C5, C6), teres major and teres minor, brachialis anterior, and supinator (C6). For C7, they involve the triceps, brachioradialis, and extensor carpi radialis muscles (Figs. 21.29–21.31).

They may also involve other muscles. In the upper limb, trigger points of local origin that are not associated with a segmental vertebral syndrome are relatively frequent, and at all levels, they are frequent in the paraspinal muscles.

Trigger point palpation is not always easy. They can be the direct result of a segmental dysfunction or be part of a segmental vertebral syndrome. Then they are located caudad to the responsible segment. They can also be the direct result of a local segmental dysfunction. In this case, they are located noticeably at the level of the responsible segment.

Tenoperiosteal Tenderness

Tenoperiosteal tenderness affects the scapular insertion of the levator scapulae, for C3 and C4; the rotator cuff tendons (infraspinatus, supraspinatus, biceps, etc.), for C5 and C6; the

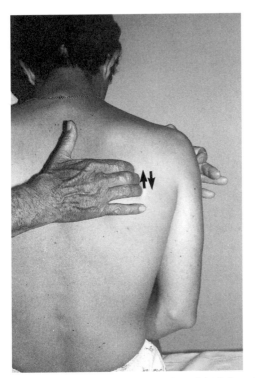

Figure 21.29. Trigger point palpation of the infraspinatus muscle (segmental vertebral syndrome of C5 or C6).

lateral epicondyle, for C6 and C7; the radial styloid, for C6; and the medial epicondyle, for C7 and C8.

EXAMINATION OF THE THORACIC SPINE

Examination of Mobility

To test thoracic mobility in all directions, it is most convenient to have the patient seated astride the end of the examining table, if possible, as though sitting in a saddle (Figs. 21.40–21.43). Otherwise, the patient can sit with legs over the side of the examining table. A chair or stool is not stable enough.

The examination can be more precise if the examiner explores the upper, middle, and lower regions with the techniques described below as techniques of mobilization (see Appendix 4). Passive assisted range of motion is applied until resistance is felt and then repeated with mobilization at end range. This allows better judgment of the mobility and flexibility of each level. Flexion, extension, lateroflexion, and rotation are studied.

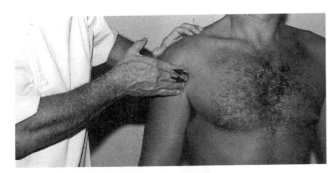

Figure 21.30. Palpation of the biceps tendon (segmental vertebral syndrome of C5 or C6).

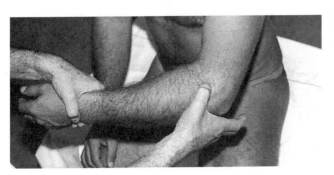

Figure 21.31. Palpation of the lateral epicondyle (segmental vertebral syndrome of C6 or C7).

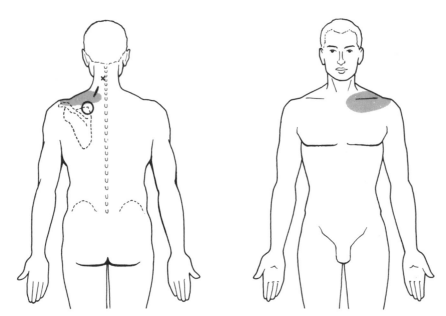

Figure 21.32. Segmental vertebral syndrome of C4. *Cellulalgia:* supraclavicular fossa, infraclavicular region. *Myalgic cords:* levator scapulae. *Tenoperiosteal insertion:* levator scapulae (which may also be related to involvement of C3 and, rarely, C5).

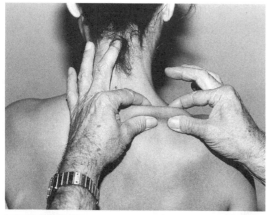

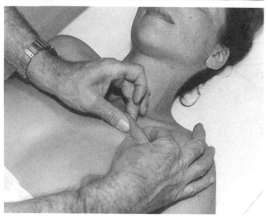

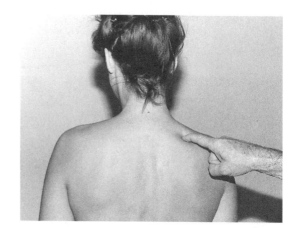

Figure 21.33. Top, Examination of cellulalgia in the suprascapular region (segmental vertebral syndrome of C4). **Bottom left,** Examination for cellulalgia in the infraclavicular region. **Bottom right,** Palpation of the insertion of the levator scapulae (segmental vertebral syndrome of C3 or C4).

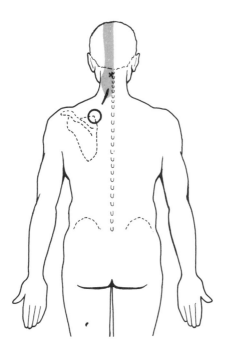

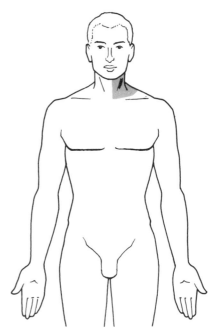

Figure 21.34. Segmental vertebral syndrome of C3. *Cellulalgia:* posterior inferior region of the neck, anterolateral neck, and at the level of the scalp. Cellulalgia is replaced by scalp tenderness that can be elicited on frictional palpation. The region where C3 is involved is the occipital paramedian region. Sometimes, this is also associated with a cellulalgic zone over the eyebrow area. *Trigger Points:* levator scapulae, sternocleidomastoid, and trapezius. *Tenoperiosteal insertion:* levator scapulae.

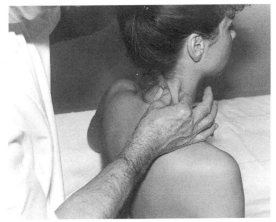

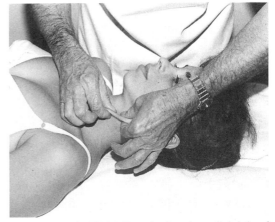

Figure 21.35. **Left,** Examination for cellulalgia at the level of the neck. **Right,** Examination for cellulalgia of the anterolateral neck (segmental vertebral syndrome of C3).

Flexion. As seen in Figure 21.40, the patient is asked to straighten the back. Is this movement painful? Is the curve of the spinous processes smooth? Is there any segmental stiffness? Then, while grasping the base of the neck and upper thoracic spine with the left hand, the examiner applies pressure, resulting in slight flexion alternating with a return to the neutral, while the right hand palpates the spinous processes, which should open like a fan, in flexion. The examiner should look for regions of hypomobility and should also check

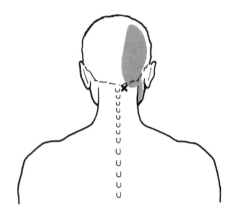
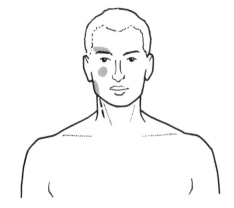

Figure 21.36.   Segmental vertebral syndrome of C2, characterized by
- *Scalp sensitivity to the friction maneuver.* At this level this finding is equivalent to findings on the pinch-roll test. The paramedian region of the scalp corresponds to the posterior branch of C2. The retro-auricular and infra-auricular region corresponds to a territory supplied by cutaneous branches of the anterior primary ramus of C2 and, to a lesser degree, C3.
- *Cellulalgia of the angle of the jaw* (innervated by the

cutaneous branches of the anterior primary ramus of C2 and C3).
- *Cellulalgia of the eyebrow region:* "eyebrow sign" of Maigne, associated usually with pain on the pinch-roll test, often associated with pain and sub-mandibular tenderness (see Chapter 48, "Head-aches of Cervical Origin"). This sign is common to the first three cervical segments.
- *Trigger points of the sternocleidomastoid muscle* (rarer for C3).

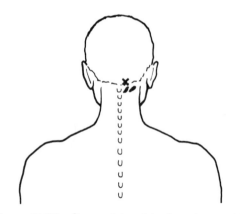
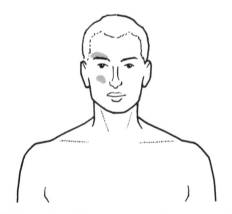

Figure 21.37.   Segmental vertebral syndrome of C1. *Cellulalgia:* region of the eyebrow and, occasionally, of the submandibular cheek. *Trigger points:* suboccipital muscles.

to see whether repetitive mobilization against resistance is painful.

Extension.   As seen in Figure 21.41, the patient's arms are crossed on top of the head. The examiner's left hand and forearm supports the patient. While applying counterpressure with the right hand at different levels of the spine, the examiner rhythmically mobilizes, with the left hand producing hyperextension of the segment on which the hand applies the counterpressure. These maneuvers are painless on a normal spine. During the maneuvers

the examiner's hand should feel an elastic resistance.

Lateroflexion.   With the patient in the same position as for the extension examination (Fig. 21.42), the examiner applies slow and repeated movements of lateroflexion to the back. With the other hand, a counterpressure is applied to localize the movement and also to prevent the maneuver from involving the lumbar segment. This movement is difficult in thick and stocky persons. *Caution:* The examiner should not displace the shoulders of the patient laterally;

otherwise the movement of lateral inclination is at the level of the lumbar spine.

Rotation.   The patient sits in the same position as for examination of extension (Fig. 21.43) but the arms can be kept crossed on the chest, especially for examination of the inferior thoracic spine. The examination maneuver is the same as for examination of extension. To examine left rotation, for example, the examiner stands behind the patient, with the left arm in front of the patient's thorax, holding the patient's right arm, and assists the patient's spine into left rotation. This rotation is done at the same time in the thoracic and lumbar

spine, though it is minimal in the latter. The examiner notes if the movement is limited globally and if it produces or exaggerates pain as it is performed first from one side and then from the other.

Then the examiner tests the mobility of each region of the thoracic spine—upper, middle, and lower—applying localized pressure with the other hand. Alternating rotation with a return to the neutral position, the examiner presses with the right hand on the right paraspinal region to assist rotation to the left and presses with the left hand on the left paraspinal region to assist rotation to the right. The hand

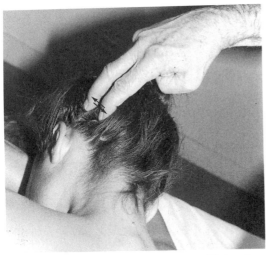

Figure 21.38.   Frictional maneuver (Maigne).

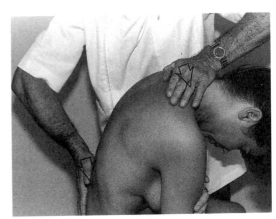

Figure 21.40.   Flexion. The examiner applies a gradual pressure at the upper thoracic spine, which causes a forward flexion of the thoracic spine.

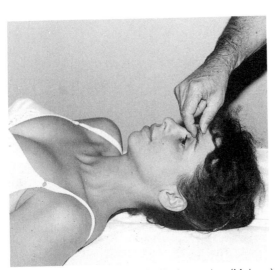

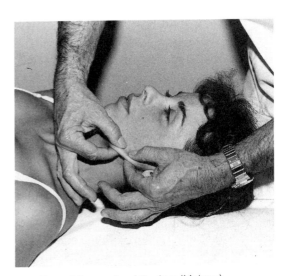

Figure 21.39.   Left, Eyebrow sign (Maigne). **Right,** Sign of the angle of the jaw (Maigne).

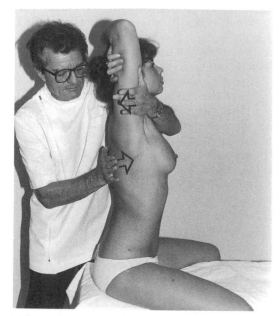

Figure 21.41. Extension. The patient sits with arms crossed over the head. With the left hand the examiner grasps the patient's arm in front and from the left. With the right hand, the examiner then places pressure on the back and applies a counterpressure with several slow movements that cause the thoracic spine to arch forward to the maximum of its extension.

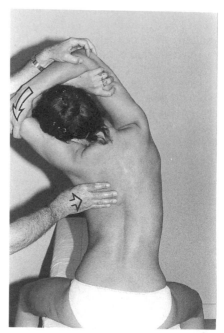

Figure 21.42. Lateroflexion. The patient sits as for the extension examination shown in Figure 21.41. The examiner, standing to the left of the patient with a hand on the patient's right elbow, pulls the patient toward him. While this is being performed, the examiner uses the right hand to put counterpressure on the lateral side below the axilla against the thorax.

pressing the spine should recognize the normal sensation of elastic resistance; this movement should not provoke any pain. The examiner should carefully note any localized stiffness or pain.

Segmental Examination

Segmental examination includes assessment for facet joint tenderness, as well as tenderness to PA pressure on the spinous process, transverse pressure against the spinous process, and pressure against the interspinous ligament.

Tenderness to PA Pressure on the Spinous Process. Pressure is applied, preferably with the thumb. This pressure should be dissociated from the superficial sensitivity of the spinous process as a result of apophysitis, frequently seen at this level. Examination for superficial tenderness due to apophysitis can be performed with gentle friction with the pad of the finger on the spinous process (Fig. 21.44). This tenderness disappears with superficial anesthesia.

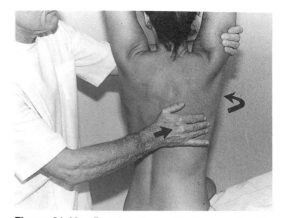

Figure 21.43. Rotation. The patient sits as for the extension examination shown in Figure 21.41. To test left rotation, the examiner takes the patient's left shoulder and pulls, bringing the back into a rotation, while the examiner's right hand assists in controlling the movement. To test right rotation, the examiner reverses the placement of the hands and the movement.

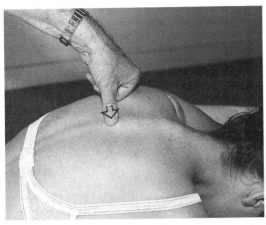

Figure 21.44.   PA pressure on the spinous process.

Transverse Pressure against the Spinous Process.   The patient should be in the prone position, face down across the table, although it is possible to examine the upper thoracic spine with the patient seated (Fig. 21.45). Pressure is applied in a slow and progressive manner to each spinous process from the left and then the right. The same precautions as for applying PA pressure to the spinous process are taken to eliminate a pain of apophysitis.

Pressure against the Interspinous Ligament.   This examination is performed with the aid of the round end of a key (Fig. 21.47).

Examination for the Presence of Facet Joint Tenderness.   The upper thoracic spine can be examined with the patient seated, back slightly

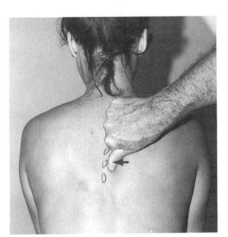
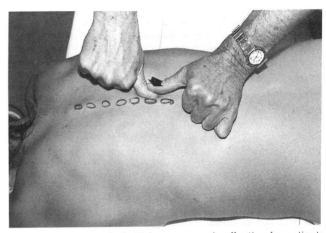

Figure 21.45.   Transverse pressure against the spinous process. **Left,** This maneuver is effective for patients who are seated for examination of the upper thoracic spine. **Right,** It can also be performed on a patient lying down, across the table, to better examine the inferior thoracic spine.

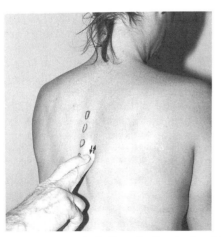
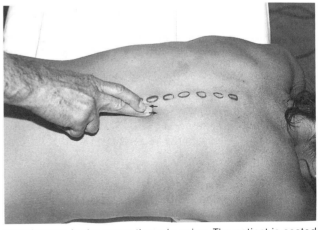

Figure 21.46.   **Left,** Examination for facet joint tenderness in the upper thoracic spine. The patient is seated. **Right,** Examination for facet joint tenderness in the inferior thoracic and midthoracic region. The patient is lying across the table.

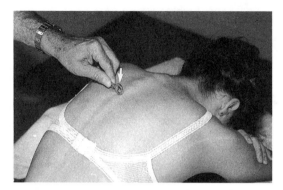

Figure 21.47.   Examination for interspinous ligament tenderness.

flexed, shoulders rounded, and elbows resting on the knees (Fig. 21.46). For examination of the middle and lower thoracic spine, however, the patient should be in the prone position, lying face down across the table.

It is better to use the pad of the finger for this examination. The middle finger is placed 1 cm lateral to the midline and slid slowly, parallel to the line of the spinous processes, stopping every centimeter to execute a to-and-fro movement vertically, in deep pressure-friction. The index finger can reinforce the middle finger by pressing on its dorsal face (Fig. 21.46).

Sources of Errors.   As we have seen in Chapter 20, some errors of interpretation are possible in the thoracic spine, particularly at the midportion.

Hypersensitivity of the Subcutaneous Tissues.   The subcutaneous tissues of the thoracic spine, particularly of the midthoracic segments, are often very sensitive to palpation (see Chapter 36, "Chronic Thoracic Pain"). Pain resulting from pressure on the spinous process or facet joints can be due to compression of skin and subcutaneous tissues that are abnormally sensitive. This hypersensitivity is detected by the pinch-roll test, which should be performed before any segmental examination at the midthoracic level (see "Sources of Error and Precautions in the Segmental Examination" in Chapter 20).

Point of Emergence of the Cutaneous Branches of the Posterior Rami.   The cutaneous branches of the posterior rami of T2, T3, and T4 become superficial very close to the midline, emerging between T5 and T8, noticeably on the line of the facet joints. The subjacent branches clearly emerge more laterally.

Thus, tenderness to longitudinal friction applied with the pulp of the finger at the level of T5, T6, and T7 does not necessarily mean that there is a particular sensitivity of the corresponding facet joints but that there is, more often at that level, tenderness over one of the points of emergence of the posterior ramus of a spinal nerve from above. This is particularly frequent at T2 (see Chapter 36, "Chronic Thoracic Pain"). The zone adjacent to the tender point corresponding to the cutaneous territory of the nerve is in that case painful to pinch-roll (Fig. 21.48).

If, on the contrary, there is truly facet joint tenderness at T5-T6 or T6-T7, the adjacent subcutaneous tissues are not tender to pinch-roll. On the other hand, three to four segments lower, the cutaneous territory corresponding to the dermatome of that nerve may be sensitive to pinch-roll (Fig. 21.48).

Detection of facet joint tenderness in the lower thoracic spine does not present the same risks. The cutaneous branches arising from the lower thoracic levels innervate the subcutaneous tissues overlying the flanks and upper buttocks; their point of emergence is clearly more lateral and cannot be compressed against a hard surface.

Examination of the Thoracic Spinal Nerves

The neurologic examination follows the same course as that of the cervical level.

Anterior Rami

Cutaneous Territory.   Anterior rami are known and unanimously accepted. The cutaneous territory of T4 corresponds to the nipple line; T6, to the xiphoid; T10, to the umbilicus; and T12, to the inguinal ligament.

The muscles are difficult to examine. The monoradicular intercostal muscles cannot be tested, and the flat muscles of the abdomen (rectus, obliquus, transversus) are pluriradicular (from T6 to T12).

The reflexes corresponding to thoracic roots are the abdominal cutaneous and abdominal muscular reflexes.

Abdominal Cutaneous Reflexes.   These reflexes are sought with a blunt point and produce a contraction of the ipsilateral abdominal muscles to the region that has been excited.

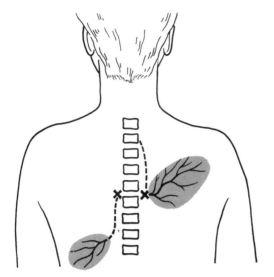

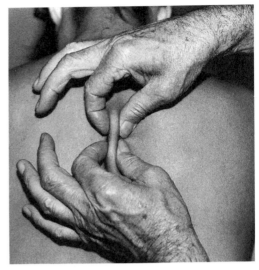

Figure 21.48. Sources of error in segmental examination of the thoracic spine. **Left,** At the midthoracic level the examiner must avoid placing pressure on painful skinfolds, thus provoking pain. The examiner should always perform the pinch-roll test before going on to the segmental examination. **Right,** Another source of error peculiar to the midthoracic region results from the superficial emergence of the cutaneous branches of the posterior primary rami of T2 and T3, perpendicular to the segment. At the T4-T5 and T6-T7 region, these branches become superficial far below those segments. In other segments the emergence

point is more lateral.

Finding a painful point or palpating the median line with the fingers can, on the right, be due to a compression of the emerging branch of the posterior primary ramus of T2 or T3 (see Chapter 36, "Chronic Thoracic Pain") or a pain on the facet joints of T4-5 or T5-6. In the first case, one will find a cellulalgic zone that corresponds to the dermatome of the branch of the posterior primary ramus. In the second case, the cellulalgic band is situated several segments below this territory and corresponds to a posterior primary ramus of T5 or T6, i.e., at the T9 or T10 level.

- Superior: excitation of the cutaneous supraumbilical region, corresponding to T6-T7
- Middle: excitation of the paraumbilical region, corresponding to T8-T9
- Inferior: excitation of the hypogastric region, corresponding to T10-T11

Abdominal Muscular Reflexes. Tapping over the symphysis pubis produces contraction of the abdominal muscles corresponding to T8-T12.

Posterior Rami

We have already pointed out the particular importance of the posterior ramus of T2, which seems to be responsible for the entire cutaneous territory of the posterior rami from C5 to T1 (Maigne). Caudally, the dermatomes course obliquely and laterally. As a general rule, T11 is above the iliac crest, while T12 is below it.

Examination for Manifestations of the Segmental Vertebral Neurotrophic Syndrome of Maigne

Cellulalgia

Superior Thoracic Spine. Cellulalgia of the supraspinous fossa corresponds to the C4 segment. The zone relating to the supraspinous fossa and the mediodorsal region corresponds to the inferior cervical segments (Maigne) and, as we have seen above (see "Posterior Branches" in Chapter 20), coincides with the very large cutaneous territory covered by the cutaneous ramus of the posterior ramus of T2 and, sometimes, of T3 (see Chapter 36, "Common Chronic Thoracic Pain"). (This large territory of T2 does not appear on the maps of dermatomes that are usually published.) Below T2, the thoracic dermatomes follow each other from top to bottom (Fig. 21.49).

Middle and Inferior Thoracic Spine. As shown in Figure 21.49, the topography of the

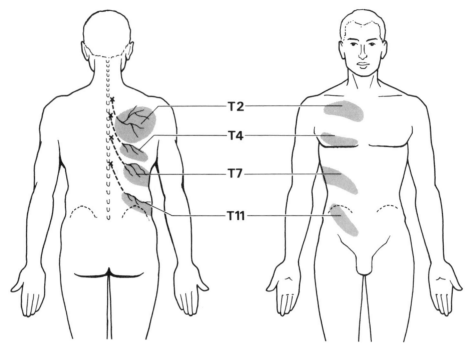

Figure 21.49. Cellulalgia of the midthoracic and subscapular regions corresponds to segmental dysfunction of the inferior cervical spine. Anatomically, the large territory is innervated by the posterior ramus of T2 and of T3 (see Chapter 36, "Chronic Thoracic Pain"). The T4 level corresponds to the territory of approximately the T8 level and, anteriorly, approximately the level of the mammary glands. The T7 level corresponds to the territory posterior to the T11-T12 level and anterior to the level of the last ribs. The T11 level corresponds to the territory just above the iliac crest and anteriorly (seen less frequently) in the lower quadrant of the abdomen.

cellulalgic zones corresponds to that of the cutaneous territory of the posterior rami for the back and of the anterior rami for the chest and abdomen. The posterior cellulalgia is practically constant in thoracic segmental dysfunction, whereas the anterior cellulalgia is less so.

Thoracolumbar Junction. For T11, T12, and L1 (Fig. 21.50), the cellulalgic zones are more or less common to the three segmental levels and correspond to the cutaneous territory innervated by their respective spinal segment:

- Posterior zone, to the upper buttocks and low back
- Anterior zone, i.e., the inferior part of the abdomen, with a small triangular zone overlying the superomedial thigh
- Lateral zone, at the level of the trochanter

According to a Chinese study done by the School of Ninghsia, very common anastomoses exist between the nearby posterior rami at the inferior dorsal and superior lumbar levels. Most of the nerves contain fibers coming from two to three vertebral segments. The anastomoses occur either between the lateral branches or between a lateral and medial branch. This would explain why the cellulalgia of the upper buttocks belongs to T12 and L1 but is sometimes identical when T11 and even T10 are affected.

Trigger Points

Trigger points are found in the paraspinal muscles but are relatively rare. When the thoracolumbar junction is involved, they can be localized to the level of the inferior part of the rectus abdominis and quadratus lumborum.

Tenoperiosteal Tenderness

Tenoperiosteal tenderness is present only when the thoracolumbar junction is affected

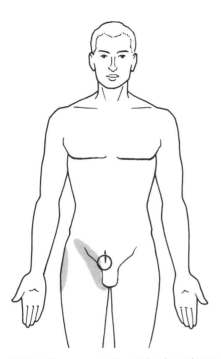

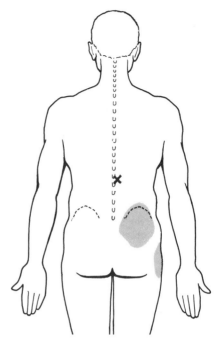

Figure 21.50. The segmental vertebral syndrome of T12 and L1 is characterized by common celluloteno-periosteomyalgic findings. *Cellulalgia:* upper buttock; anteriorly, the inferior aspect of the abdomen and superior thigh region; laterally, the trochanteric region.

Trigger points: noted less frequently and usually of minor significance; can be found in the inferior rectus abdominis region. *Periosteal sensitivity:* noted to involve the hemipubis and be homologous to the level of the insertions of the abdominal muscles.

and involves the ipsilateral hemipubis, which is often painful to palpation only, without giving the patient any pain spontaneously (Fig. 21.50) (see Chapter 60, ''Syndrome of the Thoracolumbar Junction'').

EXAMINATION OF THE LUMBAR SPINE

Examination of Mobility

Mobility is first assessed with the patient at rest. The patient stands with legs apart, in double support. The examiner looks to see if the patient's lumbar lordosis is normal, accentuated (hyperlordosis), or decreased (flat loins) or if it is replaced by a kyphosis, and if there is a scoliosis or lumbar shift and a possible unbalanced pelvis because of a leg length discrepancy.

- The degree of lumbar lordosis is generally tied to the angle of inclination of the sacral endplate with respect to the horizontal.

- Abdominal muscle weakness results in accentuation of the lumbar curvature with ante-tilting of the sacrum. It is a frequent cause of hyperlordosis and is one of the elements of the ''trophostatic syndrome of the post-menopause'' (de Sèze et al., 1961).

- In some patients, there is no accentuation of the lumbar curvature, but there is a break tied to the horizontal line of the sacrum.

- In cases of spondylolisthesis, such a break can exist, but palpation especially is used to feel the depression of the spinous process, which gives the impression of the step of a stairway. An antalgic list, often seen in cases of a disk problem, is characterized by the presence of a lumbar shift and by protective lumbar muscle guarding, causing deviation of the spine.

Active Motion Testing

Flexion.   As shown in Figure 21.51, the upright subject is asked to bend forward at the waist with the legs extended. The examiner

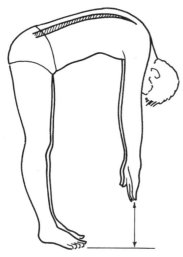

Figure 21.51.   The distance between the floor and fingers, on forward flexion, depends largely on hamstring flexibility.

should note the presence of a smooth curvature in kyphosis, of stiffness, and of a fixed incomplete reversal of the lumbar lordosis when flexion is exaggerated by a few degrees. The degree of flexion can be determined by measuring the distance between the fingertips and the ground on forward flexion, though this distance depends on several factors, especially the flexibility of the hamstrings and the mobility of the hip joints. Some subjects, even if they have a stiff spine, can touch the ground with their fingers (Figs. 20.11–20.14) if their hamstrings are sufficiently flexible, provided that their hips have enough mobility to allow this motion. Nevertheless, with all its obvious limitations, this convenient maneuver provides some very useful screening comparison from one examination to another with respect to the global flexibility and degree of pain with motion.

Schöber's test, a very good test of spinal flexibility, is described below:

- A mark is traced at the level of the spinous process of S1, and another is traced 10 cm higher (Fig. 21.52).
- At the end of flexion, the two marks should have diverged an additional 4–5 centimeters if the inferior lumbar spine has normal flexibility. In case of stiffness, these figures are lower (Fig. 21.52).

Lateroflexion.   The patient, standing with

arms at the sides, is asked to bend laterally to the right, then to the left, allowing the hand to slide along the thigh. The curvature should be smooth and symmetric. Is there a break in the lateroflexion on one side or a global stiffness? The examiner should note (*a*) the distance from the end of the fingers to the ground or the level of the inferior limb reached by the hand stretched on the bent side and (*b*) if that movement provokes a pain (Fig. 21.53). In cases of acute lumbar pain most often due to a disk lesion (acute sciatica due to a herniated disk), the patient presents with an antalgic list with marked unilateral protective paraspinal muscle guarding. This attitude is called antalgic because it tends to decrease the problem responsible for the pain by splinting the involved spinal segment and protecting against painful motion. The pseudoscoliosis thus provoked can be convex to the side of the pain; i.e., the patient can bend freely away from the pain but cannot bend on the other side. This is known as the "crossed antalgic attitude" of de Sèze. Conversely, the pseudoscoliosis can be concave to the side of the pain, and the patient can bend freely toward the painful side but not away from it. This is known as the "direct antalgic attitude" of de Sèze (see Chapter 42, "Acute Lumbar Pain").

Rotation.   The patient is seated astride the end of the table and is asked to rotate to the right and then to the left. Notice is taken of any range of motion restriction, especially when pain is produced with motion in one direction or in both.

N.B.   If the patient cannot assume the astride position, the patient can sit normally on the table, and the examiner can stabilize the patient's pelvis with both hands.

Extension.   The patient, standing or sitting, is asked to lean backward and throw out the chest. The examiner notes if that movement is possible, limited, or painful.

"Hollow Round" Maneuver.   This interesting maneuver (Fig. 21.54) tests both the lumbar mobility in flexion-extension and the muscular control of the patient who can perform, more or less easily, this simple movement. The patient, standing, partially flexed, with arms outstretched and hands placed on the edge of the table, is asked to alternately arch and hunch the back (i.e., into "kyphosis"), forming a hollow round shape. An anteroposterior stiffness can thus be observed. Many patients with lum-

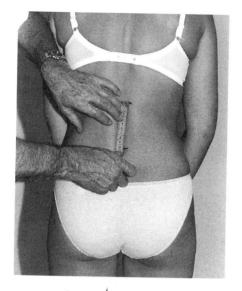

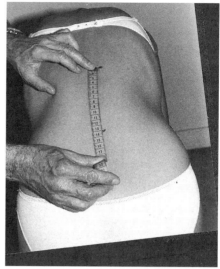

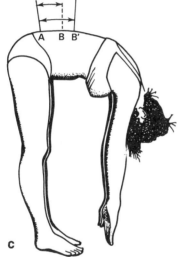

Figure 21.52. Schöber's test. **Top left,** With the patient standing, the examiner marks the S1 spine (A, **bottom left**) and then measures 10 cm above it (B, **bottom left**). **Top right,** With the patient forward flexed, if the lumbar spine has normal mobility, the spinous marks are noted to diverge, and the distance between A and B (**bottom left**) is noted to elongate by about 4–5 cm (B'). If the spine is rigid, this distance will not be modified. **Bottom left,** The results of this test seen in profile.

bar pain are unable to sustain this posture, as if this part of the body was out not under their control. Regaining conscious control of these movements and restoring the proprioceptive capability of the region can be some of the aims of physical therapy.

With the patient in this position, the examiner can also test lateroflexion of the pelvis by asking the patient to unilaterally contract the quadratus lumborum muscle. This is the "happy dog" movement of Peillon.

Passive Motion Testing

To test passive motion, the patient sits astride the end of the table or, if the hip joints do not allow the patient to assume the astride position, sits on the table, with legs dangling. The examiner moves the patient's spine to detect restricted or painful motion that may not have been apparent with active motion testing. It is not easy to test flexion in this position, but it is excellent for examination of extension, rotation, and lateroflexion.

Figures 21.55–21.57 show those maneuvers whose results can be reported on the "star diagram." As shown in these figures, the examiner first moves the patient's spine in all the ranges that are possible. Then, at the end of the movement range, the examiner performs some repetitive movements of tension to better test the flexibility and to elicit tenderness.

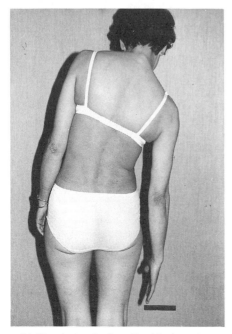

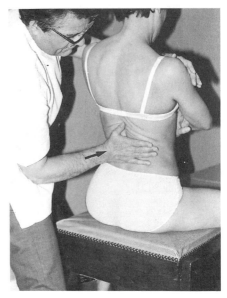

Figure 21.55.   Extension.

Figure 21.53.   Lateroflexion. On this test, the examiner can note the curve formed by the spinous processes and can visualize the presence or absence of a smooth curve. The examiner can also note the sign of Cassure and whether the movement provokes lumbar or rib pain.

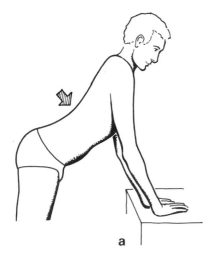

a

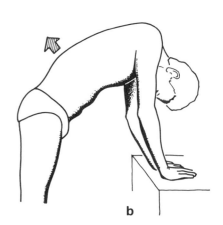

b

Figure 21.54.   The patient, standing, flexes forward slightly, placing both hands on the table. **a,** The patient is then asked to round the back. **b,** Then, the patient is asked to arch the back. Aside from any stiffness, many patients are unable to perform this maneuver. This implies a lack of control and coordination and an underlying lumbar problem.

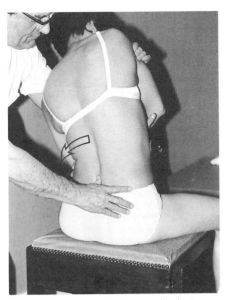

Figure 21.56.   Lateral flexion.

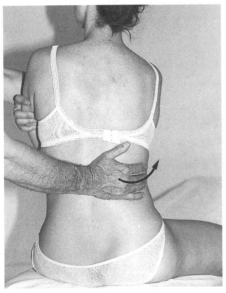

Figure 21.57.   Rotation.

Extension. The patient sits with arms crossed on the chest. The examiner's left forearm passes in front of the superior part of the thorax and grasps the patient's right shoulder (Fig. 21.55). With the right hand, the examiner applies counterpressure successively at the level of the superior, middle, and inferior lumbar regions while moving the spine in extension.

Lateroflexion. While stabilizing the patient's pelvis with one hand, as shown in Figure 21.56, the examiner uses the other hand to induce lateral inclination. To do this, the examiner grasps the front of the patient's opposite upper arm and depresses the shoulder.

Rotation. For testing left rotation as is shown, for example, in Figure 21.57, the examiner's left hand moves the patient's right arm (crossed on the chest) forward, while the examiner's right hand presses on the patient's right paraspinal region. The trunk is brought into left rotation with the examiner's left hand, while maintaining the patient in a vertical position. The right hand assists the movement by amplifying it on the zone where it receives support.

The thoracolumbar, midlumbar, and lower lumbar regions are tested this way to look for some loss of normal flexibility and for any tenderness. The maneuvers are repeated on the opposite side.

Segmental Examination

For the segmental examination, the patient lies prone, across the table, with a cushion under the abdomen, if necessary (Fig. 21.58).

Each spinal segment is examined one by one, from bottom to top or from top to bottom, from T10 to L5. The examiner should remember the causes of error in regard to the spinal process or the pinching of a painful skinfold between the thumb and spinous process.

PA Pressure on the Spinous Process. Slow, firm pressure is applied with both thumbs placed over each other (Fig. 21.59).

Transverse Pressure against the Spinous Process. This is performed with the thumb or better with both thumbs placed over each other, moving from bottom to top, then from top to bottom of the spine (Fig. 21.60).

Contralateral Pressure. This is performed as described for examination of the thoracic spine.

Longitudinal Friction overlying the Facet Joints. These articulations are deep at the lumbar level (Fig. 21.61). Nevertheless, they can be irritated by firm pressure applied with the thumbs placed over each other, with one reinforcing the other and executing small movements of deep friction. Above L2, the examiner can use (as for the thoracic spine) the

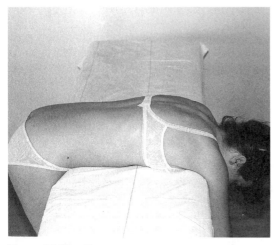

Figure 21.58. Position for lumbar and lower thoracic segmental examination (Maigne). This position is comfortable for both patient (even one with acute lumbar pain) and examiner, since it exposes the thoracolumbar region well and opens up the spinous processes. A variation of this position consists of having the patient assume a similar position at the foot of the examining table; with this position the curve of the back is less pronounced.

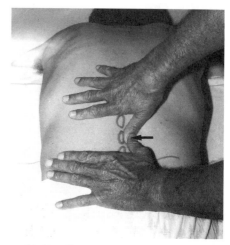

Figure 21.60. Transverse pressure against the spinous process. At this level it is good to use two thumbs superimposed.

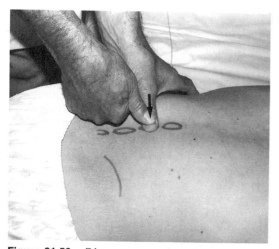

Figure 21.59. PA pressure on the spinous process.

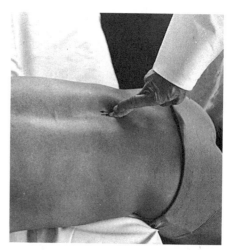

Figure 21.61. Longitudinal friction overlying the facet joint.

Examination of the Lumbar Spinal Nerves

Anterior Rami

Cutaneous Territory. There are rather pronounced differences in the cutaneous territory, depending on the authors. We do not discuss the description of Keegan and Garrett, which has been reproduced often, but discuss another one, closer to the present concept (Fig. 21.63), which takes into account our own clinical and anatomic findings.

pad of the middle finger, with the index finger pressing on its dorsal side and reinforcing it.

Pressure against the Interspinous Ligament. This is performed with the round end of a key (Fig. 21.62).

Muscular Innervation. Table 21.2 demonstrates the muscles innervated by roots T12-S2. In practice, muscular innervation can be tested as follows:

- Hip flexors (psoas iliac)—L1, L2, L3
- Knee extensors—L3, L4
- Dorsiflexors and toe extensors—L4, L5
- Tibialis anterior—L4 and, to a lesser degree, L5

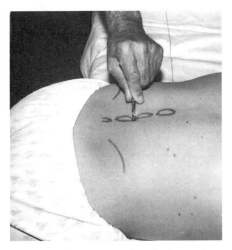

Figure 21.62. Pressure against the interspinous ligament.

- Extensor hallucis longus—L5
- Triceps surae—S1

During the examination, the patient should be standing on one foot on the tips of the toes. This maneuver can be sensitized if the examiner presses simultaneously on the shoulders of the patient to make the movement more difficult.

Reflexes. Testing of the anterior rami reflexes is performed in the following manner.

L4: PATELLAR REFLEX. Tapping the patellar tendon produces knee extension.

L5: MEDIAL HAMSTRING REFLEX. The examiner grasps the medial hamstring of the patient's flexed knee firmly with the index finger and then taps the index finger, producing adduction of the thigh and occasional, knee flexion.

S1: ACHILLES REFLEX. Tapping the Achilles tendon produces plantar flexion of the foot.

Examination for Manifestations of the Segmental Vertebral Neurotrophic Syndrome of Maigne

A segment-by-segment description provides a simpler and more logical examination for manifestations of the segmental vertebral neurotrophic syndrome of Maigne.

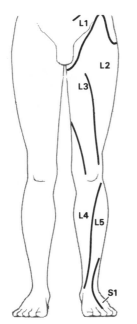
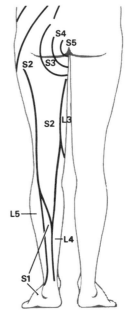

Figure 21.63. Lumbosacral dermatomes.

Table 21.2.
Muscular Innervation of T2–S2

	T12	L1	L2	L3	L4	L5	S1	S2
Quadratus lumborum	■	■	■					
Serratus posterior		□	■	□				
Iliopsoas		■	■	□	□			
Adductor longus			■	□	□			
Adductor magnus			□	■	□			
Quadriceps femoris			□	■	■			
Rectus femoris			□	■				
Tibialis anticus					■	□		
Gluteus medius					□	■	□	
Gluteus minimus						■	□	
Tensor fasciae latae						■	□	
Semitendinosus						■	□	
Semimembranosus						■	□	
Extensor digitorum longus						■	□	
Extensor hallucis longus						■	□	
Peroneus brevis and longus						■	□	
Tibialis posterior						■	■	
Popliteus					□	■	□	□
Gluteus maximus						■	■	□
Pyriformis							■	□
Biceps femoris							■	□
Gastrocnemius and soleus							■	□
Flexor digitorum longus							■	□
Flexor hallucis longus							■	□
Intrinsic muscles of the foot								■

L1.   L1 has been looked at with the thoraco-lumbar junction (T12, L1) (see "Examination of the Dorsal Spine," above) (Fig. 21.51).

L2.   For L2, the cellulalgic zone involves the anterolateral aspect of the mid and lower thigh. It corresponds to the territory of meralgia paresthetica, seen with entrapment of the lateral femoral cutaneous nerve. A small cellulalgic zone overlying the medial iliac crest can exist simultaneously.

L3 AND L4 (Fig. 21.64).   The cellulalgic zones corresponding to L3 and L4 overlap one another, but the medial aspect of the knee and the superomedial aspect of the leg belong to L4. Trigger points are located in the rectus femoris and the vastus medialis. Periosteal tenderness over the medial knee is rather frequent in disorders of L4.

L5 (Fig. 21.65).   Trigger points are located in the gluteus medius and minimus and the tensor of the fascia lata (Fig. 21.67). A tenoperiosteal pain of the greater trochanter is frequently

noted in dysfunction of the L4 and L5 segments (Fig. 21.68). In the lower limb, the manifestations exist only when there is or was an irritation of the root. For L5, this is a small cellulalgic zone of the superior anterolateral aspect of the leg, seen also in half the cases of sciatica of L5 (Fig. 21.66). Trigger points of the toe extensors and tibialis anterior are rare.

S1 (Figs. 21.69 and 21.70).   S1 trigger points involving the gluteal muscles are consistently found in all cases involving L5-S1 segmental dysfunction. Pyriformis trigger points are inconstant but can be associated with S1 segmental dysfunction. Trigger points of the biceps femoris and those of the lateral gastrocnemius and soleus are found only in cases in which L5-S1 dysfunction is associated with S1 sciatica; then, it is a constant finding (Fig. 21.72). Similarly, the cellulalgic zone of the posterior calf is not found unless there is an S1 sciatica; then, it is seen in 50% of cases (Fig. 21.71).

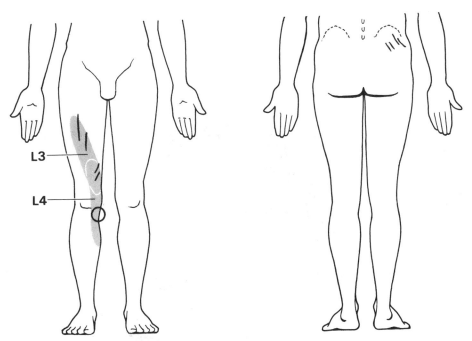

Figure 21.64.   Segmental vertebral syndrome of L3 and L4. *Cellulalgia:* seen on the anterior thigh at a higher level for L3 and at a lower level for L4. *Trigger points:* noted in the rectus femoris, vastus medialis, tensor fascia lata, and gluteus medius. *Periosteal hypersensitivity:* pes anserinus.

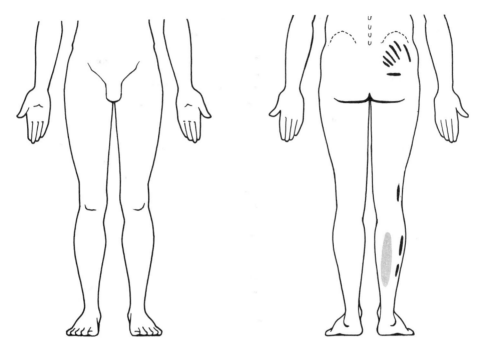

Figure 21.65.   Segmental vertebral syndrome of L5. *Cellulalgia:* anterolateral calf. *Trigger points:* the gluteus medius, gluteus minimus, tensor fascia lata, and gluteus maximus, particularly involving the upper muscle bundles throughout. *Periosteal hypersensitivity:* greater trochanter.

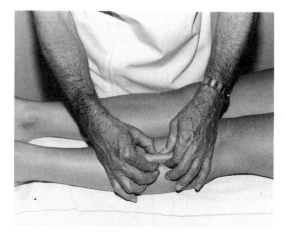

Figure 21.66.   Test for cellulalgia in the segmental vertebral syndrome of L5. This is found only in cases of sciatica or the sequelae of sciatica, involving more than 60% of cases.

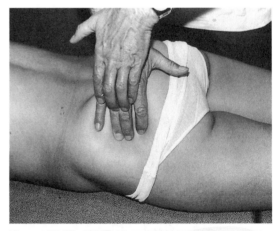

Figure 21.67.   Palpation of the trigger points of the gluteal muscles in the segmental vertebral syndrome of L5. They are always present.

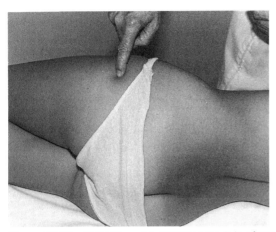

Figure 21.68.   Palpation of the trochanter. It is often painful in the segmental vertebral syndrome of L5.

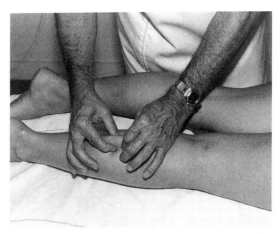

Figure 21.70.   Examination of subcutaneous tissues in the segmental vertebral syndrome of S1. As in the segmental vertebral syndrome of L5, it is generally seen in cases that simultaneously involve sciatica and is found in 60% of cases.

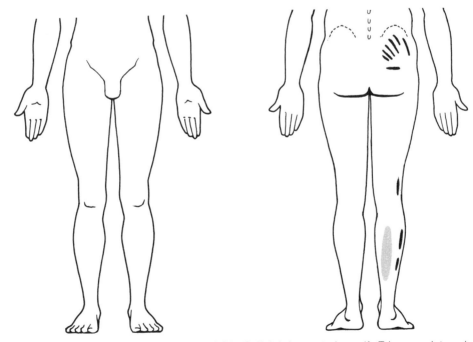

Figure 21.69.   Segmental vertebral syndrome of S1. *Cellulalgia:* posterior calf. *Trigger points:* primarily the muscles of the gluteus maximus, piriformis, gluteus minimus, and gluteus medius; also the inferior biceps femoris and the lateral soleus.

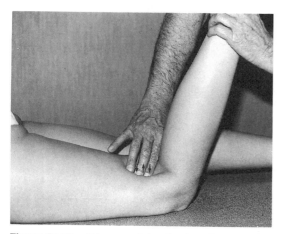

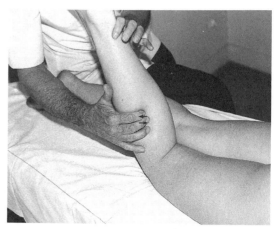

Figure 21.71. Trigger point palpation of the inferior biceps femoris. Trigger points are present in almost all cases of S1 sciatica and in cases involving sequelae of this condition. They are not found in cases of segmental distress involving L5-S1 without sciatica.

Figure 21.72. Palpation of trigger points in the gastrocnemius and soleus. The same procedure can be performed for the biceps femoris (Fig. 21.71).

TREATMENT

22

SPINAL MANIPULATION

Applied in sensibly chosen cases and well executed, spinal manipulation provides excellent treatment for numerous disorders of the spine. However, it has often acquired a bad reputation as a result of fanciful pathogenic interpretations, accidents and incidents produced in nonmedical hands, and abuses by some who wanted to use these manual techniques to treat the most varied of diseases.

Spinal manipulation has been hypothesized to be effective by acting upon "spinal subluxations," "sacroiliac subluxations," "dysfunctions of bones of the skull," "joint fixations," etc. Each maneuver was "justified" in the context of a specific paradigm by the existence of a particular lesion diagnosed empirically by means of palpation techniques whose subtlety often defied common sense. Other users of manipulative techniques limited their practice to two or three routine maneuvers that were used to treat all cases.

The use of manipulation was largely justified by some theoretical frameworks in which some perturbations of the interspinal movement, such as "hypomobility," "joint blockage," or "subluxation," were represented as interfering with the normal function of the organ, facilitating or leading to illness. These spinal perturbations known as "osteopathic lesions (or somatic dysfunction)" by osteopaths and "subluxations" by chiropractors are detected by particular techniques of palpation by the former and by radiography by the latter. For these schools, manipulation practiced according to varied modalities constitutes an essential means of restoring normal function to the spine and thus to the entire organism. This leads to the use of manual techniques, either alone (chiropractic) or in association with methods of traditional medicine (osteopathy)

to treat a diverse list of conditions. The ambition was always to treat the "entire organism." Specifically relieving a sciatica or a low back pain was not the aim; the aim was to restore some "general equilibrium."

J. B. Mennell was the first to use certain manipulative techniques, most of them borrowed from osteopathy, with the exclusive aim of treating musculoskeletal disorders. He adhered to the osteopathic concept and its diagnostic use of palpation and included an interest in blockage of the sacroiliac joints. His successor at St. Thomas Hospital of London, James Cyriax, used only a few simple manipulative techniques, which were applied routinely in some restricted indications, essentially with regard to disks.

The method proposed in this book is based on different principles, although many of the techniques used are the same. This method aims only to treat certain common pain syndromes resulting from painful mechanical dysfunctions of the spine and related to the locomotor apparatus.

These pains can be local or regional; can be cervical, thoracic, or lumbar; and occasionally are associated with neural dysfunction of radicular, sciatic, femoral, or cervicobrachial neuralgic origin. They can also be referred distally in the corresponding nerve root territory: pseudotendinous, pseudovisceral, etc., which is discussed in Chapter 18, "Segmental Vertebral Cellulotenoperiosteomyalgic Syndrome" (of Maigne).

Segmental dysfunction is sometimes due to degenerative disk disease. Most often, however, it is due to "painful minor intervertebral dysfunction" defined as a benign and painful dysfunction of the spinal segment and not as a "loss of segmental motion" appreciated by palpation. The clinical diagnosis is simple; it is based on pain elicited during the segmental examination. In this method, the choice of manipulative technique is determined by the pain provoked during the segmental examination. Manipulation is thus executed according to "the rule of no pain and of opposite movement" (Maigne).

In this system, therapeutic manipulation derives from clear clinical diagnosis and is within the capability of any physician. Its application is controlled by strict rules. Execution of the maneuvers requires long and regular training.

In France, this system of manipulations has been approved in a 1-year program of special training at the university. This program was begun in 1969 at the Faculty of Medicine of Broussais Hôtel Dieu by the author (University of Paris VI). It was the first of its kind in the world to be implemented in a traditional medical curriculum. It was followed by a program at Marseilles (taught by Professor Bardot and Dr. Guillemet) in 1976 and, in the following years, at other faculties of medicine scattered throughout France: Lyon, Renne, Toulouse, Grenoble, Strasbourg, Tours, Montpellier. Depending on the decisions made by the council of each university, this course was reserved for "physician specialists" qualified in physical medicine or rheumatology or for "physician generalists" with a year more of postgraduate study. Since its inception, the course in Paris has been widely attended by foreign physicians, often funded by scholarships from their countries.

These manipulative techniques not only are efficient therapy when they are used properly but also provide an exceptional means of studying the common pain syndromes of spinal origin. Their effectiveness provides evidence of the spinal source of numerous pain syndromes that would never have been attributed to the spine were it not for their resolution with manipulation. Performed correctly on the involved segment, they can relieve pain. When performed incorrectly or in the wrong direction, they can aggravate or produce the pain caused by these segments. In many cases, their favorable action has led us to question our fundamental understanding of common pain mechanisms. Manipulation for us has been a key—an Ariadne's thread in the analysis and the understanding of many common

pain syndromes. It has caused us to reconsider many well-established ideas.

GENERAL CONCEPTS

Basic Principles

There are three steps in manipulation:

- Position the patient and physician properly.
- Place the segment under tension.
- Perform the manipulative thrust itself.

Let us imagine a patient lying supine. The physician grasps the patient's head with two hands (Fig. 22.1). This is known as the *position set*. The physician then rotates the patient's neck toward the left as far as possible.

The rotation is increased slightly until end range is reached. This is known as *taking up the slack*.

If the physician then returns to the starting point and repeats the movement several times, it is called a series of mobilizations in left rotation. But if, after having taken up the slack, the physician suddenly applies an additional slight rotation, with a rapid, low-amplitude thrust of the right wrist, the resistance to motion yields, and the available segmental motion increases by a few more degrees. The manipulative thrust just described is accompanied by a characteristic "cracking" noise. This forced, brief, unique movement, performed only after the slack has been taken up, is characteristic of manipulation (Fig. 22.2).

The manipulative thrust should always be executed after taking up the slack as a low-amplitude movement. A large-amplitude forceful movement is violent, unmeasurable, painful, and dangerous. This movement should be perfectly controlled by the operator and, to be well executed, requires experience. The manipulation should be perfectly painless. It can be executed by a trained physician at all levels of the spine of a normal patient without being painful or uncomfortable. It should not be rough, and the operator does not have to use great force if the technique is perfect and the patient is positioned properly.

Remarks
The correct technical execution of a manipulation demands absolute attention to the three steps:

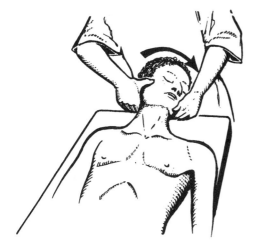

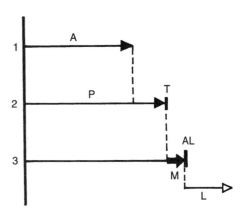

Figure 22.1. If the patient voluntarily turns his head all the way to the left, this is noted to be an active movement and is designated by line A. If the examiner turns the patient's head in rotation to the left, this is considered a passive movement and is designated by line P. At this point, the examiner and the patient have the same impression that further movement is not possible. This point is referred to as the "taking up the slack" point (T). If, after the taking up the slack phase is complete, the examiner uses a forceful brief thrust and exaggerates the movement, resistance is noted to "melt away," and a cracking sound is produced. This brief force and very limited movement, going beyond the point of tension, constitutes what is termed the manipulation or the manipulative thrust (M). If the thrust goes beyond the anatomic limit (AL), it is possible to produce a subluxation (L). By not going beyond this point, the examiner has exercised perfect control of movement.

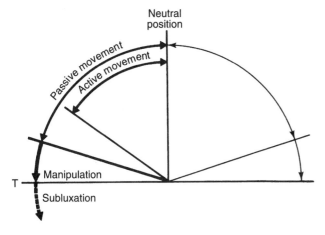

Figure 22.2. Diagram of the amplitude of movements discussed in Figure 22.1. From a neutral position, a movement can be performed in two opposite directions: rotation to the right or left, lateroflexion to the right or left, and flexion and extension. On this diagram, one can note the range of active (voluntary) movement, passive (induced) movement, and the manipulated range of movement. T marks the taking up the slack point. Beyond this normal anatomic range of motion, there is a subluxation.

1. *Correct positioning of both patient and examiner is necessary for proper execution of the maneuver. The examiner should focus completely on performing the positioning perfectly. It should be controlled from start to finish, and the examiner should always remain perfectly balanced.*
2. *The examiner should start the maneuver in the chosen direction slowly, until a resistance indicates end-range to examiner and patient. The tension is then increased slightly without coming back; thus creating a torsional pressure.*

3. *With the slack taken up and firmly maintained, the manipulative thrust is executed in the chosen direction after a brief pause (Figs. 22.3 and 22.4).*

Definitions

Manipulation

Manipulation is a very specific movement that we shall define as follows.

Manipulation is a forced passive movement that tends to bring the elements of a joint or a group of

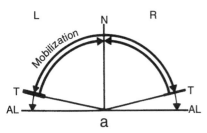

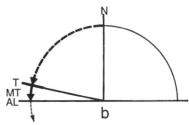

Figure 22.3.   a. Mobilization is a movement only up to the point of taking up the slack (*T*), with return to the neutral position (*N*), and is repeated many times. It can be performed in both directions (in rotation to the right (*R*) and left (*L*), in flexion and extension, and in lateroflexion to the right or left). *AL, Anatomic limit.*

b. The manipulative thrust (*MT*) is always performed in a manner that provides fine movement beyond the point of tension (*T*). The movement is brief, rapid, and not repeated. The movement must never go beyond the anatomic limit.

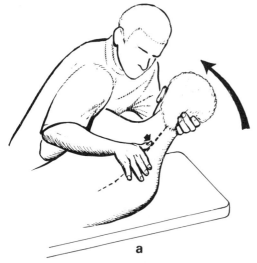

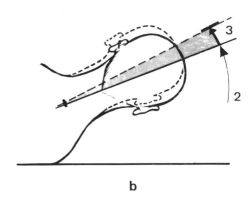

Figure 22.4.   a and **b.** Example of a cervical manipulation in left lateral flexion. The *thin arrow* (*2*) demonstrates a position that is being set in tension (*T*). The

thicker arrow (*3*) demonstrates the direction of the manipulative thrust, which is brief and limited.

joints beyond their usual physiologic range of motion. Thus, in the spine it consists of rotation, lateroflexion, flexion, or extension, isolated or combined, on the chosen spinal segment.

Thus understood, manipulation is a medical act. It is a precise movement whose coordinates are determined after a preliminary examination, and it is used for very definite indications. In the English literature, the word *manipulation* often implies the entire spectrum of manual therapy (with the possible exception of massage). Here, we distinguish manipulation as thrust techniques or "low-amplitude, high-velocity techniques" and mobilizations as articular techniques.

Mobilization

If, after having taken up the slack as described above, the examiner comes back to the starting point and repeats the same maneuver several times in a rhythmic and elastic way, we say that the examiner has executed a series of mobilizations in left rotation (Fig. 22.3). Mobilization is a passive movement, performed repetitively, which does not include any forceful or strenuous or forced movement.

"Cracking"

Cracking accompanies the manipulative thrust. It pleases the novice manipulator and satisfies the patient, who thinks (wrongly) that it is proof that "something has been put back in its place." In reality, it only means that the degree of movement has been sufficient to overcome the tonic and periarticular resistances and allow a sudden separation of the articular surfaces. This noise is proof of the manipulation, nothing else. There are cases when the manipulator should not go beyond the cracking, and there are cases when the examiner must go beyond that point. Cracking is the usual companion of the manipulation. It is not heard during supple passive mobilizations. Such cracking can be produced by the spine as well as the limbs. Even the fingers and feet can undergo cracking whenever certain mechanical conditions make the sudden separation of two articular surfaces possible.

Mechanism

In the spine, the facet joints are the source of the cracking sound, not the disk. Increasing the gap between the articular surfaces decreases the intra-articular pressure, which is already negative. In some regions, because of the degree of surface congruity and the angle of stretching, there is a thin lamina of synovial fluid between the two articular surfaces. At a certain degree of separation the phenomenon of cavitation is produced at the level of this thin layer. In a way, a void (empty bulb) is created. The gases dissolved in the synovial fluid rush in, producing the cracking noise and forming a bubble of gas (Unsworth et al.). When the joint returns to its normal position, these gases are resorbed in the synovial fluid. This takes approximately a quarter of an hour, which is why the manipulator, having produced such a cracking in a joint, should wait some time before doing it again. This *time of recharging* varies from one person to another.

Cracking does not mean that the manipulation is a success. Any "manipulation"—correct, incorrect, approximate, or useless—can produce a crack. Cracking is of interest only if the manipulation was justified and was performed on the right segment and in the right direction. Cracking is neither necessary nor sufficient and is a normal occurrence.

A good manipulator should be able to "crack" the spine of a normal person completely, vertebra by vertebra, without hurting the person at all, and this according to any of the orientations of the movement. Nevertheless, the joint that "cracks" does not have quite the same behavior as the one that does not crack, as is indicated under Mechanism of Action of Manipulation (p. 215).

DIFFERENT TYPES OF MANIPULATION

To classify, we divide the manipulative techniques into three groups: (*a*) direct, because they consist of direct pressures performed on the spine itself; (*b*) indirect, because to use them, such natural lever arms as the head, shoulders, pelvis, and legs are used to move the spine; and (*c*) semi-indirect, since during these maneuvers the examiner provides direct support to the spine.

Direct Manipulation

Direct manipulations are maneuvers executed with the heel of the hand. Generally, the pisiform is the point of pressure. The thrust employed is sudden, brief, and flat; it is applied to either the transverse or the spinous process. For example, as shown in Figure 22.5, pressure on the left transverse process of *B* will produce rotation toward the right; if, using the other hand, a counterpressure is applied simultaneously on the right transverse process of *C* as indicated in Figure 22.6, this movement will act electively on segment *BC*. The pressure given should be followed by a very quick release. These maneuvers are more difficult to execute than they may seem; the pressure is difficult to measure, and therefore, the maneuver is sometimes dangerous. In practice, however, these maneuvers offer unlimited possibilities.

Indirect Manipulation

In contrast to direct manipulation, indirect manipulations are of an infinite variety. With them, all of the spinal segments can be manipulated in all directions, always with a measurable strength; repeated and progressive mobilization can be executed, allowing excellent analysis of the segmental mobility. Indirect manipulation has an evident superiority over direct maneuvers. Briefly, the following is an

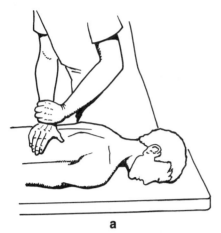

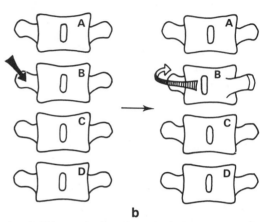

Figure 22.5.   a and **b.** Direct manipulation applied to the left transverse process of *B* with the palm of the hand. This results in a forced rotation to the right in vertebra *B*.

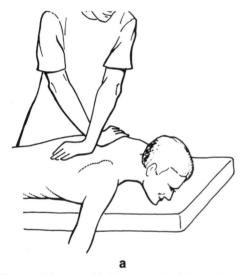

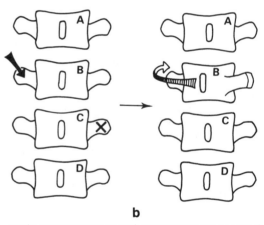

Figure 22.6.   a and **b.** Direct manipulation with counterpressure applied in the same maneuver as in Figure 22.5. In this case, however, the other hand is used to apply counterpressure to the transverse process to the right of *C* and helps to localize the movement to segment *BC*.

example of indirect manipulation that should be executed according to the three steps described above.

1. Positioning the patient: As shown in Figure 22.7, the patient has been placed in the right lateral decubitus position. The examiner stands in front of him, puts his left forearm under the patient's left axilla, and rests his right forearm on the patient's left ischium.
2. Taking up the slack: The examiner fixates the patient's left shoulder at 45° relative to the plane of the table and maintains it in this position while with his right arm, he pushes in the opposite direction on the patient's left hemipelvis, rotating the lumbar spine until there is a feeling of resistance. Manipulation is useful at this point because it is the best time to take advantage of taking up the slack to obtain a more efficacious terminal thrust.
3. Manipulative thrust: Finally, while maintaining the tension (taking up the slack), the examiner exaggerates his pressure on the

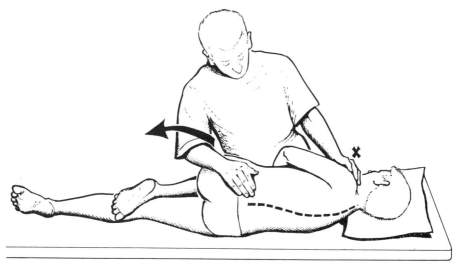

Figure 22.7.   Indirect manipulation.

ischium with a sudden and brief thrust, resulting in a manipulation.

By changing the amount of inclination of the shoulders and pelvis, by placing the lumbar spine in lordosis or kyphosis, by using other points of support, and by modifying the direction of the manipulative thrust, the examiner has within his or her grasp various maneuvers meeting the different needs of the patients to be treated.

Semi-indirect Manipulation

To obtain greater precision for some regions, semi-indirect manipulation techniques are used. In this type of maneuver, taking up the slack is always done by support at distance, but the examiner also provides direct support in the segment to be manipulated, with the hand, knee, or chest. On the spine set in tension, the manipulative thrust can be performed in two ways: either by the sudden exaggeration of the movement at a distance, with the knee or the hand applying the counterpressure to localize the manipulation—"resisting" it—or by exaggerating the local pressure that "assists" and locally accentuates the movement started by taking up the slack at a distance. Thus, we can describe manipulations that are "assisted semi-indirect" or "resisted semi-indirect."

Assisted Semi-indirect Manipulation

At the start, this type of manipulation is indirect. The examiner applies to the spinal region to be manipulated, a movement in the desired direction by an action at a distance. At the same time, with the other hand, the examiner localizes its action on the precise segment where the maneuver should act. Thus the examiner accentuates the global movement by acting in the same direction.

Consider, for example, a manipulation of the thoracic spine in which a left forced rotation of T9 on T10 is desired. The patient is sitting astride the end of the table, with his hands behind his neck (Fig. 22.8). The examiner, standing behind him, passes his left arm under the patient's left axilla and grasps the patient's right shoulder. Pulling his left hand toward the left and backward, the examiner imparts a rotatory moment to the patient's trunk while the heel of his right hand is placed over the right transverse process of T9. Taking up the slack occurs in two steps: first, by the left hand for the global movement, and then by a slow and progressive pressure of the right hand on the transverse process of T9. In practice, these two movements are simultaneous. The manipulative thrust is provided by the right hand, which increases the rotation locally by "assisting" the movement. This is why we call this technique *assisted manipulation*. In

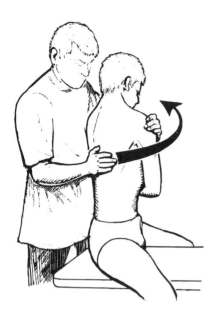

Figure 22.8. Semi-indirect assisted manipulation.

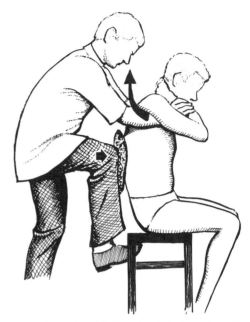

Figure 22.9. Semi-indirect resisted manipulation.

this case, it is an assisted manipulation in left rotation.

Resisted Semi-indirect Manipulation

The converse to the procedure described above, resisted semi-indirect manipulation allows the examiner to localize the action of some maneuvers to a precise point on the spine. Consider, again, manipulation of the same segment, T9-T10. To impart a manipulation that produces maximal segmental flexion, we employ the technique of manipulation that makes use of the examiner's knee, described below and illustrated in Figure 22.9.

The patient is seated on a stool, with hands crossed behind the neck. The examiner passes his forearms under the patient's axilla and grasps the patient's wrists. By the position in which the patient's body is placed and the actions of the examiner's forearms, the patient's spine is brought to a position of global flexion; i.e., the disks are "gapping" backward. To localize the maneuver, the examiner performs it in such a way that the global curvature imposed to the spine has its apex at T9-T10 and then applies counterpressure with the right knee against the spine, protected by a small pad or towel over the spinous process of T10. Taking up the slack is performed by raising the patient's axillae. Then, while firmly maintain-

ing counterpressure with the knee, the examiner delivers the thrust vertically and slightly toward himself, which produces a manipulation with the usual cracking.

Let us now analyze what happened. Figure 22.10 shows the vertebrae in maximal flexion, and the *arrow* at G is the point of counterpressure of the knee at T10. Suddenly, flexion is exaggerated, while at the same time the physician pulls the patient's whole spine toward himself; the point of counterpressure provided by the knee prevents vertebra A from following the movement. When raising the axillae, the physician brings the spine into flexion, and the maximum force of distraction is imparted to the joint between A and B. When the physician suddenly exaggerates the raising of the shoulders and brings them slightly toward himself, he has exerted a force F opposing force G of the motionless knee maintaining the spinous process, pressing on it to the front and bottom. So the knee is a fixed point of resistance toward the imposed global movement, and this is thus a "resisted" maneuver. Thus, to obtain forced flexion of a spinal segment, the examiner needs to support the spinous process of the inferior vertebra of the segment while maintaining the supra-adjacent region in forced flexion. Conversely, to produce exten-

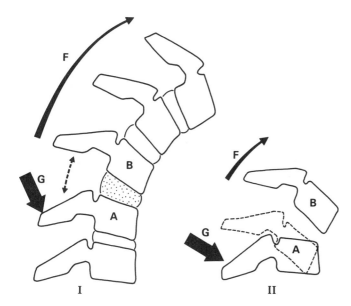

Figure 22.10.   See the text.

sion on this same segment, the region is brought into extension, then counterpressure is applied to the spinous process of T9 (superior vertebra of the concerned segment). This is considered an assisted semi-direct manipulation, since the local support increases simply the imposed global movement.

Figure 22.11 demonstrates a resisted semi-indirect maneuver used currently for later-oflexion on the inferior cervical spine or on the cervicothoracic junction. The patient is lying on his right side. With one hand (here the left one) the physician holds the patient's head and pulls the neck into left lateroflexion while applying counterpressure with the pad of his thumb to the left side of the C7 process to apply the essential manipulative impact to the supra-adjacent segment C6-C7 (Fig. 22.11).

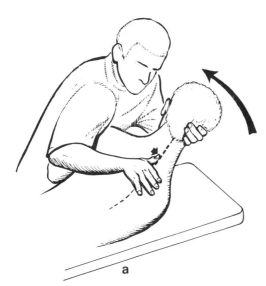

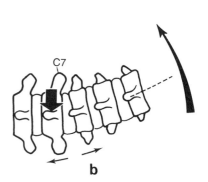

Figure 22.11.   **a** and **b.** Semi-indirect resisted manipulation in lateral flexion. Here the counterpressure is applied with the thumb to the left spinous process (here C7) that is subjacent to the segment being manipulated (C6-C7).

LOCALIZATION OF THE MANIPULATION

The semi-indirect assisted or resisted manipulation allows precise localization of the manipulation on a given segment of the spine. This localization is also a function of the technique used. Because of its particular characteristics, such maneuvers exert their effects primarily on a particular spinal region.

If the case allows, the examiner can also use the particularities of spinal physiology. For example, if a rotation of the trunk to the right or left is applied to a seated subject with the thorax in neutral position, the pivot point of the rotation is at T10-T11. But if the trunk is flexed prior to imparting rotation, the pivot point ascends a few levels. Conversely, if the trunk is extended prior to rotation, the pivot point rests at a lower point in the spinal column. If a thoracic manipulation is indicated in rotation, the precision of its localization is facilitated by the use of this particularity.

Another characteristic feature of spinal mechanics can also be used. In the thoracic and cervical spine, lateroflexion and rotation are coupled movements. If a rotational manipulation is desired at a given segment, in a given direction, the spinal region is placed into ipsilateral lateroflexion first, so that the segment to be manipulated is situated at the apex of the lateral curvature so formed. If a right rotation is desired, a right lateroflexion is performed first. If a left rotation is desired, a left lateroflexion is performed first.

This particularity can be illustrated by a metallic tape measure. Imagine a segment of that tape measure. It is maintained vertically by the examiner holding each end between the thumb and index finger of each hand. If it is then rotated, this rotation is distributed along the entire height of the tape, with maximal rotation at the midpoint. But if it is side bent slightly while maintaining the rotation, the examiner can, at will, modify these two coordinates and vary the position of the pivot point of the curvature, from top to bottom in a very precise manner. This position is the point of least resistance. A slight degree of lateroflexion results in a high pivot point, while a greater degree results in a lower pivot point. The more

marked the lateroflexion, the lower the rotation (Fig. 22.12).

When possible, it is convenient to take advantage of these particularities, although this cannot always be done. The examiner can, for example, be led to perform a maneuver combining lateroflexion and rotation of opposite direction on the same segment, thoracic or cervical, or to perform a midthoracic manipulation (T7-T8) in rotation and in extension.

Remarks

The exact correlation of the manipulative movement and its therapeutic aim with a purely physiologic movement is not possible. When there is a meniscal blockage in a knee, for example, the maneuver necessary for a possible unblocking of the affected knee cannot be chosen on the basis of the normal physiology of the knee. The necessary movement has to be based on the results of the clinical examination of the affected knee. It is the same at the spinal level and in the system that we propose. In all cases, the rule of "no pain and of the opposite movement" described below should be the guide.

INDICATIONS FOR MANIPULATION

It is absolutely necessary to be able to identify the indications for manipulation. Here, we propose a classification of manipulation according to the movement as characterized by an observer.

Usually, the manipulative techniques are described according to the "lesions" that they are supposed to correct on a given vertebra. For example, the manipulation for "a right L5

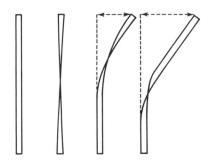

Figure 22.12.   Tape measure (see text).

posterior'' means that the fifth lumbar vertebra is rotated to the right relative to the sacrum; ''subluxed'' or ''fixated'' in this malposition for some instances or having lost its freedom of movement in left rotation for others. The maneuver will have as its aim ''restoring'' the vertebra to its proper alignment in some cases or ''restoring'' the movement that has been judged as limited in others.

Such nomenclature is, of course, extremely convenient. It explains the corrective movement and visualizes it. Everything is included in these few words, ''right L5 posterior'': the diagnosis and the direction of the maneuver to be used. Two examiners can thus communicate easily. What remains to be known is the validity of diagnoses that are based on the palpation and the reality of such ''subluxations'' or ''hypomobilities.'' To describe a maneuver intended to correct a ''left atlas posterior'' or a ''right sacrum anterior'' means that one is able to assert that the atlas has lost partial or total possibility of right rotation (it is fixated in left rotation) or that the right sacroiliac joint is blocked ''in position of nutation.''

Even if this was true, it would remain to be proven that a loss in mobility in right rotation is treated by forcing the right rotation or that a loss of extension is treated by forcing the extension. Is a blocking of the knee, whose extension is limited by a meniscal lesion, treated by a sudden extension? Or if posterior disk blocking produces an acute low back pain and extension of the concerned segment is made impossible (bringing together the spinous processes), is it logical to play ''nutcrackers'' in forcing this extension? We shall come back to this essential point. But for now, let us stress that if we describe the maneuvers as they are seen from the outside, it is because we should not judge too early what a manipulation can correct. Presently, it is the only way to proceed objectively, even if it is schematic, and it is the one we have always used (Maigne, 1959).

Manipulation is a global gesture that can be broken down in all cases to its elementary components with respect to the three cardinal planes; i.e., any manipulative movement can be defined perfectly by its coordinates, as long as the examiner takes into consideration that an element of segmental traction is practically always involved. Consequently, it can now be concluded that there is a very great variety of possible maneuvers.

Components of the Manipulative Movement

The degrees of freedom available for spinal segmental motion are flexion, extension, lateroflexion (both to the right and left), and right and left rotation. Manipulation can, therefore, be performed in all these orientations, isolated or combined (Figs. 22.13–22.16).

During extension, the posterior edges of the vertebral endplates converge, the nucleus pulposus migrates anteriorly slightly, the anterior edges of the spinal endplate diverge, and the facet joints converge.

With flexion the opposite occurs; i.e., the anterior edges of the vertebral endplates converge, the posterior edges diverge, the nucleus migrates posteriorly, and the facet joints diverge.

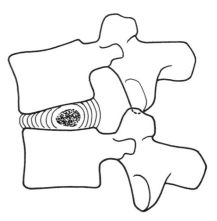

Figure 22.13.   Flexion.

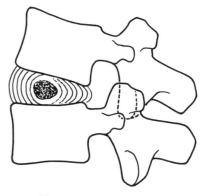

Figure 22.14.   Extension.

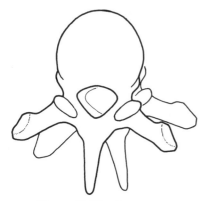

Figure 22.15. Rotation.

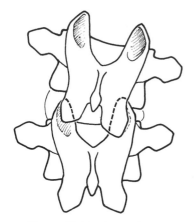

Figure 22.16. Lateroflexion.

In right lateroflexion, the vertebral end-plates and facets converge on the right side and diverge on the left.

In right rotation, the right transverse process of the concerned vertebra tends to move backward in relation to the subjacent vertebra.

By convention, spinal segmental motion is always described with respect to the subjacent segment. Imagine a male patient standing, with pelvis fixed. He rotates the trunk toward the right; i.e., his right shoulder becomes posterior in relation to the plane of the pelvis. It is a thoracolumbar rotation toward the right. Now consider the same person in the same position but this time with his shoulders fixed while his pelvis turns. His pelvis rotates to the left, and the left hip becomes posterior while the right hip becomes anterior. This is also considered a thoracolumbar rotation toward the right, because the rotation of the trunk is judged in relation to the pelvis (subjacent segment) consid-

ered as fixed. This is true even if it is the rotation of a one spinal segment only or if it is a flexion, extension, or lateroflexion movement. Thus, its relation to the subjacent segment considered fixed is the defining element.

Description of the Manipulation

To accurately and precisely describe a given manipulation so that it can be rapidly and easily conveyed to others, exactly reproduced, or recorded in the chart, the examiner should do the following.

- Designate the segmental level at which the manipulation is performed.
- Specify the exact direction given to the maneuver.
- Indicate the technique used.

Level at Which the Manipulation Is Performed

Most often, this level is the precise level (C5-C6, T3-T4, L5-S1) where a segmental dysfunction (painful minor intervertebral dysfunction (PMID)) has been discovered. In other cases, we cannot be as selective, and then the maneuver must be designated as a cervical (C), cervicothoracic (CT), thoracic(T), thoracolumbar (TL), or lumbar (L) manipulation on the superior (s), middle (m), or inferior (I) part of the region that has been considered; e.g., superior cervical spine (Sc); midthoracic spine (Mt); inferior lumbar spine (Il).

Direction Given to the Maneuver

The manipulation should be perfectly defined in the three planes: frontal, sagittal, and horizontal. Any movement, passive or active, of the spine is a combination of the elementary movements: flexion or extension, right or left rotation, and lateroflexion, right or left. It can be written as follows.

- Flexion (forward flexion): F
- Extension (backward flexion): E
- Right rotation: RR
- Left rotation: LR
- Right lateroflexion: RLF
- Left lateroflexion: LLF

Direction of the Manipulative Thrust. When an examiner writes "manipulation in right rotation," the direction of the thrust is clear. When an examiner writes "manipulation in right rotation, right lateroflexion, extension," the position of the segment during the manipulation is defined very well, but the direction of the manipulative thrust is not precisely described. The latter can be performed sometimes in a direction resulting from the three orientations, although generally it favors one of them.

In this example, however, there are three possibilities: from that position the thrust can be made either in extension, in right lateroflexion, or in right rotation. Daily practice demonstrates that the therapeutic effectiveness of each of these maneuvers is different. Note that rotation and lateroflexion are, as already seen, similar movements combined at the cervical and thoracic levels; this is true in some physiologic conditions for a normal segment. It is probably not the same in the case of the imposed, forced movement that the manipulation induces on a segment that is no longer functional.

Furthermore, these different maneuvers are going to have a powerful stretching action on different muscles, depending on the direction of the thrust. This point is essential in understanding the action of the manipulation. Nevertheless, it is convenient to limit ourselves here to mechanical notions only.

To define a manipulation and give it its identity, the examiner should describe exactly the direction of the terminal thrust. For example, in the case of a manipulation in right rotation (RR) performed on a spinal segment positioned in right lateroflexion (RLF) and in extension (E), the movement can be written down by underlining the direction of the thrust: RR + RLF + E.

Technique Used. As for the technique used, one can create a personal terminology. In the Appendices, we give a few names to some techniques: "chin free," "epigastric,"

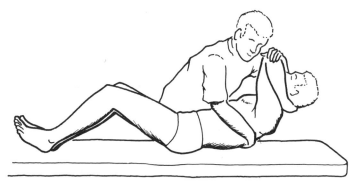

Figure 22.17. Dorsal decubitus (DD) or supine position.

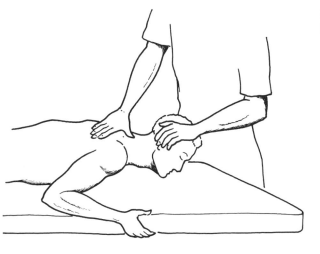

Figure 22.18. Ventral decubitus (VD) or prone position.

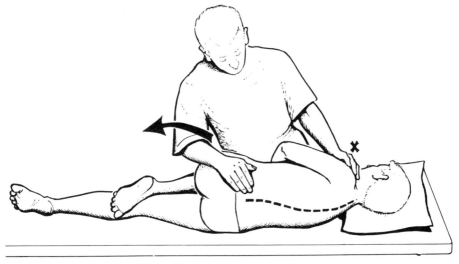

Figure 22.19. Lateral decubitus (LD) position.

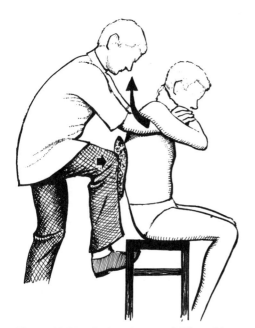

Figure 22.20. Patient in seated (S) position.

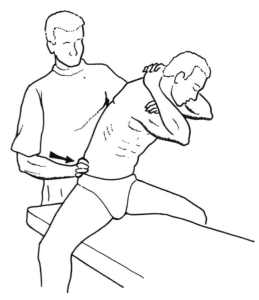

Figure 22.21. Patient sitting astride (SA) the table.

"single knee," or "dual knee" techniques, etc. A technique can also be identified by describing exactly the position of the patient during the manipulation.

• *Recumbent*
—On the back or in supine (S) position (Fig. 22.17)

—On the abdomen, or in prone (P) position (Fig. 22.18)
—On the side or in lateral decubitus (LD) position (Fig. 22.19)

• *Sitting*
—Normally, with both legs hanging over one side of the table (S) (Fig. 22.20)

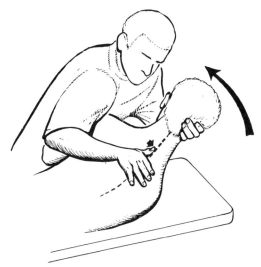

Figure 22.22. Patient in right lateral decubitus position (RLD).

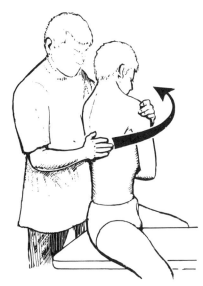

Figure 22.24. Patient seated astride (SA) the table.

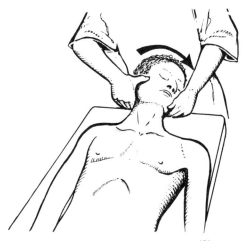

Figure 22.23. Patient in supine (S).

—Seated astride the table (SA) (Fig. 22.21)
• *Standing* (S)

Examples

Manipulation of the Lower Cervical Spine (C6-C7). The patient is lying on his right side (RLD) (Fig. 22.22), and the manipulation is performed on C6-C7 in left lateroflexion (LLF); the examiner would write down: C6-C7 (RLD) (LLF).

Manipulation of the Superior Cervical Spine (C2-C3). The patient is lying supine (S); the segment is in neutral extension and flexion and is brought in left rotation (Fig. 22.23); the examiner would write down: C2-C3 (S) (LR).

Manipulation on T12-L1 in Left Rotation. The patient is sitting astride (SA) the table (Fig. 22.24); the examiner would write down: T12-L1 (SA) LR.

Low Lumbar Manipulation on L4-L5. The patient is lying on his right side (RLD) (Fig. 22.25); the segment is in left rotation (LR), and the spine is positioned in flexion; the examiner would write down: L4-L5 (RLD) F + LR. (LR is underlined here because it is the direction of the terminal thrust.)

RULE OF NO PAIN AND OPPOSITE MOVEMENT (MAIGNE)

For any case necessitating a manipulative treatment, there are useful maneuvers, harmful and dangerous maneuvers, and indifferent maneuvers, i.e., maneuvers that are neither helpful nor harmful. The examiner should find the former and avoid the latter, determining the direction of the maneuver that gives the best results. This direction does not depend on the side where the patient feels the pain. If we look at several cases of common right sciatica, we notice that a maneuver where the left rotation is dominant relieves the condition in some cases, while the same maneuver is difficult and

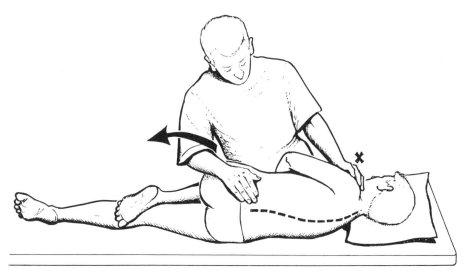

Figure 22.25. Patient in right lateral decubitus position (RLD).

aggravating in other cases, which, conversely, can be relieved by a maneuver in right rotation.

This basic problem in manipulation has been considered by very diverse authors and schools. Some ignore it deliberately, and from the moment that a manipulative treatment is decided according to their criteria, they apply the same global, stereotyped, and symmetric maneuvers, almost ritually, to all patients, which reduces notably the possibilities and indications. Such is the case with J. Cyriax, who insists especially on the associated use of traction.

Others think, with some small differences, that manipulation corrects "malpositioned joint blockage" or "loss of segmental joint play." So they use palpation or sometimes radiographic means to diagnose this "malposition" or "hypomobility." Thus they justify their manipulation and determine the adequate maneuver or maneuvers (they are often numerous) to use.

According to Mennell, restoration of "joint play" is essential. With some notable exceptions, this is the doctrine of the American school of osteopathy, as well as the doctrine of the German and Czech schools of manual medicine. For these schools, the aim of manipulation is to restore the mobility of a vertebra supposed to have lost its play of normal movement. This loss of play is appreciated by palpation of segmental motion: degree of separation and orientation of the spinous processes in flexion-extension, positions of the transverse processes in rotation, etc.

Thus, in these schools it is assumed that if such a vertebra has a normal play in extension (its spinous process comes close to the subjacent one) but has a decreased play in flexion (its spinous process does not separate well from the subjacent one), then the manipulative movement that can be applied will tend to force that vertebra in flexion. Similarly, if it is assumed that such a vertebra turns well toward the left but not well toward the right, a maneuver forcing a rotation to the right should be performed.

The system of application of manipulation that we propose is different. It is not based on the notion of spinal mobility, in which hypomobility becomes an indication for manipulation and hypermobility is treated as a contraindication for manipulation. Rather, it is based on the notion that one can locate the responsible segment by finding in which segment pain can be produced by passive movement.

It is not the loss of segmental join play that seems to us to be the fundamental element, insofar as it can be appreciated by palpation. What seems characteristic to us is the segmental pain; i.e., when a spinal segment is responsible for a local or referred pain (be it a PMID or a disk problem), it is painful when it is directly solicited by forced maneuvers that exaggerate its movement in certain directions, while it is painless in the opposite direction.

The painless directions are precisely the ones that we chose for the manipulation.

Indeed, experience has shown us that the direction of the useful manipulation is always the one opposite to the one producing the pain or the symptoms of the patient, provided that this direction is also free and painless. Note that we mean here the pain produced by the movement that has been applied passively on the concerned segment, not the pain produced by an active movement performed by the patient. Generally, there is a concordance between the two, but not always. The manipulation performed in this nontender direction we call the "rule of no pain and opposite movement" (Maigne).

The rule of no pain and opposite movement consists of forcing the passive, free, and painless movement (no pain) rather than the passive and painful movement (opposite movement). For clarity, let us take the example of a patient presenting with a cervical pain resulting from a forced movement. The C5-C6 level is painful. Taking up the slack in right rotation is free, while taking up the slack in left rotation is painful and blocked. Thus, by imparting right rotation to the involved segment, left rotation can be freed and the pain of the patient can be eliminated.

In practice, things are a little more complicated, since each spinal segment can be moved in six directions: flexion, extension, right lateroflexion, left lateroflexion, right rotation, and left rotation. The necessary maneuver can be a triplanar thrust, combining all of the available pain-free and unblocked motions; or a series of unidirectional maneuvers can be performed according to each of the free directions. Thus, it is on a pragmatic basis, constantly tested by experience, that we have proposed this rule of application of manipulation (1959). But it also has a physiologic justification. Forcing at the end of its course, with a brief and sharp thrust, the free passive movement, in the direction opposed to the one producing the pain, produces an inhibitory reflex. This reflex eliminates or diminishes the mechanisms perpetuating the painful segmental spinal dysfunction and its radicular consequences (cellulalgia, trigger points).

This rule of no pain and opposite movement implies the necessity of describing exactly the techniques and their direction that are adapted to each case. This means that we have to proscribe the standard techniques and the routine of manipulating systematically to the right and then to the left. It is fortunate that the lack of precision of most of the standard techniques, which decreases their efficiency, also decreases their possible harmfulness.

Practical Application of the Rule of No Pain and Opposite Movement

The result of the clinical examination is reported on a schema in the form of a six-branched star (Fig. 22.26), showing the directions of the spinal movement. The coordinates of the necessary manipulative movement appear clearly; the schema shown in Figure 22.26b demonstrates a case in which the passive examination has disclosed that right rotation, right lateroflexion, and extension are painful, while left rotation, left lateroflexion, and flexion are free and painless. The necessary manipulation in this case (if the clinical context favors this type of treatment) will thus be maneuvers that utilize these free directions rather than the painful or blocked directions and that are either unidirectional or combined.

It is not the side of the patient's pain complaint that determines the direction of the manipulation, but the direction of the pain produced by the passive movement. In Figure 22.27, two examples of right sciatica are presented. The clinical context and the previous examination seemed to indicate that these patients would be good subjects for the use of manipulation. In both, the sciatica was located on the right side; one presented with an antalgic scoliosis convex on the right side, while the other presented with an antalgic scoliosis concave on the right side. Results of passive lumbar movements on the patients in sitting position until the segments were set in tension showed that the free and painful movements were different in these cases; they were completely opposite. The manipulative movements required by the rule of no pain and opposite movement were also opposite. The star diagrams (Fig. 22.27) reveal this difference clearly.

As shown in Figure 22.27, the following maneuvers were performed: for patient *A* sitting astride the table, lateroflexion performed in left rotation (plus left lateroflexion plus flex-

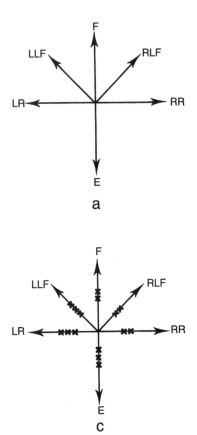

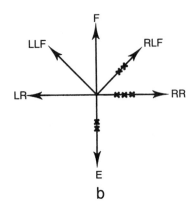

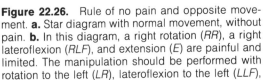

Figure 22.26. Rule of no pain and opposite movement. **a.** Star diagram with normal movement, without pain. **b.** In this diagram, a right rotation (*RR*), a right lateroflexion (*RLF*), and extension (*E*) are painful and limited. The manipulation should be performed with rotation to the left (*LR*), lateroflexion to the left (*LLF*), and flexion (*F*), utilizing maneuvers that combine these diverse orientations. **c.** Movement in all directions is painful. The rule of no pain and opposite movement cannot be applied; thus this represents a contraindication to manipulation.

ion); for patient *B* sitting astride the table, lateroflexion performed in right rotation (plus right lateroflexion plus extension); for patient *A* lying on his right side, left lateroflexion plus left rotation; for patient *B* lying on his left side, right lateroflexion plus right rotation; for patient *A* lying on his right side, a combined maneuver of left rotation plus flexion; and for patient *B* lying on his left side, a combined maneuver of right rotation plus extension.

Technical Contraindications to Manipulation

If all directions are painful, all branches of the star diagram are crossed out and no manipulation is possible (Fig. 22.26*c*). This is common in infectious, inflammatory, or tumoral lesions, etc., it can also happen in common mechanical disorders.

In this case, the nature of the disorder would normally lead to a manipulative treatment, but because of the rule of no pain and opposite movement, manipulative treatment is not possible. We say that it is a "technical contraindication" to manipulation.

In practice, the manipulative treatment will have a good chance of success when at least three degrees of freedom are available. If there are only one or two free directions, repetitive mobilization can be applied in these directions, and its effect can be estimated before manipulation is performed.

Particular Cases

Application of the rule of no pain and opposite movement is evident and simple when the examination demonstrates clearly painful and clearly free passive movements. It can, how-

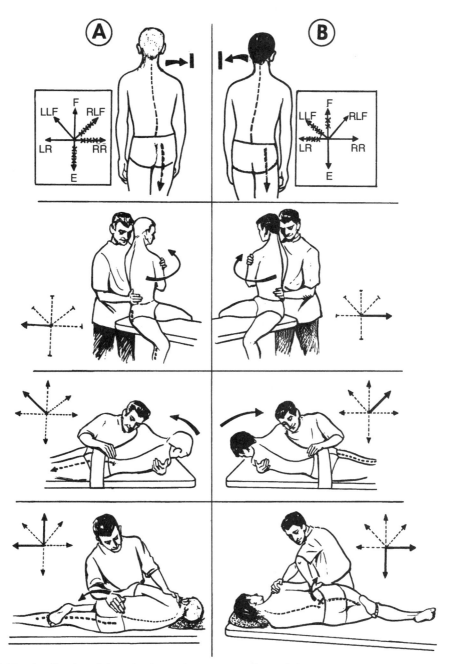

Figure 22.27.   Application of the rule of no pain and opposite movement in two cases of right sciatica. **A.** Patient with right sciatica for whom rotation to the right (*RR*), lateroflexion to the right (*RLF*), and extension (*E*) are painful movements. **B.** Patient with right sciatica for whom rotation to the left (*LF*), lateroflexion to the left (*LLF*), and flexion (*F*) are blocked and painful movements. As a result, therapeutic maneuvers are performed in the opposite direction in these two cases. The examiner will perform three maneuvers on each patient: first, rotation to the left for **A** and rotation to the right for **B;** then, lateroflexion to the left and rotation to the left for **A** and lateroflexion to the right and rotation to the right for **B;** followed by flexion and rotation to the left for **A** and extension and rotation to the right for **B.**

ever, be a little less evident and simple when these movements are less clear. For example, a PMID can exist in a segment that was painful on segmental examination, while the active and passive movements that were imposed on the region were painless in all directions. These findings are not rare. The examiner then has to face several possibilities.

- The findings of the segmental examination clearly show that the rule can be applied. If pressure on spinous process C in Figure 22.28 is painful from right to left and pressure in the opposite direction (left to right) is painless, manipulation can be performed in the painless direction, i.e., in left rotation. Remember that pressure on the spinous process from right to left produces right rotation, while pressure on the spinous process from left to right produces left rotation. If lateral pressure is painful in both directions, a rotational manipulation should not be performed.
- Occasionally, one can repeatedly mobilize the segment to end range in each direction. Performed in unfavorable directions, however, they produce a disagreeable feeling for the patient and accentuate the facet joint tenderness to palpation and the local paraspinal protective muscle guarding. Performed in pain-free directions, they decrease the facet joint tenderness and other signs.

This way of proceeding is especially useful at the cervical level where facet joint palpation is easy and where there is often some PMID responsible for chronic problems (e.g., headache) without the existence of any limitation or pain produced by the movement.

Rule of No Pain and Opposite Movement in Direct Manipulation

With direct manipulation, pressure is applied directly to the concerned vertebra. Thus the segmental examination determines the direction of the maneuver to be performed. In Figure 22.29, for example, the spinal segment BC presents a PMID. The pressure toward the left on process B is painful (Fig. 22.29a). While maintaining that pressure on B, a counterpressure in the opposite direction is performed simultaneously on the process of C, exaggerating the produced pain (Fig. 22.29c). The converse maneuver, pressure toward the right on B and toward the left on C, is painless. The manipulation chosen consists of exaggerating this last movement, which can be performed by pressure on the right transverse process of

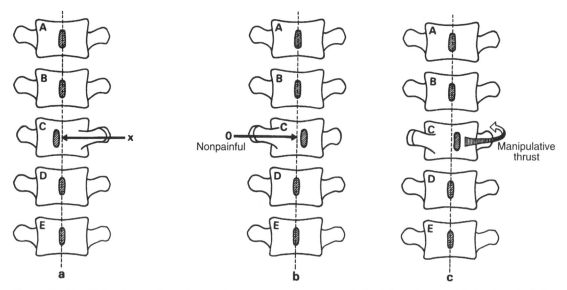

Figure 22.28. Rule of no pain and opposite movement with lateral pressure on the spinous process. **a.** Movement from right to left produces a painful right rotation of the vertebra (X, pain). **b.** The opposite movement (left rotation) is nonpainful. **c.** Manipulation is performed with a forced rotation to the left, which is free and nontender.

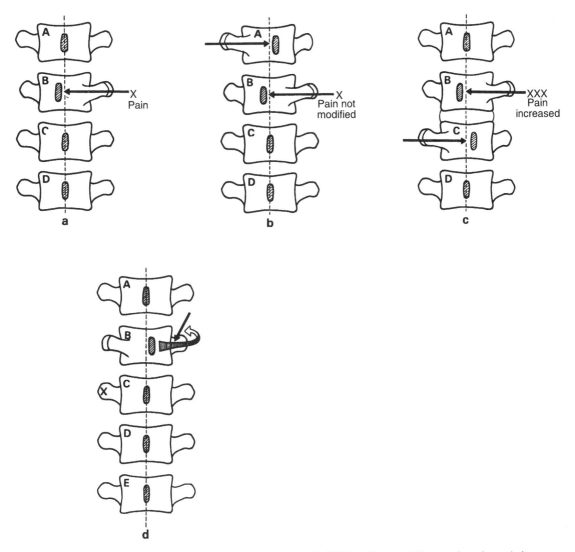

Figure 22.29. Rule of no pain and opposite movement with lateral and opposed movements. **a.** Lateral pressure from right to left on segment *B* produces pain. One would like to know if the cause of this pain is due to segments *AB* or segments *BC*. **b.** While maintaining pressure on *B* from right to left, one may simultaneously execute a counterpressure in the opposite direction on segment *A*. This does not increase the pain already produced. **c.** In contrast, the same maneuver executed on segment *C* notably increases the pain (*XXX*), which could be produced purely by pressure on segment *B* alone. Thus we are able to demonstrate that segments *BC* are the cause of the pain. **d.** As a consequence, the manipulative maneuver, directed and applied according to the rule of no pain or of the opposite movement, will consist of a movement opposite in direction to that noted in **c.** A counterpressure (*X*) is applied to the left transverse process of *C*, while pressure is applied to the right transverse process of *B*.

B and counterpressure on the left transverse process of *C* (Fig. 22.29*d*).

Remarks

When manipulation is painful but, nevertheless, produces relief, most often it is because one of the secondary coordinates has not been well chosen, while the principal coordinate was correct. This could also be due to joint or periarticular irritation or even due to an awkward or poorly performed maneuver. When spinal motion is limited by simple stiffness without the presence of a precise PMID and when the limited movements are not painful during the phase of taking up the slack, it is possible to act according to the limited direc-

tions with progressive mobilizations and to continue these up to the manipulation if the latter is easy to do.

In conclusion, we can say that the rule of no pain and opposite movement (*a*) provides a set of indications or contraindications for the manipulative treatment, (*b*) determines the maneuver to be executed, and (*c*) sets conditions for the execution of a maneuver. This rule is a valuable guide from which the examiner should not depart, but it is not sufficient to guarantee good manipulative treatment. The indication should be clearly established, and the technique should be perfectly applied, well measured, and well centered on the responsible segment.

PROTOCOL OF A MANIPULATIVE SESSION

Manipulation is a treatment just like any other treatment. It may be evident, but we should evaluate it as we would any other proposed treatment. Its correct use depends first on a proper diagnosis. The disorder should be mechanical, although not all mechanical disorders respond to manipulation. There are also many contraindications to manipulation: the patient's general state of health, state of the spine, vascular state, etc. In addition, manipulation should be technically possible; the "rule of no pain and opposite movement" should be applicable, and the spine should not be too stiff.

The selected maneuvers should be perfectly executed, and the applied force should be exactly measured. If the applied force is insufficient, it can be inefficient, too exaggerated, and traumatic. The selected maneuvers should be applied judiciously. Sometimes, one or two maneuvers are sufficient during one session; sometimes, several will be necessary. The frequency of the sessions also plays a role. What has to be performed depends on the results and on the reaction of the tissues, which can be appreciated by careful palpation. Sometimes priority should be given to mobilization or stretching and sometimes to a brief but measured maneuver. The possible association with other local or general treatment is also part of the management.

When Is a Manipulative Treatment Justified?

First Establish the Diagnosis

Any spinal pain requires clinical and radiologic assessment, with support by laboratory and electrodiagnostic data where appropriate. Remember

- Any inflammatory, tumoral, or infectious lesion of the spine may become symptomatic during an effort or a forced movement. Therefore, it is serious to miss the correct diagnosis.
- Appropriate radiographic studies of high quality that clearly reveal all the elements of the concerned region are necessary and are to be completed by dynamic studies if necessary. Sometimes, radiographic abnormalities only become apparent after a disease process is well established, as is the case with many serious disorders of the spine. If there is the slightest doubt, it is better to abstain from manipulation and try to arrive at the diagnosis by others means, such as laboratory testing, including analysis of blood and urine, electrodiagnostic evaluation with nerve conduction studies and electromyography, bone scan, computed tomography scanning, and magnetic resonance imaging.
- Finally, remember that manipulative treatment is rarely an irreplaceable therapeutic modality. It is, of course, attractive because of its rapid action and its elegance. But it is valuable only if well executed. It is better to do something else than to manipulate wrongly; "Primum non nocere." Then take all necessary precautions.

Then Take the Necessary Precautions

Once the manipulative treatment has been decided, be sure that the manipulation can be performed on the spine in question. The state of the spine has to be evaluated radiographically. The presence of a significant osteoporosis is, of course, a contraindication to manipulation, even if there is a real mechanical problem.

Cervical manipulation should be avoided in patients with an abnormality of the cervico-occipital junction. "Postural testing" should also be performed (see below) to uncover the possible presence of vertebrobasilar insufficiency that has not been recognized and which is an absolute contraindication to cervical manipulation. The neck of a patient whose general and vascular state is not sound should not be manipulated (see "Contraindications to Manipulation," below).

When Is a Manipulative Treatment Possible?

Although a manipulative treatment may be justified on the basis of the diagnosis (mechanical problem), this does not mean that it can be performed, even if the conditions discussed above are favorable.

- The rule of no pain and opposite movement is applicable.
- Manipulation is easily feasible. There are some stiff spines in which the maneuvers bump against painless and global resistances. Manipulation should be avoided on these stiff spines, with progressive mobilization treatments used instead.
- Manipulative treatment, if performed, should show rapid proof of its effectiveness. Therefore, a "starting schedule" should be performed.

How Is the Treatment Managed?

A complete starting schedule is necessary to follow the results of each treatment. All measurable or appreciable elements of the clinical examination as described above are first noted and, if possible, reported on a star diagram.

Manipulation Session

Once the premanipulative diagnosis has been established, the treatment session will consist of three phases:

- Maneuvers of general and local relaxation
- Maneuvers of oriented mobilizations
- Maneuvers of manipulation (thrust)

Maneuvers of General and Local Relaxation

With the patient in an adequate position, the examiner starts by executing slow, rhythmic maneuvers of relaxation. This allows the examiner to appreciate the quality of the patient's muscle tone and find some deep contractures that were not apparent at the beginning of the examination. These maneuvers, performed slowly, have a real relaxing effect and can result in significant improvement. It is not uncommon to see a resistant (chronic) sciatica be relieved by massage of the muscles of the external iliac fossa. Relaxation of the muscles of the supraspinous and infraspinous fossae often has a favorable effect on the sequelae of cervicobrachial neuralgias.

Maneuvers of Oriented Mobilization

After the maneuvers of relaxation, just as after each sequence of treatment, a quick examination can be performed to evaluate the improvement in the limited and painful movements. The second step of the treatment is the execution of mobilizations and stretchings that are oriented in the pain-free directions. The spinal segment should be brought slowly to end range. Then a pause is helpful, followed by relaxation of the pressure and resumption of the mobilization. These movements should be slow and elastic, with pressure well linked and well executed rhythmically. Each maneuver is repeated several times according to each of the orientations and in combination with them.

These oriented mobilizations should first be global, affecting the whole region; then they can be more specific, with manipulation techniques that will not go beyond taking up the slack, localizing its effect on the concerned spinal segment. Often, it is necessary to stop the treatment here during the first session, especially in difficult cases that are acute or very well established. It is wise also to limit these maneuvers in the treatment of frail spines. Otherwise, the session will continue until the so-called manipulative time is reached.

Maneuvers of Manipulation (Thrust Techniques)

The patient is now used to the movements executed on the spine and does not feel any more uneasiness when the spine is "pulled" a little or put under slight tension, since the painful movements are theoretically avoided. In most cases, the first manipulation can be performed in the direction opposed to the one that is the most blocked and painful. It can be monodirectional or combined with another free orientation. The result of this first maneuver is judged according to the elements given below. Depending on the result of the first maneuver, a second maneuver is executed with another free orientation as principal coordinate. After a new examination, a third maneuver can be applied, possibly using some orientations that the preceding maneuvers have freed. The examiner should not do more than three consecutive manipulations on a spinal segment in one session. Sometimes, it is necessary to limit it to one maneuver.

Experience is irreplaceable. The examiner will adjust and vary maneuvers according the patient's responses and especially the results of the palpation examination. The maneuvers can be varied in terms of the degree of pressure—light, when done with the tip of the fingers, or more forceful—and the time maintained. Sometimes they can be a little sharper to obtain a more marked reflex effect.

Evaluation of the Response to Treatment

The effect of each therapeutic gesture, such as massage, mobilization, injection, and especially manipulation, should be immediately assessed before the next therapy is begun. This assessment can be based on the following.

• A simple objective sign: Lasegue's sign, distance from the fingers to the ground, range of motion, modification in pain produced by an exactly described spinal movement, etc.
• An ordinary gesture that has been impossible or difficult to do before manipulation and that has become easier or possible later (e.g., putting on a sock).
• Manifestations of the segmental vertebral cellulotenoperiosteomyalgic syndrome: decrease in the sensitivity or disappearance of a cellulalgic zone, especially in the territory of the posterior ramus of the spinal nerve; decrease in the tenoperiosteal sensitivity (shoulder tests, epicondylar pain tests, palpation); decrease in the sensitivity of a trigger point; as many elements expressing the favorable action of the gesture that has been executed

• Decrease in the number of the local signs of the PMID; disappearance of these signs is not always immediate; decrease or disappearance of the facet joint tenderness is a very accurate test
• Subjective impression of the patient who feels better or not, with the clear limitations of such an subjective accounts taken into consideration

At the end of this manual treatment, some attenuated signs of PMID may persist, even if the patient is perfectly relieved. The "active" PMID has become a "latent" PMID. In this case, should the treatment be continued? The answer varies. Sometimes, all the treatments that can be given will not make a perturbed segment become totally painless on examination; it is often sufficient to have a later session to stop the pain (two or three times/year). Otherwise, complementary treatments, manual or other, the correction of other zones of dysfunction (see Chapter 61, "Transitional Zone Syndrome"), and a well-organized course of physical therapy will generally overcome a refractory PMID and make all the signs disappear.

Reactions following the Manipulative Treatment

In about one-third of cases, the patient can experience some reactions after the first session. After the second session, these reactions are less common and always less pronounced; they are benign and most often mild. They are characterized by stiffness or a temporary increase in the pain that has been treated, usually occurring after an interval of a few hours. They can exist even if the manipulation has been soft, done "with the tips of the fingers." They would be more pronounced, however, if the maneuvers had been more numerous and more forceful. As a rule, they do not interfere with the good result this treatment can bring unless the patient, who has been told or warned, stops treatment before undergoing the one or two supplementary sessions (without reaction) that would have relieved the problem.

Stiffness

Posttreatment stiffness is usually moderate and readily responds to anti-inflammatories and application of heat. It tends to last 6–48 hours. Cases of stiffness can be more severe.

Stiffness is generally less of a problem in later sessions, or it is very much reduced in intensity and duration, similar to postexercise soreness.

Transient Exacerbations

Transient exacerbations of the treated pain can occur immediately after the first session of manipulation in cases in which the patient will eventually experience significant improvement. In 20–25% of cases, however, patients may experience a momentary reaction characterized by a recurrence or an increase of the pain 6–12 hours after the treatment. It may last for a few hours and sometimes for 1 or 2 days. These reactions are rarely very severe but are seen, as in the following example.

Case History. Mr. C., a 26-year-old judo champion, fell on his head, which resulted in acute headache with vertigo. Radiologic, ENT (ear, nose, and throat), and neurologic examinations were normal. The manifestations persisted for 3 weeks after the incident. A segmental examination revealed a PMID of C2-C3. Only one mild and painless manipulation was executed in rotation. There was an immediate improvement in cervical range of motion with relief of pain. The following night, the headache recurred, radiating toward the ear with such intensity that in the morning the patient consulted with an ENT physician, thinking he had an acute otitis (he had had one 2 years before). The ENT examination was unremarkable. In the evening, the symptoms seemed to decrease. By the next morning, everything had disappeared—vertigo, headache, cervical discomfort. The manifestations did not recur.

This patient had been an athlete used to shocks and blows, and the manipulation had been performed with "the tips of the fingers." Nevertheless, reactions occurred. A second manipulative session thus should not be performed before the reactions of the first session, be they postmanipulative stiffness or temporary increases of pain, are gone. Reactions usually occur only after the first session, they are very much attenuated after the second, and they are rare after the third. Their recurrence at each session, with no improvement in the treated state, means that the treatment should be discontinued and the diagnosis reevaluated.

These reactions are always preceded by a free time of 6–12 hours after treatment. Their presence or absence is not prognostic of the result of the treatment. A "reaction" occurring 48 hours after the treatment is usually not a reaction; it is usually a recurrence whose cause is often related to the patient's behavior.

False Reactions or Premature Recurrence

Besides these normal reactions, many postmanipulative pseudoreactions are due to the behavior of the patient. Since patients feel very much relieved after the treatment or want to test the result, they may try to do what was difficult or impossible to do the day before or take risks, including forceful physical efforts, postural stressful positions, or exposure to climatic irritants. Often, notwithstanding explanation, the patient does not understand the nature of the ailment very well. For example, a farmer suffering from a chronic effort-related low back pain that was relieved immediately after manipulation rushed, as soon as he was home, to the heavy object that had caused his ailment. "Then I put myself exactly in the position I was when I felt pain, and this time I lifted it without pain! Doctor, one can say that your repair was good." For him, the vertebra either "was in place" or "was not in place." If it was, he believed that he had been mechanically returned to his full functional capacity.

For a few days after manipulation, the patient remains very vulnerable to recurrence, especially if the treatment has resulted in substantial relief. If the patient performs an activity such as caused the problem initially, there may be not only a temporary irritation but also a severe recurrence. Patients should understand that a session of manipulation, even if it results in a very noticeable relief, leaves them "fragile" for a while, and therefore, they should compensate for this by modifying some activities of daily living.

The session should be followed by relative rest for 48 hours. This does not mean the patient should remain in bed, and although there are some exceptions, the patient should avoid the efforts, movements, and positions that brought on the usual pain. These precautions should be followed much longer in old or difficult cases.

Sympathetic Reaction

Besides painful reactions, there are sometimes functional sympathetic reactions that can be immediate. After even minimal manipulation of the cervicothoracic region, it is not unusual for patients to experience axillary perspiration. It happens at every session, be they a few days or a few months apart. This just demonstrates the action of the maneuvers on the sympathetic system, and it has no effect on management of the treatment.

There is another type of reaction, which is rather rare but about which we should be aware. In the hours following a high lumbar or low thoracic manipulation, the patient can experience an attack of abdominal discomfort and diarrheal episodes. Modifications of menstruation can be seen exceptionally; manipulation can either start them, hasten them, or make them more profuse. One of our female patients who had manipulation of the neck four times per month for shoulder pain also experienced menstrual blood flow starting the evening of the day of treatment and lasting 4 days, absolutely the same as her normal menstruation. Seen again 3 years later, three times per month for cervicobrachial neuralgia, she experienced menstrual blood flow lasting 4 days after each treatment. Rarely, 24 hours after a manipulation session some patients (especially those who complain more or less frequently of analogous symptoms) experience a painful epigastric attack or pelvic or abdominal pain, sometimes sharp, lasting a few hours. This reaction generally indicates the disappearance, perhaps definitively, of these symptoms.

Evolution of Pain after the Manipulation Session

After the first session, with the possible reactions being lessened, there are several possible outcomes.

- There is a complete and immediate disappearance of pain, which can be permanent or transient, with pain reappearing, attenuated, the following day. This is the most frequent occurrence and is a good prognosis for the rest of the treatment. There may be no change in the intensity of pain. The signs remain the same. After two or three sessions, the treatment can be discontinued.
- Sometimes, immediately after manipulation, the patient may not note a significant improvement but, 1 or 2 days later, notices a distinct improvement of the painful state. In some very chronic cases, the improvement is seen only a few days after manipulation, after a moderate reaction mixed with stiffness and exacerbation of the usual pain or of the dysfunction being treated.
- Rarely, the patient experiences an increase in pain. This is quite rare if the indications are appropriate and the treatment well executed. The diagnosis should be reviewed but only after finding out what the patient did after the treatment. Most often we learn that the patient, feeling "miraculously" cured of low back pain, for instance, drove several hundreds miles, stood for an extended period of time, carried heavy packages, or was exposed to cold. It can also be due to an acute synovitis, which appears coincidentally and is unrelated to the treatment.

Number and Frequency of Sessions

Sometimes, a single session is sufficient; other times, several sessions are necessary. Three sessions are the average, and in some chronic cases, five or six sessions are necessary. It all depends on the case being treated and on the partial results obtained at each session. In general, if there is no improvement in the spontaneous pain and especially in the signs of the examination after three sessions, it is useless to continue.

These sessions are the "acute" intervention. A maintenance treatment (i.e., a session every 3 or 6 months) that, with some simple maneuvers, reduces pain in the neck or flank is perfectly justified in some chronic low back pain syndromes or cervical pain syndromes.

There is no problem when the patient is relieved completely right away. Nevertheless, if it is a chronic case, the patient should be reexamined 3 or 4 weeks later to be sure the signs have disappeared.

When several sessions are necessary, their frequency will vary depending on the case and the findings on subsequent examinations. One or two sessions each week is a reasonable average. Some patients will react better to short intervals between sessions; others will react better to longer intervals between sessions. In cases of an acute low back pain or torticollis (wryneck), for example, which usually can be cured spontaneously in 3–7 days, it is certainly not necessary to do four manipulations in 7 days; one or two manipulations can be performed at 2- or 3-day intervals.

With a subacute disorder such as refractory sciatica, the first manipulation can be performed, and its result assessed 4 days later. Depending on that result—a sharp or mild reaction—the manipulation can be performed 3 or 4 times, at intervals of 3–4 days, with a pause as soon as relief is obtained. The patient is seen again 1 month later.

In the case of a chronic disorder such as low back pain or cervical headache, one manipulation a week for 3 weeks will allow better evaluation of the results of different techniques. If a result is not obtained, two or three additional sessions can be tried at 2- or 3-day intervals. When the spine is very stiff but is tolerating the manipulation, sessions performed at very short intervals will give a result that sessions performed with long intervals would never bring.

The dosage of maneuvers (i.e., the frequency of the sessions) is very important in manipulation. Patients do not all tolerate these treatments in the same way. The stiff brachymorphic type of patient generally tolerates stronger treatments at short intervals. The hyperrelaxed lanky type of patient does not tolerate this type of treatment very well. With them it should be sufficient to perform the minimum of manipulation, with a long interval between sessions. Otherwise, they may develop a true painful spinal syndrome with some misleading improvements after the sessions, which may eventually contribute to worsening of their condition.

Should we just content ourselves with treating the segment responsible for the pain that brought the patient to consultation? Yes, as a first step. If the result is easily obtained, maybe a certain balance has been reached in the spine whose regional mobility is perturbed. But this is not the case if there is a recurrence. Then it is necessary to relax the stiffened zones of the spine and to treat the latent PMIDs that could exist at other levels, especially if they are located in the junction zones (see Chapter 61, "Transitional Zone Syndrome").

Age Considerations with Respect to Manipulation

It has often been written that manipulation should be reserved for young patients, with the indication of choice being acute low back pain. This is incorrect. The acute low back pain of the young is less regularly relieved than is that of patients in their 40s and 50s. If this disorder is often a good indication for manipulation, it is neither the only one nor the best.

Manipulation can be used in most individuals, with the execution of the maneuvers varied according to the person's age. Many maneuvers should be performed very gently. If the indications of manipulation are limited to the sensible ones, it is rare to have to treat children, but it can be done with positive results. With children, only the necessary movement is to be performed, very gently; there is no other concern than the difficulty of precision.

Quite often, however, it is necessary to treat the elderly. They often receive a great deal of relief from gentle mobilization. It gives them greater ease of movement and can also help relieve the small minor nuisances brought by paraspinal protective muscle guarding perpetuated by segmental stiffness. No forceful, strenuous, or sharp maneuver should be used. It is remarkable how some aged spines can be helped considerably by a few gentle movements, where according to clinical and radiologic studies, these patients could be considered to be beyond all possible help.

Quality of Results

Among the criticisms of manipulative treatment, a common complaint is that the results do not last. Sometimes this is true, although many good results are long lasting in spite of the apparently bad condition of the patients with poor static, poorly conditioned, or weak muscles, with severe multilevel disk degeneration, etc. In the case of manipulation relieving reversible dysfunctions, it would seem logical that such a "dysfunction" could recur easily or it would not recur with frequency. The result of the manipulation, however, depends on the accuracy of the diagnosis and largely on the quality of the execution (i.e., the examiner). This is evident but should be emphasized, as many think that from the moment a region has "cracked" and a certain relief occurs, all has been done. There is a world of difference, however, between an elective manipulation or mobilization that is forced and approximate, with some sessions of cracking that are repeated systematically every 2 or 8 days (even if, to the unskilled observer, all the maneuvers seem to be the same) and a well-organized treatment protocol with sessions that are appropriately dosed, progressive, and with an appropriate frequency. If the maneuver has not been sufficiently precise (i.e., sufficiently "pushed"), the relief it produces may have little chance of lasting.

It is the same if one neglects to relax the stiff spinal segments that are supra-adjacent and subjacent to the painful zone. This "reharmonization of the segmental movements" (Lescure) is a very important part of the treatment by manipulation, which should not be limited to the painful segment. When good reharmonization is obtained, the quality of the result is generally such that certain manipulators neglect completely the physical therapy that is often indispensable. Indeed, muscular insufficiency and poor muscular synergy or, even more, the lack of muscular control are greatly responsible for spinal fragility. Recognizing these factors and designing an effective therapeutic exercise program to correct them is essential for the patient's total rehabilitation. Finally, let us repeat the need for a maintenance session 1, 2, or 3 times per year in disorders such as cervical spondylosis, in which there is a normal tendency to "reblocking" and where manipulation as part of a comprehensive rehabilitation strategy, although not curative, can give temporary relief, sometimes of long duration, that no other therapeutics can give as well.

Good training in palpation of tissues enables the examiner to appreciate the persistence or the disappearance of the local changes generally accompanying "the painful minor intervertebral dysfunctions." If these changes persist after the manipulative treatment, it means that the problem is not completely solved, even if the patient is relieved and the other symptoms have disappeared. One should not forget that manipulation does not change the anatomic state of the treated segment. It makes the PMIDs tolerable and painless, but does not always make them disappear completely. Of course, in these conditions, the state of the organism has an essential role. Certain subjects with a very low pain tolerance threshold are significantly incapacitated by slight dysfunctions that others cannot discern.

GENERAL INDICATIONS FOR SPINAL MANIPULATION

Used judiciously, manipulation is a useful and rapidly efficacious therapeutic modality. It is the principal treatment for "painful minor intervertebral dysfunctions" (PMID) as we have defined "benign and painful dysfunctions of the spinal segment," which represent the common denominator of most spinal pain syndromes that are called "common." Spinal manipulation acts also on the cellulalgic, myalgic, tendinous, and periosteal manifestations that result from these PMIDs. This explains the often favorable action of manipulation on some referred pain syndromes that seem to have no ties with the spine.

Thus the indications for spinal manipulation are pain syndromes tied to these PMIDs. These can be local (cervical, thoracic, lumbar), radicular, or referred pain. But manipulation can also be useful in some cases of herniated disk or stiffness commonly associated with spondylosis. In this last case, progressive mobilization is often preferable. All PMIDs are not systematically amenable to manipulation, however. There are instances in which manipulation can be inefficient and even contraindicated. Often it is beneficial to use manipulation in combination with other therapeutic modalities, physical or pharmacologic, in the context of a multidimensional rehabilitation program, aiming at the local irritation resulting from the PMID or at the manifestations of the segmental spinal syndrome whose persistence can create a secondary vicious cycle that impedes the patient's rehabilitation.

There is no irreplaceable therapeutic modality in the treatment of common vertebral pain syndromes. If there are cases that only manipulation can cure or relieve, they are infrequent. Other therapeutic approaches can often lead to good results—maybe less brilliant, but satisfying—if they are applied properly where necessary. It is always better not to manipulate than to manipulate poorly. The remedy should not be worse than the disorder being treated.

What is unique to treatment by manipulation is the elegance and the rapidity of the result, which is sometimes instantaneous, in general needing two or three sessions, but occasionally needing more than six. We now survey the principal indications for manipulative therapy. The chapters on the principal common disorders of spinal origin detail its place in their treatment.

Cervical Region

Chronic posttraumatic, postural, or static cervical pain and pain in which spondylosis fosters stiffness and intervertebral dysfunctions are the usual indications.

In acute cervical pain, manipulation can only be applied if it is of micromechanical origin. Very rarely is that origin seen, however, even if a forced movement seems to have been the cause.

Cervicobrachial radiculitis is a frequent indication when it is mild or is chronic and mechanical. In addition, there is a whole pathology whose cervical origin is usually unrecognized and which will benefit from manipulative treatment. As far as the superior cervical spine is concerned, headache is the problem. Headache of cervical origin is much more frequent than is noted in the classical literature. Its own semiology has been described (Maigne). It is considered in detail in Chapter 48, "Headaches of Cervical Origin."

Some cases of vertigo, nausea, or minor cognitive problems seen as sequelae of cervical trauma can also respond favorably to a cervical treatment.

Many cases of pseudotendinitis of the shoulder with pain and limitation of movements have a cervical component and are the manifestations of a segmental spinal neurotrophic syndrome due to C4-C5 or C5-C6 PMID. Spinal treatment is then very useful. It is often the same for the pain syndromes of the lateral epicondyle (C5-C6, C6-C7). The cervical factor is less frequent in the pain syndromes of the medial epicondyle (C7-C8).

Thoracic Region

In cases of "common thoracic pain of the adult," the inferior cervical spine has to be examined with most attention. Eight of 10 times, it is an "interscapular pain of cervical origin" (Maigne), with an interscapular para-T5, very specific tender point. Another less frequent form of cervicothoracic pain is due to the dysfunction of the levator scapulae. It can be associated with a PMID of C3-C4 or C4-C5. Common thoracic pain of thoracic origin is less common. Some pain syndromes are indications for manipulative treatment. Costal sprains, especially of the false ribs, give misleading pain syndromes; their diagnosis requires an adequate manipulative treatment.

Lumbar Region

Manipulation is an excellent treatment for numerous acute and chronic low back pain syndromes referred to as "common." Half of the acute low back pain syndromes are relieved after the first manipulation. The chronic low back pain syndromes do not all originate from the inferior lumbar spine. In chronic low back pain of low lumbar origin, manipulation is often a useful treatment, even if the radiologic findings show significant discopathy, osteophytosis, etc. The effect can be long lasting, but it is always better to complete the treatment with an appropriate therapeutic exercise prescription to stabilize the result.

A number of low back pain syndromes have their origin in the thoracolumbar junction (T11-T12 or T12-L1) (Maigne). They can be acute or chronic. An adequate manipulative treatment can most often be applied to these types of "low back pain of thoracolumbar origin" with excellent results. Physical modalities seem to be less effective in this condition. Sciatica resulting from disk involvement is a good indication when it is of moderate or average intensity. Manipulation does not seem to have a noticeable effect on the results obtained in sciatica of recent onset or in recurrent cases; however, the latter seems to react better and more quickly than the former. It has often been written that manipulation should be reserved for sciatica of recent onset in the young patient. Based on our experience, however, the results of manipulation are less effective in patients 20–30 years of age than in patients 40–50 years of age.

The femoral neuralgias react noticeably like sciatica. Meralgia paraesthetica is often well relieved, because in contrast to generally accepted opinion, it most often contains a spinal factor.

Coccyx

Coccydynia of traumatic origin resulting, for example, from a fall or from delivery is relieved regularly in one to three sessions with the technique that we propose. This is not the case with the coccydynia of nontraumatic origin resulting from local pathology (see Chapter 46).

Visceral Disorders and Functional Disorders

We do not consider visceral disorders to be an indication for spinal manipulation, even if manipulation sometimes influences certain functional problems. The use of manipulation for prevention or treatment of visceral disorders is a major concern for most of those who (with some variations) use manual techniques aimed at "restoring a normal joint play," correcting "spinal subluxations," or curing "mechanical dysfunctions" of the spine. This is evident with the chiropractic school and to some extent the osteopathic school and some medical authors.

According to Korr, one of the best-known neurophysiologist of the American osteopathic school, any functional perturbation—muscular, spinal, articular, myofascial, or other "somatic dysfunction"—facilitates the corresponding spinal cord segment, which can produce a perturbation of any of the neural elements arising from that segment. This interrelation between all the physiologic systems is the basis of the osteopathic concept.

Thus the osteopathic lesion, now called "somatic dysfunction," whose definition includes any dysfunction of the musculoskeletal apparatus, is capable of creating adverse somatovisceral reflexes. This concept is based on some real findings. It is known that such reflexes exist. Such a mechanism can be responsible for some functional visceral pain

syndromes that the spinal treatment can sometimes suppress or attenuate.

Indeed, it is not unusual to have some patients who have been manipulated for low back pain notice that their habitual constipation has resolved or that their gastrointestinal discomfort has abated after a thoracic manipulation. But to affirm that these viscerosomatic reflexes play an important role in organic pathology is a leap of faith. Conversely, visceral disorders can present with certain cutaneous or myofascial manifestations (Mackenzie). There are instances in which anesthetizing these zones brings relief or decreases the visceral pain; this is well known. For some, however, this could mean that there is occasionally a facilitative reflex arc acting favorably on the disorder, although this has not been proved.

The spectrum of manipulation is sufficiently broad and well established in the domain of musculoskeletal pain without trying to apply it blindly to pathologic phenomena in which the role of the spine, if it exists, is uncertain. It is also true that those who tend to use manipulation as a general therapeutic modality are those whose medical education is the weakest.

CONTRAINDICATIONS TO MANIPULATION

A distinction must be made between clinical and technical contraindications. The former are disorders of a nonmechanical nature for which manipulation should not be used and, moreover, could be dangerous, as in cases in which osseous or vascular conditions prelude its use. The latter are cases in which manipulation appears to be a feasible means of rational treatment in problems of a mechanical nature, but is contraindicated because the rule of no pain and opposite movement cannot be applied.

Clinical Contraindications

Clinical contraindications depend on the nature of the disorder. Some contraindications are positive. Spinal fractures and pain due to infectious, tumoral, or inflammatory disorders are, of course, absolute contraindications. Some of these conditions have occult presentations and are only discovered when the patient presents with what seems initially to be a mechanical problem that began during a physical effort or a traumatic episode. Thus treatment by manipulation is desirable only after an exact diagnosis has been made on the basis of clinical and radiologic examinations, confirmed if necessary by complementary examinations as mentioned previously. It is necessary to have high quality radiographs, for it is more dangerous to have bad ones than to have none. A bad radiographic study of the neck in a patient with a head trauma can lead to misinterpretation of a fracture of the odontoid or atlas. Anomalies of the cervico-occipital junction present contraindications as does significant osteopenia.

The most frequent and serious accidents of manipulation are vascular accidents, occurring most often in patients with a vertebrobasilar insufficiency. If there is the least doubt, this diagnosis should be eliminated and neurologic advice obtained. We discuss below the signs that can point to this vertebrobasilar insufficiency, which is the major trap of the spinal manipulation (see "Errors of Manipulation").

Technical Contraindications

Even when the mechanical nature of a spinal problem is clearly established, manipulation can be used only if the rule of no pain and opposite movement is respected. As indicated above, manipulation is contraindicated when all directions of movement are painful. In practice, however, this is also true when only one direction is free. When two directions are free, a few mobilizations can be tried in the free directions, and then the result is assessed. Three degrees of freedom should be available to maximize the chance of success with manipulation.

Even when there are three free directions, manipulation is contraindicated when a painless resistance is encountered in taking up the slack. For instance, when flexion, left rotation, and left lateroflexion are painful, while right rotation, right lateroflexion, and extension are painless, a manipulation is still contraindicated if the examiner feels a painless resistance while taking up the slack.

Another contraindication to manipulation exists in the case of a patient who has a stiff spine or demonstrates marked tonic resistance to passive motion. Even if the patient is well relaxed and the examiner is well trained, only

mobilization and stretching should be performed. The increase in soft tissue resistance may be temporary and disappear by the next session.

Patient fear of the manipulation is a contraindication to manipulation. The patient might, for instance, suddenly contract during the thrust, and the maneuver could be dangerous. If the examiner has complete control of his or her own maneuvers, however, with progressively insistent and painless mobilization (which might be found to be sufficient), the patient may gain enough confidence to allow the examiner to go beyond taking up the slack and perform a manipulative thrust if indicated. This should be done only with the patient's consent.

Manipulation is contraindicated if the examiner has not perfectly mastered the techniques of manipulation. Acquisition of the manual skills necessary to competently perform manipulation takes a long time. In a whole year of daily work, only the basic techniques and how to apply them in basic cases can be assimilated. From this indispensable beginning, the examiner must have daily practice, and just as in sports such as tennis or golf, several years are necessary to really master a sufficient number of techniques. Even then, there will always be important differences between the average practitioner and those specialists who take care of a small proportion of difficult cases. It is a matter of skillfulness. A maneuver that is forced or held too long or a slight difference in the points of support or in the orientation of the movement can transform a failure into success.

Improperly performed manipulation is contraindicated. It is better not to manipulate than to manipulate incorrectly. This is also true for a trained examiner when the necessary material (table, stool at right height) is not available. A manipulation executed on a bed or a sofa is a dangerous acrobatic maneuver for the patient and sometimes for the examiner.

ERRORS OF MANIPULATION

The relief of acute low back pain in a few seconds or improvement, by application of a simple maneuver, of a painful neck that has been limited for months, is not unusual with manipulation. Because it works rapidly, the experienced examiner is tempted to apply manipulation when faced with a pain whose origin seems benign and mechanical in a patient who has had a previous good outcome with manipulation and insists on its use upon experiencing a similar pain. Some patients do not hesitate to alter their story slightly just to persuade the examiner or themselves that the pain for which they come to consultation has certainly started after a forced movement or an effort. The errors in the use of manipulation are numerous. A patient with a history of several spinal incidents of a mechanical nature can have a new disorder of quite another nature that manifests itself by spinal pain, reminding him or her of a previous incident. An infectious or tumoral disorder can become painful for the first time following a strain or trauma. Sometimes, the symptomatology is so similar to the one met every day that the examiner can be tempted to use the remedy that seems most useful, manipulation. Some of these errors are more frequent than others. Let us examine them successively.

Errors in Diagnosis

Errors in diagnosis are essentially due to the absence or poor quality of radiographic studies or to views that are insufficient for evaluating the region in question.

Case History. Mr. B. is 69 years old. His son, a physician, sent him to us for a possible manipulative treatment. Mr. B. has had occipital pain syndromes. Two weeks before, he had been hit on the head by a heavy board. The radiographic studies were of rather good quality (except for the open mouth view, which could barely be interpreted) and showed no spinal lesion. But because of the continuous discomfort, the symmetry of the blockage, and the suboccipital protective muscle guarding, tomographic studies were requested, which uncovered a fracture of the atlas.

One can imagine what result a blind manipulation would have yielded in the following case.

Case History. Mr. C. is 30 years old. A few weeks before, he had a trivial cervical trauma while stopping suddenly at a red light. The force of deceleration resulted in cervical pain that was not improved by analgesic medication and was irritated by massage. The cervical radiographic studies he brought with him seemed normal. Dynamic views were requested, which showed a subluxation of C5 on C6; in flexion, C5 translated almost completely on C6.

Errors in Rheumatology

Errors in rheumatology result most often when there is a delay in the radiologic evaluation in relation to the clinical evolution. The physician-manipulator should fall into this type of trap less frequently than do others. With rare exception, inflammatory arthritides are detected by the premanipulative assessment that shows that movement applied to the involved segment is painful or limited in all directions, making the manipulation technically impossible if the rule of no pain and opposite movement is respected.

Errors in Neurology

Errors in the neurologic domain certainly provide most of the errors of manipulation. Many neurologic disorders can, at their inception, mimic a benign spinal pain. Mechanical treatments in these cases can aggravate the problems dramatically, even the simple spinal examination described in the following case history reported by Held.

Case History. A young boy 12 years of age was hit on the neck while playing. Torticollis (wryneck) and cervical discomfort developed during the next several weeks. A physician performed a physical examination, testing simply the cervical mobility. Suddenly, a tetraplegia occurred, diagnosed as a spinal cord vascular accident. If the patient had been manipulated, it would have sparked a formidable medicolegal dilemma! But what if the physician-examiner had been known to practice manipulation? Would anyone be convinced that it was only an examination?

This case is similar to the next one, the case of a patient whose cervicobrachial neuralgia was severely and suddenly aggravated during an examination that was absolutely normal and performed by her rheumatologist. Subsequent examinations uncovered a cervical tumor. Conversely, manipulation can oddly improve some symptoms whose origin is certainly tumoral. Meningiomas and neurinomas are very misleading. They often present as local pain (neck pain in the case of cervical meningioma, most often seen in women) or radicular pain syndromes with a very slow evolution and with remissions, and the interval between the appearance of the pain and the appearance of the motor problems can be months, even years. The following case history reported by Held is particularly demonstrative.

Case History. A 40-year-old woman with cervicobrachial pain radiating to the interscapular region was seen by her physician, who prescribed traction and manipulation, which brought about improvements in the patient. Several months later, a more intense relapse occurred, with anorexia, weight loss, and depression. Her general state of health and gastrointestinal tract were normal. She was subsequently admitted to the hospital, where she underwent electroconvulsive therapy (ECT), followed by a sleep laboratory assessment that was prematurely discontinued by the patient. Another series of manipulation followed; the patient improved, gained weight, and had no more pain. Two years later, there was a relapse; the same manipulation had no effect. Progressively, new problems appeared: leg spasms and sensory problems in the left hand (she burned herself without feeling it). The neurologic examination demonstrated a subtle deficit of the right lower limb, a right Babinski's sign, hyperreflexia of the right upper limb, and hypoesthesia to touch, with analgesia in a C4 distribution on the left. A diagnosis of an ependymoma of the spinal cord was made. Following a surgical intervention, she was left with impaired neural function in all four limbs including spasticity and a sensory deficit.

This case history underlines the difficulty in diagnosing these tumors. The peculiar improvement, obtained twice by manipulation and retained for long periods, delayed the diagnosis. Some patients with syringomyelia can present with cervicobrachial neuralgia or acroparesthesia. This diagnosis is easier to make when the pain syndromes have a lancinating quality, like pain produced by burns or intense cold. The most formidable error is the one set up by the vertebrobasilar circulatory dysfunction, which causes the most frequent severe accidents and is sometimes the most difficult to foresee in manipulation (discussed below). Cervical manifestations rather similar to those of the vertebrobasilar dysfunctions are frequently seen in neuropathies such as pseudovertigo, headache, visual fatigability, and fainting tendency.

It is, of course, much less dangerous to use manipulative therapy on a patient whose manifestations are the expression of a neurosis rather than a vertebrobasilar dysfunction. But it is not harmless to condition such patients until they become "obsessed with the idea of the blocked vertebra" or "the displaced vertebra." The particularities of manipulative therapy, especially when it is performed in a context of illegality, have been described very well by Grossiord.

It is a very particular therapy whose apparent ease of administration has something magic in it to which patients are extremely sensitive. The myth of the "spinal displacement," the revealing of "microdisplacements" by views of the whole spine, the prestige of a foreign diploma, the external apparatus of the maneuver, the spirit of its execution, the authority of the examiner, its theatrical elements, all create a climate that does not correspond very well with the slow, cautious and unrewarding approaches that mainstream medicine and therapy impose on us in general. In these patients, the illegitimately performed manipulation creates the "consciousness of blockings" or of spinal displacements [that] repeat and that should be put back in place. Thus the multiple experiences of manipulative treatments can create a supplementary point of attention and of anxiety.

It is what Lescure has called "the obsessional neurosis of the spinal displacement" maintained unconsciously (?) by some persons under the cover of infantile or mythical conception of the illness.

The physician who is conscious of these problems must make every effort to dissuade patients who are conditioned by a vocabulary now commonly used by the public or by dubious theories presented in books that seem quite serious to the layman and which the media like to promote. Even after lengthy explanations that the physician has not "put back a displaced vertebra" and that "vertebrae do not displace themselves," but that the physician simply "unwedged a disk fragment" or "relaxed its spine," the patient will ultimately remind the physician that he or she, for instance, "put back to its place the fifth lumbar that was displaced." It is not very serious when this is limited to terminology. But it is much more serious when patients become truly obsessed by this myth of displacement and, to be manipulated, go constantly to practitioners who are more or less qualified or manipulate themselves. The result is that their neurotic fixations continue to increase, with the unavoidable risk that one day an amateur may manipulate vertebrae and produce a spinal sprain or a disk lesion.

The fashion of "spinal displacements" seems for now to be in full regression. But it is being replaced by other terminologies well received by the public with the help of the media. For example, how many problems are due to "dysfunction of the cranial sutures." Some of these practitioners pretend even to treat cerebral palsy and Down syndrome by normalizing the positions of the sphenoid and the temporal bones, while others, with the help of various maneuvers, will put back into balance the "vital circuits."

Vertebrobasilar Insufficiency

Vertebrobasilar insufficiency (VBI) is a formidable source of error. Although rare, it is the most frequent cause of the dramatic accidents associated with manipulation. It is all the more misleading because the manipulative accidents can happen in a patient who never complained before and who comes complaining of headache or vertigo, symptoms that are frequently tied to "painful minor intervertebral dysfunctions" and are often relieved by manipulation. In the case of VBI, however, cervical manipulation can have disastrous consequences, especially if the maneuvers are forced, repeated, or maintained. But accidents have also followed maneuvers that seemed to be mild. In fact, two types of VBI can be distinguished: thromboembolic VBI and hemodynamic VBI described by Rancurel.

Thromboembolic Vertebrobasilar Insufficiency

The existence of thromboembolic vertebrobasilar insufficiency has been admitted by all. From the physiopathologic point of view, it is analogous to carotid vascular accidents.

There can be (*a*) thrombosis affecting the spinal subclavian trunk, resulting sometimes in permanent and transient neurologic deficits, or (*b*) platelet emboli or thrombi coming from the neck or from an ulcerated atheromatous plaque, producing transient or permanent vascular accidents. Depending on the affected artery, it will produce a lateral homonymous hemianopia, the Wallenberg syndrome, or complex attacks of the brainstem, characterized by a unilateral or bilateral pyramidal syndrome, sensory problems, cerebellar syn-

dromes, peripheral paralysis of one or more cranial nerves, and possibly dysphasia or dysarthria. A well-developed collateral circulation can avoid or limit these infarcts, but the two principal anastomotic systems are often insufficient. The posterior communicating arteries (which unite the carotid and vertebrobasilar systems) can be nonfunctional, and the basilar trunk is sometimes supplied by only one spinal artery, with the other ending in the inferior cerebellar artery. In view of their brainstem involvement and potential for producing tetraplegia, these infarcts with posterior circulatory topography are the most serious neurologic accidents and the most typical (but rare) accident seen with cervical manipulation. The treatment is anticoagulation, after ruling out the possibility of hemorrhage. The systematic practice of postural testing, the execution of gentle and precise maneuvers, and their contraindication in those suspect of harboring atheromata, constitute the best and most effective means of preventing these types of accidents.

Hemodynamic Vertebrobasilar Insufficiency

Rancurel describes a second type of vertebrobasilar insufficiency, the hemodynamic VBI. It has some special characteristics because of the very particular anatomy of the vertebrobasilar system. The spinal arteries behave like peripheral arteries, with systolic-diastolic pulsation and a low diastolic pressure. The inferior part of the basilar arterial trunk is hemodynamically fragile because it is a zone where the vertebrobasilar and carotid pressures are about equal. From that zone emerges a symmetric and paired artery that is particularly vulnerable because it is long and thin and supplied by a weak pressure; it is the middle cerebellar artery, which supplies the internal ear.

"Hemodynamic VBI" will manifest clinically if there is a decrease in the blood volume in the spinal artery, in general resulting from a spinal or subclavicular atheromatous stenosis. Its neurologic manifestations are brief, always the same in the same patient, and also "posturosensitive," happening only in the standing position when the diastolic pressure is lower than in the supine position as well as with abnormal neck posture (hyperextension, rotation). When these abnormal postures are performed passively, as is the case during postural testing, performed prior to any cervical manipulation, certain symptoms indicating relative ischemia in the territory of the middle cerebellar artery may be produced, even if the patient is lying down (Fig. 22.30):

- Central vestibular dysfunction, especially vertigo, whose pathologic characteristic is recognized if it is associated with other disorders
- Visual problems, diplopia, or blurred vision
- Brief loss of consciousness or poorly defined discomfort; signs that may not be recognized as a VBI unless there are other associated symptoms
- Hypoacusis with tinnitus and buzzing, which should be unilateral
- Amnesia
- Rarely, "drop attacks"

These attacks are usually brief (a few seconds to 5 minutes maximum). They are always stereotyped and disappear in the supine position. In 105 cases reported by Rancurel's group (Vitte et al.), with patients with an average age of 62 years, the following problems were noted: acute dysequilibrium (98%), visual problems such as amaurosis and amblyopia (23%), diplopia or blurred vision (36%), problems of vigilance or of consciousness (40%), drop attacks (19%), dysphasia followed by dysarthria (18%), and attacks of hypotonia or

hypokinesia (15%) along the way that are exceptionally isolated.

Spontaneous reproduction of these signs by "postural testing" (see below) presents an absolute contraindication for any manipulative treatment and requires an evaluation for the existence of a hemodynamic VBI. Four clinical elements are particularly suggestive:

- Posturosensitive character of the symptomatology
- Occurrence in brief and repeated attacks
- Presence of a supraclavicular bruit
- Reproduction of the syndrome by the compression of the spinal artery (Rancurel)

This compression at the triangle of Tillaux in the suboccipital region is performed with the thumbs, moving from right to left, and then, if necessary, to both sides for 20 seconds maximum, with the patient standing. The test is positive when the symptoms of the patient are reproduced (Fig. 22.31). The validity of this test has been aided by the use of Doppler ultrasonography.

Compression should be stopped immediately once symptoms are reported. The test can then be performed safely.

Electronystagmography is of diagnostic interest when it is performed with spinal compression. The typical abnormalities are (*a*) appearance or increase of saccadic movements on visual pursuit, (*b*) hypermetria of the saccadic movements (two-thirds of cases), or (*c*) their hypometria.

This examination supports the diagnosis of VBI and allows the selection of patients having to undergo an angiographic exploration. Doppler ultrasonography is a useful screening tool for the detection of spinal atheromata, carotid stenosis, or subclavian steal syndrome, but only angiography can show the exact location and the severity of that stenosis. Such lesions are, in some cases, amenable to surgical cure by bypass or endarterectomy. Published postoperative results are very satisfactory. Mixed forms can exist, as in thromboembolic VBI with hemodynamic VBI.

Vertebrobasilar Insufficiency due to Osteophytes Compressing the Spinal Artery

Even if vertebrobasilar insufficiency due to osteophytes compressing the spinal artery is

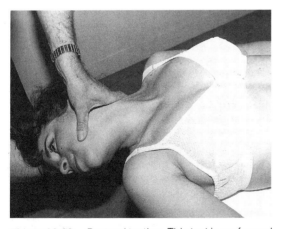

Figure 22.30. Postural testing. This test is performed with the patient supine, but it should also be performed with the patient seated (see text).

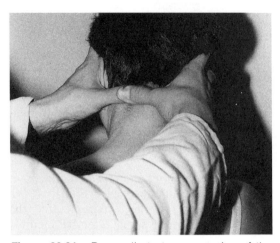

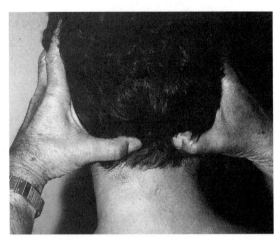

Figure 22.31. Rancurel's test: compression of the spinal artery in the triangle of Tillaux (see "Hemodynamic Vertebrobasilar Insufficiency," above). This test is performed with the patient standing. First, one side is examined, then the other side is examined (*left*). Finally, both sides are examined at the same time (*right*).

relatively rare, the mid or lower cervical spine can be directly responsible for circulatory compromise of the spinal artery caused by articular or uncinate process osteophytes compressing it. During some neck movements, paroxysmal attacks can be produced if compensation is not supplied by the rest of the vascular system. Arteriography will show the possible obstacle, and in some cases, surgical intervention (Jung) can free the artery and reestablish normal blood flow.

ACCIDENTS AND INCIDENTS OF SPINAL MANIPULATION

Reading the medical literature and the long chapters on "errors" and "accidents" in this book could lead one to believe that manipulative accidents happen frequently. In fact, manipulation practiced in a medical setting is a treatment with very few risks. In 25 years, with about 200,000 manipulations performed in our hospital, we have never had any significant or serious accident. For many years, manipulation was mentioned in the medical literature only as responsible for dramatic accidents. The literature sometimes emphasized the nonmedical status of the practitioner but always emphasized the association between manipulation and the accident.

Fortunately, things have changed, at least in France, thanks to the development of this therapeutic system in hospitals and to university teaching. There is no useful therapeutics without risks, and in some particular cases, some movements that are usually harmless can have dramatic consequences. Manipulation, when applied to old and frail spines, is not inoffensive if the examiner does not have perfect

---

Signs of Vertebrobasilar Insufficiency

Vertebrobasilar insufficiency is an absolute contraindication to the use of cervical manipulation. Its signs (listed below according to Rancurel and Vitte) should be very well known.

- **Headache:** benign, often occipital
- **Vestibular problems**
  —Positional rotary vertigo
  —Episodic vertigo of central origin
- **Visual problems:** often temporary
  —Blurred vision
  —Diplopia
  —Amaurosis
- **Concentration and loss-of-consciousness problems**
  —Syncopal episodes
  —Temporary periods of coma
- **Motor problems**
  —Drop attacks
  —Transient hemiparesis
- **Auditory problems**
  —Deafness
  —Hypoacusis

technique or cannot measure the maneuvers properly.

Dramatic Accidents

In the French experience, dramatic accidents are mostly the results of maneuvers executed by nonphysicians. Common to most dramatic accidents, some of them fatal, is a mistake in the diagnosis or an absence of diagnosis. It is the brutal manipulation of a cervical spine with Pott's disease, with metastases, or with a fracture that will lead to sudden death or quadriplegia. It is the forced manipulation of a thoracic or lumbar spine with spondyloarthropathy or of a spine that has become frail due to disease that will result in paraplegia. Such are the most frequent, although rare, dramatic accidents.

Besides the accidents in which the error of diagnosis is flagrant, however, we are aware of the possibility of postmanipulative vascular accidents happening even in the absence of any predisposing factors that could be clinically or radiologically discovered (Cambier). In general, these are due to thrombosis of the trunk of the spinal artery or of the posteroinferior cerebellar artery (Wallenberg syndrome), whose evolution can be fatal or result in significant sequelae. These vascular accidents happen in patients with a VBI whose signs can be very subtle initially. The initial lesions affect the spinal artery: intimal tears, subintimal hematomas, pseudoaneurysm. It is possible that the manipulation produces a transitory protective muscle guarding that is the initial occurrence; then, either by migration of an embolus, resulting from intimal lesions, or by parietal edema, or by a process of an aneurysm dissection, the occlusion of arteries downstream occurs.

The consequences of these dramatic accidents are serious: death in 25% of cases and severe neurologic sequelae in 50% of cases, with only mild sequelae or a complete cure in 25% of cases (Ali Cherif). The victims are often women under 40 years of age, which means that atherosclerosis plays a less prominent role than had been thought. The contributory role of the birth control pill has been emphasized; 70% of vascular accidents due to the pill happen in the first year of its being taken. In these patients, a progressive headache can be the warning sign of a thrombosis. Most of the observations that have been reported take the following course. During the manipulation, malaise or nausea occurs; then there is a free interval; then the picture is formed rapidly and progressively, revealing an extensive thrombosis, with spinal cord, brainstem, or cerebellar symptomatology. The Wallenberg syndrome is the typical picture of these accidents and is characterized by the following.

- Ipsilateral to the lesion: cranial nerves IX and X are affected, resulting in a ipsilateral paralysis of the muscles of the palate, pharynx, and vocal cords; the descending root of V and the sympathetic fibers are affected, producing a hemianesthesia of the face and Horner's syndrome; and a cerebellar disorder producing hemiataxia and vertigo.
- Contralateral to the lesion: the spinothalamic tract is affected, producing a decrease in the pain and temperature sensation of the trunk and limbs.

At higher levels, the "locked-in syndrome" (i.e., motor deafferentation) may occur, usually corresponding to a lesion of the brainstem, due to infarction or basilar thrombosis. In this syndrome, there is association of quadriplegia and paralysis of the last cranial nerve with conservation of ocular movement in the vertical direction. Consciousness is also preserved. The prognosis for such patients is very poor. A typical observation (Ali Cherif) is reported in the following case history.

Case History. A 51-year-old male presented with brief episodes of vertigo and a temporary diplopia. Cervical manipulation was followed by nausea. Over the next 24 hours, his condition worsened, progressing from right hemiplegia to quadriplegia and then coma. He was hospitalized, and the examination revealed a lesion of the brainstem. Death followed. The postmortem examination demonstrated an old occlusion of a spinal artery and a recent thrombosis of the other spinal artery.

But here is the often-cited observation by Ford and Clark.

Case History. A 37-year-old bacteriologist, coming home one evening, found that his wife was twisting her head from side to side with her hands, which were placed on either side of her head. She claimed that her neck was stiff and that this made it feel better. He asked her to do the same for him. She twisted it strongly to one side. He then said, "That feels better.

Do it again." She did so, and he staggered and fell. Vertigo occurred, with vomiting, ocular and auditory problems on the right side, stiffening of the left arm, and sphincter dysfunction. The next day, he was admitted to Johns Hopkins Hospital where examination revealed an obtunded level of consciousness with dysphasia and dysphagia, no weakness but a tendency to fall to the left, an ataxia of a cerebellar type, an inequality of the pupils with a ptosis of the left eyelid, and horizontal nystagmus. His condition deteriorated rapidly. The patient died 60 hours after the accident. The autopsy revealed thrombosis of the basilar artery, of the left posterior cerebral artery, and of the left posteroinferior cerebellar artery.

Treatment consists of anticoagulation started as soon as possible. Such particularly serious accidents have occurred most often in patients who were treated for a benign disorder having nothing to do with the spine. As a rule, these accidents are due to powerful maneuvers, usually repeated. But softer maneuvers, especially if they are repeated and maintained, can have similar consequences. Besides, in some people, activities performed in a prolonged and awkward head position (e.g., a plumber working under a sink or an automobile mechanic working under a dashboard) can produce vascular accidents of the cerebral trunk (Alajouanine et al.). When ipsilateral neck hyperextension and rotation are performed simultaneously, there is an interruption to flow in the contralateral spinal artery (Kleyn and Nieuwenhuyse). This has been confirmed by angiography. Tatlow and Bammer were able to be more precise, noting that the interruption occurred at the atlanto-occipital joint. This did not occur in normal subjects, as the regional circulation is, fortunately, easily supplied. But in the case where there is only one spinal artery and it is thrombosed, the blood supply is compromised and the accident occurs. This is a very serious accident, and even when there is recovery, usually it is slow and incomplete. The accident can be fatal.

Other neurologic complications have been reported; for example, thrombosis of the carotid (Boldrey, Maas, and Miller) or compression of the spinal cord, producing quadriplegia or paraplegia. Manipulation can also unmask or aggravate preexisting occult lesions (neoplastic, Pott's disease, unrecognized fracture, etc.)

Serious Accidents

Serious accidents are not rare in the hands of ignorant or awkward examiners. They are due to a lack of diagnosis and often a technical mistake (e.g., a lever arm that is wrongly applied, a forced maneuver performed blindly, or manipulation in the wrong direction). They can also be due to aggravation of the treated disorder: torticollis or low back pain sciatica becoming hyperalgic or refractory. They can also transform torticollis into cervicobrachial neuralgias, or low back pain syndromes into severe sciatica, or benign sciatica into paralysis during the same session. Rib fractures without displacement are often due to awkward examiners, but they can also be seen in the work of good practitioners, as the 11th and 12th ribs are very fragile under some angles of pressure. Costal sprains, produced by some maladapted maneuvers, are more frequent and often foster refractory pain syndromes. More rarely, there is the possibility of purpura after manipulation (Tomlinson). We have seen such a case—a very extended purpura on the legs, the day following a lumbar manipulation for a benign traumatic low back pain that had otherwise been very well relieved.

Incidents

Incidents are extremely frequent if the examiner is not well trained. We should emphasize the inconvenience they cause some patients as a result of their durability, duration, and refractory character. Wrongly performed manipulation can create all the symptoms that examiners are able to treat.

Maneuvers performed on the cervical spine can result in a refractory headache absolutely identical with the one that is an indication for manipulative therapy. Patients are frequently seen who complain of cervical pain, low back pain, and thoracic pain that occurred during a session of manipulation and from which they did not suffer before the session. Such pain can be due to a benign incident that is easy to correct at the next session or can be due to a maneuver that was a little too forceful. Most often, however, these incidents are due to spinal sprains, costospinal sprains, or disk injury that is refractory and that has resulted from a maneuver performed with use of the wrong supports and in the wrong direction. These incidents, produced because of forced maneuvers, are difficult to treat. The examiner needs a great deal of patience and the use of very soft and progressive movements, as the patients, already alerted, fear any passive movement.

Prevention of Accidents: Postural and Rancurel's Tests

Almost all accidents due to manipulation can be avoided if the diagnosis is correct, the indication is well chosen, the correct direction of the manipulation is respected, and the execution of that manipulation is technically perfect.

Obviously, only an examiner who is totally educated in spinal pathology and in manipulative techniques and their use can practice this therapeutic system without risk and with regular results for the patients. As far as the delicate problem of vascular accidents of the vertebrobasilar trunk is concerned (whose diagnosis is not always easy to make), these accidents should be avoided if the history and physical examination have not uncovered the suspect signs that we have described, by using postural and Rancurel's tests as we propose, and most importantly, by abstaining from any manipulative treatment when in doubt.

Postural Testing

The postural test consists of maintaining the superior cervical spine of the patient in a position of hyperextension, with first right then left rotation for a few seconds, interrupted immediately at the least feeling of vertigo or nystagmus (Fig. 22.30), whose occurrence calls for the greatest caution. This test is performed with the patient in the supine and the sitting positions.

Rancurel's Test

As discussed above, Rancurel's test (Fig. 22.31) consists of compressing the spinal arteries in Tillaux's triangle, with the patient standing.

Medical Responsibility

The physician's responsibility in the matter of manipulation has been very well analyzed by Roussat from the point of view of French law. It is no different from the other acts a physician is called upon to practice in this domain, but some experts have a totally hostile attitude to this form of treatment. However, a physician who prescribes spinal manipulation to be performed by a nonphysician or who covers the activity of a nonphysician could be charged with "illegal exercise of medicine" (Cass. Crim. 10 April 1964, Bull. Crim. n105, p. 236). In case of accident, the physician is responsible. Manipulation is a delicate and often difficult therapy to perform; it is a typical medical act in which the physician, in deciding and then in performing the act, engages all of his or her knowledge and takes all of the responsibility. It is not simply an act of prescribing; besides, prescribing is impossible, qualitatively and quantitatively.

MECHANISM OF ACTION OF MANIPULATION

If there is still some mystery about the way manipulations work, it is because we still do not know enough about most of the disorders that they relieve. What do we know about the exact pathogenesis of acute torticollis, postural thoracic pain, benign low back pain, and coccygodynia, to cite only a few of the current indications of manipulation?

The responsibility for this ignorance is not to be ascribed to the therapeutics or to those who use it. The other treatment modalities used in these disorders often result in less effective results and are no better justified. The classical concepts in spinal pathology do not help one to understand the action of manipulation that relieves some pain syndromes quickly and well.

That is why it is necessary to appeal to the hypothesis of a reversible disorder; i.e., a wrong movement creates it, and a right movement corrects it. It is from this perspective that the "displaced vertebra" of the bonesetter (a "folk" manipulator often found in rural areas), the "subluxation" of the chiropractor, and the somatic dysfunction of the osteopaths have been cited. Most schools of manual medicine in the world, such as the school of osteopathy, consider that this reversible mechanical disorder is due to hypomobility of the concerned vertebra, restored by manipulation. There is nothing more apparently logical.

Unfortunately, this perturbation cannot, except in rare cases, be demonstrated by radiographic or dynamic cineradiographic examinations. It is detected and analyzed by a refined system of palpations whose validity is unproven not because of the reality of the modification of the tissues palpated but because of the interpretation of the examiner.

It is the critical analysis of these facts that brought us to the concept of "painful minor intervertebral dysfunctions" (PMIDs), in which only the pain of the segment is considered when it is produced by exactly described palpational maneuvers, with these maneuvers being painless on the other segments. When the manipulation results in a satisfying effect, the segment returns to its painless state and simultaneously the patient is relieved of the local or referred pain that was the cause for the required treatment.

Therefore, to discuss the mode of action of the maneuvers for most of their indications requires an understanding of the mechanism of segmental dysfunction, about which we can only hypothesize (see Chapter 17, "Painful Minor Intervertebral Dysfunctions"). Not only is manipulation a treatment for PMIDs, it also produces relief in disorders such as common sciatica, where the role of disk lesions has been described. One can, in that case, ask whether the mechanism of action is then different and, if it is, wonder when the manipulation relieves a coccygodynia or a costal sprain. Disk pathology has been widely studied, and its lesions are perfectly well known. But the mechanism of pain relief by manipulation in sciatica is unclear. Let us first look at the effects of manipulation on a spine that is considered normal.

Effects of Manipulation on the Normal Spine

By normal spine, we mean a spine in which no movement is limited or painful and no vertebra or paraspinal region is experiencing any spontaneous pain, with the radiographic studies also being normal. If, for example, cervical maneuvers are executed on such a spine, there can be no action and no reaction; sometimes, however, axillary perspiration can be seen immediately.

Thus on a normal spine, a well-performed manipulation (the risk of a wrongly performed manipulation is not to be neglected) does not cause any particular phenomenon, any more than a manipulation performed to unlock a blocked meniscus would have any effect on a normal knee.

The localized perspiration suggests action of manipulation on the sympathetic system. There are also other actions such as abdominal disturbances and alterations of menstrual periods. Manipulation can have mechanical and reflex effects. Its mechanical effects are

- To restore normal mobility in a stiffened joint as is performed, although less efficiently, by classical mobilization, when the joint has lost a part of its joint play.
- To treat a reversible mechanical dysfunction, articular or periarticular, as, for example, release of a meniscal blocking of the knee. Its reflex effects are to produce a reflex or vasomotor action by the forceful or strenuous stretching of the muscles, tendons, articular capsule, and ligaments.

Possible Mechanical Factors

Disk Lesions

In the case of disk protrusions and the related acute low back pain syndrome, one can imagine that manipulation tends to reinstate the center of the disk to the displaced disk fragment. On the other hand, in the case of a herniated disk that causes a sciatica, it is less likely that the manipulation can "put back" the hernia. Chrisman et al. have studied 39 patients with sciatica who were relieved by manipulation. They found no change in radiologic images performed before and after the treatment, even when the latter showed a marked compression and relief was maintained for 3 years or longer. Farfan thinks that 30–40% of patients relieved of sciatica by manipulation show the same radiologic findings before and after the manipulative treatment. We have made the same observation. One might imagine in these cases that manipulation slightly alters the relation of the herniation and the nerve root in a favorable way, without leading to even partial resorption of the herniation. The truth is that it is difficult to put the toothpaste back into the toothpaste tube!

But even admitting that attenuation or suppression of the impingement of the disk upon the nerve root or posterior longitudinal ligament could be possible, one would think that it could not last and that the painful phenomena would come back very quickly. However, the relief is often lasting.

The logical hypothesis is that manipulation, by separating even very temporarily the antagonists, makes it possible during that short period to obtain a decrease or a disappearance of the inflammatory phenomena responsible for pain.

Is the mechanism that results in pain as quickly reversible? The manipulative practice offers, in a little different domain, the demonstration that it is possible to have a rapid change in some physiopathologic phenomena. When a manipulation is performed in the treatment of a thoracic PMID with cellulalgia in the dermatome of the corresponding posterior ramus, one can notice (sometimes in less than a minute) the clear decrease and even the disappearance of the pain on the "pinch-roll maneuver" and of the thickening of the fold. This fold, which was thick and edematous, rapidly becomes supple and painless.

Although the inflammatory reaction of discoradicular impingement differs from reflex cellulalgia, though the role of the inflammatory mediators is credible in both cases, this example demonstrates the rapidity with which some phenomena can regress. There was also the hypothesis that manipulation acted on some intradiscal blockings, releasing a painful dysfunction of the segment, or on some facet joint "blockings" or "rubbings."

Some authors believe that there may be some incarcerated nuclear fragments in annular fissures, which would not compress any sensitive element and would not produce any direct symptom. But by leading to dysfunction of the mobile segment, these intradiscal blockings could make it less mobile and cause acute or chronic dysfunction of another part of that segment, especially at the facet joint.

By modifying the position of the fragment that was displaced, the spinal segment would again have a normal play. This mechanism, if it exists, can involve only a fraction of the cases that are treated and can be considered only at the inferior lumbar level or at the inferior cervical level, the most common location of disk herniations.

Facet Joint Lesions

With the facet joints, we are in a domain that is much more hypothetical than that of the disk lesions, even if it seems that the perturbations start especially at their level—perturbations that manipulation treats very efficiently. A certain number of authors have tried to explain the action of the manipulation in "a facet joint blockage."

The intra-articular blocking of a meniscoid formation has been consider by some; Zuckschwerdt et al. were the first (1955) to express this hypothesis. The "theory of incarceration" had some supporters (Keller, Hadley, Kos, and Lewit), but others were against this explanation (Terrier, Dörr, Penning, Töndury, etc.).

Kos showed that the cartilage lining the facet joints can easily be deformed. He experimentally made imprints on its surface by pressing steel marbles, other materials, and hairs on the cartilage. The prints he obtained were clear but temporary (5 minutes for the hairs). On the other hand, he noticed that the top of the meniscoid formations was thicker and harder than the rest (chondroid zone) (Fig. 2.6). He then suggested that during an excessive movement, the meniscoid formation could be entrapped in the joint. The free and hard extremity compressing the cartilage would create a socket in which it could be retained. There would then be excessive traction on the joint capsule where the base of the meniscoid formation is inserted. Irritation of the capsular mechanoreceptors would produce a reflex muscular contraction that would increase the pressure while maintaining the blocking. Only a manipulation aiming at separating the two articular surfaces could free the included fragment.

Bogduk, who later studied the anatomy of the meniscoid formation, thought that only a few of them have a form that would allow such a mechanism. He also thought that such a wedging could not be produced because the base of the formation is loose and that sufficient pulling on the capsule would be necessary to produce pain.

Can the role of the meniscoid formations be considered in chronic cases? For Emminger, these meniscoid formations could show all the "possible effects of wear, be the seat of spondylosis, be the victim of trauma, etc. Some of them could remain wedged." Manipulation could free them "if there was not already some fixed chronic problems." Töndury could not find convincing evidence proving the evolution because of age, but "during the wear of the cartilaginous covering, the meniscoid formations undergo stress from a mechanical point of view, and thus wear considerably. Small fragments can even slip into the joint." But because of their usual thinness, it does not seem to cause blockage.

Other mechanisms could predispose to a facet joint blockage. Gillot has noted the frequency of the irregularities of the cartilaginous surface of these joints. He noted, as did Freudenberg, the frequent presence of transverse crests in the inferior lumbar spine. Farfan thought that they were the consequence of a progressive dysfunction of the mobile segment and were linked to disk deterioration, but he does not believe that they have a role in blockage (see "Possible Role of the Discal or Facet Joint Pathology" in Chapter 17).

The Reflex Factor

The purely mechanical action of manipulation is a convenient hypothesis for now. But even in the cases where it seems probable, one should also consider a reflex effect to understand all of the observed phenomena. The supporters of the theory of facet joint blockage due to a lesion of the meniscoid formations also give an essential role to the reflex contraction in maintaining the vicious cycle.

But is the presence of a permanent mechanical lesion in the facet joints a necessary condition for its pain and the starting point of the excitation of the neural receptors? A benign sprain of the fingers remains painful for a long time to the least pressure and the least torsion, while flexion-extension is free and often painless, and there is no detectable mechanical le-

sion. This can also be the case in the facet joints.

Any dysfunction of the innervated elements of the spinal segment, particularly the posterior longitudinal ligament, facet joints, interspinous ligament, and muscles, produces a reflex action that tends to immobilize or, better, to limit segmental motion. In this reaction, one would think that protective muscle guarding plays an essential role. As we have seen in Chapter 17 on PMID, a temporary dysfunction of a spinal segment can, in some conditions, become chronic because of the very particular and strictly automatic character of the functioning of the spine.

The facet joints can be the starting point of that dysfunction; and if the facet joint is not, itself, the initial cause, it is the victim. Moreover, this maintained protective muscle guarding strains the intrinsic segmental muscles, which then become a source of nociceptive influx. We have previously emphasized the particular relationships between the muscular bundles of the intertransverse muscle and the internal and external branches of the posterior ramus of the spinal nerve. These branches penetrate the bundles of that muscle and course around the transverse process. They innervate them after giving off some articular branches. A mechanism of discomfort in the neural foramina as a result of muscles permanently in protective muscle guarding is possible, as the medial branch passes through an osseofibrous tunnel (see Chapter 8, "Innervation of the Spinal Structures").

This explains the fact that the cutaneous area of the posterior ramus is almost always the source of modifications in texture and sensitivity when there is a segmental dysfunction, by PMID in particular. This cellulalgia localized in the area of the posterior dermatome is, indeed, the manifestation, the most frequent and the earliest of the "segmental spinal neurotrophic syndrome."

Whatever is the mechanical support considered to explain a reversible blockage of the mobile segment, the reflex muscular dysfunction plays an important role. Besides, in some cases, relaxing a tense muscle by using manual techniques or local anesthetic injection relieves an acute or chronic spinal pain. Manipulation or stretching the muscle can also achieve the same goal, but it also produces a sharp traction on tissues that are rich in proprioceptors: tendons, ligaments, articular capsule. When performed in the correct direction, it produces a powerful inhibitory reflex at the spinal cord level. It is thought that it is a presynaptic inhibition of nociceptive impulses in the posterior horn of the spinal gray matter. But, to us, this inhibitory reflex seems possible only if the directed traction is performed in the direction of "no pain," opposite to the painful direction, producing an intense stimulation of the corresponding mechanoreceptors.

Articular Cracking and Gapping

Manipulation is, indeed, a very particular movement. Unsworth et al. (see "Cracking," above) have studied the mechanism of the articular cracking and have concluded that it was the result of the phenomenon of cavitation. But some other conclusions can be drawn from their studies. They showed that the manner in which joint gapping was produced determined a difference between the "cracking" joints and the ones that do not "crack" when they are submitted to identical forces of traction.

The noncracking joints have a progressive gapping proportional to the power of the traction. The cracking ones, on the other hand, do not separate during the traction until a point at which, nearly instantaneously and suddenly, this separation becomes maximal, which is equal to that obtained by a progressive gapping. The sudden separation corresponds to the noise of the cracking.

In both cases, when the traction stops, the return to the normal position follows the same progressive curve. The terminal articular gapping in both cases is slightly greater than it was at the start. This experiment, though it did not have that aim, demonstrates well that the ultrarapid, explosive stretching obtained when the joint cracks—the manipulation—thus has an effect on the periarticular and muscular structures that is different from the progressive stretching produced by mobilization. Without doubt, this particular reflex effect gives manipulation the essential aspects of its effectiveness.

23

SPINAL TRACTION

Spinal traction is a therapeutic modality that is applied via an apparatus that exerts a distractive force in line with the axis of the spinal column. The use of spinal traction dates back to the time of Hippocrates, Galen, and Aesculapius, with very exact descriptions of the technique in their writing. Some illustrations show patients who are firmly attached to the apparatus while axial traction is applied by the use of ropes, winches, and levers. In most of these drawings, one of the operators also applies simultaneous pressure to what appears to be a hump.

Traction is a treatment modality used in the treatment of mechanical pain of spinal origin. Although they have some common indications, the indications for traction are more restrictive than are those for manipulation. However, traction is less frequently useful, and its action is clearly slower.

The operator who can master manipulations finds that traction has very limited application, which is unfortunate because traction is much less difficult and tiring for the operator!

MODE OF APPLICATION

Lumbar traction is usually performed on a specifically designed traction table. Under specific conditions, it can be performed with the patient in bed. Cervical traction can be performed with the patient on a table, on an inclined plane, in bed, or in sitting.

Traction can be continuous; with the patient in bed, it is performed for periods of several hours per day. Most often, it is intermittent. A typical session lasts 10–30 minutes, with a frequency varying from twice a day to twice a week. Traction can be maintained continuously during the whole session or applied intermittently, with the maximal traction maintained for only a brief period. The traction is thus applied in a cycle, gradually increasing the distractive load and gradually releasing it until no tension is applied. The choice of method is case dependent.

Traction Table

A typical traction table is depicted in Figure 23.1. It is composed of a stationary surface (to which the thorax has been fastened by straps) as well as a lumbar surface that is mobile. Movement of the inferior surface will create traction of the lumbar spine. This traction can be applied in different ways: with weights or by rolling up a rope on a windlass. With these procedures, there is an inconvenience: the traction and especially the detraction are irregular.

It is preferable to have the surfaces spaced by a crankshaft, or better, by an hydraulic system or by a motor. The results are independent of the system's mechanics. An automated system is more regular than a manual one, maybe a little less measurable, but easier for the operator. The traction speed should be variable; it should be weak, especially at the end of the traction (an average of 3 mm/min for the lumbar spine and 2 mm/min for the cervical spine).

CERVICAL TRACTION

Application

The patient's head is held by a collar with occipitomental support, such as Sayre's collar (Fig. 23.2) or Maigne's cervitractor (Fig. 23.2), which has the advantage of applying pressure

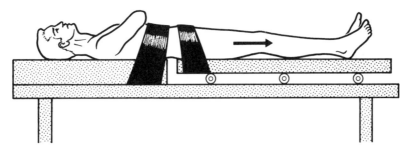

Figure 23.1.   Traction table.

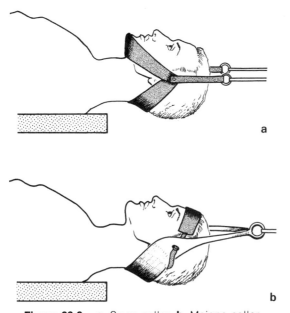

Figure 23.2.   a, Sayre collar. **b,** Maigne collar.

neither to the chin nor to the temporomandibular joints, but which does not adjust to patients who are too brachycephalic or whose occipital prominences are too flat. Under these conditions it tends to slip during traction. In spite of this inconvenience (not frequent in practice), it is more comfortable because it allows the patient to talk and does not require removal of dental apparatus.

Traction on an Inclined Plane

On an inclined plane, the weight of the body supplies the force of traction. Since the force of traction is limited by the friction of the body against the table, the table should be as smooth as possible. Varying the inclination of the plane varies the force of traction. This simple system is convenient, the patient is generally relaxed, and the traction is rather easily measured (Fig. 23.3).

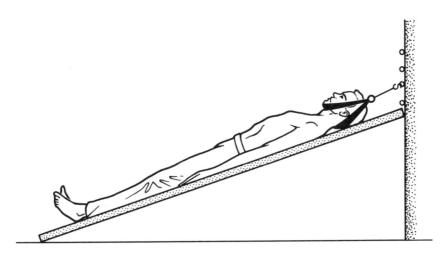

Figure 23.3.   Cervical traction on an inclined plane.

Traction on a Special Table

The patient lies supine with the shoulders maintained by straps. Traction is performed either by weights or by a crankshaft or hydraulic system. Here the traction becomes efficacious quickly; therefore, it should be very slow, very progressive, and very well controlled (Fig. 23.1).

Traction in Sitting

The patient is seated on a special table, fastened either at the pelvis or the shoulders. The collar is fixed on a pole just above the patient's head. This is a very comfortable position.

LUMBAR TRACTION

In lumbar traction, the thorax and the pelvis should be fastened.

Fastening the Thorax

There is no perfect way to fasten the thorax, and generally, a corset is used to help. It is a complex problem because the thorax is elastic and compressible, and a strong compression is uncomfortable. Strong pressure is applied to the epigastrium, which can be uncomfortable. Traction should not be performed immediately after a meal. At the start of traction, there is always a certain slippage that is difficult to avoid and which should be limited.

Fastening the Pelvis

There are fewer difficulties with fastening the pelvis. Several systems of corsets are used, but obese patients create some problems that are difficult to overcome. The table we have designed (1959) has a very convenient system that readily fixates the iliac crests and increases this grasp in proportion to the traction (Figs. 23.4 and 23.5). The attachment should be comfortable and not be able to slip. It should be easy to put on and remove.

Application of Traction

Traction should be applied slowly, progressively, and if necessary, gradually. The patient should feel relieved under traction. In no case, should pain increase; if it does, the treatment should be halted. The maximum amount of traction applied is determined by the tolerance

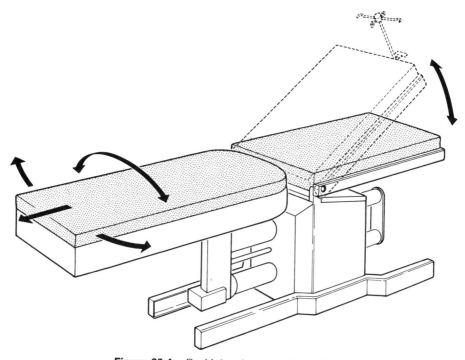

Figure 23.4. Dr. Maigne's examining table.

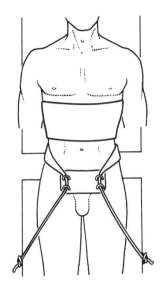

Figure 23.5. System for lumbar traction (Dr. Maigne's table).

of the patient and the resulting relief. The rate of release of traction (detraction) should be gradual, slower than the traction. If pain recurs during detraction, the rate of detraction should be slowed and sometimes followed by enough mild traction to suppress the pain.

Traction in Bed

Bed rest is often prescribed for treatment of acute lumbar pain and sciatica. It is tempting to increase the effect of the rest by continuous traction to suppress or decrease pain. Continuous traction in bed is tolerated poorly, and patient compliance is low. Chantraine et al. have devised a simple apparatus that is easy to carry, which they called the "automotor frame." The patient, lying in bed, performs au-

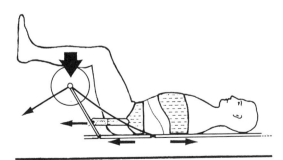

Figure 23.6. Chantraine's apparatus for applyiing lumbar traction.

totraction by pushing the legs, which are flexed on a roller. This allows autotraction to be performed in bed comfortably for 15–30 minutes, repeated during the day (Fig. 23.6).

MODE OF ACTION OF TRACTION

Most authors seem to think that the aim of traction is to increase the intervertebral spacing. It is true that with sufficient traction, the vertebral end plates can be separated measurably. However it would be simplistic to believe that the relief is due to the induction of intervertebral disk separation. Furthermore, traction can occasionally increase the pain. It is more sensible to consider two possible complimentary modes of action: a mechanical action and a reflex action.

Mechanical Action

The traction separates the involved spinal segments.

Reflex Action

The stretching that is performed, if it is not painful, reflexively relieves the protective muscle guarding by stimulating segmental mechanoreceptors.

Thus the goal of traction is not to stretch to the maximum, but rather, in a manner that causes the pain to disappear. Maintenance of painless traction may decrease the degree of inflammation and vasocongestion, and in some favorable cases, they do not completely return when the traction is loosened. Conversely, if traction is painful, it should be discontinued immediately; if it does not bring relief during the session, it is useless to continue.

We thought that orientation of the traction (1959), which could maintain the minimal optimal traction on a given spinal segment, might have a better effect and would relieve a greater number of patients. With this in mind, we designed a suitable table. The thoracic surface can be raised or lowered; the pelvic surface is mobile laterally and in rotation. One finds the position of lateroflexion and flexion in which the patient is best relieved using minimal traction. This traction is then progressively increased and is maintained for about 10 minutes; then the pelvic surface is slowly put back into its normal position. The axial traction is increased for 3–4 minutes, and the detraction is performed very slowly. This has produced good results in cases in which the axial traction was inefficient. This table brings better relief to the patient, especially because of the system of pelvic positioning (Fig. 23.5) and the ability to slightly incline the thoracic surface of some acute lumbar patients who cannot sustain the strict lying position.

INDICATIONS FOR TRACTION

The usual indication for traction is radicular pain of spinal origin. We have had the best results with cervicobrachial neuralgia, femoral neuralgia, sciatica (to a lesser degree), cervical pain, and lumbar pain.

Cervical Spine

Before prescribing traction, a manual test must be used to determine whether traction on the neck relieves the patient or increases the pain. Manual traction is performed according to the technique shown in Figure 23.7. If the maneuver increases pain, no traction is performed; if it clearly relieves the pain, then traction is a valuable treatment.

A certain number of cases of cervicobrachial neuralgia cannot be treated by manipulation, because the rule of "no pain and of the opposite movement" cannot be applied. They are relieved by manual traction and can thus benefit from that treatment.

On the other hand, one can use both manip-

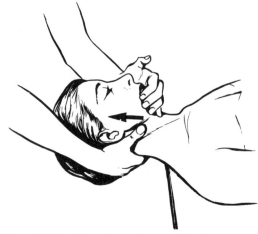

Figure 23.7. Manual traction test. It is important to perform this test before prescribing cervical traction. Traction is indicated if it helps reduce pain, and it is contraindicated if it exacerbates pain.

ulation and traction. These treatments can be performed separately; for example, traction daily and a manipulation once or twice a week for 2 weeks. They can also be performed together in the same session, but then it is better to minimize the manipulative maneuvers. In the upper cervical spine, traction is rarely useful.

Lumbar Spine

Continuous traction in bed has been used historically for severe sciatica treated in hospital. Intermittent traction can be used when manipulation cannot be performed because of contraindication or because of a lack of an experienced manipulator.

24

MASSAGE

Massage is a very effective modality for treating pain of spinal origin, when used appropriately. Lately, however, it has been much maligned. First there were the orthopedists who thought it was necessary to use an active physical modality in the osteoarthritic and traumatic conditions, and they did not consider massage to be a useful treatment. Then there was a lack of scientific evidence to validate its efficacy. This gap appears difficult to fill, since massage is performed by many different techniques, for various indications, and the choice and the execution of these techniques is highly operator dependent. But the main reason for a lack of interest in massage is that most masseurs, physiotherapists, and especially their teachers are no longer attracted to this form of treatment. Too many of them do not consider it useful, but simply tiring and of little value.

A good massage, it is true, is difficult to perform. It is useful only if it is well tailored to the patient, which requires some knowledge and experience. It means that a massage is only as good as the masseur who does it, which does not make it amenable to scientific study according to present criteria. In any event, a well-executed "massage," with the appropriate indications, is an extremely valuable therapeutic modality that is far too often neglected. For pain of spinal origin, massage relaxes the paraspinal muscles and relieves the cellulomyalgic manifestations of local or spinal origin.

MASSAGE FOR PARASPINAL MUSCLE RELAXATION

Acute Muscle Spasm

In torticollis (acute wryneck) and low back pain syndromes, massage can noticeably decrease the muscle spasm or protective muscle guarding. In some cases, it can even make it disappear completely and halt the vicious pain-spasm cycle.

Executing the maneuver is a matter of experience. It produces a kind of "dialogue" between the hand of the masseur and the muscle of the patient (Dolto). The hand should sense the reactions of the muscle and thus find the maneuver that is most useful. Relaxing maneuvers are always slow and progressive and are usually associated with stretching the muscular fibers that are hypertonic, with a slight mobilization in the pain-free direction.

Chronic Muscle Spasm

In any chronic spinal pain, there is always protective guarding of the paraspinal muscles. Palpation is facilitated if the skin has been lubricated beforehand. Two techniques are used: maneuvers that employ "deep gliding" parallel to the line of the spinous processes, and maneuvers that employ transverse stretching. These maneuvers are performed in a mea-

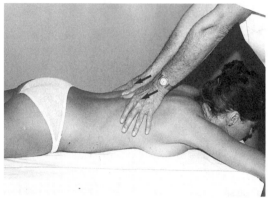

Figure 24.1. Massage to relax paraspinal muscles. This maneuver is performed in a gliding fashion, with pressure continuously applied from the upper back to the lower lumbar region.

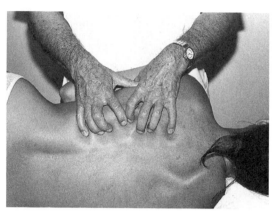

Figure 24.2. Petrissage and stretching of paravertebral muscles, with the patient lying on her side.

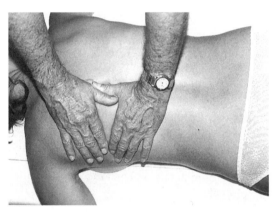

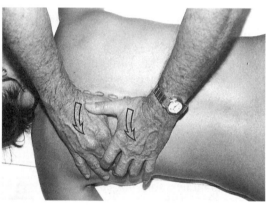

Figure 24.3. Petrissage and stretching of paraspinal muscles. Note the position of the thumb that "kneads" the muscles. *Left,* starting position. *Right,* terminal position. The maneuver should be performed slowly and rhythmically with resting periods.

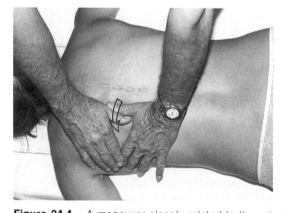

Figure 24.4. A maneuver closely related to the prior point of contact in applying the massage. maneuver. Here the thenar eminences are used as the

sured way, slow, rhythmic, and progressive, which is adjusted to the reaction of the muscles. They are useful before manipulative therapy. They can also be used alone. They are especially useful in cases of persistent deep muscle spasm after a treatment by manipulation or injection (Figs. 24.1–24.4).

The most useful techniques are described for each region, with the techniques of manipulation, as "maneuvers of relaxation" (see "Appendices of Manual Techniques").

MASSAGE AND CELLULOTENO-PERIOSTEOMYALGIC MANIFESTATIONS

Massage is a useful treatment of cellulalgic edema and trigger points. It can also be indicated in some ligamentous and tenoperiosteal pain syndromes.

When these manifestations are part of a spinal cellulotenoperiosteomyalgic syndrome, their local treatment is indicated only after the spinal treatment has been performed; the latter often suffices to resolve these manifestations.

Cellulalgia

First the cellulalgic zone is mobilized gently in all directions, as if it had to be detached. Then, very progressively, the operator executes some gentle superficial "kneading" maneuvers, superficially, without using too much force on the most painful zones and nodules. Finally, the maneuvers become more forceful, and the nodules can be progressively kneaded.

The most used maneuvers are the ones derived from Wetterwald's techniques: rolled, stretched, broken, and compressed skinfolds, which are very well known thanks to Dolto (Figs. 24.5 and 24.6). These alternate with superficial and relaxational maneuvers. For instance, prolonged and progressive subcutaneous tissue massage can be performed, paying particular attention to the peripheral zones and alternating with muscular maneuvers aiming at the bulk of the muscle and the tenoperiosteal insertions.

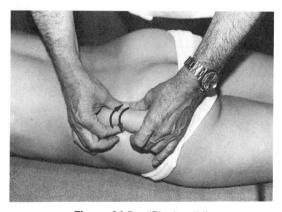

Figure 24.5.   "Pinch roll."

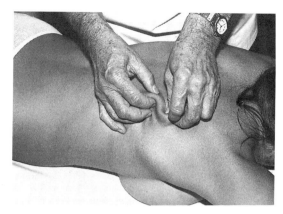

Figure 24.6.   "Skin folding."

Trigger Points

In the limbs, the most useful and most adequate maneuvers are the ones that use deep gliding. Often it is beneficial to alternate stretching with these maneuvers (Fig. 24.7).

The most sensitive indurated zone should not be approached directly, but progressively. The maneuvers should be progressive, with very little pressure in the beginning; they should not provoke acute pain.

These trigger points are found most often in the muscles of the external iliac fossae. They usually result from dysfunction of the lower lumbar spine. Here the best technique is deep kneading (Fig. 24.8); the maneuvers should be slow, with progressive pressure. They can occasionally be painful, but the pain subsides when the operator stops. During the session, pain should decrease progressively; besides, it is a particular pain that the patients like to call "a pain that feels good." If pain increases despite adjustment of the technique, that maneuver should be stopped.

Rhythm and pressure are measured by the muscle response. If favorable, the taut bands relax under the finger. Postural stretching is performed with the massage. Subsequent sessions reveal that the taut muscle fibers are smaller and have less tonicity, indicating that they will disappear with a few treatments.

If no improvement is noted with these maneuvers, it is useless to continue; their cause persists.

Pressure maintained for up to 90 seconds on a trigger point can be useful. It is an interesting technique in some acute cases, and it can also

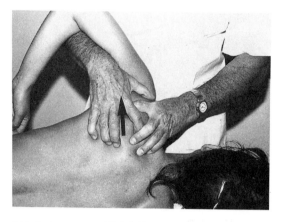

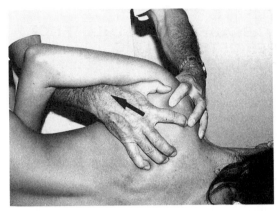

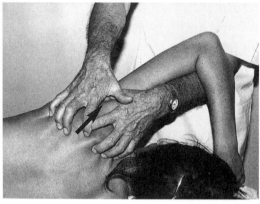

Figure 24.7. Petrissage and stretching of the muscles of the shoulder girdle in different directions.

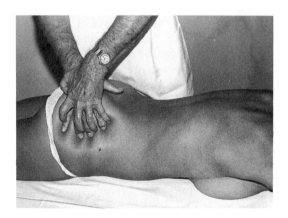

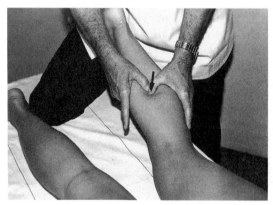

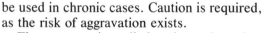

Figure 24.8. Petrissage of the gluteal muscles.

Figure 24.9. Ischemic compression of a calf trigger point.

be used in chronic cases. Caution is required, as the risk of aggravation exists.

Firm pressure is applied on the tender point, progressively increased with the thumb, and reinforced if necessary with the other thumb, without ever reducing the pressure. Thumb pressure can be replaced by elbow pressure in large muscles (glutei) (Fig. 24.9).

The muscle under pressure should be perfectly relaxed. This may not be easy, because the pressure should reach the maximal pain that is bearable. By palpation, one checks whether the tender point has resolved. If it persists, the same pressure technique can be repeated again, once or twice, with each sequence interspersed with a few active movements of the muscle or the application of heat. Brief pressure can also be used, for 5–10 seconds, and repeated several times a day; this can be performed by the patient. In most cases, the result is clearly not as good as it is with the preceding technique.

Shiatzu is a technique that replaced the needle implantation of traditional acupuncture with pressure applied on the acupuncture points with the pad of the finger. Its efficiency seems to us, with some exceptions, to be very relative.

Tenoperiosteal Pain, Tenalgias, Tendinitis

Spinal treatment usually decreases or relieves the tendinous or tenoperiosteal tenderness caused reflexively by a segmental vertebral syndrome, so that it will not be symptomatic. When spinal treatment is impossible or inefficient, local treatment can be started. Injection is very convenient, but if corticosteroids are contraindicated, massage becomes the best treatment. The deep transverse massage proposed by Cyriax is then the most efficient technique.

DEEP TRANSVERSE MASSAGE (DTM)

Cyriax used DTM in the treatment of tendinitis. He believed that the technique freed adhesions formed between sheath and tendon. It should be performed on a tendon placed under tension.

Whatever its mode of action, DTM is a disagreeable technique but a useful one. Troisier recommends its use for the following: rotator cuff tendinitis, forearm extensor tenosynovitis, lateral epicondylitis (the epicondyle should not be rubbed), medial epicondylitis (the epicondyle can be rubbed), and patellar tendinitis, as well as tendonitis of the tibialis anterior, tibialis posterior, peronei, and extensor digitorum longus muscles.

Massage is performed with the fingertips, the thumb, or the middle finger, with reinforce-

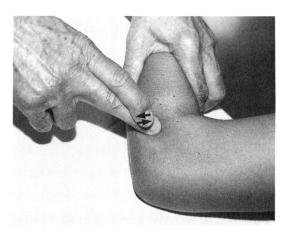

Figure 24.10. Transverse massage of the common extensor tendons.

ment provided by the index finger pressing on the dorsal side of its phalanx (Fig. 24.10). To be useful, it should be performed according to the following principles (Troisier):

- The finger should be at the precise site of the lesion, perpendicular to the soft tissues.
- Movements should be back and forth, of short amplitude, perpendicular to the fibers of the ligament or the tendon, with a pressure that is sufficient and constant.
- The finger should move the skin as it moves itself; it should not slide on the skin. The treated element thus receives firm pressure and transverse friction.

The start of the treatment is painful, but the pain generally decreases during the session. A session lasts 5–15 minutes. Its frequency varies from once daily (recommended by Troisier in forearm tenosynovitis) to twice weekly, usually, as too-frequent massages are not well tolerated. The number of sessions varies from 6 to 12. After the first session, improvement should occur in spontaneous pain, in the tests against resistance, and in range of motion. If pain increases in proportion to the treatment, the treatment should obviously be reconsidered. If no improvement is noted despite good massage technique, the diagnosis should be reevaluated.

25

STRETCHING

Stretching techniques are of great interest in painful musculotendinous conditions. They can be performed longitudinally, parallel to the muscle or tendon fibers, or transversely, with one or more fingers that stretch the muscle or the tendon perpendicularly.

LONGITUDINAL STRETCHING

As the name indicates, a longitudinal stretching technique tries to lengthen a muscle or a tendon. This maneuver can be performed manually, posturally, or by active exercises. It is performed slowly and progressively.

Manual Stretching

As an example, let us take a patient with trigger points in the triceps surae and biceps. The patient is positioned in supine with legs extended. The examiner raises slowly the leg in question as if to elicit Lasègue's sign, locking the knee in extension and the foot in dorsiflexion (Fig. 25.1). At a certain degree of inclination, 60° for example, the patient may feel pain with stretching of the involved muscles. By palpation, the examiner should determine whether the pain that is provoked is from the muscle, the stretching, or irritation of the sciatic nerve with dural tension. Elevation is stopped if the pain becomes too severe, and the level is maintained. After a while, the discomfort disappears, allowing an increased stretch range. In a few minutes, a level is reached that cannot be surpassed, but the elevation of the leg, which was painful and impossible beyond 60° becomes easy and painless at 80°. At the same time, the trigger points become less sensitive and less hypertonic. The

maneuver is repeated several times, depending on the result. This treatment can be performed every day or every other day. During these maneuvers, the patient should be instructed not to resist, to remain well relaxed, and to breathe calmly (Fig. 25.1).

Global Stretching of the Extensor Muscles

The same maneuver can be performed on both legs together. The result is a stretching of the extensor muscles (extensors of the spine and hips). The patient's shoulders should be on the examining surface, with the arms pulled caudad and the head in flexion (chin in), resting on the examining surface on the inferior part of the occiput (Fig. 25.2). Performed gradually with good respiratory control and good patient relaxation, this posture can relieve irritable protective muscle-guarding of the paraspinal muscles and stretch the hamstring and triceps surae muscles, which are often "shortened" in patients with low back pain and a source of trigger points. This stretching technique can be performed on all muscles or muscle groups; the technique to be used depends on the trigger points to be treated.

Stretching of the gluteus medius and tensor fascia lata is often useful. The technique is shown in Figure 25.3. The many techniques described in this book can be used at the vertebral level as stretching techniques for specific regions of the spinal column, by placing the tissues under tension and maintaining it for 10–30 seconds or more.

Postural Stretching

In some cases, stretching can be obtained posturally (e.g., by use of a system of pulleys and gradual steps), but these procedures nei-

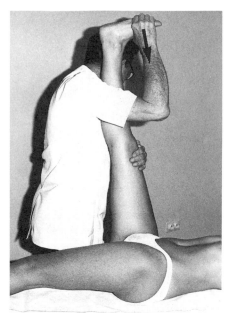

Figure 25.1. Stretching of the triceps surae and hamstrings.

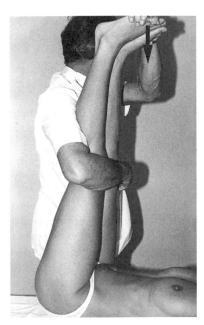

Figure 25.2. Global stretching of the extensor muscles.

ther give the same control nor allow as fine an adjustment as do the manual procedures.

Stretching Exercises

Patients can perform their own stretching, using exercises or even some postures inspired by yoga.

VAPOCOOLENT SPRAY AND STRETCH

Travell, Mennell, and Simons developed this technique for the treatment of "trigger points" that produced local or referred pains. As we have seen, these trigger points often correspond to a segmental vertebral syndrome and thus have a spinal origin. In these cases, spinal treatment should be given first. Those that persist can have the treatment described below, just as the ones whose origin is local.

The patient's position depends on the region to be treated. After applying vapocoolant spray to the skin overlying the region to be stretched, the physician passively stretches the muscle to its end range, gradually and slowly. During the stretching, the patient is asked to relax and take deep breaths. With

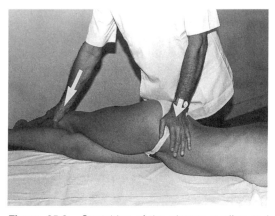

Figure 25.3. Stretching of the gluteus medius and the tensor fascia lata.

each expiration, the slack is taken up, and further range can be gained with subsequent stretching.

The vapocoolant currently in use is Flurimethane, which replaces the previously used ethyl chloride. The stream of vapocoolant is directed on the skin at an angle of 30° and a distance of 45 cm. Several passes of spray are applied in the direction of the muscle fibers in question. The whole muscle is sprayed as well as the zone of pain referral.

The authors call this technique "stretch and spray," because they consider the stretching to be essential. Spraying facilitates the stretching; the cooling of the subcutaneous tissues results in an inhibitory reflex of muscle tone (Travell, Mennell). This light cooling likely acts as a counterirritant that allows the muscle to relax reflexively.

TRANSVERSE STRETCHING

Transverse stretching is one of the basic maneuvers of the traditional bonesetters (a "folk" manipulator usually found in the French Countryside). The principle is simple, as is the correct execution. They are brief stretching maneuvers. For example, consider a patient with a hard, strained, taut band of muscle. This can be a trigger point due to a segmental spinal dysfunction or due to a reflex contraction of some muscle fibers. The taut bands are oriented in the direction of the muscle fibers in question. The maneuver consists of grasping the taut muscle fibers with the pad of the thumb and stretching it perpendicularly to its fibers. The thumb places the fibers under maximum tension and then suddenly releases them, as if plucking the strings of a musical instrument. After the maneuver, the taut muscle fibers are less sensitive to palpation, sometimes they are insensitive, but in any case, they are less hypertonic than at the start (Fig. 25.4).

This maneuver is really not as simple to execute as it seems. One must know exactly where the bundle to be treated is. The thumb should

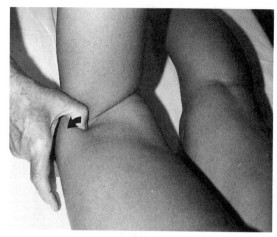

Figure 25.4. Transverse stretching of the biceps femoris.

probe normal muscle before contacting the concerned muscle. The speed of execution should be slow, and the constant pressure of the thumb is indispensable in the success of the maneuver—how much pressure is a question of experience. Bellon has demonstrated this very well.

This technique can be applied to the muscles of the limbs, trunk, and neck. Application of this technique to the paraspinal muscles is sometimes very effective, but it is difficult. The maneuver is easier if the trigger point can be stretched over a bony prominence where the grasp is easier to obtain (e.g., iliac crest or the spine of the scapula). If performed with improper technique, this maneuver can often exacerbate the painful tissues.

26

THERAPEUTIC INJECTIONS

Therapeutic injections are a convenient and efficacious means of precisely introducing a medicinal substance, usually a local anesthetic or a cortisone derivative or both, into a specific tissue site. They are used to act on neural elements, joints, peri-articular structures, tendinous sheaths, muscle, a subcutaneous tissue, etc. Thus an extreme variety of possibilities is offered by this technique whose efficiency will depend on the choice of indications, choosing the appropriate tissue to be injected, the substance injected, and the technical expertise of the examiner.

SPINAL INJECTIONS

The techniques used are epidural, intrathecal (or into the subarachnoid space) or facet joint, and ligamentous and selective neural blockade. Asepsis of the skin should be strict; the hands of the examiner should be disinfected or gloved. Syringes and needles should be disposable; one needle should be used to aspirate the liquid (if this is done through a rubber cork that has been carefully disinfected) and another one for the injection.

In a patient on anticoagulants, certain injections are relatively contraindicated. The articular and epidural injections should not be performed if the prothrombin rate is greater than 25.

Epidural Injection

Epidural injection is useful in the treatment of lumbar pain and radicular pain due to a disk disorder at L3-L4, L4-L5, or L5-S1. The substance injected in the epidural space penetrates the dura, including the dura mater of the last lumbar and sacral roots, and the superficial layers of the lumbosacral disks and the posterior longitudinal ligament.

Three routes of administration are possible:

- Via the sacrococcygeal hiatus
- Via the translumbar route
- Via the first sacral foramen

Sacrococcygeal Hiatus

This technique was described in 1901 by Sicard. At present, it is used infrequently, with the translumbar route the method of choice. A 20-mL syringe is filled with 15 mL of 0.5% lidocaine and 2 mL of a corticosteroid solution (e.g., 80–120 mg of methylprednisolone acetate). A 2- to 3-inch, 20-22 gauge needle is appropriate.

The patient is positioned in prone (Fig. 26.1) or in lateral decubitus. The two sacral cornua bordering the hiatus are carefully identified. Local anesthetic is injected subcutaneously, followed by insertion of the needle into the hiatus. The needle is initially angled at 45° to the skin, and once inserted, is redirected tangentially (Fig. 26.2). Once in place, it is essential to be certain that no cerebrospinal fluid appears at the hub of the needle, as can occur with an inadvertent subarachnoid puncture. Fortunately, this is an extremely rare occurrence with this method.

If not already in place, a syringe is then connected to the needle, and a second check is performed by aspiration. There is almost never a problem with needles of 40–50 mm, but there can be with longer needles. In the event of accidental cerebrospinal fluid (CSF) puncture, the needle should be removed and the injection aborted. In most cases, the dural sac descends to S2, but it can sometimes be located lower. During the injection, a hand is placed over the

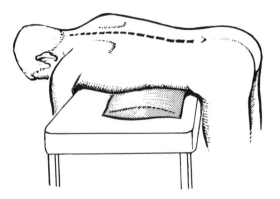

Figure 26.1.   Patient position for epidural injection.

posterior aspect of the sacrum to palpate for any subcutaneous fluid or air as a result of malpositioning of the needle behind, rather than in, the sacral canal. Even with appropriate needle placement, this occasionally occurs when there is a developmental malformation of the sacrum (partial spina bifida) (Fig. 26.3). If there is abnormal permeability of an anterior sacral foramen, the liquid can escape anteriorly.

During epidural injection, the patient may experience a spontaneous recurrence of pain, brought on by dural stretch. This pain resolves spontaneously after a few moments, once the

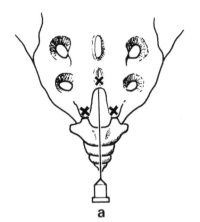

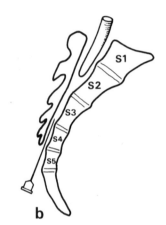

Figure 26.2.   Injection via the sacrococcygeal hiatus. **a.** Frontal view. **b.** Lateral view.

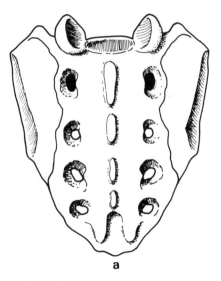

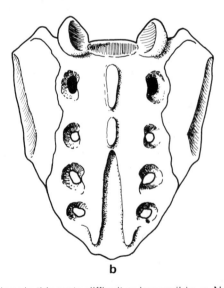

Figure 26.3.   Sacral anomalies can exist which make injection via this route difficult or impossible. **a.** Normal sacrum. **b.** Anomaly of the hiatus.

injection is halted. Following the procedure, patients are reexamined after lying on their backs for a few minutes to evaluate the effectiveness of the injection. The postprocedural assessment should try to elicit signs of root tension that existed prior to the injection. It is also useful to ask the patient about his general feeling, then to attempt some functional tasks that were impossible or difficult to execute before the injection, such as for instance putting on his socks. In some cases, O. Troisier uses much larger quantities of liquid (at least 50 mL). He used a solution of 0.5% betoxycaine chlorohydrate. He was convinced of the favorable mechanical effect of a larger volume of injectate that acted to lavage the epidural space and temporarily separate any adhesions between the dural sheath and the bulging disk. The level of the anesthetic block is at a higher level with this increased volume.

Translumbar Route

The translumbar route is the most commonly used route at present. The patient is seated and slumped forward to open the interspinous space. If the supine position is preferred, place a pillow underneath the abdomen. Then the spinous processes of L4 and L5 are located. A 20- to 22-gauge spinal needle with a short bevel, is inserted between the two processes. At a depth of 4–5 cm, the resistance of the ligamentum flavum is felt, preventing the injection. Then the needle is advanced 1 or 2 mm more, and injection into the epidural space is easily performed. Before the injection, the absence of CSF is verified by aspiration. Then 3 mL of the corticosteroid solution is injected, pure or mixed with a solution of 0.5% lidocaine (3–5 mL) (Fig. 26.4). If the dura has been perforated because of an adhesion of the

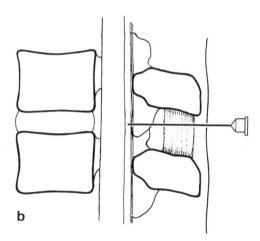

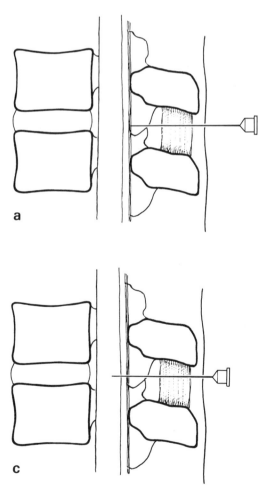

Figure 26.4. Epidural injection via translumbar approach. **a.** The needle encounters resistance produced by the ligamentum flavum. **b.** The needle penetrates the ligamentum flavum and makes its way to the epidural space. It is in this area that one should infiltrate, after aspiration, for an epidural injection. **c.** The needle has entered the dural sac. Aspiration results in the ability to draw back cerebral spinal fluid. The injection should not be performed in that space.

dural sac to the ligamentum flavum or because of a mistaken maneuver, the needle must be pulled back slightly, checked by aspiration for CSF, and if there is none, then the corticosteroid solution is injected without anesthetic.

First Sacral Foramen

This technique was proposed by Lievre in 1955. The patient is seated or prone with a pillow under the abdomen. The spinous process of L4 is located at the level of the iliac crests. From there, the spinous processes of L5 and S1 are located, as well as the posterior superior iliac spines. From the latter, a triangle is outlined whose apex is S1. The line joining the two iliac spines forms the base. The injection is performed at the middle of the line connecting the process of S1 to the posterior superior iliac spine, at right or left (Fig. 26.5). This point is opposite the first sacral foramen.

A 20- to 22-gauge 2- to 3-inch needle is directed perpendicularly until it comes into contact with the periosteum; it is slightly advanced until it penetrates the sacral foramen from outside. It is preferable not to inject any anesthetic solution because if there is any anomaly of the dural which is lengthened around the root, there is the risk of performing a subarachnoid injection resulting in spinal anesthesia. After verification by aspiration, 2–3 mL of corticosteroid is injected.

Remarks

Other locations can be used. A vertical line is traced one finger's breadth lateral to the spinous process of L5. Then a horizontal line is traced a thumb's breadth below the inferior edge of that process. The injection is performed at the intersection of the two lines (Fig. 26.5).

Intrathecal Injection

This technique was described by Luccherini. It consists of the intradural injection of a solution of 1–2 mL of a corticosteroid derivative. It is the same technique as for the lumbar puncture the same precautions have to be taken (Fig. 26.4).

Here it is better to use a smaller gauge needle so that a CSF leak is minimized through the puncture site. After injection, the patient remains prone for 1 hour, with large pillows under the abdomen if necessary. The patient remains recumbent for 24 hours.

This technique is indicated in selected lumbar pain syndromes with sciatica. It also provides an opportunity to draw some CSF prior to injection. CSF examination, which has been too long neglected, can help avoid many diagnostic errors.

It is inadvisable to repeat this type of injection more than two or three times, especially if the result of the first injection is equivocal.

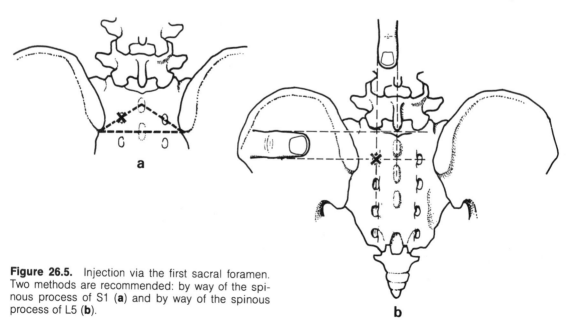

Figure 26.5. Injection via the first sacral foramen. Two methods are recommended: by way of the spinous process of S1 (**a**) and by way of the spinous process of L5 (**b**).

It is essential that the substance injected is suitable for intrathecal usage; corticosteroid derivatives should be used in solution, avoiding whenever possible dexamethasone, whose solvent is irritating.

Adverse Effects. A very painful spinal headache can follow intrathecal injection of corticosteroids. It may be due to leakage of CSF related to the puncture site; hence the need for a smaller gauge needle and the recumbent position for 24 hours. Occasionally, an inflammatory reaction is noticed a few days after intrathecal injection of corticosteroids, associated with an increase in CSF proteins. The best treatment then seems to be the administration of 30 mg of hydrocortisone orally for 3–4 days.

Accidents. Meningitis can occur when sterile technique is poor in performing a spinal puncture and even more so when there is an injection of corticosteroid derivatives. The use of single-use preservative-free materials considerably lowers these risks.

Facet Joint Injections

In this book, we have emphasized the role of the facet joints. Facet joint dysfunction is a constant in PMIDs. Injection is often useful, especially for the treatment of a PMID that has been insufficiently improved by manipulation, when manipulation is contraindicated, or during acute synovitis.

A good segmental examination should be performed as well as a careful search for the "facet joint point." The injection is justifiable only if the articulation is found to be tender on examination.

It is performed with 0.5 mL of corticosteroid derivative; an anesthetic should not be used at the cervical level. A short-bevel needle is inserted perpendicularly to the skin until contact is made with periosteum. The substance is injected after the needle has been withdrawn 1 mm without changing its direction and after aspirating to be sure there is neither blood nor CSF.

When first starting to perform these injections, it is best to do them under fluoroscopic guidance; experienced physicians often find this unnecessary. However, if the injection performed in this fashion is inefficient and if the clinical examinations continue to point toward the involvement of the facet joint, it is

then advisable to perform another injection under fluoroscopic guidance. The point of injection is marked in case other injections are necessary; they will then be performed with the patient in the same position as when the mark was made.

Lumbar Region

The patient is flexed forward across the table, with a cushion placed under the abdomen. Even when there is a thick layer of overlying subcutaneous tissue, it is usually possible to locate the "facet joint point" by the pressure-friction of the pad of the middle finger. The finger slides in short movements back and forth, parallel to the spinous processes (see "Segmental Examination," in Chapter 21). The injection is performed exactly over the tender point that has been located and perpendicular to the skin, with a 2.5- to 3-inch 20- to 22-gauge needle. The point of injection is slightly more lateral to the midline for L5-S1, L4-L5 than for L1-L2, L2-L3 and L3-L4 (Fig. 26.6). The injection is performed after aspiration, always keeping contact with periosteum and aiming toward the lateral aspect of the capsule where it is more lax.

Remarks
Skin markings can also be used:

- *For L5-S1, a horizontal line is drawn tangent to the superior edge of the spinous process of S1. The point of injection is on this line, about 2.5 cm lateral to the midline.*
- *For L4-L5, the same tracing is done with the process of L5. The point of injection is 2 cm lateral to the midline.*

It is understood that these tracings vary with the morphology of the subject. They should always be correlated with the provoked tender paraspinal point. When in doubt, the injection should be performed under fluoroscopic guidance.

Thoracolumbar Junction

Except in particular cases, T12 is a transitional vertebra; its superior articular processes are thoracic, and its inferior articulations are lumbar (this role is given sometimes to T11).

The location for the facet joints is the same as for L2-L3. It is much easier to locate T11-

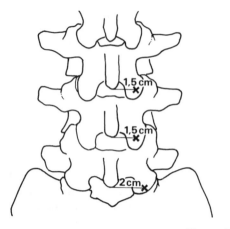

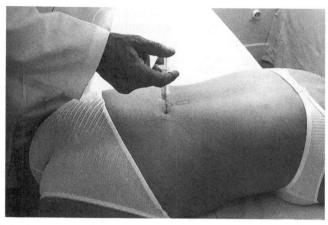

Figure 26.6.   Lumbar facet injection.

T12 and T10-T11 with precision using palpation friction performed with the pad of the middle finger, over the sensitive facet joints. The injection can be performed at the level of this point, perpendicular to the skin, until contact is made with the bone. But at that level, it is better to push the needle 1 cm lateral of the midline, then go on until in contact with periosteum, and from there inject while maintaining contact with the bone, going from medial to lateral until the needle loses contact with the bone. In this way, the target is the external part of the articular mass (Fig. 26.7).

Thoracic Region

Same technique as above (Fig. 26.8).

Cervical Region

As with the thoracolumbar region, cervical dysfunction is frequently an indication for

Figure 26.7. Thoracolumbar facet injection. It is good to verify the disappearance of pain noted on the "pinch roll" test in the territory of the posterior primary rami to which that territory corresponds. This test helps to verify the efficacy of the injection.

facet joint injection. To locate the tender facet joints, the patient lies supine, which is the best position for palpating these joints. The injection can be performed with the patient sitting on a stool, with the neck in flexion and the head resting on a table. Careful palpation is necessary, performed by pressure friction with the pad of the middle or index finger. A median vertical line is drawn corresponding to the line of the spinous processes. The site of needle insertion is located 2 cm lateral to the midline. The needle is inserted perpendicularly to the skin until in contact with periosteum.

This contact should be clear. Then the needle is moved slightly laterally and medially to verify the contact. The injection should be performed with a corticosteroid derivative without anesthetic (Figs. 26.9 and 26.10).

As always, it is performed strictly on contact with periosteum, after being sure that the aspiration is clear of blood or CSF. It is advis-

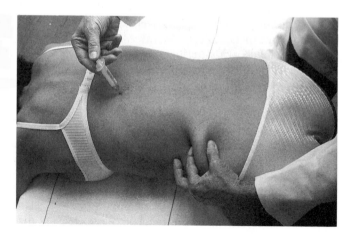

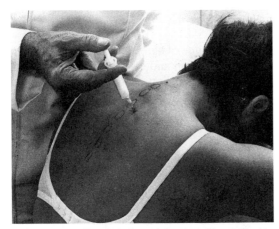

Figure 26.8. Thoracic facet injection. The patient is positioned lying across the table for the low thoracic region. For the upper thoracic region, the patient can be seated, bent forward, with the arms folded in front. The head is laid on top of the crossed arms on the table during the procedure.

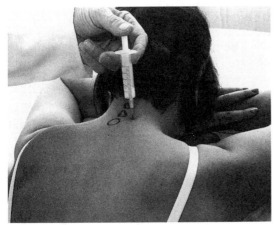

Figure 26.9. Low cervical facet injection. The same position is used as for upper thoracic vertebrae.

able to use corticosteroid derivatives that are suitable for the CSF, as it lessens the risk to the patient in case of error. In fact, there is no risk if one carefully follows the rule to inject only on contact with periosteum at the posterior aspect of the joint and to aspirate and withdraw a little just before injecting.

The effect of the injection occurs rather quickly. In case of success, movement that was limited and painful moments before becomes less painful and freer, even totally painless.

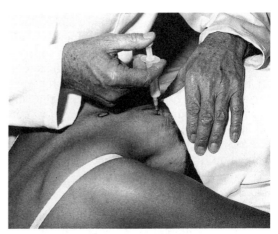

Figure 26.10. Upper cervical facet injection.

Ligamentous Injections

Interspinous Ligaments

The interspinous and supraspinous ligaments are often sensitive to pressure in a "minor interspinous disorder" (key sign). Most often, this sensitivity is discovered during a systematic examination; it does not produce any discomfort or any spontaneous pain. However, there are cases in which the ligament is responsible for a painful spinal syndrome. It can be demonstrated by a simple test: anesthetic injection that makes the discomfort and pain disappear. However, if the sensitivity of the ligament does not disappear after a manipulation, then it has to be treated locally. In cases with only ligamentous pain without any sign of a PMID, injection is the treatment of choice, and it is performed with a mixture of anesthetic and corticosteroids.

For resistant cases, the solution recommended by Hackett is the best. This author attributes almost all spinal or articular pains to "ligamentous laxity" or tendinous origin and treats them with sclerosing injections. This concept is questionable, but the treatment is sometimes effective. Barbor uses the same procedure on more limited indications and proposes the following mixture, favored also by Troisier:

phenol 0.50 g
glycerin 5 g
glucose 5 g
distilled water to a total volume of 20 mL

This solution is mixed with an equal volume of lidocaine 1%. A few drops are injected onto the periosteum, trying to contact the superior and inferior insertional points of the ligament, at multiple points (1/3 mL usually for each space) (Fig. 26.11). There is sometimes a very painful reaction lasting 1–3 days. It is performed again 3–4 times at weekly intervals, depending on the degree of improvement. One can go up to 6 injections if necessary.

Iliolumbar Ligament

Several authors have noted the frequent existence in common lumbar pain of a sensitive point at the junction of the middle and medial thirds of the iliac crest, 7–8 cm lateral of the midline, and also the fact that anesthetic injection at this point relieves some patients. It has been thought that this point represents the insertion of the "iliolumbar ligament."

But it is not certain. The point that is usually painful is localized on the posterior surface of the iliac crest; however, the ligament is inserted largely on the anterior surface and is not accessible to palpation. In fact this point, as we have shown, usually corresponds to the cutaneous branch of the posterior ramus of L1, sometimes L2. This is the "crestal point" of the "low back pain of thoracolumbar origin" described by R. Maigne. It disappears with injection of the facet joint causing the irritation (T12-L1 or L1-L2) and the cellulalgic zone frequently adjacent corresponding to the der-

matome of the nerve (see Chapter 41. "Lumbar Pain").

The presence of ligamentous calcification at the iliac insertion and osteophytes at the level of the spinal insertion, visible on radiographs, does not confirm that the iliolumbar ligament is the cause of a lumbar pain.

SELECTIVE NEURAL BLOCKADE

Injection of the Anterior Primary Rami of the Spinal Nerves

These injections are rarely useful. One has to be careful when the sheath of the nerve extends beyond the interspinal foramen, as their injection can result in CSF puncture producing dramatic risks. For the cervical nerves, the needle is advanced a fingerbreadth lateral to the spinous process. For C5, it is advanced until it contacts the tubercle of Chassaignac, which is easily found by palpation; it fills the external extremity of the transverse process of C6. The point of the needle is moved slightly upward. For C6, the needle abuts against the transverse process of C7, one then passes under and injects. For C7, same technique is used; one goes under the transverse process to reach the anterior branch of the 7th cervical nerve root.

Injection of the 5th lumbar root can be useful when medical treatment or epidural injections have been ineffective in relieving pain. The patient lies across the table, and the needle is advanced at a point 4 cm lateral to the midline at the level of the inferior pole of the 5th lumbar vertebra. Advanced perpendicularly, it meets the transverse processes of L5, then it is withdrawn slightly and passed below to reach the L5 root.

Injection of the Posterior Primary Rami of the Spinal Nerves

A facet injection need not be performed intra-articularly as it almost automatically involves the posterior branch of the spinal nerve that courses around it. If one wants to examine the role of the posterior ramus in a pain syndrome, the painful zone should be carefully located, using the "pinch-roll" test in the area of its dermatome.

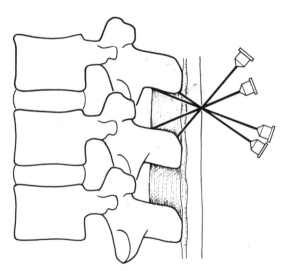

Figure 26.11.   Injection of the interspinous ligament.

After having located precisely the facet joint that was painful on examination, a few drops of a local anesthetic are injected at the articular contact, at the thoracic and lumbar regions. The result obtained on the painful cellulalgic zone is then rechecked with the pinch-roll test. If it is successful, this zone quickly becomes painless and even sometimes supple. Then the corticosteroid derivative is injected with the needle still in place. Otherwise, the position of the needle should be slightly modified and a few more drops of anesthetic solution injected. This procedure is repeated two or three times until the expected result is obtained. In case of failure, one checks, in the same way, whether the supra-adjacent or the subjacent joint is responsible for the irritation. Recall that injection of anesthetic should be avoided at the cervical level.

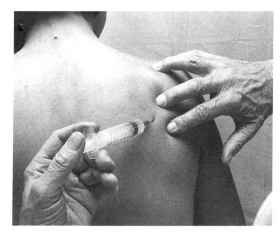

Figure 26.12.   Injection of an infraspinatus muscle trigger point.

TRIGGER POINT INJECTIONS

Trigger points can be the source of both local or referred pain and tenderness. Some are manifestations of a segmental spinal cellulotenoperiosteomyalgic syndrome, while some are isolated and have a local cause. In both cases, anesthetic injection of the trigger point is a valuable test to determine whether it is responsible for the painful syndrome. The injection often momentarily exacerbates the pain, which disappears afterward. If the trigger point is part of a segmental spinal syndrome, it is better as always to first treat the responsible spinal segment. Local treatment is indicated if no result or a poor result is obtained.

The injection of trigger points should be thorough. It is sometimes difficult. A few milliliters of 1% lidocaine are injected into the most painful point of the muscle. Thus, the trigger point should be very well localized and isolated; then it is grasped between the index and the middle finger of the left hand (Figs. 26.12–26.14), or in some cases, pinched between thumb and index. Several successive examinations are necessary to localize the most painful point. While introducing the needle, the needle is aimed at an acute angle, and one drop is injected as soon as the skin is penetrated. While maintaining the needle underneath the skin, the muscle is repeatedly probed in a circumferential manner. Contact

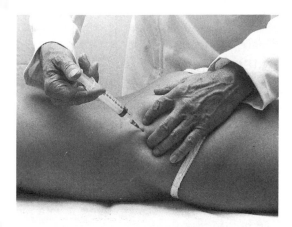

Figure 26.13.   Injection of a gluteus medius trigger point.

with the trigger point produces a brief contraction, a characteristic feature of trigger points known as a local twitch response (LTR). This indicates to the examiner that the target has been reached. The LTR is sometimes quite sharp and often reproduces the original pain referral pattern. At each occurrence of an LTR, a few milliliters of lidocaine are injected. Often one injection is sufficient; sometimes two or three more may be necessary with an interval of a few days.

When the trigger point is of local origin, and especially if it has a tendency to recur, the postural or static problem that may be a perpetuating factor should be sought. One can also use the dry needle (acupuncture) technique, ad-

Figure 26.14.   Injection of a sternocleidomastoid muscle trigger point.

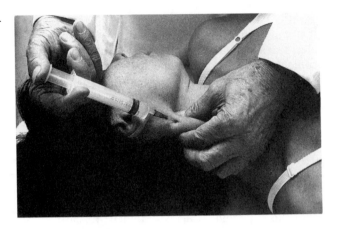

vanced in the most sensitive point and left until it can be easily removed, as in the beginning that needle seems to be held firmly by the tissues. The results are interesting but not as reliable as tests with lidocaine.

INJECTION OF SCARS

It is not rare to see that a scar, or part of it, is responsible for unrecognized pain referral, rarely attributed to their cause. They are not always local and can be distantly referred, generally in the homologous spinal segment. In these cases, the scar can be demonstrated to be painful by pinching it between the thumb and the index finger or by rubbing it with the pad of the index finger.

The painful part is injected with a few drops of a local anesthetic. This is both diagnostic and therapeutic. The test is positive if the spontaneous pain disappears after the injection, and it is a treatment if the relief persists after the injection, which can occur immediately or after three to four injections performed at intervals of a few days. The relief generally persists, but sometimes it is useful to add scar massages. Of course some scars may simply be sensitive to palpation without being a source of spontaneous pain for the patient.

ACCIDENTS ASSOCIATED WITH INJECTION OF LOCAL ANESTHETIC

Serious accidents are rare in the use of local anesthetic in spinal pathology.

Allergic Reactions.   Severe allergic reactions are rare. The reactions are usually a rash or respiratory in nature, such as asthma. They are chiefly due to the action of the esters in lidocaine.

Toxic Accidents.   These are especially due to lidocaine. The injection should be stopped as soon as the patient demonstrates signs of general malaise, anxiety, paresthesia around the mouth and of the tongue, sensations of vertigo, or dizziness. They occur very rarely at the concentrations used to treat spinal or articular pathology; the quantities and the concentrations are usually not strong. Nevertheless, anaphylactic shock or a convulsion can occur. That is why it is absolutely necessary to have resuscitation equipment on hand, including an appropriate intravenous solution to facilitate the administration of adrenalin, or Valium in the case of convulsions (Favarel-Garrigues).

Diffusion of the Local Anesthetic toward the Neuraxis.   Several delayed reactions have been reported after an injection of triamcinolone or of dexamethasone with lidocaine performed at the level of a cervical joint. In these cases, it seems that the lidocaine was injected in the subarachnoid space; so it is absolutely necessary to always check by aspiration before injecting and to inject only at the bony level.

Sanchez reports that according to some literature, a local anesthetic introduced by paraspinal injection is capable of reaching the spinal cord by simple diffusion and without any penetration of the needle into the spinal canal or the intervertebral foramen, for the following reasons.

- The meningeal coverings can brim over the intervertebral foramen for several centimeters.

- Some arachnoid villi occasionally herniate through the dural sheath and perforate it. They particularly permit the anesthetic to reach the subarachnoid space.
- It has been experimentally demonstrated (radioactive isotope dyes) that a substance injected into a nerve can undergo retrograde diffusion into the spinal centers.

COMPLICATIONS OF STEROID INJECTION

Steroid injections can produce local reactions, which occur most often immediately after the injection and sometimes after a delay of several hours. These reactions last 24–48 hours, and they can be relieved by the application of ice.

With an articular injection, the greatest complication is septic arthritis. G. Ziegler et al. reported 19 cases of septic arthritis seen in their hospital service, of which 7 were iatrogenic. This complication is rare provided aseptic precautions have been taken (1 of 25,000 injections for Pouletty and Besson). But an acute infection can result from an injection performed in an already infected joint. The prognosis of septic arthritis depends on the rapidity of the diagnosis and treatment. Most resolve without any sequelae, unless the treatment is started late and the cause of the infection remains undetermined.

Corticosteroid injections, periarticular or articular, should not be performed if there is a hemarthrosis or cardiac prosthesis.

Repeated corticosteroid injections in the same joint are responsible for the degradation of different articular and periarticular structures.

Intratendinous injections in the Achilles tendon, as practiced in the past, have been associated with tendinous rupture. With superficial injections, some depigmentation of the skin or local atrophy of subcutaneous tissue can occur, which produces a dimple that disappears over time. We have used facet joint injections for more than 25 years, and we have never had any accidents.

Meyer et al. have reported a case of delayed paraplegia after some epidural injections performed too soon after one another, using corticosteroid derivatives in microcrystalline suspension. Remember that injection of corticosteroid, even local, is still an injection of corticosteroid. One should keep in mind the well-known contraindications of this therapy.

HYDROTHERAPY, THERMOTHERAPY, CRYOTHERAPY

HYDROTHERAPY AND THERMOTHERAPY

Hydrotherapy has been used a great deal in many countries. In France, it was very popular and fashionable during the last century, but later it was mostly used in thermal spas. Although physicians and patients who used it were very enthusiastic about it, its efficacy and utility were always questioned by the medical profession. The use of these modalities was reawakened by the development of physical therapy, and the vogue of thalassotherapy helped to better elucidate its potential.

Hydrotherapy with all its modalities is certainly a great asset in the treatment of spinal disorders. Unfortunately, its use is limited by the need for significant investment in the equipment needed to perform this type of therapy. We will describe the technique we use in performing hydrotherapy and thermotherapy in our department of orthopedic medicine at Hotel Dieu, which we consider most useful in the management of some cases.

Hotel Dieu Method

We inherited a very old tradition of hydrotherapy in our department, and the technique that we use most often in spinal pain and radicular pain disorders originated from it. The treatment consists of a heat bath, followed by rest in the supine position, then followed by a general shower, which can be focused on the affected region, performed three times a week. The traditional name of these heat baths is "bath of light."

The therapy is performed with the patient sitting on a wooden stool and enclosed entirely in a hexagonal box. Only the head, which is covered with a cold wet towel, and part of the neck are outside the box. On the walls of the box, there are tubular infrared lights that expose the body to radiant heat. The disposition of the lights is such that there is no danger of burns by contact. The inside temperature reaches 60°C.

Each session lasts 10 minutes, but this can vary depending on the subject. Most find this treatment agreeable. Some adverse effects can occur, such as lipothymia, tachycardia, and pallor, but they are rare. With experience, they can be easily avoided (neurotic, "spasmophilic" patients). During the session, the blood pressure remains stable while the pulse increases slightly, on the order of about 10 pulses per minute.

Afterward, the subject remains recumbent for 8 to 10 minutes, protected by blankets to prolong the perspiration provoked by the stay in the heat box.

The third part of the treatment is a jet shower, at 5-m distance, at 38°C. The temperature can be changed slightly according to the reaction of the subject. The shower should not last more than 5 minutes. From experience, the operator chooses a full jet or a "broken" jet. In general, for a lean patient, the broken jet is preferred. For a stocky individual, a more powerful full jet may be selected. The "Scotch" shower is good in sciatica, and it is performed as follows: full jet at 39°C for 6–8 minutes, followed by a cold shower at 11°C in broken jet for 30 seconds. The feet are always kept warm.

Results

To evaluate this treatment, we followed 56 patients with severe discopathy associated with sciatica of at least 2 months duration who were unresponsive to the usual treatments or bed rest, and for whom surgery was contemplated. Of these 56 patients, 16 were completely relieved in 9 sessions (20 days) and the result was maintained for the following months; 12 patients were very much improved and could be relieved by procedures that had previously been ineffective; 28 had little or no improvement, and among those, 15 went on to have surgery; the remaining 13 were lost to follow-up after the last treatment test.

Results were much better in mild cases. The best indications were persistent acute lumbar pain syndromes with symptoms of sciatica, including chronic vertebrospinal pain with stiffness and diffuse muscle spasms prior to a more specific treatment pain due to acute attacks of synovitis.

Usually nine sessions are given, at a frequency of three times a week. Usually the improvement is noticed in the sixth or seventh session. In some cases, the treatment can be extended by three additional sessions. The safety and efficacy of this treatment should be emphasized.

Contraindications

This treatment is certainly contraindicated in patients who are fragile, those who have venous insufficiency, patients with heat intolerance, and those with hypertension.

CRYOTHERAPY

In France, cold is not often used in the treatment of spinal or articular pain, though it is efficacious in some acute cases.

Ice Application

The application of ice often produces rapid relief of acute shoulder pain, periarthritis of the hip, acute torticollis (wry neck), or low back pain. In all cases, the skin should be protected by wool or flannel placed between the skin and the ice bag. "Icing" is also indicated in the acute treatment of muscle strains and joint trauma related to athletic activities.

Ice Massage

A good therapeutic approach for many musculotendinous disorders, ice massage should be tried in cases that are refractory to other treatments. An ice cube the size of a mustard jar (about 5 cm in diameter) is taken in the hand protected with a cloth, and slowly massaged into the affected muscle, from one end to the other. If the tendinous insertion is affected, it should be included also.

Initially the patient feels the cold, followed by brief acute pain, after which generally there is a feeling of anesthesia lasting 3–5 minutes after the massage. At that point, the treatment is stopped. Then some slow stretching movements are applied progressively to the muscle, or postural exercises are performed.

This treatment can also be used in chronic periosteomyalgic pain syndromes, which have their origin in refractory spinal articular disorders.

Cold Pulverization

In the past, cold pulverization was a popular treatment for sciatica. It was usually performed with ethyl chloride or fluorimethane, which was sprayed on the painful area. It is used by J. Travell and J. Mennell in the treatment of the "myalgic points" "trigger points" to facilitate stretching (see "Vapocoolent Spray and Stretch" in Chapter 25).

28

ELECTROTHERAPY IN PAIN OF SPINAL ORIGIN

Electrotherapy is used in different ways and is certainly beneficial in the treatment of pain of spinal origin. It is used in cases where other forms of medical or manual treatments are contraindicated and also in cellulotenoperiosteomyalgic manifestations.

THE SPINE

During inflammatory arthritic episodes, low-frequency (10–25 Hz) short wave diathermy is often effective. Higher frequency (200 Hz) short waves, continuous, with thermic effect, can be used in persistent facet joint pain or stiffness. However, continuous short waves should be avoided at the cervical level. Continuous thermogenic short waves are applied to the region of pain referral in cases of sciatica, femoral pain, or cervicobrachial neuralgia. Afterward, short waves at low frequency are applied at the spinal level.

Ultrasound can be used in pain of the interspinous ligament. Two to three sessions, lasting 3–5 minutes each, generally suffice. Microwaves are useful in refractory cervicoscapular pain after trauma or in some lumbogluteal pains.

Midfrequency currents also have an analgesic action.

It is sometimes useful to use longitudinal iontophoresis with calcium or anti-inflammatories. One pole is placed at the root of the limb, the other at the extremity, on the path of the pain.

MANIFESTATIONS OF THE NEUROTROPHIC SPINAL SEGMENTAL SYNDROME

Cellulalgia. Iontophoresis (galvanic current) can be performed with noninjectable products such as α-chymotrypsin or with anesthetic products before localized kneading sessions.

Tendinous Pain. Ultrasound is often prescribed, though in our experience good results are infrequent. Iontophoresis with salicylates, ketoprofen, or corticosteroids often leads to good results (Teyssandier). Pulsed short wave diathermy also has a beneficial action (8–10 sessions).

Trigger Points. This is the best indication for ultrasound. Pulsed short waves at 200 Hz can be associated with the diadynamic currents of Bernard. Iontophoresis of muscle relaxants seems to have little efficacy.

Periosteal Pain. Pulsed athermic magnetic short waves are useful in the treatment of periosteal pain.

29

LUMBAR ORTHOSES

The use of a rigid lumbar orthosis to immobilize or give support to the spine is useful in managing some forms of low back pain. It can offer valuable relief and can prevent or shorten the need for bed rest (Fig. 29.1). It is also useful in the treatment of certain chronic low back pain disorders.

INDICATIONS

Acute Low Back Pain

A lumbar corset can be indicated as a first measure in patients with acute lumbar disk pain who must remain mobile because of external demands that do not allow their level of activity to be interrupted, when anti-inflammatory treatments are contraindicated, and when manipulation does not help.

It can also be prescribed for a patient who is relieved by medical treatment but still feels vulnerable and wants to return quickly to work. The support is usually worn for 8–15 days, depending on the case.

In acute low back pain of thoracolumbar origin (Maigne), it is less efficacious. However, in severe cases, when injection and manipulation are contraindicated or ineffective, it can be of use. In such cases, one uses a thoracolumbosacral (TLSO) orthosis of sufficient height to limit trunk rotation and lateroflexion. This orthosis can be difficult to tolerate because it can compress an irritable posterior ramus against the iliac crest and exacerbate a zone of gluteal cellulalgia. The means used to avoid these complications are not always effective.

Sciatica

A lumbosacral orthosis (LSO) can be used in conditions that cause low back pain while standing. It can then be worn 15–30 days.

Chronic Low Back Pain

In some refractory and severe chronic low back pain syndromes, a custom-molded rigid lumbosacral orthosis gives temporary relief to the painful region. When LSOs are used, it is frequently noted that after a variable time (1–4 months), other treatments that were previously ineffective, become efficacious. Sometimes the patient is relieved only while wearing the LSO, and the pain recurs when it is removed. If wearing an LSO does not produce relief and the benign nature of the low back pain and its lumbosacral origin is certain, a spinal fusion should be considered as it may have a good chance of success.

FABRICATION OF A RIGID LUMBAR ORTHOSIS

To facilitate fabrication, the subject should be able to stand for 15 minutes. The fasting patient stands up and holds a high bar or leans against a wall. The antalgic attitude should always be respected and should not be corrected. The patient is naked during the casting process. The skin is sprinkled with talc, then the patient puts on a jersey (or better two). The iliac spines and any other vulnerable bony prominences are protected by felt padding.

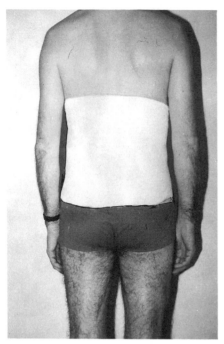

Figure 29.1.   Plaster lumbosacral orthosis.

Five to 6 rolls of plaster of 20-cm width are used. With the first two rolls, the cast is applied circumferentially from inferior to superior, starting at the pubis, then up around the abdomen to the xiphoid process.

The lateral and posterior parts of the orthosis are reinforced with the next two rolls. During the entire process, the patient is asked to pull in the abdomen.

The final rolls are applied circumferentially, overlying the first four rolls. After each application, the plaster is well smoothed. Using a paring knife, one makes an indentation in front to avoid having the plaster compress the groin in the sitting position. The edges are folded back to reinforce them.

Finally, the jersey is cut 5–6 cm above and below the plaster, and is folded back on the superior and inferior edges. A small roll of plaster, or adhesive tape, often suffices. The patient should feel at ease in the cast; sometimes there is relief. If the orthosis does not lead to improved symptoms in the days immediately following its fabrication, it should be modified or refabricated. When the antalgic posture is severe, it is better to make a new orthosis every few days; as the antalgic list

diminishes, the old orthosis is no longer comfortable.

In the case of low back pain of thoracolumbar origin (T11-T12), the orthosis should sit higher in the back and on the sides, often to the level of the inferior scapular border, while the anterior part rests below the xiphoid.

In most cases, the orthosis is left closed and is worn night and day for 2–8 days. Then a vertical paramedian incision is performed, which allows its removal. To put it back on, the two sides are fixed with large sticking plaster, or better, with Velcro, so the patient can take it off during the night, take a bath, and shower. Usually, it is worn 2–4 weeks in cases of acute low back pain or sciatica and up to 2–4 months for severe chronic low back pain.

Fabrication of an LSO with plaster is quick, easy, and very economical. But the thermoplastic materials now on the market can be used to fabricate lighter orthoses that are more convenient for the patient and should be used if the patient will be wearing the orthosis for long periods of time or for esthetic reasons, as they are less bulky. The plaster LSO increases the waistline a great deal, forcing the patient to wear loose-fitting clothing.

Plaster Orthosis Syndrome

Plaster orthosis syndrome occurs infrequently, but it can lead to a fatal outcome (Boegli et al.). It has been especially observed after spinal surgery or spinal trauma and in cases in which the cast was made for the treatment of scoliosis or kyphosis. It has also been noted with cases of femoral fracture.

It starts with a sensation of gastric fullness and nausea, progressing to acute gastric dilation with painful abdominal distention and painful flatulence. Gastric decompression by nasogastric suction usually suffices to relieve symptoms, though some patients go on to require surgical intervention. This syndrome is due to high duodenal obstruction, with acute secondary gastric distention. Most authors believe that the "the mesenteric artery compression syndrome" is the primary cause. It is felt that the anatomic disposition facilitates partial or complete obstruction of the duodenum, which may narrow the space between the duodenum and the superior mesenteric artery.

MODE OF ACTION

Numerous authors have studied the mode of action of spinal orthoses. It seems logical to look at the effects of the spinal immobilization that they produce, but radiologic studies have shown that this immobilization is just relative, which is what made some conclude that LSOs produce no real effect. These considerations can be expressed in the form of a well-known syllogism.

- Spinal orthoses are designed for immobilization.
- However, it has been proven that they do not completely immobilize the spine.
- Therefore, their effect is that of a placebo and is of no therapeutic interest.

However, daily experience demonstrates very well their utility and efficacy on pain. Therefore it is unnecessary to completely immobilize the spine to achieve beneficial results, and the mode of action of a spinal orthosis is much more complex than one thinks. One should give consideration to the possibility that

- It restricts all movements and suppresses extreme movements;
- It provides a passive support to enable the patient to maintain postures that are comfortable with minimal effort and avoid postures that habitually produce pain;
- It decreases the pressure on the involved spinal segment and therefore lessens the degree of irritation imposed upon its elements.

LUMBOSACRAL CORSETS

Lumbosacral corsets are considered a poor substitute for the natural support of the lumbar spine, which is derived principally from the supporting musculature. In spite of this, many competent practitioners think otherwise and often prescribe this form of therapy.

INDICATIONS

The use of the lumbosacral corsets is indicated in the treatment of low back pain but does not replace a therapeutic exercise prescription, as they are complementary treatment modalities.

Before prescribing the use of a lumbar corset, the indication should be thought out. It is unnecessary to prescribe it for patients who suffer from a low back pain that is present only in the morning and gets better as the day goes on. It should be prescribed only for those who suffer continuously and whose pain increases with fatigue. It is indicated in the following circumstances.

- In a patient with an acute attack who is recuperating slowly. In this case, it is used as a temporary adjunct while physical therapy is performed and providing results.
- In elderly patients or in patients for whom a therapeutic exercise program is contraindicated. In these cases it is prescribed as a permanent measure.
- In patients with osteopenic lumbar spines or weak muscles. In this case it is worn only occasionally, when the patient feels vulnerable or when the lumbar region is going to be stressed (e.g., a long trip).

TYPES

There are many types of lumbosacral corsets.

- A belt for lumbar support with two or three steel ribs, thoracic, vertical (Fig. 30.1).
- The lumbar corset with a more or less reinforced armature, called "closed cage" or "open cage." The terms open and closed depend on whether the lateral supports on the iliac crests are connected (closed cage) or not (open cage) to the thoracic support by steel blades (Fig. 30.2).

Depending on the case, one can decide between a very rigid lumbar corset with a closed cage or a belt with lumbar support. Particular attention should be given to the abdominal bearing (Fig. 30.3), especially in older women with large, soft, protuberant abdomens (belt of Atlas type) (Fig. 30.4).

MODE OF ACTION

The patient should feel comfortable in the lumbar corset. Norton and Brow, Million et al., and Revel and Armor have proved that the lumbar corset does not really limit the movements of the spine, it is just a reminder to the patient. It modifies the usual movements; the patient becomes used to being supported by the corset and so modifies the normal muscular support and zones of vertebral stress. Further, there is warming produced on the lumbar regions. In fact, in many subjects, simple and

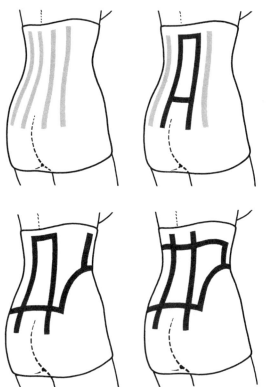

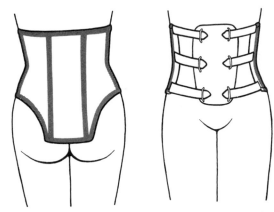

Figure 30.2. Lumbosacral corset with caged reinforcement.

Figure 30.1. Lumbosacral corset with different types of reinforcement.

supple belts can do the same thing and are very satisfactory.

Lumbosacral corsets can be prescribed at three levels: T12, T9, T6. The case of the "low back pain of thoracolumbar origin" (Maigne) is very particular (see Chapter 41, "Low Back Pain of Thoracolumbar Origin (T11, T12, and L1). Here frequently the lumbar corset is not well tolerated by the patient, and it can increase the pain as the superior transverse bar

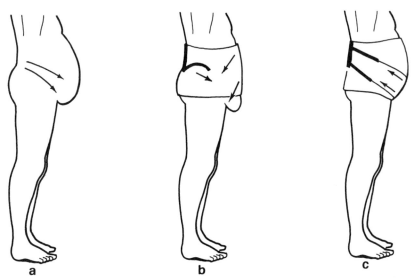

Figure 30.3. Abdominal corset. The abdominal corset is indispensable for the patient with obesity and low back pain, particularly if the abdomen is pendulous.

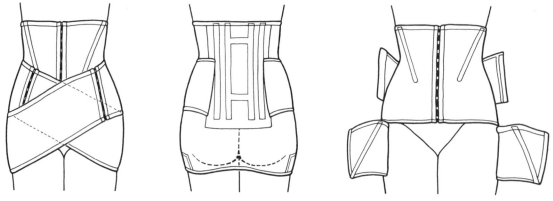

Figure 30.4.   Dr. Leven's support belt. This flexible support belt called an "atlas," helps to support the abdomen remarkably well, and supports the lumbar region.

pushes on the responsible segment while the inferior bar compresses the region of the iliac crest. It therefore presses on the cellulalgic zone and on the cutaneous branch of the posterior ramus of the irritated spinal nerve. Sometimes there is a problem in the choice of lumbar corset when a low back pain of lumbosacral origin is associated with a low back pain of thoracolumbar origin, especially in the elderly. In this situation the corset should be high (T9) and should not have any rigid element supported on the iliac crest (Fig. 30.5).

CONTRAINDICATIONS

There are not really any absolute contraindications, but there are instances in which the lumbar corset is not well tolerated for extraspinal causes; for example, patients unable to tolerate abdominal pressure (colitis, cholecystitis, gynecologic problems, vesical or genital prolapses, etc.). The lumbosacral corset should not be prescribed after an attack if an antalgic attitude persists. This situation will change over time; however, a lumbar corset should not be used during this time. During this phase, a rigid lumbosacral orthosis may be indicated and of greater utility. The patient should feel absolute relief in the lumbar corset, not "tolerate" it. If it bothers the patient or there is no decrease in the low back pain, then the prescription for this type of therapy should be reconsidered.

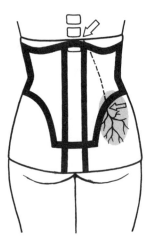

Figure 30.5.   In cases of low back pain of thoracolumbar origin, the lumbosacral corset is often poorly tolerated because the superior reinforcement of the lumbar corset can press on the painful spinal segment. Pressure on the iliac crest can induce pain by compression of the posterior ramus, which is irritated by the compression in the cellulalgic zone.

It is sometimes difficult to convince a patient to wear a lumbosacral corset; but sometimes it is more difficult to get a patient who feels comfortable with one to take it off.

The exercise prescription should start early. As soon as it becomes effective, the patient should take off the corset from time to time, then completely, and wear it only for the occasional painful exacerbation, in instances of prolonged standing, or if there is a fear of a painful attack.

31

CERVICAL COLLARS

Cervical collars are a harmless and useful means of treatment of acute cervical pain and cervicobrachial neuralgia.

TYPES OF COLLARS

The different types of cervical collars include flexible (soft) or semirigid providing limited immobilization, rigid, and minerva (Fig. 31.1).

Flexible Collars

Flexible collars are made of felt or polyethylene, enveloped in fabric. They come in different heights and lengths.

Collars with Rigid Reinforcement

These collars are reinforced by varying amounts of rigid materials, usually made from polyethylene. Their height can be adjusted by different procedures and they are fixed by Velcro attachments.

Mini Minerva

These collars have a chin support (Fig. 31.2). Some have only an occipital and chin support, others also have a sternal support for improved immobilization.

INDICATIONS

Cervical Trauma

In acute cervical trauma, a cervical collar is put on immediately both for patient relief and for safety. Radiographic and tomographic examinations such as CT or MRI are then used to assess the cervical spine for evidence of bony or soft tissue trauma. After the full evaluation, it can be decided whether the collar will be worn for a few days or be replaced by a minerva collar for more prolonged immobilization. A plaster minerva is for maximum immobilization in orthopedic services.

Acute Cervical Pain

All acute torticollis (wryneck) can be relieved by immobilization, and the soft collar is

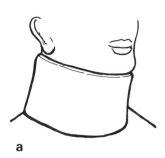

a

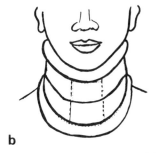

b

Figure 31.1. Different types of cervical collar. **a.** Soft foam. **b.** Plastic construction with variable height.

253

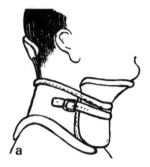 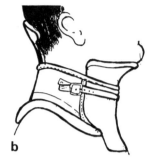

Figure 31.2. Collars with chin support. **a.** Chin and occipital support. **b.** Chin, occipital, and sternal support.

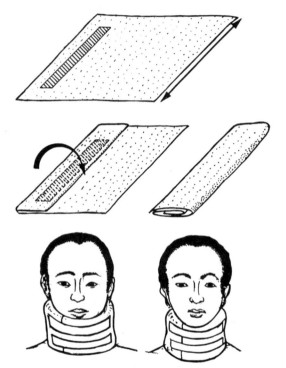

Figure 31.3. A cervical collar can be easily made using a towel and a piece of cardboard. On the *left*, supporting the chin; on the *right*, without chin support.

usually the most effective for this. An emergency collar can be made in a few minutes (Fig. 31.3).

With a Terry Towel. For satisfactory immobilization, the towel should support the chin. A long towel is folded to make a band about 20 cm high and put around the neck including the chin; it is then fixed with an adhesive band. The back part can be reinforced with a small piece of cardboard placed in the towel.

With a Newspaper. The paper is folded in a band, placed in a thin towel, and attached with an adhesive band. Some cotton can be inserted at the level of the maxillary and clavicular region for the comfort of the patient.

Cervicobrachial Neuralgia

Cervicobrachial neuralgia is a good indication for treatment with a cervical collar, even though the acute phase may last only a few days. In the cases associated with severe pain, complete immobilization is desirable. A minerva made of rigid plastic material, with an occipital and chin rest, should be used.

Chronic Cervical Pain

Some patients have their cervical pain increased or precipitated by travel (e.g., long trips by car). In such cases, it is useful to wear a cervical collar. A collar is also helpful during acute attacks of cervical arthritis.

32

THERAPEUTIC EXERCISE

Covering fairly the subject of therapeutic exercise for spinal pain would require a whole book; we present here what we think are the most important indications relating to the therapeutic system proposed in this book.

Physical modalities such as massage are often considered in the systematic treatment of patients having benign mechanical spinal pain. It is essential in most cases, which emphasizes the important role of the physiotherapist, but it is not always indicated and can at times be contraindicated. In some cases, it can perpetuate the pain.

Most subjects with spinal pain need to have postural reeducation. The physician and therapist will usually evaluate and correct the mechanical aspects of typical daily activities such as getting in and out of bed, standing, sitting, and other postures that may be associated with activities of daily living and daily work. That is what back schools try to do.

CERVICAL PAIN

If the techniques of massage, mobilization, and postural advice are indispensable in treating cervical cases of "painful minor intervertebral dysfunction," the same cannot be said for reconditioning exercises, except in the case of fracture, where it is indispensable.

However, in some cases, therapeutic exercise can be very useful, particularly in young women with a long neck and a slim musculature who have developed pain because of static postures at work over long periods of time and in certain benign traumatic cervical discopathies. Isometric contraction against manual re-

sistance is often very useful. The contraction is maintained for 5–10 seconds, followed by complete relaxation.

Sometimes, some micromovements performed in the same conditions give better results, but excessive active exercise should be avoided. In all cases, the contraction or the micromovement should be strictly painless. Later, certain exercises can be performed by the patient to retain permanent dynamic and static cervical muscular protection.

THORACIC PAIN

Thoracic pain of low cervical origin is not often improved by an exercise prescription. One should insist on the importance of physical exercises in two cases: with the scoliotic patients, young or old, where it is necessary to maintain and develop the abdominal and paraspinal musculature, and in juvenile- and adult-onset kyphoses, where contraction of spinal muscles against an isometric resistance can be prescribed as well as some active stretching and autostraightening exercises to fight against the tendency toward accentuation of the physiologic curvatures.

LOW BACK PAIN

Low Back Pain of Lumbosacral Origin

Low back pain of lumbosacral origin, due to disk or facet joint disorders, is the best indication for a comprehensive reconditioning and stabilization program. However, it should be tailored to the patient's needs.

One should not try to correct a lordosis or a kyphosis or to excessively develop the paraspinal or abdominal muscles because they "maintain" the spine. The aim of the therapeutic exercise program is to help the patient with low back pain to lead as normal a life as possible with a minimum of inconvenience.

Therefore, the patient should be advised and helped to regain conscious control of the lumbopelvic mechanism and to learn to control it; (the simplest exercise for this is learning how to tilt the pelvis). On the other hand, it is equally important to learn what types of activities to avoid and how to reduce stress on the lumbosacral junction during those activities. To do this, the patient should learn how to lock the spine in a neutral position while maximizing use of the legs for the performance of physical activity. Maintenance of neutral spine position is the basis of the dynamic stabilization program that is often the cornerstone of physiotherapeutic intervention in low back pain.

These two elements may be supplemented to the patient's advantage by other techniques such as muscle conditioning by isometric or isotonic exercises (in cases of progressive degenerative disk disease) "postural adjustments," and proprioceptive adjustments in patients with exertional low back pain (e.g., those resulting from athletic activities). In these cases, the aim is to provide protection for the affected segment and relative loosening of the region with a program that teaches how to avoid extreme or stressful movements.

Therapeutic exercises for low back pain have traditionally been categorized as either extension or flexion programs. The rule of no pain and opposite movement should dictate which of these exercises is to be used.

Low Back Pain of Thoracolumbar Origin

Low back pain of thoracolumbar origin is generally not a good indication for therapeutic reconditioning exercises. In these cases, priority should be given to postural advice, sometimes with the use of a proprioceptive retraining of that region.

Nevertheless there are two instances in which reconditioning is necessary: in subjects who have frequent recurrence of pain and in athletes. The syndrome of the thoracolumbar junction of Maigne (see Chapter 60) is indeed frequent in athletes and can present as low back pain or pubic pain. Rehabilitation is directed toward protecting the thoracolumbar transitional zone by exercises (Ledoux and Halmagrand) that

- Will improve the segmental spinal mobility of the super adjacent regions (thoracic)
- Will release the paraspinal soft tissues and the thoracolumbar fascia (lumbar region and the hamstring muscles)
- Will improve the dynamic action of the quadratus lumborum and the abdominal obliquus muscles
- Will develop proprioceptive function

Rehabilitation of the Lower Limbs

It is fundamental in all cases of low back pain that reconditioning exercises for the quadriceps are essential. The patient should learn to squat easily (instead of bending forward at the waist) and use the buttocks instead of the spine. The patient should be taught to perform daily flexion and extension exercises of the knees, squatting and getting up while keeping the torso straight.

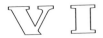

CLINICAL ASPECTS
OF PAIN OF
SPINAL ORIGIN

33

CHRONIC NECK PAIN

There are pains that in their usual forms are always recognized as being of spinal origin, such as cervical pain, thoracic pain, low back pain, and radicular, cervicobrachial, femoral neuralgia or sciatica. For some pain, the spinal origin is rarely considered, such as headache, for example, or for which it is never considered, as in limb joint pain or pseudovisceral pain.

Before accepting a spinal origin, according to the classical concept, the diagnosis should be supported by diagnostic imaging including radiographs or other forms of radioimaging searching for pathology of the segment or segments that may be responsible. However, it is well-known that significant pathology can be painless and areas with pain may show unrelated pathology or no pathology at all.

The concept of "painful minor intervertebral dysfunction" (PMID) that we propose and the concept of "segmental cellulotenoperiosteomyalgic syndrome" (CTPM) that we describe complete the classical semiology and allow objective examination of the role of the spine in many common pain disorders, either as an originator or as an aggravating factor. A combination of clinical examination techniques and radiographic examinations permits diagnoses of conditions that previously eluded both proper diagnosis and management; for example, the frequent cervical origin of common thoracic pain and the thoracolumbar origin of some low back pain syndromes, cervical-origin headache, epicondylar pain syndromes due to segmental spinal dysfunction, pubic pain syndromes, and hip and knee pain syndromes similarly due to segmental spinal dysfunction. In addition, some pain syndromes appear as the result of interacting factors, usually one local (often related to a local compression) and

the other more distant, involving a spinal mechanism.

Finally, unexpected associations of diverse pain resulting from the same PMID are considered; a typical example of this is the "thoracolumbar junction syndrome." Multiple PMIDs can produce a typical clinical pain syndrome of which the "syndrome of transitional zones" is a good example. Neck pain can be found in many contexts and can have variable characteristics. The pain may be mild yet be associated with serious pathology.

Diagnostic Errors to Be Avoided

The diagnostic mistakes that should be watched for include intramedullary tumors (meningiomas, neurofibromas, ependymomas), which can produce symptoms of chronic cervical pain for a long time. The pain can be localized or associated with occipital or brachial referral patterns. Tumors of the posterior fossa may, for a period of time, produce only local cervico-occipital pain.

Congenital anomalies of the cervico-occipital junction can become painful after trauma, even a trivial one, because of development of arthritic lesions or spontaneously. Sometimes, metastatic lesions, primary spinal cord tumors both malignant and benign, syrinx or cysts of the spinal cord, can initially present with findings suggesting benign neck pain. When the cervical spine is affected by inflammatory conditions, the diagnosis is rarely difficult to make, as the patient has had similar episodes in the past. The anterior subluxation of the atlas is a known entity related to the destruction of the alar ligament. Nontuberculous infectious discitis is not very common in the cervical spine; however it is not difficult to diagnose, as it usually presents with pain, inflammation, and, in some cases, evidence of spinal cord compression. Pott's disease is more discrete, and the radiographic studies can be confused for a while with degenerative discopathy. In elderly patients, a fracture of the odontoid may not be recognized when there is an associated benign cervical pain appearing after minor trauma.

CLINICAL SIGNS OF NECK PAIN SYNDROMES

The level of the cervical spine that is affected determines the symptomatology and the possible referral patterns of the pain. When the superior cervical spine is affected, pain radiates toward the mastoid or the occiput. Usually, headache is also present, and more rarely, some manifestations of the "cervical syndrome" (see Chapter 50).

When the midcervical spine is affected, pain radiates toward the supraspinous fossa, and if the inferior cervical segments are affected, it radiates toward the interscapular region. All these pain syndromes are usually also associated with a variable degree of painful limitation of movements. It is usually this limitation of movement that causes the patient to seek medical consultation (e.g., a patient who has difficulty backing up a car because of a problem maintaining the head in a turned position).

History

A good history should document the precipitating causes of the pain, its date of onset, progression, conditions that ameliorate or aggravate it, its location and pattern of radiation, and the effects of movements and daily activity patterns on the pain. Associated manifestations such as headache, dizziness, thoracic pain, or shoulder pain should also be noted.

Range of Motion Assessment

To test active motion, the patient is seated; for the passive movements, the patient is examined in supine. Attention is given to range of motion restriction, to movements that produce pain, and to where in the arc of motion they produce it. The result of these examinations can be summarized in a "star diagram," which

allows one to follow the progression of the condition graphically in subsequent examinations. It also helps in determining which manipulative techniques may be useful and in assessing the effects of these techniques on the underlying condition.

Segmental Examination

The segmental examination allows one to determine which spinal segment or segments are responsible for the pain. Three signs should systematically be looked for:

1. Facet joint tenderness, a consistent sign found in all cervical segmental pain syndromes and often unilateral. For this examination, the patient is placed in the supine position (Fig. 33.1).
2. Pain on PA pressure applied to the spinous processes. The patient is seated for this examination (Fig. 33.2).
3. Interspinous ligament pain, which can be found by pressure with the pad of the finger index or with a key ring. Transverse pressure on the spinous process is not used at the cervical level, except in certain patients in whom it is possible for C2 and C7.

Evaluation of Cellulotenoperiosteomyalgic Manifestations of the Segmental Vertebral Syndrome

These manifestations are looked for systematically. They are constant, with or without the presence of referred pain.

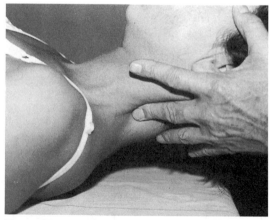

Figure 33.1.   Segmental examination. Evaluation for facet joint tenderness.

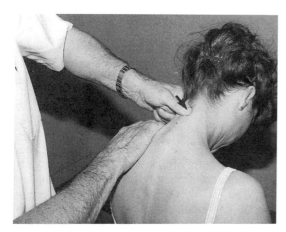

Figure 33.2. Segmental examination. Palpation of the spinous processes.

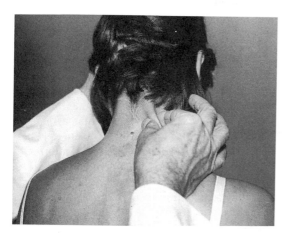

Figure 33.3. Throughout the cervical spine, it is important to examine the subcutaneous tissues of the neck and of the supraspinous fossa and medial thoracic region by means of the pinch-roll test.

The subcutaneous tissues of the interscapular region (between T2 and T6) are carefully studied with the "pinch-roll" test. A cellulalgic zone, especially if it is unilateral and a painful point by T5 or T7 (the "cervical point of the back" of Maigne), usually proves that there is pain in the inferior cervical spine (C5 to C7) (see Chapter 36, "Thoracic Pain of Cervical Origin"). In the same way, the supraspinous fossae (C4), the posterior and anterior regions of the neck, are examined. In the face and scalp, we also look for the signs of "pinch roll of the eyebrow," " the skin overlying the angle of the jaw," and the "friction of the scalp" (Maigne). They are usually the results of upper cervical involvement (see Chapter 48, "Headache of Cervical Origin") (Figs. 33.3 and 33.4).

Palpation of the cervical muscles is performed to find trigger points. Pressure on these points may reproduce the usual pain or symptoms. The most affected muscles are the shoulder girdle muscles including the levator scapulae, scalene, sternocleidomastoid, trapezius, and the supra and infraspinatus (Fig. 33.5). Examination of the shoulder muscles against isometric resistance can reveal tendinous pain, the possible consequence of a CTPM syndrome involving C4-C5 or C5-C6. Palpation of the lateral epicondyle is often painful ipsilateral to the facet joint tenderness when segments C5-C6 or C6-C7 are affected.

Radiographic Examinations

Radiographic studies should include an anteroposterior view of the whole cervical spine

Figure 33.4. The cellulalgic manifestation of cervical segmental dysfunction. At the level of the scalp, the pinch-roll test is replaced by the "friction sign test."

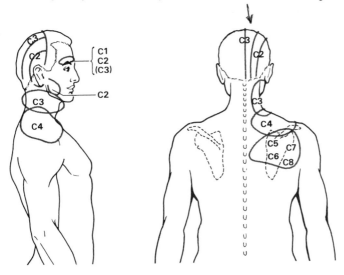

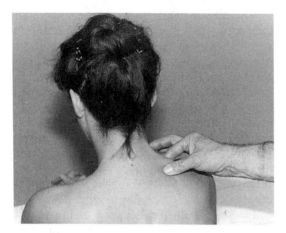

Figure 33.5. The search for trigger points should be systematic, palpating the muscles of the neck and shoulders. Here the examination of the trapezius is depicted.

(usually C3 and inferiorly), an open mouth view demonstrating the C0-1-2 segments, and a standard lateral view, making certain (especially in cases of suspected cervical spine trauma) that C7 is well seen. Occasionally it is necessary to apply traction to the upper limbs caudally, either with an assistant or with Bogy straps, to clear the shoulders from obstructing the view of the cervicothoracic junction. Occasionally a "swimmer's view" is necessary in difficult cases. Oblique views can be ordered to better visualize the neuroforamina.

In posttraumatic cervical pain, "pillar views" should be obtained by inclining the x-ray tube 30°, so as to be able to visualize the articular pillars. Dynamic views in flexion and extension performed later in the trauma workup are also necessary. If further studies are needed, CT or MRI of the upper cervical spine can be performed.

DIFFERENT ORIGINS OF NECK PAIN AND THEIR TREATMENT

Origins of neck pain include

- Acute inflammatory arthritic spondylitis
- "Painful minor intervertebral dysfunction" which is by far the most frequent cause, the spine being radiologically normal or arthritic
- Muscular caused by myalgic or trigger points
- Ligamentous pain
- Diffuse cellulalgia of the nape of the neck

Cervical pain with psychologic manifestations is not included here, but there is a psychologic element in cervical pain, especially when it is accident related.

Cervical Spondylosis

Spondylosis often does not produce pain, so the patients are able to ignore it until they have an inflammatory attack, an accident, a forced movement, or when it becomes so inconvenient that they have to see a physician. Then radiographs reveal the "spondylosis." From that moment, any pain in the neck may be wrongly attributed to it. Therefore, the patient should know what is due to the spondylosis and what is not.

Inflammatory Attacks

The pain of inflammatory attacks is not due to the spondylosis, but rather to the inflammatory involvement of the facet joints or uncinate processes. The pain can be subacute, acute, episodic, or of variable duration. Motion testing generally demonstrates pain in all directions of movement. Manipulative treatments are contraindicated in this condition.

Treatment. If the acute inflammatory arthrosis affects only one or two facet joints, which is a frequent finding, then an articular injection with a corticosteroid derivative is an excellent treatment. This treatment is, of course, impossible if the uncinate process is the source of the inflammatory reaction, in which case anti-inflammatory medications should be given and possibly a cervical collar be prescribed.

In some patients, inflammatory attacks continue for long periods, in which case "ultrasound therapy" may prove useful. After the acute inflammatory arthrosis, a persisting pain and stiffness may be noted because of the stiffness of the segment, which progressive mobilization and physiotherapy can improve.

Arthrotic Stiffening

Spondylosis can cause a progressive stiffening of the neck, which is painless and occurs often without the knowledge of the patient, except when accompanied by painful inflammatory attacks. This is often associated with a diffuse cellulitic edema of the nape of the neck and the supraspinous fossae.

At the level of the cervicothoracic junction, this cellulalgia can produce a "buffalo's hump," especially pronounced in women, which decreases after a few sessions of mobilization produce improved joint mobility.

Treatment. The treatment of the stiff spine should consist of attempts to increase segmental mobility and soft tissue flexibility by use of progressively firmer mobilizations without manipulation (Fig. 33.6). Treatment of the paraspinal muscles is very important: relaxing massage, with deep gliding, in the longitudinal direction and with transverse stretching.

The results of this form of therapy are excellent and do not depend on the degree of radiologic impairment. A very arthritic spine can be improved rapidly and regain nearly normal articular laxity, while another, less affected, may prove resistant to therapy. When spondylosis affects the facet joints, the results of mobilization are less effective and these take longer to improve than does degenerative disk disease arthritis or an uncinate process spondylosis.

Pulsed magnetic short waves (PMSW) are useful in this condition, as we have shown in our department, with G. Van Steenbrugghe, in a double-blind placebo-controlled study of 58 patients. In 10 biweekly sessions, PMSW therapy resulted in 70% good results, versus 28.5% with placebo. Using placebos is easy with

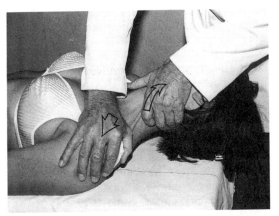

Figure 33.6. Mobilization with stretching and rotation to the right, and right lateral flexion. Mobilization and muscle stretching have a special place in the treatment of neck pain.

these waves, as they have no thermogenic effect that could be felt by the patient.

Spondylosis and PMID

Arthritic segments can produce PMID more frequently than do normal spines.

Painful Minor Intervertebral Dysfunctions

When a cervical pain occurs in a patient with a radiologically normal or arthritic spine after trauma or without apparent cause, it is often due to PMID.

Localization of the PMID

When the spine is arthritic, PMID is not always localized to the level of the radiologically most affected segment, and often it affects only one level, even when the spondylosis affects several segments. PMID of the superior cervical spine can produce occipital pain and cervical pain, but in most cases, patients do not complain of cervical pain, but rather of headaches. The headaches are described as having an occipital topography, but are more often described as supraorbital (see Chapter 48, "Headaches of Cervical Origin," and Chapter 50, "Cervical Syndrome").

PMIDs of the midcervical region (C3-C4, C4-C5) generally produce cervical pain that radiates toward the supraspinous fossa or the shoulder, producing a painful discomfort or a clear limitation of rotation and of lateroflexion of the neck on one side, associated often with trigger points of the levator scapulae and tenoperiosteal tenderness of its scapular insertion.

PMIDs of the lower cervical spine can be responsible for a low cervical pain, often postural, radiating sometimes to the shoulder, the arm, and between the scapulae. Many PMIDs are manifested only by an isolated interscapular thoracic pain (see Chapter 36), sometimes by a pseudotendinous pain in the shoulder (C4, C5) or by an epicondylar pain (C5, C6). These muscular, tendinous, or tenoperiosteal hypersensitivities are often revealed by systematic examination; they are never found clinically.

Treatment of PMID. Manipulation is usually the best treatment for PMID, except for some contraindications often related to the state of the spine (anomalies of the cervico-occipital junction, etc.), to the vascular state (postural tests), or of technical form (cases for which the rule of no pain and of the opposed movement would not apply) (Fig. 33.7).

If the response to manipulation is incomplete (i.e., if the facet joint remains tender to palpation), one or two injections of a corticosteroid derivative usually relieve the patient completely. When manipulation is contraindicated, injections are the treatments of choice, with or without mobilization and electrotherapy (pulsed short waves). In case of persistent ligamentous pain, a local injection of lidocaine with a corticosteroid is indicated.

The efficacy of the treatment can be judged not only by the subjective improvement of the patient and the amplitude of the movements, but also by the elements of the CTPM syndrome discovered at the initial examination. Their disappearance should be sought, if necessary finishing the cervical treatment with a local treatment.

Patients should learn to guard the neck, especially in rotation, in positions used at work and with activities of daily living. They should also be taught to avoid all fatiguing positions, such as reading in bed, watching television while sitting in a poorly adjusted seat, and sleeping prone. Education is essential to reduce recurrence.

A Particular Case: Posttraumatic Cervical Pain

The frequency of cervical trauma has increased in direct proportion to the use of the automobile. We do not refer here to trauma with neurologic or osseous repercussions, but to those traumas classified as minor.

The resulting cervical pain is usually attributed to "benign sprains" of the spine. The ligamentous system remains intact, and the dynamic x-rays are normal or show only minor static disorders of the spine: segmental stiffness, loss of the cervical lordosis, and slight axis alteration of the odontoid processes in relation to the lateral masses of the atlas. Rotation of the atlas on the axis compensates for the abnormal mechanics of the subjacent segments to maintain the horizontal orientation of the eyes. Convexity of the articular surfaces also gives an aspect of false pinching and of false axis alteration. There exists also a func-

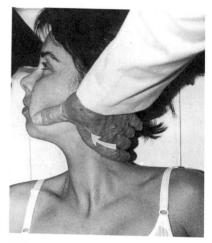

Figure 33.7. A manipulation in right rotation on C5-C6. The indication for manipulation should be well thought out.

tional block (Wackenheim) of the superior spine, either an atlanto-occipital block or atlantoaxial block. The former is characterized by an atlanto-occipital space that does not move at all in flexion or extension, the latter by a constant atlantoaxial or inferior cervical spine pinching producing a supra-adjacent hypermobility. The curvature abnormalities generally persist even if the patient is relieved of pain and the spine has clinically regained its suppleness.

Treatment. These cases have to be treated with great caution during the first weeks because the trauma produces ligamentous microlesions, capsular and muscular microlesions that contraindicate manipulative treatment. In the first days, a cervical collar is useful, with analgesic, anti-inflammatories and some muscle relaxants. The cervical collar should not be worn for a long time since the patient might become dependent on it and refuse to discontinue its use. However, it can be worn for a while during the night if the position of the neck produces pain.

Maneuvers of muscular relaxation without mobilization can be useful, as can electrotherapy. Manipulation should not be considered until 1 month after the accident. Then it should be performed carefully, after a series of mobilizations to end range; it consists of one or two maneuvers. Sometimes the result can be spectacular. As always, its use depends on negative postural tests.

Sometimes therapeutic exercise is started

very early, with isometrics. We prefer to use it when the cervical mobility has returned and the pain is much decreased. Its use should always, as in manipulation, be determined by the rule of no pain and opposite movement. The extensor muscles are treated initially, then the flexors, which are often neglected. It consists of multidirectional isometric contractions to stimulate and readjust the musculature whose traumatization has inhibited and perturbed function.

This physical therapy should not have the patient focus too much on the spine, especially when a psychologic element is involved. It is even better to do without if it is not indispensable, reassure the patient that the pain is benign, and explain how to avoid harmful positions.

When the patient is seen late in the course of the disorder, the usual treatment of PMID and of the CTPM manifestations can be provided.

Persistent pain on hyperextension or hyperflexion of the neck is usually due to the interspinous ligament, which can be treated by injection with lidocaine and corticosteroid derivatives.

Cervical Pain of Muscular, Subcutaneous, or Ligamentous Origin

Muscular Origin

The muscles of the neck can be a source of cervical pain. It can be due to trigger points, secondary to an articular or disk pain, or occur as a result of spinal segmental dysfunction. It can also be due to trigger points occurring after exertion or because of postural problems that result in excessive fatigue of the muscle, which should be stretched or injected. The trapezius muscle or the levator scapula is often the one affected.

Subcutaneous Origin

Some patients have cellulalgic zones affecting the entire nape of the neck and the supraspinous fossae. These form a "buffalo's hump" at the level of the cervicothoracic junction. These regional infiltrates differ from the localized infiltrate, are usually unilateral, and belong to the CTPM segmental syndrome. They are often well tolerated, though patients are very sensitive to cold and drafts, but they are sometimes the only cause of the cervical pain. The best treatment is massage, which can be combined with electrotherapy (iontophoresis).

Ligamentous Origin

In cervical pain syndromes that are tenacious, especially those resulting from cervical trauma, the possible involvement of the supraspinous ligament should be considered and sought. This can be done by palpation with the tip of the index finger, which can produce an acute pain between two spinous processes. The examination is often positive between C4-C5 or C5-C6. This interspinous pain is usually connected to a PMID, but if it persists despite treatment and despite the disappearance of the facet joint pain, it should be treated locally by injection with a corticosteroid derivative, lidocaine 0.5%, or procaine 0.5%. If no results are noted, then careful sclerosing therapy can be considered (see "Interspinal Ligaments" in Chapter 26).

Cervical Pain and Psychologic Disorders

The problem of cervical pain, especially when it is posttraumatic, is that it often has a psychologic element that is uncovered under different conditions. The patients are often anxious and distressed, with a tendency toward hypochondriasis—the kind of patients who have other neurotic manifestations, revindication, or compensation neurosis. No treatment can improve them, except of course a satisfactory indemnification. In some cases, the pain may be purely psychogenic; patients project onto the cervical level the conversion symptoms of their neurotic state, which of course no cervical or antalgic treatment can improve, but which can be aggravated by multiplication of paraclinical investigations.

34

TORTICOLLIS (WRYNECK) AND ACUTE CERVICAL PAIN

The most frequent cause of acute cervical pain is "benign torticollis (wryneck)," a distressing disorder, usually of short duration. However, it can be chronic if linked to an inflammatory arthritis or to a herniated disk. On rare occasions it can also be due to severe pathology. For example:

A progressive or acutely painful torticollis seemingly triggered by a mild trauma or sudden movement can actually be due to an underlying benign or malignant spinal tumor.

Patients with acute cervical pain should always be examined for possible fracture, utilizing radiographic studies liberally followed by tomographic studies such as CT or MRI if there is the least suspicion.

Episodes of acute cervical pain can be seen in the anomalies of the cervico-occipital junction as transient episodes of painful blockage of the neck.

Osteomyelitis (due to TB or other infectious agents) can take the form of a torticollis associated with fever and other signs of infection.

In the child, in the presence of fever and acute torticollis, a calcific nucleopathy (ochronosis) should be considered.

Acute stiffness of the neck in a patient with rheumatoid arthritis can be due to an atlantoaxial subluxation, and this possibility should be sought.

BENIGN ACUTE TORTICOLLIS

In the medical literature, torticollis is described as an inclination of the head on the neck—an involuntary, irreducible, constant, generally painful inclination of deforming appearance. In current language, the word *torticollis* means the benign torticollis, an acute and painful locking of the neck in rotation and lateroflexion, generally lasting a few days.

This condition is frequently blamed on cold drafts or sudden forced movements. Pain upon awakening is frequently reported. In very severe acute cases, the neck is "frozen" in side bending, and any movement, however small, exacerbates the pain. The neck is only locked on one side, with the other side being normal; in some cases, rotation can be blocked in both directions.

These common forms of torticollis can be due to PMID or be of muscular origin. It is sometimes difficult to distinguish which is responsible because acute PMID can cause a severe protective muscle guarding.

Torticollis due to PMID

Torticollis is generally the result of a rapid movement of the neck. Motion is usually free on one side, impaired and painful on the other. A segmental examination can localize the responsible level, and the facet joints can be found to be quite tender to palpation (often C2-C3).

Treatment

In general, manipulation is possible, but it should be preceded for a long time by mobilization maneuvers and progressive stretching in the pain-free directions. Manipulation should be mild and well planned and can help to reduce the protective muscle guarding. If manipulation is not possible (rule of no pain), a cervical collar can help to relieve the patient and shorten the acute phase. Facet injection is also useful.

When torticollis appears after cervical trauma, high quality radiographs are necessary to document PMID and confirm that no other pathologic explanations exist. In the immediate posttraumatic phase, the only treatment recommended is the cervical collar; manipulation should not be performed. After the 4th week, depending on the condition of the patient, manipulations may be considered.

Torticollis of Muscular Origin

In some cases of acute torticollis, examination does not reveal any particular segmental sensitivity. In these cases only the muscles seem to be affected, especially the sternocleidomastoid, the splenius, or the levator scapula. Their palpation is very painful. A cold draft is often thought to be the cause by the patient; however, a viral origin is thought possible by some investigators.

Treatment

The basic treatment for this condition is the use of a cervical collar, anti-inflammatory medications, analgesics, and muscle relaxants. Injection of the trigger points can bring quick relief. Acupuncture sometimes helps, as does stretching of the affected muscle.

Torticollis of Mixed Origin

Sometimes the two mechanisms (i.e., articular and muscular) seem to be associated. In such cases, the muscular factor should be treated first, followed by injection of the affected facets. Mobilization can be performed with great caution and only if strictly painless.

ACUTE CERVICAL PAIN

Due to Acute Synovitis

Acute cervical pain due to synovitis can produce moderate or acute pain. In the latter case, the neck is not locked or stiffened by pain but may have a loss of range of motion, with motion being painful even at rest. It is not unusual for acute cervical pain to be present with radiographic studies that fail to demonstrate significant pathology while the segmental examination demonstrates swollen facet joints.

Treatment

When only one or two articulations are affected, an articular injection with corticosteroid derivative is the treatment of choice. In other cases, anti-inflammatories can be used. The cervical collar can help bring about significant relief.

As a Result of a Herniated Disk

A herniated disk can cause acute neck pain and can appear after a violent shock while in hyperflexion. It can sometimes also appear after a simple forced movement in rotation. Initially, the condition presents with acute cervical pain, severe protective muscle guarding, and almost always associated interscapular pain. Typically, the pain increases with coughing or sneezing, and postural positions connected with supine. The patient can assume less painful positions such as head flexed forward and on the side. Progressively, the pain will reach the shoulder, then the arm.

The cervical herniated disk often evolves into a chronic phase, with the patient having low-level continuous pain, with episodic exacerbations lasting a few weeks to a few months at a time.

Treatment

Treatment during acute attacks should consist of immobilization with a Minerva cervical collar and the use of anti-inflammatories. Cervical traction is sometimes efficacious, but it is indicated only when the manual traction test relieves pain and does not exacerbate it (see Fig. 23.7), as it is not always well tolerated.

Cyriax advocates manipulation that involves both rotation and very strong manual traction. We are not convinced of the benefit of this approach.

35

CERVICOBRACHIAL NEURALGIA

Cervicobrachial neuralgia (CBN) is a pain referred to the upper limb as a result of an irritation or compression of a cervical nerve root (C5, C6, C7, or C8). This compression is usually the result of osteophytosis, uncarthrosis (disco-osteophytic nodule or "hard hernia"), or, rarely, to a herniated disk. The herniated disk is seen in young people, while the osteophytosis is not seen before the age of 40. In some cases of common CBN, none of these causes may explain the pain.

When there is no clear explanation, PMID or an acute synovitis of a facet joint spondylosis may be the cause. The pain in these cases is not due to nerve root compression; it is referred pain from any of the segmental spinal elements. In some cases, the cervicobrachial pain is the result of a serious lesion, which can pose significant diagnostic challenges.

PAIN

In general, the pain of CBN starts progressively and involves a painful stiffening of the neck with interscapular or precordial referral. Pain in the arm will occur a few hours to a few weeks later. For most practical purposes, this pain sums up the clinical picture. The pain can be replaced by paresthesia in the distribution of the affected root down to the hand, ending at one or several fingers with tingling. It is generally distressing, with nocturnal attacks sometimes triggered by movement of the neck, coughing, or sneezing. The pain can be almost unbearable. The neck may be held in antalgic postures or demonstrate simple stiffness with limitation of movements. Such cases often demonstrate no objective neurologic findings. Objective findings of other types are seen in only about 50% of cases. The reflexes are rarely abnormal, nor are motor problems usually seen.

EXAMINATION OF THE NECK

Examination of the neck starts with an evaluation of the neck range of motion with the patient seated, followed by a reassessment in supine with the head slightly past the end of the table, in a position of maximum relaxation.

The angle of the neck at which movement triggers pain is determined; an increase in this angle usually signals an improvement in the problem.

Examination of the Affected Level

The main sign of the segmental examination is pain on palpation in the corresponding articular pillar. This sign is constant in CBNs of mechanical origin. Pressure on the spinous process is also painful. An "anterior doorbell point" can reproduce or increase the spontaneous pain.

Axial compression over the vertex, with the patient sitting, can provoke an exaggeration of pain. Conversely, traction on the neck can relieve the patient.

Test of Manual Traction

The patient is in supine position; the physician takes hold of both the chin and occiput and applies progressive traction on the neck. If this maneuver relieves the pain in the arm or in the shoulder, a treatment by mechanical traction or suspension can be planned (Fig. 35.4). If it exacerbates the pain, any manual or mechanical traction should be avoided.

INTERSCAPULAR PAIN

CBNs are often associated with interscapular pain. It can precede the attack, come with it, or survive it. The epicenter of the pain is usually a fingerbreadth lateral to T5 or T6 and is painful on palpation. This is what we describe as the "interscapular point of cervical origin," or "cervical point of the back" (Maigne 1968). It is not specific to CBN; it is our impression that it is the thoracic mirror of the pains of the inferior cervical spine.

This "cervical point of the back" is common to the inferior cervical segments (see Chapter 36, "Thoracic Pain of Cervical Origin").

CLINICAL EXAMPLES BY SEGMENTAL LEVEL

Each cervical root when affected has a unique clinical syndrome.

C5 Syndrome

Sensory deficits: varying degrees of paresthesia or hypesthesia over the anterior shoulder to the lateral border of the elbow

Motor deficits: deltoid, supraspinatus, teres minor, sometimes biceps, leading to impairment of abduction and external rotation of the shoulder

C6 Syndrome

Sensory deficits: varying degrees of paresthesia or hypesthesia over the anterolateral shoulder, lateral arm, to the thumb (Fig. 35.1)

Reflex deficits: decreases or absent biceps, brachioradialis, and pronator teres reflexes

Motor deficits: weakness and atrophy of the biceps, brachioradialis, and thenar muscles, resulting in impairment of elbow flexion and pronation

C7 Syndrome

Sensory deficits: varying degrees of paresthesia or hypesthesia over the cervicothoracic junction, posterior shoulder, arm, forearm,

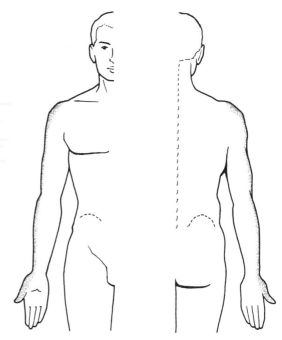

Figure 35.1.   C6 topography.

dorsum of the wrist, index and middle fingers, and occasionally, the ring finger (Fig. 35.2)

Reflex deficits: decreases or absent triceps reflex

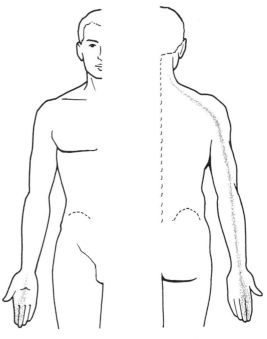

Figure 35.2.   C7 topography.

Motor deficits: weakness and atrophy of the triceps and long finger and wrist extensors, resulting in impairment of extension of the elbow, wrist, and fingers

C8 Syndrome

Sensory deficits: varying degrees of paresthesia or hypesthesia over the medial arm, forearm, wrist, hand, and 4th and 5th fingers (Fig. 35.3)

Reflex deficits: decreased or absent finger flexor reflex

Motor deficits: weakness and atrophy of the hand, especially the intrinsics and hypothenar eminence

ETIOLOGIES

Cervicobrachial Neuralgia Due to Cervical Spondylosis

CBN is considered one of the clinical expressions of cervical spondylosis. It usually affects people in their 50s, and women more than men.

Cervical radiographs show the degenerative changes, especially of the uncovertebral

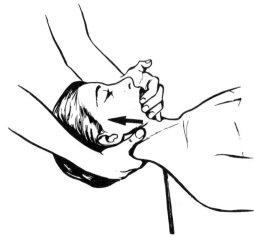

Figure 35.4.   Manual traction test. If this maneuver reduces cervical brachial pain, then cervical traction will be effective. If it induces pain, it is then in contraindication to the use of cervical traction.

joints, with osteophytes encroaching on the intervertebral foramen. Inflammation related to a disco-osteophytic nodule is felt to be the cause of the CBN.

The pain often decreases, then disappears in 3–6 weeks, sometimes resulting in persistent paresthesia. There are some chronic and refractory forms for which CT/myelography or MRI may be necessary.

CBN Due to Disk Herniation

In young people, CBN can be the result of a herniated disk following trauma or a violent effort; the antalgic attitude and the stiffness of the neck are usually pronounced. Radiographs of the cervical spine may show a relative gap, laterally or posteriorly. Diagnosis is made with the aid of MRI or CT studies. Most often, medical treatment is sufficient. When pain persists or motor deficit or pyramidal signs are found, surgery may be indicated.

CBN Due to PMID

CBN can occur in a patient with no spondylosis (e.g., after an accident or a forced movement) with less marked signs than with a herniated disk. The segmental examination in these cases reveals pain at the corresponding vertebral level. PMID should be considered as a diagnostic possibility in cases that have no significant pathologic findings on cer-

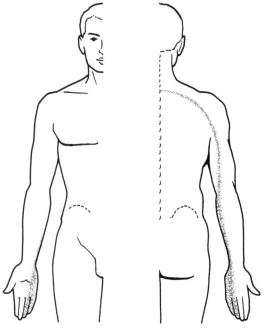

Figure 35.3.   C8 topography.

vical x-rays, CT, or MRI. In these cases it is more likely that the pain is referred from an articular disorder as opposed to pain due to nerve root compression.

DIFFERENTIAL DIAGNOSIS

The diagnosis of cervical spondylosis is usually not difficult to make. In spite of this, diagnostic errors occur on occasion, as the symptomatology is not always typical and complete.

Entrapment Syndromes

This radicular syndrome should not be confused with an entrapment syndrome involving the more distal neural segments such as the plexus or peripheral nerve; for example, in the median nerve in the carpal tunnel or the ulnar nerve in the cubital tunnel or Guyon's tunnel. A cervical rib can be involved in a thoracic outlet syndrome resulting in a C8-T1 syndrome, characterized by paresthesia and motor and vasomotor dysfunction of the hand.

Referred Pain Syndromes

Some tendinous pains of the shoulder and elbow can lead one into making a diagnosis of moderate chronic pseudoradicular pain. Many of these tendinous pains are the result of a cervical PMID. In the acute form of the syndrome of the levator scapula, there can be a brachial referral simulating a CBN, the thoracic pain being put in the background. But there are more serious causes.

Intramedullary Tumors

The glioma is by far the most frequent intramedullary tumor. It results in a refractory CBN, exacerbated by the supine position. Initially, only local involvement is noted without spinal cord signs. Radiographic studies performed in the 3/4 oblique position for visualization of the intervertebral foramina may show enlargement of the neural foramen. Diagnosis is greatly aided and facilitated by the use of CT or MRI.

Meningioma is less common, as are malignant intramedullary and epidural tumors.

Infectious Discitis

As a result of infection by various agents, both tubercular and nontubercular, cervical discitis can occur, which can induce a CBN. The diagnosis can be made on the basis of cervical stiffness in association with an infectious syndrome with abnormal radiographic findings. However, the value of the clinical examination should not be overlooked, nor should the utility of bone and gallium scans be forgotten.

Spinal Metastases

CBN of metastatic origin can result in extremely severe pain that evolves rapidly with progressive neurologic signs. The monoradicular disorder becomes pluriradicular. The pluriradicular syndrome soon gives way to a spinal cord syndrome with spinal cord pain and findings consistent with an extradural compression (metastatic, hematologic, etc.).

Pancoast Tumors

An intense cervicobrachial pain is often the first sign of tumors of the pulmonary apex often associated with interscapular pain. Motor and sensory deficits in a C8-T1 or lower plexus distribution are seen, associated with Horner's syndrome. The diagnosis is confirmed by pulmonary radiography that shows the opacity of the apex, which in the beginning is sometimes only a simple decrease in transparency.

TREATMENT

In the acute phase, especially if the pain is intense, a brief (6 days) course of corticosteroid therapy is of use, starting with a high dose then gradually tapering off. One can start with smaller doses using the Luccherini technique: an intradural injection of 2 mL of hydrocortisone acetate, which necessitates a brief hospitalization.

In milder forms, nonsteroidal anti-inflammatory medications are sufficient. Analgesics are used but are not effective unless used concurrently with a medication such as diazepam.

In the subacute or refractory forms, immobilization of the neck with a well-adapted minerva is indispensable. In milder forms, the use of a cervical collar decreases pain and helps the patient to avoid exacerbating postures, particularly at night. Surgery is rarely needed for this condition. Mechanical treatment, such as manipulation and traction, can also be used.

Manipulation

In some cases, manipulation can bring quick relief to the patient. Generally, they are not useful in the acute phase, where the rule of "no pain and opposite movement" is not applicable. Manipulation is most indicated in the subacute form. They are applied only if previous mobilizations resulted in the patient's having the impression of relaxation and relief.

They are executed in each of the nonpainful directions. If the result is good, two or three can be performed, one especially on rotation, and on lateroflexion. The third can be in flexion and extension, depending which one of them is free. Between each mobilization and after each manipulation, the patient is reexamined so as to see if progress has been made, and will decide, so to say, what maneuvers are to follow. If the final result is going to be good, a relief is frequently already seen at the first session (Figs. 35.5–35.7). In one out of three cases, the patient may have a more or less disagreeable reaction the following night after the first session. He/she should be warned about this possibility. This reaction, however, does not change the prognosis as far as the final result is concerned.

After three sessions without any improve-

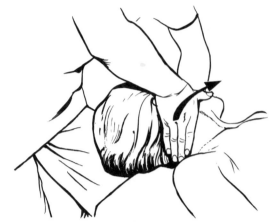

Figure 35.6. Technique for rotatory manipulation to the left.

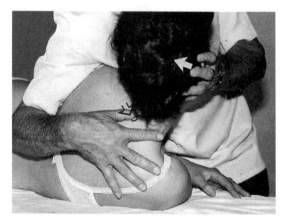

Figure 35.7. Manipulation technique in left lateral flexion.

ment, the manipulative treatment should be terminated.

Spinal Traction

Spinal traction can be very useful. If the manual traction test is favorable (Fig. 35.4), suspensions on an inclined plane or traction on a table can certainly bring significant improvement. The head of the patient is maintained with a Seyre collar (Fig. 23.2a) or with Maigne's apparatus (Fig. 23.2b).

Manipulation and Traction

It is interesting to try both manipulation and traction during the same treatment session; however in general, it is better to do them dur-

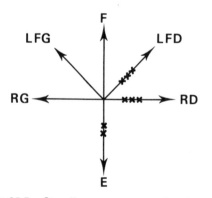

Figure 35.5. Star diagram corresponding to a right C6 cervical brachialgia.

ing separate sessions. If they are performed during the same session, it is better to start with the manipulation.

Manipulation under Traction.   A manipulation is performed in rotation under traction. The physician grasps the chin and occiput of the patient in the cup of the hand and applies progressive traction to the cervical spine. If this maneuver is painless, it can be executed as a manipulation in rotation of the pain-free side. For herniated disks, Cyriax recommends manipulation under very strong traction, with an assistant holding the patient's feet.

Residual Pain and Cellulotenoperiosteomyalgic Manifestations of Spinal Origin

After the acute phase is over, the cellulotenoperiosteomyalgic manifestations are often responsible for persistent pain, which may appear to be pseudoradicular or tendinous. A more or less annoying interscapular pain is rather frequent.

In such cases, the subcutaneous tissues and muscles that are most often affected should be carefully examined by palpation, and trigger points should be sought and evaluated for a possible role in the maintenance of persistent pain referral to the shoulder, upper arm, or elbow. The target muscles frequently noted are the infraspinatus, teres major and teres minor (C5-C6), triceps (C7), and the common wrist extensors. The trigger point that originates the persistent pain is sharply localized and painful on palpation. An injection of Xylocaine is necessary to stop the radiating pain. This injection may be sufficient to treat this condition; otherwise, stretching, massage, or ultrasound therapy should be used. The tendinous sensitivities especially affect the supraspinatus (C5-C6), the biceps (C5-C6), and the lateral epicondyle (C6-C7).

36

CHRONIC THORACIC PAIN

The "benign" or "common" thoracic pain of the adult is certainly the most neglected aspect of spinal pathology, in spite of its frequency. The literature concerning this entity is sparse. Most of the literature remarks on the paucity of clinical findings and tends to relegate this condition to the functional area, stressing psychic factors that certain authors consider to be the essential cause.

Thanks to the segmental examination set out in this book and the study of cellulomyalgic manifestations, we can demonstrate that most pains in the midthoracic region present with a characteristic clinical picture and have an origin in the inferior cervical spine (Maigne, 1964). The psychic factors and the state of the organism are, of course, not to be neglected, but they only participate in the cause of the pain without explaining it. Other causes of common thoracic pain exist, such as thoracic vertebral, muscular, or rarely ligamentous origin.

Diagnostic Errors to Be Avoided

Visceral disorders, even when they are not yet recognized, can be the cause of misleading thoracic pain. Pancreatic lesions, especially cancer, can produce refractory thoracic pain, as can certain ulcers of the stomach or of the duodenum. Pleuropulmonary and cardiac disorders and aortic dissection can produce, for a certain time, isolated thoracic pain. D. Belaiche observed a paradoxical case of thoracic pain linked to a gastric ulcer that could be relieved only by indomethacin! (personal communication). Also spinal lesions due to multiple myeloma, metastasis, discitis, or osteoporotic vertebral compression fractures can produce a temporary thoracic pain with many aspects in common.

INTERSCAPULAR THORACIC PAIN OF LOW CERVICAL ORIGIN (MAIGNE)

Most common thoracic pains are felt in the midthoracic interscapular region. Though pain in this region may originate in the thoracic spine, in our experience, the vast majority of pains in this region originate from the lower three cervical spinal segments (1964). In spite of the cervical origin of this pain, the patient feels pain in the neck only exceptionally; instead, it is projected to the thoracic level. It disappears with the cervical treatment. On examination, this pain at the thoracic level demonstrates constant and characteristic signs and symptoms.

Clinical Picture

The pain is felt between the shoulder blades; some patients describe a highly circumscribed point, such as a right or left paraspinal point. Sometimes it is localized to a more diffuse region, which may be unilateral or involve the midback. The pain may even be described as intrathoracic.

The patient likens the pain to a "red hot iron," a "cramp," or an "intense and localized fatigue." It can appear after trauma, a poorly performed manipulation, or an uncorrected postural stress, etc. The pain usually has an insidious onset.

Though the pain is chronic, there are episodes of worsening, often associated with periods of fatigue, overwork, or postural or psychic stress. Persons in certain types of occupations (e.g., typists, keyboard operators, sewing) at times suffer from this pain. In general, it is decreased by rest. In some cases, the reverse is noted, with increased pain in the morning upon awakening. This is felt to be due to poor postural positioning of the neck during sleep, especially in people sleeping prone, which forces the neck into full rotation.

The pain can start out as an acute pain due to a strenuous effort or sudden movement (see Chapter 37, Acute Thoracic Pain).

Clinical Examination

Examination of the Back

At the thoracic level, two signs are characteristic of thoracic pain of cervical origin:

- A remarkably constant painful point, localized to the paraspinal levels of T5 or T6 "the cervical point of the back"
- A cellulalgic zone adjacent to this point and spreading laterally toward the acromion

Cervical Point of the Back (Maigne). There is a painful point about 2 cm from the median line at the level of T5 or T6. This vertebrointerscapular point is constant and seems to reflect the pain of the lower cervical spine. The pain can have any type of origin: benign, malignant, articular, discogenic, or tumoral (Fig. 36.1). The examination should thus be as thorough as possible.

The patient is seated with the head flexed, hands on lap, in complete relaxation. The examiner uses the middle or index finger to glide slowly, following a line parallel to the line of the spinous processes, one fingerbreadth lateral to the midline. The examiner applies firm, continuous, and constant pressure with the pad of the finger while at the same time executing small frictional to-and-fro movements repeated every centimeter, just as if the examiner wanted to mobilize the subcutaneous tissues over the underlying muscles. This maneuver is performed several times. It is exactly the same maneuver performed in the segmental examination during the evaluation of facet joint tenderness.

At T5 or T6, usually 1–2 cm lateral of the midline, a very tender point is found. Mild pressure on this point and on it alone will reproduce the patient's usual pain, even if it had been reported to be higher, lower, or even at an intrathoracic point (Fig. 36.2).

Localization of that point is remarkably fixed. We did a radiologic localization in 150 patients and found this point opposite T5 or T6 in 138 cases, opposite T4 in 7, and opposite T7 in 5.

N.B. The "cervical point of the back" can be confused with facet joint pain of T5-T6 or T6-T7 (Fig. 36.5). This occurs much less frequently in clinical practice, and it is usually quite easy to distinguish the two. If it is really a "cervical point of the back," there is a cellulalgic zone adjacent to it overlying the ipsilateral scapula and spreading laterally (Fig. 36.3). If the tenderness is due to an irrita-

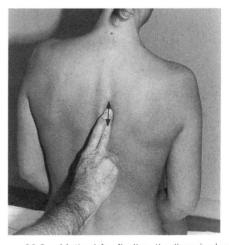

Figure 36.2. Method for finding the "cervical point of the back." This painful point is found exactly next to T5 or T6, approximately 1 or 2 cm lateral of the median line (see X on Fig. 36.1). This is the same maneuver used to find the painful facet joint during the segmental examination.

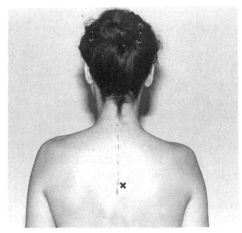

Figure 36.1. The "cervical point of the back" (Maigne). In cases of thoracic pain of cervical origin, pressure on this point reproduces the spontaneous pain of the patient.

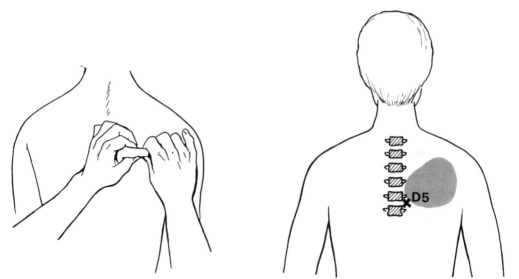

Figures 36.3 and 36.4.   Next to the "cervical point of the back," the pinch-roll test can detect a cellulalgic zone that extends laterally.

ble thoracic facet joint resulting from segmental dysfunction at T5-T6 or T6-T7, the corresponding cellulalgic zone is located lower, toward T9 or T10 in the dermatomal territory of the posterior ramus of T5 or T6 (Fig. 36.5).

Midthoracic Cellulalgic Band.   The "cervical point of the back" usually has a large cellulalgic zone adjacent to it that is demonstrable by means of the pinch-roll test. It spreads lat-

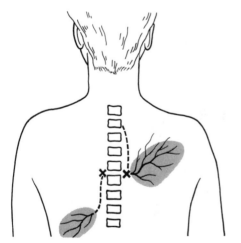

Figure 36.5.   The "cervical point of the back" (*right*), can be confused with thoracic facet tenderness due to the T4-T5 or T5-T6 segment (*left*). In this case, the cellulalgic band that would correspond to the posterior ramus of T5 would be situated much lower, nearer the T9-T10 level.

erally from the "cervical point of the back" toward the acromion, a height of 6–8 cm. It is larger laterally than medially and is sometimes limited to a smaller surface. The cutaneous and subcutaneous tissues of that zone are thickened and painful to pinch-rolling. The thickening can be very significant in some chronic cases. Sometimes, the changes are mild and may only involve a portion of the possible area, while it is painless on the opposite side or in the sub- or supra-adjacent regions (Figs. 36.3 and 36.4).

One or two taut bands of muscle sometimes occur with the cellulalgia. They are localized in the paraspinal muscles and sometimes at the level of the lateralmost iliocostalis muscle. Palpation should be performed very thoroughly with the pads of the fingers, which are held in the manner of hooks, perpendicular to the direction of the bundles, which are very sensitive and the size of a small pencil or a match.

Radiologic Signs.   The radiologic examination is generally normal; however, minor benign abnormalities may be found that are not causally related to the pain, though one is often tempted to blame these lesions, as though this were a case of "guilt by association." Examples of these pathologies noted but not causally related include scoliosis, hyperkyphosis, thoracic arthrosis, and the sequelae of Scheuermann's apophysitis of adolescence. Sometimes thoracic x-rays may be very misleading. We have seen patients with old traumatic compression fractures of T5 or T6, to which chronic refractory thoracic pain was wrongly attributed. In these cases the pain was, in fact, found to be due to a cervical PMID that had occurred during the same accident. The evidence for this was the disappearance of the pain after cervical treatment.

N.B. With chronic thoracic pain, the "cervical point of the back" and the cellulalgia remain on examination, even when the patient does not suffer, as in all the cases of chronic PMID.

Examination of the Neck

Most often, the patient does not complain about the neck. If the patient feels pain, the cervical pain and the back pain do not seem to be related.

The examination sometimes demonstrates some impairment in the movements of the neck. In a few rare cases, forced rotation, forced hyperextension, or both produce the thoracic pain. In general, the neck movements are free and painless.

The segmental examination demonstrates that one of the last three segments of the inferior cervical spine is affected. The segmental examination reveals facet joint tenderness (Fig. 36.6), sometimes with pain on palpation of the spinous process and the interspinous ligament. The "cervical point of the back" and the cellulalgic zone are always ipsilateral to the cervical facet joint tenderness.

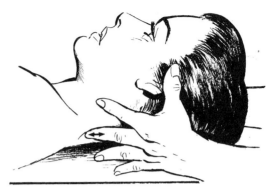

Figure 36.6. Segmental examination of the inferior cervical spine (C5-T1) demonstrating facet tenderness ipsilateral to the "cervical point of the back."

Among common thoracic pain syndromes, cervical segmental dysfunction is often due to a PMID and is sometimes the result of synovitis.

The "anterior doorbell sign," which we described in our first publications, consists of provoking the patient's usual thoracic pain by applying pressure with the thumb at the responsible level and at the anterolateral part of the spine (Fig. 36.7). This maneuver demonstrates the link between the cervical spine and the midthoracic pain. This sign is inconstant, and it is not always easy to demonstrate. There are cases in which this "cervical doorbell point" should be looked for carefully by modifying the point at which pressure is applied by a few centimeters. It is found in about 6 of 10

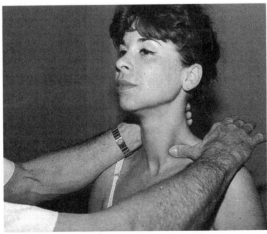

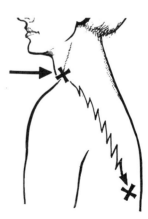

Figure 36.7. The "doorbell sign" (Maigne). Pressure is applied to the anterolateral aspect of the cervical spine. In most cases, such pressure applied to an involved segment produces a painful referral toward the thoracic spine.

cases of thoracic pain of cervical origin. However, it is not necessary to find it to prove the cervical origin of a thoracic pain when other signs are present and are localized to the same side.

Cervical spine radiographs are indispensable to rule out all serious lesions (just as thoracic spine and thorax radiographic studies are also needed). The responsibility of the cervical spine cannot be asserted or invalidated by the existence or absence of signs of spondylosis or of degenerative discopathy, just as the thoracic spine cannot be held responsible because there is spondylosis, a sequelae of Scheuermann's disease, or scoliosis.

Cervical Spine and Thoracic Pain

The link between thoracic pain, the painful point para-T5, the adjacent cellulalgia, and the cervical spine can be demonstrated by the following therapeutic test: any treatment that makes the painful cervical segment painless on segmental examination is tried, and the thoracic pain and signs are then reevaluated for persistence or disappearance. The treatment can take the form of manipulation or facet injection. If this test successfully reduces the pain, the cervical origin of the midthoracic spine pain should be considered confirmed.

Conversely, any treatment that makes the cervical segment more painful on segmental

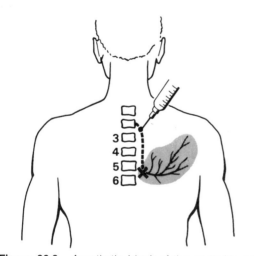

Figure 36.8. Anesthetic block of the posterior primary ramus of T2 at the point where it traverses the T2-T3 facet joint can relieve spontaneous thoracic pain, the "cervical point of the back," and pain on the pinch-roll test.

examination increases the thoracic pain, the "cervical point of the back," and the cellulalgia. This may be due to performing the manipulation for the PMID in the wrong direction.

This type of thoracic pain is currently seen often as a result of poorly performed manipulations of the inferior cervical spine. These patients complain little or not at all about their necks, but a great deal about their backs.

No Simple Anatomic Explanation. There is apparently no anatomic explanation for this painful projection. The posterior rami of the last spinal cervical nerves might make it possible, but no anatomist sees their territory as so low; most even think that they do not have any cutaneous branches.

Thoracic Pain and Cervical Herniated Disk. Most authors do not view thoracic pain as being due to the cervical spine, as we do, and the point para-T5, which we call the "cervical point of the back," has not been proven to be a sign of cervical dysfunction. Nevertheless, some authors have been intrigued by the sometimes acute interscapular pain preceding and associated with cervical herniated disks.

Stookey and Michelsen and Mixter on one hand, Elliot and Kramer on the other, report it without giving any explanation. Wedell and Feinstein noted the constant "irritation" of the paraspinal muscles of the thoracic region seen on electromyography in patients with cervical herniated disks; they concluded that "the protective muscle guarding at that level is not due to the lesion of the spinal nerve compressed by the herniation, but by another source of unknown pain."

Cloward's Experiments. During interventions for cervical herniated disks performed under local anesthesia, Cloward irritated, electrically or mechanically, different elements of the spinal segmental levels. He noted that irritation of the superficial anterolateral annular fibers produced acute pain in the ipsilateral periscapular region that reproduced or exacerbated the usual referral pattern. He obtained the same effect by irritation of the motor root at the same level. He reinforced the muscular nature of that pain with electromyographic evidence. He attributed it to the irritation of the muscles of the shoulder girdle, which are innervated by the lower cervical roots: rhomboideus muscle (roots C4-C5), infraspinatus muscle (roots C5-C6), and latissimus dorsi and subscapularis (C6-C7). He noted also that the patients felt pain at the level of the superiomedial angle of the scapula for C4-C5, over the midscapula for C5-C6, and the inferior scapula for C6-C7.

This experiment deserves comment.

- It demonstrates definitely that a cervical lesion can produce a thoracic pain, which is essential for our thesis.
- The electromyographic evidence is less convincing in the explanation of the pain mechanism. It is normal for muscles that are innervated by a nerve root that is compressed by a herniated disk to show some electromyographic disturbances. It does not prove their responsibility for the pain.
- Our observations do not agree with Cloward's about the level at which the pain is perceived according to the cervical height affected. When patients are asked about it, the various answers obtained do not depend on the responsible cervical level.

If the patients are examined, we learn that pressure on the "cervical point of the back" and on it alone always reproduces their pain, even if they have the impression of feeling it higher or lower. In numerous cases of cervical radiculopathy due to C6, C7, or C8 that we have examined, we have always found the "cervical point of the back" at the same place, para-T5 or para-T6, whatever the responsible level. We have made the same observation in cases of lower cervical PMID without radicular pain syndromes.

Cloward did not note the existence of this point, the real epicenter of the thoracic pain, nor the existence of the adjacent cellulalgic zone. Therefore, the pathologic explanations that he proposed must be reconsidered.

Pathogenic Mechanism: A Personal Hypothesis

To analyze the mechanism of thoracic pain of cervical origin, it is first necessary to know to what the "cervical point of the back," para-T5 or T6 and the cellulalgic zone associated with it, corresponds. That is what we have first tried to establish.

Posterior Primary Rami of the Second Thoracic Nerve Root.   The anterior primary rami of C5–T1 constitute the brachial plexus. Their cutaneous branches innervate the skin of the upper limb. But the posterior primary rami of

C6, C7, and C8, like the ones of L4 and L5, have no cutaneous branches. The posterior ramus of C5 and T1 is inconsistent and small when it exists (in 25% of cases, according to Lazorthes).

If, as everything seems to point clinically, the "cervical point of the back" and the adjacent cellulalgic zone show the distress of the inferior cervical spine, the question remains about what link might exist between the cervical and thoracic spinal regions. The "cervical point of the back" seems to correspond to the superficial emergence of the cutaneous branch of the posterior primary ramus of the 2nd thoracic spinal nerve root (Maigne, 1966). Indeed, if this ramus, when it goes around the facet joints T2-T3, is injected with 1 mL of 1% lidocaine, it produces temporary disappearance of

- The spontaneous pain of the patient, which is marked in the acute case
- The "cervical point of the back"
- The adjacent cellulalgic zone, which becomes flexible and painless on "pinching-rolling"

According to Hovelacque, the size and location of the posterior ramus of T2 are important. The branch extends up to the acromion, covering a large surface (Fig. 36.9). The maps of the posterior dermatomes commonly accepted by most authors are presented schematically in two ways:

- Some, like Keegan and Garret, attribute an equal horizontal band to each of the dermatomes from C4 to T3. According to them, this is why C4, C5, and C6 cover the suprascapular fossa and T1 and T2 are noticeably at the level of the 5th and 6th (Fig. 36.10).
- Others, like Töndury or Brugger, pass directly from the dermatome of C4 to the dermatome of T2—as for the anterior dermatomes; Lazorthes attributes a small paramedian zone between these two territories to C5 and C6 (Fig. 36.10).

No author accords a particularly extended territory to the posterior dermatome of T2. However, according to our clinical results, we should consider the existence below C4 of a large common territory representing C5, C6, C7, C8, T1, and T2. This territory corresponds well to the one of the posterior primary rami of T2 as described by Hovelacque, and as we

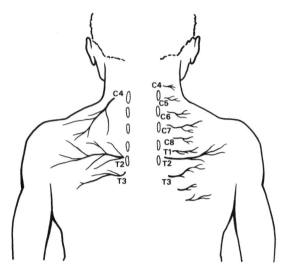

Figure 36.9.   The cutaneous branches of the posterior primary rami. On the *right* after Hovelacque, note the stress placed on the cutaneous branch of T2. But he acknowledges the presence of cutaneous branches for C5, C6, C7, and T1. On the *left*, for most anatomists, C6 and C7 are not felt to have cutaneous branches. C5 and T1 are noted to have one in four cases (Lazorthes). Our dissections confirm the significant presence of the cutaneous branch of T2. The cutaneous branch of C4 assures the innervation of the whole region and the supraspinous fossa. This diagram is closer to our clinical experience.

have found it on a few dissections. The posterior primary rami of that level present, in the first part of their path, some usual anastomoses with their neighbors (Hovelacque, Niray-

ana). It is as if the cutaneous ramus of T2 (and maybe also of T3) incorporated the complement of inferior cervical and cutaneous branches that were missing.

This hypothesis provides a satisfactory framework for understanding the clinical phenomena and our anatomic observations. The "cervical point of the back" and the adjacent cutaneous zone are the favored sites of pain referral from the inferior cervical spine, whatever their nature—benign or malignant, disk or facet joint (Fig. 36.11).

A Few Particular Cases

The interscapular dorsalgia that we have described affects women more often than men. Usually, it presents as a tenacious postural thoracic pain, more or less distressing, without any particular radiographic signs, but there are more disconcerting cases. The three cases below demonstrate the variety of conditions in which this cervical thoracic pain can be seen. The first two teach us that we should not rush to attribute a thoracic pain to a severe scoliosis or to a severe epiphysitis. The third demonstrates the errors to which misdiagnosis of this interscapular thoracic pain of cervical origin can lead.

Case 1.   M. D., a 39-year-old secretary seen for the first time at the age of 22 was referred to us by the Orthopedic Department because of severe thoracic pain attributed to severe Scheuermann disease, af-

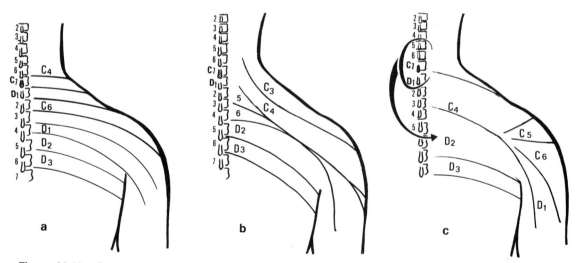

Figure 36.10.   Posterior dermatomes. **a.** According to Keegan and Garret. **b.** According to Lazorthes. **c.** According to Töndury. (The *arrow* is added by Dr. Maigne to demonstrate what has been verified).

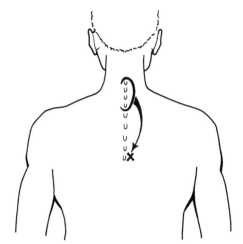

Figure 36.11. "The cervical point of the back" (Maigne). This is a reflection of a dysfunction of the inferior cervical spine, which may be due to either disk or facet disorders. It can be benign or malignant and corresponds to the emergence of the posterior primary rami of T2.

fecting particularly the 4th, 5th, 6th, and 7th thoracic vertebrae, the site of the spontaneous pain. She could not write or type for more than 1 hour. Numerous treatments such as massage, therapeutic exercise, and thoracolumbar orthoses tried over many years had changed nothing, and the pain had become so overwhelming that the orthopedic surgeon treating her had decided to perform a fusion. A consultation was requested at the Rheumatology Department, and the conclusion was the same.

Examination revealed a left para-T6 interscapular point showing extreme sensitivity and an adjacent and very thickened cellulalgic zone. Examination of the neck revealed a C7-C8 PMID, with an ipsilateral tender facet joint at that level. There was an anterior cervical "doorbell" point reproducing the thoracic pain. The cervical radiographs were normal.

Four cervical manipulations, one per week, improved the patient enough to allow her to resume her work immediately. A maintenance treatment was performed every 3 months for 1 year. Since that first treatment, 17 years ago, she had three children and never interrupted her work as a secretary. From time to time, she feels a vague point in the back when she is fatigued or has overworked herself.

Case 2. M. C. V., a 27-year-old secretary, presented with a severe thoracolumbar scoliosis at 48° and had been seen regularly in a specialized department since the age of 13.

She never had pain. In the 2 years before we saw her, she developed thoracic pains that became more and more unbearable and had interrupted her work for the last 6 months. The beginning of the pains coincided with a change in her work, which, interestingly,

she preferred to her prior job. She had two series of "massage and physical therapy," which were performed without success for 10 months. The pain was most severe at the apex of the thoracic curvature near T7.

After several consultations with the Departments of Orthopedics and Rheumatology, it was decided to try a fusion. It was then that she was seen in our department for consultation. She described her pain as being "in the two sides," "throughout her entire back." Examination uncovered an "interscapular point," para-T6 on the right, which responded to applied pressure by recreating "all her pains"; also uncovered was a significant adjacent cellulalgic zone. The cervical spine was radiologically normal. The segmental examination revealed a typical C5-C6 PMID with right facet joint pain. No "anterior doorbell point" was found. After the first cervical manipulation, she was very much relieved; after four sessions, she felt well and went back to work. In the new job, she repeatedly performed cervical rotation to the right and took, for example, some documents behind her, to the right, which she did by mechanically stretching her arm toward the back. This repeated maneuver resulted in a decompensation of the cervical PMID, which was perfectly tolerated up to then. She modified her place of work, and she now works without any inconvenience. The pain has not recurred for the past 2 years.

Most of the patients who present with this interscapular pain feel it moderately and intermittently. That pain is sometimes distressing, but it rarely has the hyperalgic and durable character of the pain seen in the next case.

Case 3. M. P., a 57-year-old patient, had a lobectomy for a massive pulmonary infarct. The day after the intervention, he complained about a thoracic pain on the side of the intervention. The surgery went without complication, and the result was excellent. But the thoracic pain persisted, preventing sleep, and being refractory to any treatment to the point that after 2 years, a rhizotomy at T3-T4-T5 was performed. The failure was total. A few months later, because of the refractory pain, the pulmonologist, neurologist, and the neurosurgeon agreed on a chordotomy. At that time, the patient consulted us at Hotel Dieu.

The thoracic examination uncovered an acutely painful point, para-T5, on the side of the scar. A slight pressure on it and only on it reproduced the usual pain. As the patient said, it was the first time in 5 years that that point was found and "his pain" reproduced. A large band of cellulalgia adjacent to that point extended up to the acromion. The cervical examination demonstrated, besides some limitation in rotation and lateroflexion on the side of the pain, a relatively acute pain of the ipsilateral C5/6 facet joint. Thoracic and cervical radiographic studies revealed a minor degree of spondylosis.

Cervical manipulation was begun. At the first session, in a spectacular manner, the thoracic pain disappeared, and the cervical movements became free and painless. The "para-T5 point" became hardly sensitive to firm pressure. The cellulalgia was more supple and hardly painful. After a second session 1 week later, the patient was without pain for a year, until the day he lifted a heavy weight, and the thoracic pain returned, disappearing again after two cervical manipulations.

Treatment

The treatment of interscapular pain of cervical origin is essentially cervical. If it is due to PMID, the most frequent cause, cervical manipulation is the treatment of choice when the state of the spine allows it and when it is technically possible. It is preceded by progressive mobilization.

It should be precise, soft, strictly unilateral, and performed according to the rule of no pain and opposite movement. Generally, the most useful maneuvers are rotation with the patient in supine, lateroflexion with the patient in lateral decubitus, and the "chin pivot" with the patient in prone position (Figs. 36.12–36.14).

Manipulation can, if necessary, be replaced or supplemented by a facet joint injection that is designed for painful cervical articulation uncovered by the segmental examination of C5-C6, C6-C7, or C8-T1. On the side of the thoracic painful point, 0.5 mL of a corticosteroid derivative is injected (Fig. 36.14) (see "Facet Joint Injections" in Chapter 26); the treatment is repeated two or three times. Cervical electrotherapy (pulsed short waves) can be useful when the two preceding treatments cannot be used. In acute synovitis, anti-inflammatory medications can be useful.

In patients who have more pain in the morning, the reason is often postural malpositioning of the neck during sleep (people sleeping on the abdomen). A cervical collar or (sometimes better tolerated) a collar made of a thick towel folded with a soft cardboard inside, worn during the night for 3–4 weeks, often can bring

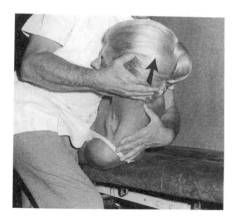

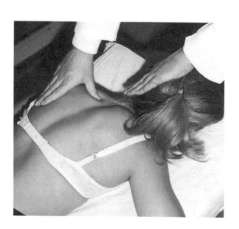

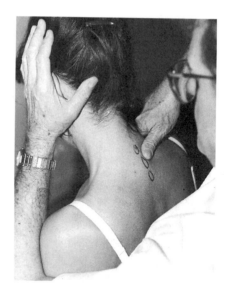

Figures 36.12–36.14. Examples of manipulative techniques used in the treatment of intrascapular pain of cervical origin (all performed according to the rule of no pain and free movement).

relief. In chronic cases, it is sometimes necessary to treat the residual cellulalgic manifestations and more rarely the taut muscle bands.

Massage. If the cellulalgic zone does not disappear completely with cervical treatment, massage using a pinch-roll or "kneading" technique performed superficially is often quite useful. This treatment is often quite painful, and it is better to try it after an anesthetic injection either on the posterior ramus of T2 or directly on the subcutaneous tissues. This injection is followed immediately by kneading maneuvers.

Psychologic Factors

Depressive or simply neurotic factors frequently exaggerate thoracic pain. In these patients, the signs of spasmophilia (Chvostek's sign, electromyogram) are often present. Suitable treatment of these cases starts with an attempt to reduce the muscular hypersensitivity producing a PMID that other subjects would tolerate perfectly or not feel at all. Relaxation can be a useful adjuvant in these cases.

Psychologic Disorders. In depressed or very anxious patients with typical clinical pictures of a thoracic pain of cervical origin, a brief cervical treatment should be performed, and its effect judged. If the result is neither good nor rapid, it is better not to insist. It is imperative to treat the psychologic state.

Physical Modalities

Physical modalities should not ignore the cervical origin of thoracic pain because doing so may cause the thoracic pain to persist or aggravate it. Modalities will bring relief to the patient only if the therapist pays particular attention to massaging the cellulalgic zone, which persists after the acute episodes.

Used after cervical treatment, it can be a double-edged sword, helping in some cases and causing acute decompensation of the patient in others through a sudden or forceful movement. All cases must be individualized.

We reserve modalities for recurrent cases. Remember that this is a cervicothoracic disorder, not thoracic, and that often it is associated with postural problems. It is necessary to have a very competent physical therapist.

Swimming for relaxation is often useful

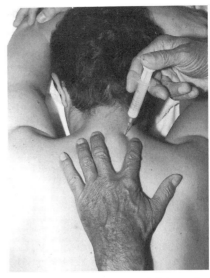

Figure 36.15. Injection of a painful cervical facet joint can sometimes replace manipulation or contribute to its effect.

(breast stroke with snorkel to allow swimming without raising the head or swimming on the back or side).

Prevention

Prevention is essential in the management of these disorders. Patients must be taught to avoid extreme neck rotation (as in backing a car, sleeping in the prone position, etc.), especially on the side of the cervical articular point; placing something behind the back, with retropulsion of the arm, especially when seated; closing the back door of the car while sitting in front; putting something on the back seat, or taking it, or taking maps from behind without getting up; and seats that are too low and too soft, which induce cervical fatigue resulting in thoracic pain. It is indispensable to study the postural issues of the work environment.

THORACIC PAIN OF THORACIC ORIGIN

Thoracic pain of thoracic origin is less frequent than is pain of cervical origin. Its principal origins are PMID, acute inflammatory arthritis, and muscular causes (i.e., myalgic cords, trigger points). At the midthoracic level, there are frequent causes of error in the segmental examination. They are due to

- Frequent cellulalgic edema of the subcutaneous tissues of the midback region, which gives "false positives" when searching for segmental tenderness to transverse pressure against the spinous process or for facet joint tenderness (see p. 141).
- The fact that the superficial emergence of the cutaneous branch of the posterior ramus of T2 occurs 2 cm lateral of the median line, and corresponds to the level of the facet joints of T5-T6 (Fig. 36.5) (see p. 276).

Thoracic Pain Due to Thoracic PMID

Thoracic pain due to thoracic PMID is the consequence of forceful activities, forced movements, trauma, or poor posture. The pain produced by PMID is generally felt at the level of the cellulalgic zone that is induced in the cutaneous territory of the corresponding posterior ramus. It is low thoracic for a T6 or T7 PMID and midthoracic for a T3 or T4 PMID.

Treatment

Manipulation is the logical treatment, respecting the usual rules. But it often involves stiff spines, so the manipulation should be prepared or replaced by flexible mobilizations and performed progressively.

Massage results in paraspinal muscular relaxation and can treat the cellulalgic zones that do not always disappear completely with treatment of the responsible PMID.

Thoracic Pain of Discogenic Origin

Benign thoracic pain has always puzzled clinicians, as most radiographic evaluations offer no explanation. This does not surprise us; we consider this pain to be of cervical origin in the great majority of cases.

Nevertheless, Bruckner et al. (1989) incriminated disk deterioration that was detected by MRI. In 10 patients with that kind of pain, 9 of them had isolated disk deterioration, while in a control series of 15 patients, they found such deterioration only twice. But in only 4 cases did the disk lesion correspond exactly to the clinically painful spinal segment, and in 5 cases, there was no coincidence.

Because of the benign nature of the degener-

ative lesions at the thoracic level, confirmation of this etiology will need more demonstrative studies involving more patients. It seems to us that the segment found to be pathologic on MRI scan must be painful on segmental examination.

Thoracic Pain Due to Thoracic Arthrosis

Thoracic arthrosis is very common and is painful only occasionally. The pain usually originates in the cervical spine if it is a "common" pain. When evaluating someone with what is thought to be thoracic arthrosis, it is best to first make certain that the pain does not have a neurologic or visceral origin or result from other conditions such as malignant illness in the older patient, spondyloarthropathy in the young, and discitis in all ages.

Treatment

In painful acute synovitis, anti-inflammatory medications are usually useful. If the patient has gastric intolerance to these medications, electrotherapy can be very useful.

Thoracic Pain and Scheuermann's Disease

"Growth apophysitis" is rarely painful at onset during adolescence. The later episodic painful attacks are often relieved by rest and anti-inflammatory medications. Rare severe forms require wearing a thoracolumbar orthosis.

In the adult, the sequelae of the Scheuermann's disease are sometimes responsible for the thoracic pain, especially when there are also some arthritic lesions fostered by dystrophic alterations, but they are rarely the cause. More often, pain in these cases are referred pains of cervical origin.

In patients with stiff and round backs, dysfunction of the cervicothoracic junction is frequently seen. Because it is necessary to keep the head horizontal, the subject straightens the neck. The inferior cervical articulations are subject to increased loading and may cause PMIDs, which facilitates a facet joint spondylosis with inflammatory attacks causing thoracic pain.

Thoracic Pain and Osteoporosis

Osteoporosis after menopause affects one woman in four. It is not painful, but when advanced, it produces such spinal fragility that even a minor trauma can produce compression fractures that appear to have no apparent cause, producing thoracic pain that starts abruptly, with a thoracolumbar localization. The pain can be severe, constant, and increased by coughing, defecation, or movements. It can also be moderate to the degree that the patient does not recall an acute onset but rather notes a progressive pain that becomes chronic and is relieved by rest and increased by activity. Diagnosis is made by radiographic demonstration of the vertebral wedging, which does not always affect the posterior wall.

Thoracic Pain and Interspinous Ligaments

The examination sometimes reveals an acute pain affecting only the interspinous ligament of one or two levels. Often this is post-traumatic. Relief and proof of the origin is generally brought by injection of 0.5% lidocaine with a corticosteroid derivative.

CHRONIC THORACIC PAIN OF MUSCULAR ORIGIN

Some muscles can be responsible for thoracic pain, such as the scalenus, trapezius, rhomboideus, iliocostalis, levator scapula, and serratus anterior. The muscle may not seem painful to the patient, but its thorough palpation (Fig. 36.6) reveals a firm taut band with a "trigger point" that under pressure reproduces the usual pain. These trigger points can

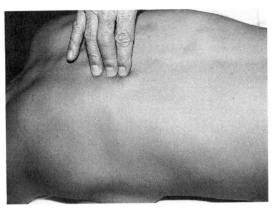

Figure 36.16. Evaluation for trigger points in the examination of the back.

be part of a spinal cellulotenoperiosteomyalgic syndrome or be a direct result of muscle fatigue because of excessive use or an incorrect position.

When the levator scapulae is affected, it can cause either a low cervical pain or a high thoracic pain. When the rhomboideus is affected, there are pains in the interscapular region. If the iliocostal muscle is affected, there is a very distinct picture of a subacute pain simulating a tenacious pleuropulmonary or one that recurs. The responsible trigger point can be as big as a match, localized most often at the level of the 7th, 8th, or 9th, 8–10 cm lateral to the midline. Fatigue or muscle cooling are the usual causes of the painful trigger points. In some cases, the pain is acute (see next chapter); the responsible cause is more rarely found in the paraspinal muscles.

Treatment

Treatment consists of injections of the cord with 1% lidocaine. Ultrasound therapy can also be quite useful.

ACUTE THORACIC PAIN

Just like chronic thoracic pain, common acute thoracic pain can be of cervical, thoracic, or muscular origin.

ACUTE INTERSCAPULAR THORACIC PAIN OF CERVICAL ORIGIN

Acute thoracic pain most often takes the form of acute "interscapular" pain of cervical origin (Maigne) (see "Interscapular Pain of Low Cervical Origin (Maigne)" in Chapter 36). It has the same signs as chronic thoracic pain. It can be the first manifestation of cervicobrachial neuralgia, which will occur a few days later, or can remain isolated.

On examination, at T5 or T6, one fingerbreadth lateral of the midline, is the "cervical point of the back" (described above). Examination of the cervical spine will reveal the responsible segment: C5-C6, C6-C7, or C7-T1. Usually, it is a cervical mechanical pain (disk herniation or "acute spinal disorder") or facet inflammation. Very rarely, pain can be due to a spinal cord tumor, visceral tumor, or other intramedullary lesion.

Treatment

Cervical immobilization with a collar or minerva is the best means to relieve the thoracic pain. Cervical manipulation is rarely possible. If it is, it can bring spectacular relief. A facet injection is useful in case of an acute PMID or facet joint inflammation. Injection of the posterior ramus of T2 at its emergence between T2 and T3 can sometimes decrease the acute pain.

ACUTE THORACIC PAIN OF THORACIC ORIGIN

In the back, there can be an acute painful manifestation similar to torticollis (wryneck) or a lumbar pain. It usually results from forceful activity or a wrong movement. de Sèze called it a "dorsalgia," emphasizing the similarity with low back pain and its discogenic origin. This is evidently possible, but the extreme rarity of thoracic discogenic disorders is well known. This type of manifestation, which we have encountered rarely, generally concerns the lower or midthoracic segments (T6–T9), and it seems to us to be an example of an acute PMID or thoracic sprain.

Treatment

If a manipulation performed according to the principle of no pain and opposite movement is possible, it can bring relief. Anti-inflammatories, analgesics, and muscle relaxants are useful.

ACUTE THORACIC PAIN DUE TO DISK CALCIFICATION

Acute lower thoracic pain with associated inflammation and fever has been observed in women over 40 years of age and has been attributed to calcification of the annulus fibrosis. These patients often have a history of similar episodes in the recent or remote past. Anti-inflammatory treatment is useful.

ACUTE THORACIC PAIN OF MUSCULAR ORIGIN

In general, acute thoracic pain of muscular origin is due to a trigger point of a muscle, which has been activated by cold, fatigue, or wrong movement. The pain is sharp, often poorly localized by the patient. Palpation of the "taut bands" of the trigger point, often difficult to find, reproduces the pain and can increase it. Relief can be obtained with injection of a few milliliters of 0.5% lidocaine at that point.

The levator scapulae and the iliocostalis muscles are most often affected. The levator scapula produces the pain of a low torticollis with acute referral to the upper limb. However, the pain may remain high thoracic (see Chapter 51, "Levator Scapulae Syndrome"). The iliocostalis sometimes reveals one or two trigger points in cases of thoracic pain of cervical origin, but they can exist in an isolated form also (postural fatigue). They can be the source of very acute pain, either fixed, simulating pleuritic pain and increased by deep respiration, or occurring with sharp and sudden releases produced by deep breathing and sometimes spontaneously.

Though we did not yet know of the muscular origin, we had already described this form in an earlier book under the name of "acute thoracic pain and lightning pains." The observation in the first patient in which we noted it, is here reproduced as it is quite typical of this condition:

Case History.   M. C., 45 years old, had felt a violent pinching in the lower thoracic region 3 days earlier, while slipping his arm in the sleeve of his vest. This pinching lasted a few minutes, then decreased, as long as he did not move at all, breathing as softly as possibly because deep inspiration or expiration caused a violent lightning pain. A few minutes later, he felt relieved and again started his normal movements, when suddenly, a similar attack immobilized him. From then on he noted a succession of calm periods followed by acute attacks lasting a few seconds to a few minutes and produced by movements or positions that varied from one moment to the next.

On examination, the spine was flexible, and analytic examination of the movements did not show any limitation, pain, or segmental dysfunction. During the examination, an unforeseen gesture produced an attack, but there was no systematization in the movement that produced it. A movement that had been performed earlier without pain would suddenly, a few minutes later, spark an acute attack. Often, deep inspiration would trigger it. Radiographs obtained the same day as the attack showed no abnormality. There was relief or exacerbation by different maneuvers of mobilization or manipulation that could be tried in this case.

An intramuscular injection of 8 mg of thiocolchicoside produced quick relief (muscle relaxation). This patient had three similar attacks in 4 years. No radiologic or clinical sign had been uncovered during the attacks. Knowing better after the first attack, the other two were treated by intravenous injection of thiocolchicoside as soon as possible, and relief came quickly, on the first day for one and on the second day for the other.

A few years later, he had a fourth similar attack for which he received a different treatment. In the meantime, we had observed similar cases, and a thorough examination of the muscles of the back revealed that the trigger points of the iliocostalis muscle were responsible. Local anesthetic injection of one or more trigger points brought some relief immediately. He was advised to refrain from exposing his back to the cold.

38

COSTAL SPRAINS

Costal sprains often present with features of thoracic or lumbar pain. They may occur after local trauma, forceful activities, or a faulty movement. On examination, no tender spinal point is found. The tenderness to palpation is localized to only one rib, while the adjacent ribs or the ribs from the opposite side are painless. Pressure produces or increases the spontaneous pain.

They usually resolve in a few days. Occasionally, these sprains become chronic, resulting in chronic pain that can lead to diagnostic errors, especially when the false ribs are involved, as is most frequently the case.

CLINICAL PRESENTATION

Costal "sprains" can be seen in different conditions.

Faulty Movement or Forceful Effort

In most cases, sprains from faulty movement or forceful effort result from abnormal rotation, sometimes very slight, as may occur in making the bed, turning back to close the back door of the car, at the start of a 100-meter dash, etc. In other cases, the condition can be produced by a violent muscular contraction during heavy lifting or sneezing.

Direct Trauma

A thoracic contusion due to a fall can cause a posterior sprain or an anterior chondrocostal sprain. It can also be associated with a vertebral or costal fracture. Occasional pain persisting after fracture of a rib is due to residual costal or vertebral sprain, often relieved by manipulation.

CLINICAL PICTURE

Sprains due to a faulty movement most often affect the false ribs. During a quick rotation of the trunk, the patient feels a pain like "a stab with a knife" in the side and bends forward and lies down immediately.

In a few hours or days, the pain decreases and disappears. It can persist longer, with pain on awakening after a forceful or strenuous movement of the trunk or coughing. These episodes become more annoying over time and lose their clear producing cause.

Most of these patients ultimately undergo renal evaluations. One of our patients had five violent attacks in 4 years. He was hospitalized three times and had five intravenous pyelograms, all negative. He had a sprain of the last rib and was relieved after the first treatment. Several other patients in our series had various interventions (appendectomy, renal surgery). Others were diagnosed and treated for lumbar pain and massages. Physical therapy treatments prescribed for these patients regularly aggravated their pain.

DIAGNOSIS

Posterior Costal Sprains

Posterior costal sprains are the most frequent. Pressure or percussion on the affected rib can be painful. The most sensitive test for this condition is "the rib maneuver" (Maigne).

The patient is seated with the physician standing behind. The patient is asked to laterally flex the trunk to the side opposite the pain, with the hand on the painful side resting on the head. With the pad of the thumb, the examiner grasps the superior edge of the painful rib and pushes it downward (Fig. 38.1B); then, grasping the inferior edge with the pads of the fingers, pushes it upward (Fig. 38.1). In costal sprains, one of these maneuvers increases the pain, while the other is painless. This sign is rather characteristic of this disorder; indeed, in costal fractures, both maneuvers are painful. Conversely, they do not modify the pain if it is due to a radicular irritation of spinal origin or if its origin is muscular or visceral. In some renal or pleuropulmonary disorders, there are pains in the last ribs, and in some hepatic disorders, pain is felt at the level of the last right rib.

In certain obese patients, it can be difficult to grasp the rib fully. Lateroflexion of the patient's trunk contralateral to the painful side should be exaggerated to free it. The integrity of the rib and the adjacent spine is confirmed by radiography. For the middle ribs, examinations can be performed on patients lying down on their sides.

N.B. During the examination, the subcutaneous tissues, which are painful and cellulitic, should not be pinched between the operator's finger and the rib; they should be examined first by the pinchroll test.

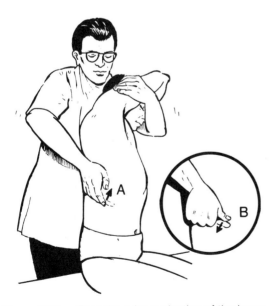

Figure 38.1.   Technique for evaluation of the lower ribs. **A.** The rib is grasped by the fingertips and pulled upward. **B.** Then the rib is pushed downward with the pad of the thumb.

Anterior Costal Sprains

There can also exist chondrocostal "sprains" localized to the chondrocostal junction, resulting from trauma or a faulty movement. They are sometimes confused with Tietze's syndrome.

Manipulation usually provides good results. The principle of the examination is the same. The patient is supine, and the operator, with thumbs opposed end to end, grasps the upper edge of the rib and pushes it downward (Figs. 38.2 and 38.3), then grasps the inferior edge of the rib and pushes it upward (Figs. 38.4 and 38.5).

IS IT REALLY A SPRAIN?

The term *sprain* is probably not quite perfect, but it seems difficult to call it a "subluxation," which is what the clinical context brings to mind in the absence of any radiologic proof. Where does this sprain occur? For the false ribs, there can be no question. As for the other ribs, we can think of two types of sprains: those at the costovertebral joint and those at the costotransverse joint. In each case one joint would act as the fixed point while the other acts as a mobile point. Such mechanisms do not seem likely on anatomic grounds.

TREATMENT

If well performed, manipulation is remarkably helpful, but it is not always easy. The useful maneuver consists in progressive exaggeration of the movement to be examined in the pain free direction, using the respiratory movements. The result is often instantaneous. Three to four sessions are sometimes necessary. Injection of the costovertebral joint is difficult, even with fluoroscopic guidance. Manipulative techniques are described in Appendix A6.

"HOOKED RIB"

When the costal covering of the inferior ribs (from the 7th to the 10th) becomes hypermobile, occasionally, flexion or torsion of the trunk can result in pinching or hooking of a rib

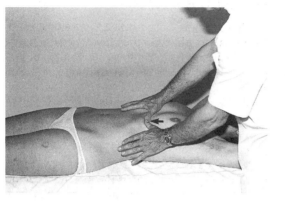
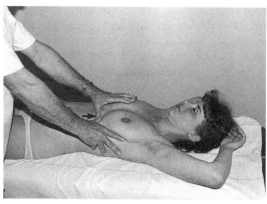

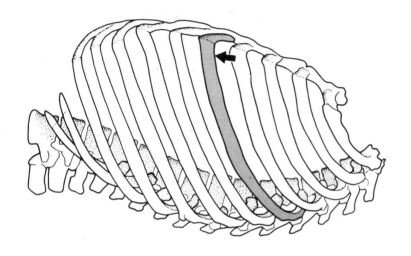

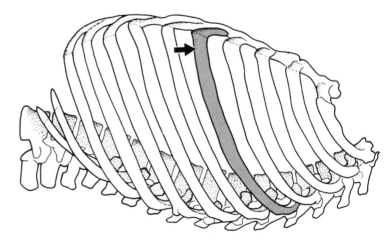

Figures 38.2–38.5. Examination of anterior rib sprain. The patient is supine. The examiner applies pressure against the superior border of the rib in a caudal direction (Figs. 38.2 and 38.3). The reverse is then performed. Pressure is applied to the anterior border in a cephalic direction (Figs. 38.4 and 38.5).

onto the cartilage of the superior rib, which creates a painful and palpable notch or indentation. In general, this hypermobility is posttraumatic; however, the trauma can be forgotten or old (E. F. Cyriax). This dysfunction can cause tenacious chronic abdominal pains. As alarming as these pains are, they can be present for many years before the diagnosis is made.

One of our patients had such a syndrome for 8 years, with many examinations and hospitalizations. Pain involved the posterior region on the left abdomen, radiating toward the rear, with occasional nausea. On palpation of the edge of the last ribs, there was a painful point and a small notch.

Passive mobilization of the rib that hooked elicited a recurrence of the usual "pain." A local injection of an anesthetic brought temporary relief. A few injections of lidocaine with a corticosteroid derivative decreased the pain significantly, but not completely. The acute pain was produced by certain movements producing a slight flexion of the trunk forward with rotation. The treatment should have been a resection of the costal end of 6–7 cm. But the patient, reassured about the cause of the pain, refused the intervention.

CHRONIC LOW BACK PAIN

Chronic low back pain is the most frequent reason for consultation regarding spinal pathology. In France, low back pain problems constitute 5% of the total budget of the Assurance Maladie (health insurance) and are a leading cause of absenteeism from the work place. Different international statistics indicate that low back pain problems are responsible for a loss of 1% of working days.

Common low back pain has always been thought to be connected with lesions, usually discogenic, of the inferior lumbar spine (L4-L5, L5-S1). We have shown that some have their origin higher, at the thoracolumbar junction (T11-T12, T12-L1) (Maigne, 1972). Strangely enough, the pain is never felt at that thoracic level but lower, in the lower lumbar, sacroiliac or gluteal region, just as in low back pain of lumbosacral origin (L4-L5, L5-S1), with which it has always been confused and which only a thorough examination can differentiate.

But before describing the different types of low back pain of lumbar or lumbosacral origin, we will discuss the principal causes of low back pain with an origin above the lumbar spine, with which it is sometimes confused. Mistakes are numerous and need a thorough examination.

The radiologic examination is important for this diagnosis as are the results of laboratory tests, because many causes of low back pain are not included in the common pain syndromes (see p. 297). There is also the possibility of low back pain of visceral origin, usually of ovarian or uterine pathology in young women and of renal, gastrointestinal, or vascular (an aortic aneurysm) origin in either sex. Furthermore, low back pain syndromes are seen in patients with a strong psychogenic component.

EXAMINATION OF THE PATIENT WITH LOW BACK PAIN

The examination starts as soon as the patient enters the room. The gait is assessed, as are the static and dynamic postures, including the ease with which the patient changes from sitting to lying. The preexamination inspection can give a great deal of information.

Clinical History

It is better to listen to the patient initially, and then ask questions. The history should inquire into

- The location of the pain and its referral pattern
- The time course of the current episode
- Any precipitating factors related to the patient's spine or general health
- Whether or not the pain is improved/worsened with movement, cough, straining, or sneezing
- The effect of posture on the pain (e.g., better or worse with standing, lying down, sitting, stooping)
- Whether the current episode is improving, worsening, or plateauing
- Whether the present pain has had a significant effect on the patient's activities of daily living including occupational and leisure activities?
- Whether there have been any previous episodes of low back pain, with or without scia-

tica, and how long they lasted, the treatments given, and their results

The patient's spontaneous expression in the beginning and the manner of answering the various questions can be of great help in drawing a psychologic profile.

Physical Examination

The physical examination is performed with the patient naked or wearing undergarments. Note is made of the patient's physique—obese, slim, muscular, etc. The presence of an antalgic attitude or asymmetry of the spine, pelvis, or lower limbs is also noted.

Active Range of Motion Assessment

The patient is standing with legs extended and feet 20 cm apart. The legs should remain extended at the knee during the entire examination.

Forward Flexion

The patient is asked to bend forward at the waste, maintaining the knees in extension. The lumbar lordosis should reverse completely by end flexion; its persistence indicates lumbar segmental stiffness. Following reversal of the lordosis, flexion continues at the hips, consistent with a normal lumbopelvic rhythm. The degree of lumbar segmental flexibility is readily assessed by Schöber's test (Fig. 21.52), which may remain unchanged even after a treatment that has relieved the patient completely. In addition to both the quality and quantity of motion, it is important to observe the point in the arc of motion at which pain is reported (the distance from fingers to floor) (Fig. 39.1).

Hamstring Muscle Tightness. Stiffness on forward flexion can be due to spinal stiffness or hamstring inflexibility, frequently seen in patients with low back pain. It can be measured in a simple way: with the patient standing, then in forward flexion, the distance between the posterosuperior iliac spine and the popliteal line is measured. A change of less than 5 cm between the two extremes is evidence of subpelvic stiffness.

Using an intriguing device called a "rachiometer" (spinometer), Badelon showed that in a normal subject, during anterior flexion of the

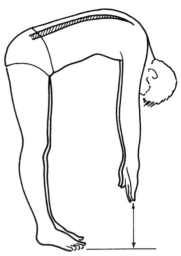

Figure 39.1. Examination performed with the subject standing and in forward flexion. One should note the stiffness, the limitation of movement, and the point at which low back pain appears. An approximate measure of this can be obtained by measuring the distance between the fingertips and the floor, with the individual flexed as much as possible.

trunk with the legs extended, the spine accounted for 47% of the range of motion, while the hips and pelvis accounted for 43%. He also noticed that in 40% of children (12 years old), there was a significant decrease in the amount of motion at the hips, which he attributed to the greater degree of hamstring inflexibility in this population. He followed these youngsters for a few years and noted a much higher proportion of low back pain problems in those with poor hamstring flexibility than in those with good flexibility. This has important obvious implications in the prevention of low back pain in susceptible subjects.

Primary and Secondary Stiffness. Is the lack of hamstring flexibility primary, linked to static problems of the lower limb, or is it of reflex spinal origin, due to spinal problems that are still painless? The "muscle spasm" of the hamstrings may be its first manifestation. In young subjects with stiff hamstring muscles, we have noted thoracolumbar PMIDs (T12 to L1) and lumbosacral PMIDs producing no low back pain yet; and often, by manipulation of the affected region, we could briefly eliminate the stiffness of the hamstrings.

Extension

The patient is asked to lean backward. The examiner notes whether this is possible as well as whether the lumbar lordosis increases smoothly and normally and whether the movement is painful or not.

Lateroflexion

The patient is asked to bend to either side, alternately, with the legs extended at the knee and slightly apart, and slide the hand along the lateral thigh to the knee. The spine should form a smooth C curve, with an ipsilateral concavity. Note is made of any signs of a "break," in the C curve, or a "bent stick deformity," whether this break elicits pain, and where the hand stops in relation to the knee or the floor (lateral distance fingers to floor) (Fig. 39.2).

Rotation

With the patient standing, the pelvis is fixed by the operator's hands, and the patient is asked to rotate the trunk to either side to test the range of motion. This technique is very approximate. The study of rotation by passive movements should be made with the patient sitting, or better, astride the end of a table, so that the pelvis is immobilized (Fig. 39.3, *left*). This is also an excellent position for testing extension (Fig. 39.3, *right*).

Functional Assessment

Patients are asked to perform some functional activities that are difficult for them, such as putting on socks, turning over on the table, or sitting on the table with the legs together. These maneuvers are sometimes more valid than the classical tests for measuring the progress obtained with a certain treatment, particularly after injection or manipulation. They also provide the opportunity, by varying

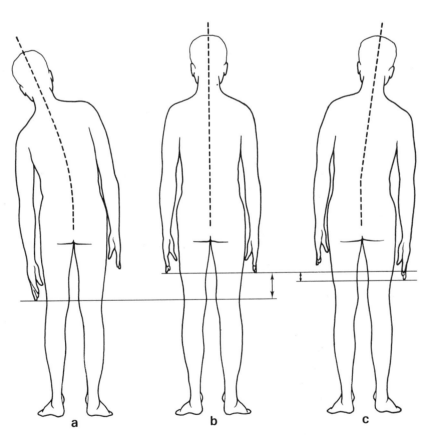

Figure 39.2. Examination of a standing and a lateral flexed position. In the standing position one notes the presence or absence of antalgic posture, any spinal stiffness, and the distance between the fingers and the floor on each side. One also examines movements that can produce the pain and when the pain appears.

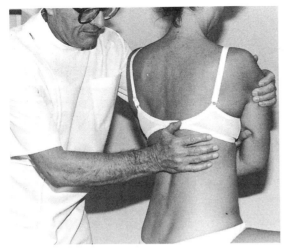

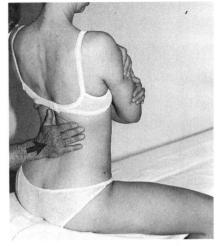

Figure 39.3. One can best test rotation (*left*), lateral flexion, extension (*right*), and flexion for evaluation of stiffness with the patient in the seated position, preferably astride the end of the examining table. The table should be narrow enough and comfortable enough to accommodate this position. One should note any limitation or position in which pain is produced.

the tests in some cases, to find out whether patients are malingering or (as some accident victims do at times) exaggerating their conditions.

Segmental Examination

The patient is in prone position across the table, with a cushion under the abdomen. Each vertebral level from T9–L5 as well as the coccyx is thoroughly examined. First, a slow and insistent PA pressure is applied to the spinous process. Then facet joint tenderness is sought, as well as pain produced by transverse pressure against the spinous process. If the latter is positive, contralateral pressure is applied to the supra- and subadjacent vertebral levels. Finally, interspinous ligament sensitivity is assessed to localize the painful levels (Fig. 39.4, *top* and *bottom*).

The transverse pressure maneuver is usually positive in one direction only. It is used to determine the rotational direction of manipulation, if this treatment is to be performed.

Palpation of the Lower Ribs in Cases of Low Back Pain

The lower ribs should always be examined because lower costal sprains can present with chronic unilateral low back pain.

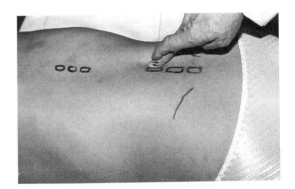

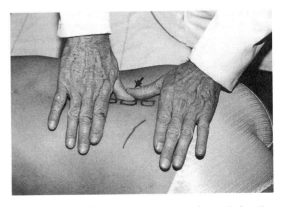

Figure 39.4. Two maneuvers performed in the course of the segmental examination, which should be performed from T8 to L5. This examination evaluates the facet joint (*top*) and transverse pressure against the spinous process (*bottom*). Note that the patient is lying on the chest across a table.

Examination of the Subcutaneous Tissues

The subcutaneous tissues should be examined systematically and meticulously with the pinch-roll method. The whole lumbar and superior gluteal region is explored. If there is a zone of cellulalgia (thickened and painful skinfolds), the subcutaneous tissues of the corresponding ipsilateral inferior abdominal and trochanteric regions should be examined (Fig. 39.5).

A diffuse regional cellulalgic infiltrate is usually of little interest. However, a localized zone of cellulalgia, in a bandlike distribution, especially when unilateral at the inferior lumbar or superior gluteal level, most often suggests that a segment of the thoracolumbar junction is a probable source, which will require more investigation. This finding is often noted in low back pain of thoracolumbar origin (TL).

Occasionally, the thickening of the cutaneous and subcutaneous tissues is such that it looks like a screen over the medial aspect of the thighs and so thickened that it is impossible to grasp a skinfold between the thumb and index finger. This special form of low back pain is discussed below.

Examination of the Muscles

Paraspinal Muscles

The paraspinal muscles are often tight and usually very tender to palpation (Fig. 39.6). They can also be the site of taut bands with or without trigger points that only a systematic and thorough palpation would find. If pressure on these trigger points (usually without the patient's knowledge) reproduces the usual low back pain, then it probably is of muscular origin.

These trigger points usually result from segmental dysfunction at the level of their motor innervation, generally at a level superior to their location, but they can also have a local origin (fatigue, physical efforts).

Muscles of the Lumbar Fossa

The quadratus lumborum is sometimes the source of one or two very painful trigger points (L1-L2).

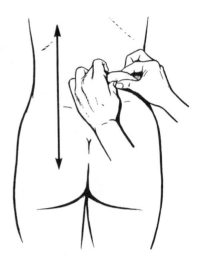

Figure 39.5. Examination of the subcutaneous tissues by the pinch-roll test should explore the entire back, from the lower ribs to the upper gluteal region.

Muscles of the External Iliac Fossa

The muscles of the external iliac fossa always have trigger points (Maigne) in low back pain of low lumbar or lumbosacral (L4-L5 or L5-S1) origin. They are often unilateral, even if the low back pain is more diffuse (Figs. 39.7 and 39.8).

Lasègue's Sign

Lasègue's sign is the classic sign of sciatica: radicular pain is produced or increased when the straightened leg is elevated. It is normally negative in low back pain without dural irrita-

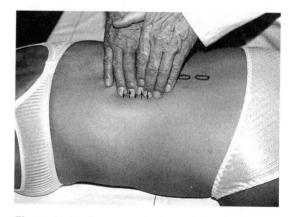

Figure 39.6. The paraspinal, quadratus lumborum, and iliocostal muscles should be attentively palpated when searching for trigger points that may eventually play a role in low back pain.

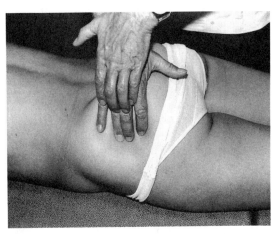

Figure 39.7.   Muscles of the lateral iliac fossa are systematically examined by deep palpation, which is performed perpendicular to their fibers from the most lateral aspect to the sacrum.

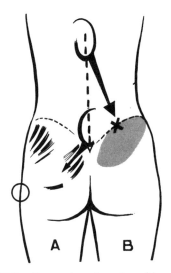

Figure 39.8.   Two main categories of low back pain can be differentiated: (*A*) low back pain of lumbosacral origin, associated with trigger points of the gluteal muscles, and (*B*) low back pain of thoracic lumbar origin (Maigne) associated with a cellulalgia of the lumbar or superior gluteal region.

tion, but its presence can reveal the onset of a moderate sciatica not noted by the patient.

This maneuver can also reveal stiffness of the hamstrings and produce or increase an isolated low back pain. Lasègue's sign can be used to follow the evolution of the sciatica as well as the response to treatment. Mobility of the hips and knees should also be tested.

Neurologic Examination

The neurologic examination of the lower limbs will reveal whether there is a motor deficit, a disorder of sensitivity, or a change in the Achilles, medial hamstring, or patellar tendon reflexes. This examination and the problem or low back pain itself must be analyzed in the context of the general clinical examination of the patient.

Radiographic Examination

Radiographs of the lumbosacral spine that include the pelvis and the thoracolumbar junction are necessary to rule out serious pathology and to appreciate the state of the spine. CT imaging may be useful if spinal stenosis is suspected.

Discography, either as an isolated procedure or followed by CT, can reveal a disk lesion in refractory low back pain. But in general, CT and plain radiography are not very helpful in benign low back pain, because many patients with disk and facet degeneration are asymptomatic, while others with normal examinations can have an organic low back pain.

If there are radiologic lesions, they must be correlated with the clinical and segmental examinations.

CONCLUSIONS OF THE CLINICAL EXAMINATION

At the end of this examination, which has been complemented if necessary by laboratory and electrodiagnostic examinations, and after having ruled out the possibility of *low back pain of visceral origin* (uteroadnexitis, renal, gastrointestinal, vascular, as aorta aneurysm, etc.) or of psychiatric origin, there can be the following.

- Either *atypical low back pain* whose most frequent causes are ankylosing spondylitis, discitis with Koch's bacillus or other organisms, compression fracture, a metastatic lesion, or multiple myeloma with a low back pain as its first symptom
- Or *common low back pain*, which can be
  —Low back pain linked to dysfunction of one of the lower lumbar segments; in gen-

eral, it is associated with unilateral or bilateral gluteal trigger points; we call it *lumbosacral lumbago* (LS)

—Low back pain linked to dysfunction of the segments of the thoracolumbar junction is associated with pain on pinch-rolling and with a cellulalgic thickening of the subcutaneous tissues of the iliac crest; we call it *low back pain of thoracolumbar origin (TL)*

—A form with the association of the two origins, LS and TL: *mixed low back pain*

—More rarely, low back pain of musculoligamentous origin, cellulalgic edema, or sprain of the false ribs

40

LOW BACK PAIN OF LUMBOSACRAL ORIGIN

Disk lesions at L4-L5 or L5-S1 are traditionally held responsible for low back pain. The role of the facet joints was considered for a long time to be insignificant, but it seems now to be a major question. Certain authors consider ligamentous or muscular origins to be a possible source of pain, but most frequently, it seems that low back pain is the consequence of a *painful minor intervertebral dysfunction* affecting one of the inferior lumbar segments.

LOW BACK PAIN DUE TO DISK LESIONS

For many years, the intervertebral disk was thought to be the only source of low back pain, and very few authors disputed this exclusivity. Discovery of the discogenic origin of sciatica, the role of the disk in spinal mechanics, its frequent involvement in pathology of the lower lumbar levels, and other often repeated arguments have contributed to diagnostic importance bestowed upon it. These arguments were as follows.

- Chronic low back pain often follows an episode of acute low back pain, often considered to be an accident of "blockage" during disk degeneration. It is often associated with episodes of sciatica, the known consequence of a radicular impingement by a disk fragment.
- Chronic low back pain that develops in a patient with no prior history of low back pain or sciatica has the same characteristics as one whose discogenic origin is proved by the association with low back pain or sciatica.
- Patients who were operated on for refractory sciatica, in whom a herniated disk was found

at surgery, suffered also from tenacious low back pain.

It is easy to counter these arguments with the mediocre results of disk surgery as done up to now in cases of pure low back pain. Some of the newer innovative techniques may change that. However, disk surgery that sufficiently relieves the radicular pain of patients with sciatica often leaves a persistent low back pain.

Still, we must admit that even if the disk does not play a direct role as has frequently been asserted, its lesions result in dysfunction of the mobile segment, including the posterior elements. Thus, both the facet joints and the interspinous ligament can be a source of low back pain.

Among the low back pain syndromes in which the disk plays a role are the following:

- Discogenic low back pain in which a disk lesion such as internal disk disruption is directly responsible for pain; this is the true discogenic low back pain.
- Low back pain due to segmental instability caused by disk degeneration. They have different clinical aspects and variable severity. The facet joints and possibly the interspinous ligament become a source of associated or isolated pain.

Discogenic Low Back Pain

In true discogenic low back pain: the discogenic lesion results in irritation of the posterior superficial annular fibers and the posterior longitudinal ligament, the only elements of the region that are richly innervated (Fig. 40.1, *A*).

Clinically, discogenic low back pain is rarely isolated. The patient has episodes of acute low back pain or sciatica, which occurs intermittently. The low back pain can be episodic or somewhat permanent and is exacerbated by coughing, sneezing, defecation, straining, and sudden gestures. Certain positions are not well tolerated or are impossible; according to Troisier, they are immediately painful, while other positions relieve them. These are the usual features, but they are not specific to discogenic low back pain. On the other hand, epidural injection by the sacrococcygeal hiatus, which is inefficient in low back pain of thoracolumbar or facet joint origin, usually brings clear relief, even if it is only transient.

In refractory cases, CT or discography, or better both together, can visualize the discogenic lesion responsible for the pain; but many disk protrusions and herniations are asymptomatic and often ignored by the patient.

Low Back Pain Due to Segmental Instability following Disk Degeneration

Disk degeneration modifies the normal biomechanics of the mobile segment and affects the facet joints, which may also start to deteriorate. Dysfunction of the posterior elements then plays a significant role in the clinical course of low back pain.

Farfan observed two mechanisms:

1. Initially, there is excessive axial loading which results in rupture of the cartilaginous endplate and intravertebral herniation. Then anteroposterior translation results during extreme flexion or extension.
2. Secondarily, excessive rotation results in radial fissuring of the disk and increased facet joint pressure on one side, with a herniated disk on the opposite side. This evolves toward a spondylolisthesis due to facet joint arthrosis, and a narrow canal. Often the facet joint dysfunction is dominant.

This severe evolution is seen from time to time, but cases in which disk degeneration does not bring such serious disorders are much more frequent. It is not uncommon to see an almost silent evolution, even if there is significant radiologic evidence of disk degeneration and facet joint arthrosis.

Usually the evolution is moderate, which can be difficult for the patient and handicapping nevertheless, resulting in low back pain in various positions and with exertion. Sometimes this evolution is completely silent, as demonstrated by Wiesel et al. They found significant discogenic or facet lesions in radiographic imaging studies, consistent with those thought to produce low back pain syndromes in patients who never experienced pain.

Dupuis and Kirkaldy Willis describe the evolution of the degenerative process in three successive phases.

1. Dysfunction, in which the initial lesion alters the normal segmental biomechanics.
2. Instability, which results in excess and abnormal segmental mobility.
3. Restabilization by fibrosis and osteophytes, which results in a decrease in intervertebral movement.

During the instability phase, abnormal segmental mobility occurs both in quantity and quality. This is best appreciated by dynamic radiologic examinations. It can be asymptomatic or symptomatic without having a direct link between the degree of instability and the severity of symptoms.

ROLE OF THE FACET JOINT IN LOW BACK PAIN

As we have seen, segmental instability linked to disk degeneration fosters facet joint lesions that contribute to the low back pain. But there are cases in which these facet joint lesions seem to be the principal cause.

Before 1930, facet joint lesions were considered to be one of the principal causes of low back pain and sciatica. Then, after the publications of Mixter and Barr, lesions of the disk were held responsible. Except for a few authors, facet joint lesions were completely forgotten before making a comeback. Certain authors even denied any role of the lesions in low back pain. In 1927, Putti attributed low back pain and sciatica to facet joint lesions of the inferior lumbar segments (essentially arthritic lesions) as well as to the asymmetry of the orientation of their articular processes. Ghormley (1933) used the term *facet syndrome* to describe the compression of the sciatic nerve (lumbosacral nerve root) in the intervertebral foramen narrowed by facet joint arthrosis. He presented the first radiographic studies depicting this narrowing of the foramen intervertebralis.

In 1971, Rees published, in Australia, an impressive series of approximately 3000 cases of low back pain in which he "denervated" the inferior lumbar facet joints by debriding them with a scalpel, blindly (percutaneously). He reported a success rate of 98%. But did Rees in fact produce a denervation or a myofasciotomy? It seems that the procedure described did not allow contact between the scalpel and the articular pillars of the posterior elements.

Maigne (1971) brought attention to "the role of the facet joints in spinal pathology" and insisted on their frequent involvement not only at the lumbar level, where they could be the origin of low back or pseudoradicular pain, but also at the thoracic and cervical levels. He emphasized their treatment by injection or manipulation (report presented at the 3rd Congress of the International Federation of Manual Medicine in Monaco in 1971) (see p. 12).

He also proposed "segmental examination" to expose clearly the dysfunction of the facet joint. The responsibility of that articulation is proved by relief brought by its anesthetic injection. Facet joint pain can be due to inflammation, but most often it is the consequence of a painful segmental dysfunction without any radiologic abnormality, which the author calls "painful minor intervertebral dysfunction."

Shealy (1975) suggested the use of rhizotomy, performed by thermocoagulation, analogous to that used in the treatment of neuralgias of the trigeminal nerve. Thermocoagulation rhizotomies were performed systematically on the articulations of the three last lumbar segments on both sides. The first published results were excellent, 80% and more; but it was soon apparent that these figures had to be modified. In most present reports, they are about 40% (Lora and Song, 40%; MacCulloch, 40%; Privat, 40%; Ignelzi, 41%; Y Lazorthes, 39%).

Burton diagnoses "facet syndrome" by the clinical examination and radiologic findings (the term *facet syndrome* has a different meaning here than the one used by Ghormley). According to Burton, pain of facet joint origin is increased by activity and relieved by rest: "getting out of bed is painful, the sitting position is not well tolerated, straightening out

after total flexion of the flank can result in sharp pain, but coughing and sneezing are painless." The best candidates for thermocoagulation (still according to Burton) are patients with radiological evidence of congenital abnormalities of the lumbar spine: "a deembedded L5 (the iliac line passes through the body of L5), facet tropism and spina bifida occulta."

All these signs seem a bit nonspecific. To verify the connection between the articulation and the pain syndrome, Mooney and Robertson (1975) proposed also using the test of articular anesthesia; thermocoagulation is applied to the articulation in question as well as the supra- and subjacent articulations to obtain as complete a denervation as possible. The author thinks that one can consider a facet joint origin for low back pain under the following conditions.

1. If segmental examination reveals segmental tenderness at L4-L5 or L5-S1 (L3-L4 is rarely affected), with a particularly clear facet joint point
2. If there are trigger points in the muscles of the external iliac fossa ipsilateral to the facet joint point
3. (Especially) if a discogenic origin does not seem to be likely

The role of the facet joint will be affirmed only if epidural injection does not modify any of the signs and if the facet joint injection, on the contrary, brings even momentary disappearance of the signs and relieves the patient.

LOW BACK PAIN OF LIGAMENTOUS ORIGIN

The origin of low back pain can be ligamentous (Fig. 40.1, *C*). According to Hackett, ligamentous "laxity" causes most articular or spinal pain. He treats low back pain syndromes by injecting sclerosing agents into the interspinous, sacroiliac, and iliolumbar ligaments. Barbor has accepted a part of these theories and has proposed a sclerosing solution that is better tolerated than the one used by Hackett. The interspinous ligament is painful in spinal instabilities of discogenic origin (described above), but its role in the pain syndrome seems weak in general. It is also often

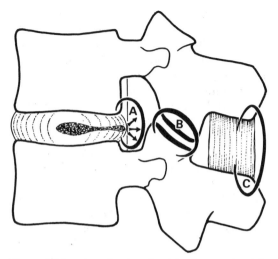

Figure 40.1. Low back pain of lumbosacral origin can have three origins that involve the mobile segment: *A,* superficial fibers of the annulus fibrosus, and the posterior longitudinal ligament; *B,* facet joints; *C,* interspinous ligament. Additionally, both the muscles that directly power the segments in question and pressure by the disk lesion on the dura may be sources of pain.

painful in painful minor intervertebral dysfunctions (PMIDs), but usually the pain disappears or decreases with manipulation.

Occasionally, ligamentous tenderness may be the principal origin of low back pain. An anesthetic injection of the ligament demonstrated its role by momentarily suppressing the painful syndrome.

LOW BACK PAIN SYNDROMES OF LUMBOSACRAL ORIGIN AND PAINFUL MINOR INTERVERTEBRAL DYSFUNCTION

To classify low back pain syndromes according to a well-defined origin, as "discogenic, facet joint, or ligamentous," is convenient but only applicable to a minority of cases. In most of the low back pain syndromes that are seen daily by physicians, the pain is due to a PMID (see "Definition," in Chapter 17). Indeed, lumbar segmental dysfunction is similar to that seen at other levels of the spine, and it is generally reversible. Moreover, the concept of PMID that we propose is independent of the radiologic state of the segment in question, which could be normal or show some signs of degeneration.

However, even in a patient with low back pain with marked radiologic lesions and significant postural asymmetries, it is not uncommon to achieve lasting relief by a simple medical treatment, such as manipulation, that is identical to the one that relieves the same pain in a person with a radiologically normal spine. Conversely, a patient who presents initially with a PMID that responds well to the usual treatments may eventually not be relieved by these treatments, suggesting possibly that a disk, facet, or ligamentous lesion may become the dominant cause of pain.

LOW BACK PAIN OF LUMBOSACRAL ORIGIN AND THE CELLULOTENOPERIOSTEO-MYALGIC SEGMENTAL VERTEBRAL SYNDROME

Periosteomyalgic manifestations of the segmental vertebral syndrome are, as we have seen, always present in low back pain syndromes of lumbosacral origin, as trigger points of the gluteal muscles. The latter can play an important role in low back pain, for these cellulotenoperiosteomyalgic (CTPM) reflex manifestations can maintain reflex loops that perpetuate the pain (Fig. 40.2).

Treatment

The treatments must first relieve the responsible segmental dysfunction, then the CTPM reflex manifestations that it produced, which often persist and perpetuate the pain. Some postural precautions will avoid some recurrences, and therapeutic exercise will stabilize the result.

Spinal Treatment

Manipulation. If manipulation is possible, it is a good treatment for segmental dysfunction. Its result can be appreciated immediately at the first session. On average, two to six manipulations are sufficient. However, if three sessions do not bring any improvement, it is better not to persist.

The basic technique is a lumbar manipulation performed in lateral decubitus, and de-

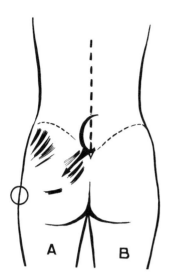

Figure 40.2. Low back pain of lumbosacral origin is almost always associated with trigger points of the gluteal muscles (L5, S1) and sometimes with hypersensitivity of the trochanter to palpation (L5) (Maigne).

pending on the case, done in relative degrees of spinal flexion or extension (Fig. 40.3, *left*). Other maneuvers are tailored to the particular needs of each patient: "belt" and "astride" techniques (Fig. 40.3, *right*) etc. (see "Manipulations" in Appendix A5).

Mobilization. Mobilization is an excellent method to prepare for a manipulation and sometimes even to replace it. In difficult cases, they are techniques of "first intention." The most useful maneuvers are described on page 472, but all techniques described as techniques of manipulation can be used in mobilization. The maneuvers are pushed until there is ten-

sion without giving the terminal thrust, and they are repeated.

Epidural Injection. When there is a discogenic component, epidural injection is indicated. It relieves the patient and often facilitates incorporation of other treatments such as manipulation and a therapeutic exercise prescription (see Chapter 26, "Injections").

Facet Joint Injection. The only treatment for facet joint inflammation is facet joint injection (Fig. 40.4). It is also indicated in chronic articular dysfunction linked to a PMID or to discogenic pathology and when manipulation is contraindicated or will not normalize facet joint functioning.

Rhizotomy. If the articular injection consistently produces definite but temporary relief, a percutaneous thermocoagulative rhizotomy may be indicated.

Injection of the Interspinous Ligament. When the interspinous ligament seems to be the source of pain, injection of a mixture of local anesthetic and corticosteroid is indicated. This is used only in a limited number of cases. If the relief is definite but temporary, then sclerosing agents recommended by R. Barbor and O. Troisier (Fig. 40.5) are indicated for use by injection (see "Ligamentous Injections" in Chapter 26).

Intradiscal Injection. In certain cases of discogenic low back pain that do not respond to treatment, intradiscal injection of aprotinin (Kraemer et al., Degrave), hexatrione (triamcinolone hexacetonide), or hexamethasone acetate, have given good results.

Physical Modalities. Electrotherapy (pulsed short wave diathermy, ultrasound, TENS,

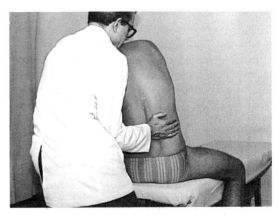

Figure 40.3. Two manipulative techniques used in the treatment of low back pain of lumbosacral origin. *Left,* Manipulation with rotation to the left in kyphosis.

Right, Manipulation with rotation to the left and lateral flexion to the left.

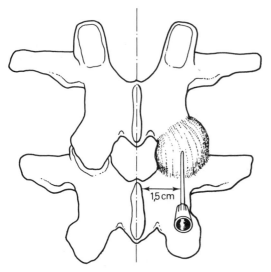

Figure 40.4.   Injection of a facet joint.

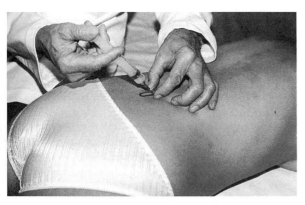

Figure 40.5.   Injection of the interspinous ligament.

Treatment of Manifestations of the Segmental Vertebral Syndrome

The CTPM manifestations that persist despite spinal treatment can be effectively treated by massage, stretching, injection, or ultrasound.

Massage.   Massage is used on the taut bands in the gluteal muscles. They are deep, slow, progressive kneading maneuvers (Fig. 40.6).

Stretching.   Stretching that takes advantage of postural or postfacilitation techniques can be used effectively to treat the affected muscles and is complementary to massage.

Injection.   The injection of the trigger points is sometimes sufficient, but it can also complement the massage and stretching.

Ultrasound.   Ultrasound has been used effectively on trigger points, and the reaction to treatment is usually rapid.

Postural Reeducation and Corrective Actions

Often neglected, postural reeducation and corrective actions are essential and must be introduced to the patient *at the beginning* of treatment. If the patient suffers from morning stiffness, a firm bed is advised; a plywood board, 1 cm thick, can be placed beneath a good quality mattress. The patient must learn to bend at the knees (both or only one) rather than stoop. Training to bend at the knee is the first step in reeducation. It can start at the beginning of the treatment. If the patient is symptomatic in sitting or standing after sitting for a

high-voltage pulsed galvanic stimulation, etc.) is an effective adjunct in chronic cases, in elderly patients, and when other treatments are contraindicated.

Cryotherapy, Thermotherapy, and Hydrotherapy

These well-known therapeutic modalities still have their place in the therapy of low back pain. The use of "sauna baths" associated with hydrotherapy, often helps to decrease chronic protective muscle guarding and the CTPM manifestations.

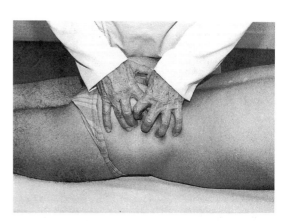

Figure 40.6.   Petrissage of the gluteal muscles containing trigger points is often useful.

while, the height of the seat must be adjusted, but it should have a firm cushion and lumbar support, at home as well as in the work place and in the car.

In many cases, a few treatments such as manipulation and/or injection, associated with postural reeducation and corrective actions, will be enough to give the patient a lasting relief. A "booster" treatment is often useful, such as manipulation performed two or three times a year. It is best to end the treatment with an exercise prescription that includes two or three stabilization techniques, which the patient will perform carefully a few times each day.

Lumbosacral Corsets and Rigid Lumbar Orthoses

The reinforced lumbosacral corset is indicated for patients who have pain when standing or with prolonged sitting. It is worn until treatment, especially therapeutic exercise, precludes its continued use. Then it is worn only occasionally. It should be worn permanently by elderly patients for whom it is the only convenient solution and by patients with atonic abdomens who, for various reasons, cannot tolerate any reconditioning.

Low back pain syndromes that are difficult to treat and that handicap the patient sometimes necessitate wearing a rigid lumbosacral orthosis during the day. It is taken off for the night, and used for 3–6 weeks. If it relieves pain, the orthosis can be replaced by a reinforced lumbosacral corset with a closed cage. Then, depending on the case, the treatments described above can be started.

Therapeutic Exercise

Therapeutic exercise is the fundamental treatment of chronic low back pain, especially low back pain syndromes that tend to recur (Fig. 40.7). Therapeutic exercise is prescribed after thorough patient evaluation, in keeping with the rule of no pain. Its aim is to restore normal muscular balance and to develop a dynamic muscular corset (abdominal, gluteal, and spinal extensor mechanism) that will protect the spine in concert with the acquisition of new habits that will enable the patient to respond to imposed demands.

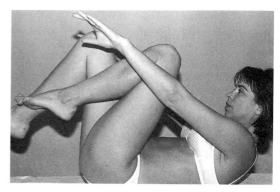

Figure 40.7. Once the patient shows improvement, a therapeutic exercise prescription is essential in the management of low back pain of lumbosacral origin. It should be adapted to the particular needs of each patient.

The following are necessary to reach these objectives.

- The lower limb muscles must be sufficiently developed to enable the patient to squat and rise and to rotate the body while maintaining the trunk in neutral position. Mobilization techniques and soft tissue release treatments are used to ensure optimum flexibility at the hips, knees, and ankles, and a home maintenance program is reinforced.
- The patient is taught how to avoid extreme movements and to "lock" the spine in neutral position while changing positions. Neutral spine is defined as the position of modified lumbar lordosis that produces optimal symptom relief. Neutral spine position, the foundation of most of the exercises taught, varies from patient to patient.
- The patient is taught how to stretch the muscles, especially the hamstring group, which is often contracted in patients with low back pain. Spinal extensor stretching is also taught.
- Abdominal exercises are taught. This is important because of the role of the abdominal muscles in unloading the spine; isometric exercises are taught initially, followed by isotonics when appropriate. Finally, exercises that condition the muscles of the perineum and the diaphragm are taught.
- Paraspinal muscle strengthening exercises are introduced. These muscles play an essential role because, depending on their state of relaxation or contraction, they can transform

the spine from a rigid cylinder to a flexible series of links that permit force absorption. A well-developed spinal extensor mechanism is necessary to allow one to assume the infinite number of positions constantly imposed on the spine.

• The patient must acquire habits that allow the muscles to dynamically respond to any and all situations of imbalance while protecting the spine.

Surgery

Surgery is rarely necessary for low back pain and is reserved for cases in which there is a total failure of medical managements. Spinal fusion has some rare but good indications. The pain must indeed come from the region to be fused (be careful in low low back pain syndromes of thoracolumbar origin). Low back pain must be relieved by a rigid lumbar orthosis. Before the decision, a careful psychologic examination is necessary.

Discectomy performed by means of classic techniques has resulted in many disappointments and has no definite indication. However, many of the newer techniques that are still in the developmental stage, (e.g., percutaneous discectomy and microdiscectomy) may show promise in certain refractory discogenic low back pain syndromes.

LOW BACK PAIN OF EXTRASPINAL ORIGIN

Low Back Pain of Myofascial Origin

Certain authors, especially J. Travell, have attributed myofascial causes to low back pain. In these cases, careful palpation of the paraspinal muscles reveals one or several particularly painful points that are located in firm taut bands. Pressure on these points reproduces the usual pain. Their injection with local anesthetic relieves pain, and the result can be lasting. The "trigger points" that are responsible for low back pain are most often located in the iliocostalis muscle, at the level of the last ribs. Pain is felt in the lumbar fossa or in the gluteal region. The longissimus and quadratus lumborum muscles can sometimes be affected.

J. G. Drevet studied similar trigger points located in the lumbar paraspinal region with ultrasonography. He noticed that they often correspond to an hypoechoic zone (41 of 62 patients), sometimes are hyperechoic (4 of 62 patients), but do not show any abnormal echoes in some patients (17 out of 62). Certain patients had had pain for a long time and many treatments without success; most were relieved with local treatment.

In four patients with hypoechoic zones, a biopsy was done and it showed that these muscular bundles were brownish and retracted. Microscopic examination revealed significant endo- and perimysial adiposis, fibrosis, and some atrophic muscular lesions; the muscular fibers were of irregular diameter and angular. It is difficult to understand these lesions, as they could be of neurogenic origin. In three cases of the four, surgical excision of this zone (in patients who were not relieved by local injections and electrotherapy) brought a total disappearance of the low back pain.

Low Back Pain of "Cellulalgic Sheeting"

After observing about 30 patients, we believe we can isolate this particular form of low back pain. In general, this low back pain is refractory to treatment. It is increased by fatigue, by certain movements, and by exertion, but it is not always decreased by rest. Forward flexion, usually limited and painful, is done with a "fixed" lumbar lordosis. The patient cannot round the back.

Examination by palpation reveals the characteristic features of this low back pain syndrome. Maneuvers of the segmental examination seem painful at all lumbar levels; transverse pressure is painful on both the right and the left, as is the facet joint.

The diagnosis is made with the pinch-roll test. It is impossible to grasp a skinfold between the thumb and index finger. The superficial soft tissues seem to cling to the underlying fascial planes in a solid block, forming a true symmetric cellulalgic sheeting overlying the lumbar region that is especially marked in the midline. These subcutaneous tissues do not seem to extend during flexion; they cannot creep freely with segmental motion, as shown by a positive Schöber's test (see "Active Motion Testing'' in Chapter 21). The tension produced by forward flexion is painful.

Treatment

Treatment consists of injecting the layers of the region with dilute local anesthetic, followed immediately by mobilization of the superficial planes on the deep planes. Then progress to kneading maneuvers, which help to mobilize them and make the tissues more supple. The second step is lumbar segmental mobilization. This seems to be a local neurotrophic reaction promoted by certain organisms.

Low Back Pain and the Iliolumbar Ligament

According to certain authors (Hackett, Hirschberg et al.), the iliolumbar ligament is responsible for certain unilateral low back pain syndromes. Diagnosis is made by finding a painful point under pressure on the iliac crest, at 7–8 cm lateral to the midline, a site that seems to correspond to the iliac insertion of the superior fibers of this ligament. An anesthetic injection at this point often relieves the patient.

In fact, this point located on the *posterior surface* of the iliac crest cannot correspond to the iliolumbar ligament, which inserts on the anterior surface of the crest and thus separated by thickness of the iliac crest. We shall see below (Chapter 41) that this point corresponds to the cutaneous branch of the posterior ramus of L1 (60% of cases) or L2 (40% of cases), which crosses the iliac crest at that precise level as it traverses a fibro-osseous tunnel (R. and J. Y. Maigne). This point disappears if the superior branch is infiltrated with an anesthetic at its emergence from the spine at the level of L1 and L2, which could not happen if the point was in fact the iliolumbar ligament.

41

LOW BACK PAIN OF THORACOLUMBAR ORIGIN (T11-T12-L1) (MAIGNE)

Low back pain of thoracolumbar origin (TL) is the most frequent manifestation of the "thoracolumbar junction syndrome" (Maigne), which also includes pseudovisceral abdominal pain and pubic and trochanteric tenderness (see Chapter 60, "Thoracolumbar Junction Syndrome"). For the sake of clarity and because the low back pain is often the only symptom that patients complain about, it is described here. It is also the first of the painful manifestations that have been attributed to the TL junction (Maigne, 1972). As we have shown, low back pain can have its origin at one or more segments of the TL junction, usually T11-T12 and T12-L1 and occasionally T10-T11 or L1-L2.

Low back pain of TL origin can be acute or chronic. It is common, and the pain is very similar to that of low back pain of lumbosacral origin, with which it is often confused. Patients never complain of spontaneous pain at the TL junction (Figs. 41.1 and 41.2).

This form of low back pain is more frequent in people over 45 years of age, but it can also be seen in young people. It can be associated with low back pain of lumbosacral origin (LS) in variable proportions.

TL low back pain shows some precise and constant clinical signs that must be sought thoroughly, which requires a certain level of experience. The diagnosis is confirmed by a response to an injection or manipulation performed on the responsible thoracic or TL segment, which is sometimes spectacular and immediate.

After a short anatomic review of the particu-

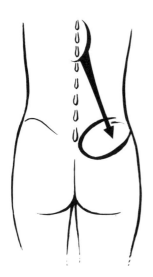

Figure 41.1. Low back pain can have a thoracolumbar junctional origin (Maigne). It may only be felt at the lower lumbar level and gluteal region.

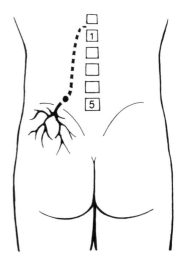

Figure 41.2. Pain of the cutaneous branch of the posterior ramus of the thoracolumbar junction.

lar characteristics of the TL junction, we describe the clinical signs and treatment of this syndrome.

___

ANATOMIC REVIEW

Facet Joints

The form and orientation of facet joints change at every level of the spine, which facilitates certain movements and prevents others. The thoracic articular processes are oriented at an angle of 60° from the horizontal, while the lumbar processes are oriented at 90° (Fig. 41.3). In the thoracic spine, the articular processes lie more or less in the frontal plane; in the lumbar spine, they are in the sagittal plane. This means that the thoracic spine allows mobility in rotation, while at the lumbar spine, this rotation is essentially impossible (Fig. 41.3).

It follows, therefore, that the TL junction is a transitional zone subjected to significant rotational strains. It is also a common site for vertebral compression fractures.

Transitional Vertebra. Anatomically and physiologically, T12 is a transitional vertebra. Its superior articular processes behave like the adjacent thoracic ones, while its inferior articular processes behave like those of the lumbar spine. Thus there is a certain disruption in the harmony of the movement, which could lead to segmental dysfunction. Normally, most of the trunk rotation occurs at the TL junction, as this motion is limited above by the ribs and made difficult or impossible below by the orientation of the lumbar articular processes (Fig. 41.4).

This role of transitional vertebra can be played by T11 in certain people. In a CT study of 32 patients with TL low back pain, T12 was transitional in 25 cases, T11 in 6, and L1 in only 1 patient. Interestingly, in the 32 patients, the lower ribs articulated with the T12 vertebral body (J. Y. Maigne et al.). In fact, this region appears to be associated with a certain degree of anatomic variation that may impact on the biomechanics of the region and on its pathology. In a Finnish study, T11-T12 was found to be the most frequent transitional segment (Malmivaara et al.).

Posterior Rami of the Thoracolumbar Spinal Nerve Roots

At the superior lumbar and inferior thoracic level, the posterior ramus emerges from the mixed spinal nerve root at almost a right angle. It courses around the articular pillar, pressing its path on the prominence of the superior articular process of the subjacent vertebra (G. Lazorthes). It divides immediately behind the interior portion of the intercostalis muscle into lateral and medial branches. The lateral branch has both motor and sensory fibers and becomes subcutaneous approximately three vertebrae below its origin. The medial branch is composed almost exclusively of motor axons and courses inferiorly, posteriorly, and medi-

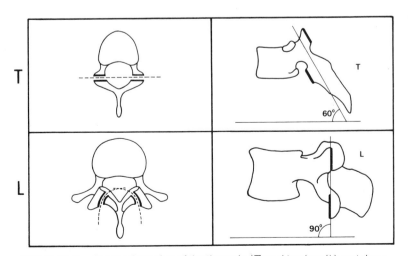

Figure 41.3.   Facet orientation of the thoracic (*T*) and lumbar (*L*) vertebrae.

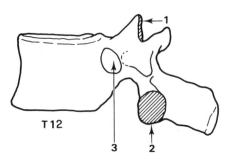

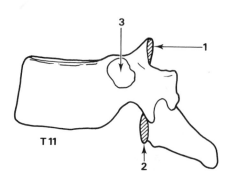

Figure 41.4.   T12 is a transitional vertebrae. *1,* Superior articular facet; *2,* inferior articular facet; *3,* articular rib facet. The superior articular processes (*1*) have the same orientation as the thoracic spine articulations (up until T11). The inferior articular processes (*2*) are oriented in a lumbar fashion.

ally before terminating in the multifidus and spinalis muscles and supplying them.

Innervation of the Subcutaneous Tissues

Classically, the cutaneous and subcutaneous tissues of the superior half of the buttock are innervated by the posterior rami of L1-L2-L3. Some authors, like Keegan and Garett, even attribute part of this innervation to L4 and L5 in their dermatome maps. However, all the anatomists agree that the posterior rami of L4 and L5 have no cutaneous branches.

Therefore, to confirm our clinical findings, we relied on studies performed by Hovelacque that clearly reveal that the innervation of the subcutaneous tissues of the superior part of the buttock is innervated by T12, L1, and L2. A few dissections that we performed with Le Corre and Rageot confirmed that these rami indeed cross the iliac crest at a right angle.

In 1976, Barrie and I noticed in 25 dissections that the primary cutaneous innervation of the superior gluteal region was provided by L1 and T12; these two rami, which are very close to each other, often cross the iliac crest at a distance of 7–8 cm from the midline, corresponding to the usual location of the "crestal point." More recently, J. Y. Maigne and I went back to these studies so that we could better describe the entire superior gluteal cutaneous innervation. The study involved 30 dissections and showed the following (Figs. 41.5–41.7).

- In 19 cases, T12 and L1 accounted solely for the innervation of the gluteal area. L1 crosses the iliac crest 7–8 cm lateral to the midline, and T12 crosses it 1–3 cm more laterally.
- In 8 cases, the innervation was provided by L2, medially, and L1 and T12, laterally.
- In 3 cases, the picture was the same as the above, but L2 received a branch arising from L3 prior to crossing the iliac crest.

This confirms that there are no cutaneous branches of the posterior rami of L4 and L5, and they are rare in L3.

Iliac Crest Crossing Point

We have noticed that the most medial cutaneous branch (L1 in 19 cases, L2 in 11 cases) always crosses the iliac crest at a point 7–8 cm lateral to the midline after having perforated the aponeurosis of the latissimus dorsi near its insert on the iliac crest. At this point, the nerve passes through a fibro-osseous tunnel restricting the nerve's free movement when traction is applied to it. This tight passage is a potential site of entrapment and may be a source of discomfort in some cases (Fig. 41.6). During some dissections, J. Y. Maigne noticed a typical case: the nerve ramus uncovered at that level demonstrated evidence of a severe stenosis with supra- and substenotic swelling.

CLINICAL SIGNS

In acute, as well as in chronic cases, pain is always felt in the sacroiliac joint, low lumbar, or gluteal region. Sometimes, it refers to the thigh, laterally or posteriorly. It is practically never felt at its origin, that is, at the TL

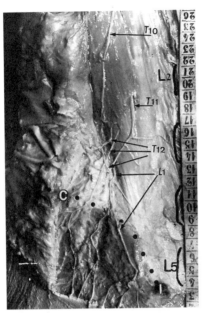

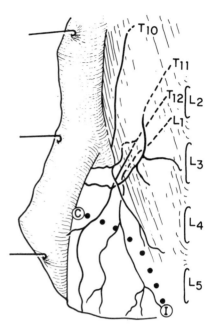

Figure 41.5. In this example (dissection J. Y. Maigne), innervation of the skin overlying the superior gluteal region is supplied by T12 and L1. One can see the crossing over the iliac crest of these nerves.

It should be noted that in this case L1 divides just before crossing over the iliac crest. This diagram demonstrates the actual paths of the nerve branches. The iliac crest is represented by dark dots.

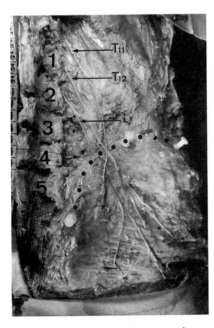

Figure 41.6. Individual variations are frequent. In this case the cutaneous branch of T11 takes a medial direction exactly where it crosses over the iliac crest and thus innervates the more medial aspect of the gluteal skin region. The iliac crest is demonstrated by the black dots.

junction. It is generally unilateral but sometimes bilateral.

This pain can be acute (see Chapter 42) and occurs often after exertion or forced rotation. Most often, it is chronic. It seems that nothing can differentiate it from chronic LS low back pain, with which it is often confused.

Clinical Examination

Clinical examination reveals the physical signs of this disorder and demonstrates the relationship between low back pain and its TL origin (T11-T12, T12-L1, or L1-L2; exceptionally, T9-T10 or T10-T11). When the patient is standing, it is common to see that lateroflexion on the side opposite the low back pain produces or increases the pain. The examination should be performed with the patient lying forward flexed across the table, with a cushion under the abdomen (Fig. 41.8).

Examination of the Lumbogluteal Region at the Iliac Crest

The index finger of the physician follows the iliac crest from medial to lateral, rubbing it

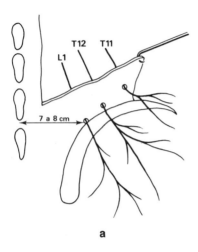

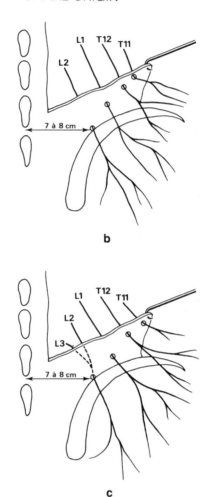

Figure 41.7. The three principal distributions of the cutaneous branches of the nerves that cross over the iliac crest (J. Y. Maigne). The medialmost branch always crosses over the iliac crest at a distance of 7–8 cm. This corresponds to L1 (**a**), L2 (**b**), or a branch composed of both L2 and L3 (**c**). It goes through a fibro-osseous tunnel in which there is only slight mobility. Occasionally it can be compressed. The cutaneous branch of T12 does not generally cross over the iliac crest in type c. It crosses irregularly in type b. These distributions essentially represent 60% (**a**), 25% (**b**), and 15% (**c**) of the cases noted.

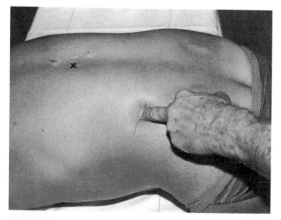

Figure 41.8. Evaluation of the posterior crestal point. The examiner slides slowly along the iliac crest exerting a mild frictional pressure, evaluating each centimeter. Note that the patient is lying forward flexed across a table.

over the skin with small transverse and vertical movements in a back-and-forth manner. At an exact point, usually 7–8 cm lateral of the midline, the examiner's finger encounters a very tender point that corresponds to the site of compression of the irritated cutaneous branch. This point is referred to as the *crestal point* (Figs. 41.8 and 41.10) (Maigne). It may be absent if the concerned ramus does not cross the iliac crest (T11, sometimes T12). It is usually unilateral.

Adjacent to that point, the subcutaneous tissues of the buttock or lumbar region are painful to pinch-rolling (Fig. 41.9). They are infiltrated by cellulalgia, which is thick and extends over an area usually about the size of the palm of the hand, sometimes covering almost all of the superior part of the buttock or the inferior part

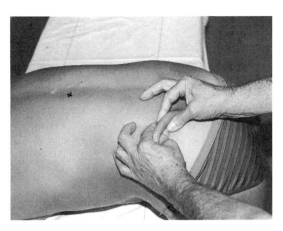

Figure 41.9. Pinch-roll test examining the superior gluteal region.

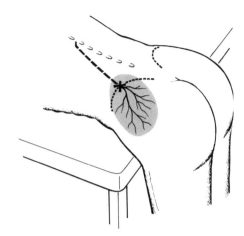

Figure 41.11. The cellulalgic zone corresponds to the territory of the posterior rami of the TL junction. This zone may be supplied by two or three segments from this region of the spine.

of the lumbar region, or covering only a few square centimeters over the the iliac crest (Figs. 41.10 and 41.11).

The degree of skinfold thickening varies greatly from one subject to the other. Sometimes it is mild; sometimes it is very thick, tight, granular, and impossible to fold. In all cases, the pinch-roll test is very painful, compared with the opposite side and the adjacent zones. The cellulalgic zone often seems to be common to the different levels of the TL junction, probably because of the frequent anastomoses that exist and the mechanism of the cellulalgia.

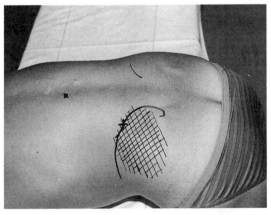

Figure 41.10. The zone that is characteristically painful to the pinch-roll test and low back pain of TL origin usually overlies the iliac crest. If the T9 and T10 segments are involved, the cellulalgic pain will be located above the crest.

Examination of the Thoracolumbar Region

At the the TL junction, the sensitivity of one or more segments appears clearly. For this segmental examination, the patient assumes the prone position across the table, with a cushion under the abdomen. The two essential maneuvers are transverse pressure against the spinous processes and the search for the facet joint point. The facet joint pain is unilateral and is always located on the side of the low back pain (Figs. 41.12, **left** and **right**). It can be bilateral if the low back pain is so.

The segmental tenderness that is uncovered is usually seen on one segment (60%), sometimes on two (25%) or three segments (15%). With rare exceptions, these segments are adjacent to each other. Tenderness to PA pressure on the spinous process and over the interspinous ligament may also be noticed, but is not as consistent.

Confirmation of the Thoracolumbar Origin of the Low Back Pain

Confirmation is obtained by anesthetic injection performed at the facet joint point of T11-T12 or T12-L1, where it was found to be tender on examination. This injection results in the disappearance of the pain as well as the clinical signs.

The needle is advanced perpendicularly about 1 cm lateral to the midline until contact

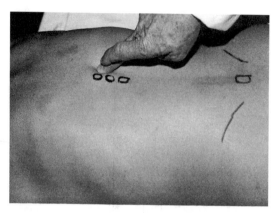

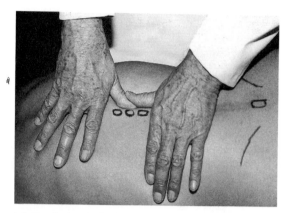

Figure 41.12. Segmental examination of the TL junction for facet joint tenderness should be performed from the right and the left. As a rule, it is found on the same side as the low back pain. It is sometimes found bilaterally (as in the following case). **Left,** Transverse pressure against the spinous process. This is systematically performed from right to left, and from left to right (**right**).

is made with periosteum. After verification by aspiration, 1–2 mL of lidocaine is injected. This can be performed under fluoroscopic guidance. With experience, it will be noticed that the point that is painful on palpation corresponds as a rule to the facet joint (Fig. 41.13, **left**). In a few moments, the following can be observed:

- Disappearance of the patient's pain and stiffness with restoration of pain-free range of motion
- Disappearance of the crestal point

- Decrease or even the disappearance of the "cellulalgic zone," which has become painless to pinch-rolling

During this injection, which affects the posterior ramus as well as the facet joints, the needle should remain in place for 1 minute, while waiting for the disappearance of the sensitivity of the crestal point on palpation and of the pain to pinch-rolling (Fig. 41.13, **right**). If this does not happen, placement of the needle should be modified slightly upward, downward, or laterally to render the injection use-

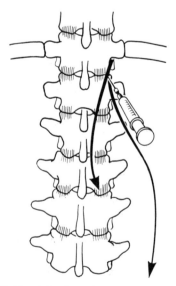

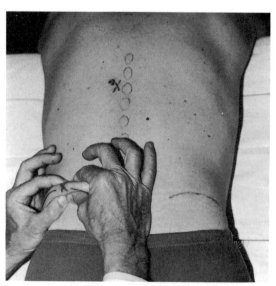

Figure 41.13. Injection of local anesthetic at the facet joint tenderness can relieve the patient's discomfort, tenderness on pinch-rolling (**right**), the cellulalgic zone, and crestal point pain. The needle (**left**) should remain in place until the signs disappear and be moved only slightly if there is no improvement.

ful. One should be sure that the injection has affected the appropriate level, as two levels can be affected, but rarely three.

When examination has revealed dysfunction of two or three segments, it might be necessary to inject all of them. This depends on the result of the procedure. In recurrent cases, it is a good idea to mark the point of injection that helped, to verify whether the same segment is affected. But even if there are two or three painful TL segments on examination, it is not uncommon to find that only one is responsible for the referred pain.

Placebo Injection.   If the injection, lidocaine or saline, is performed at a distance from the facet joint point or on an insensitive segment (with the patient unaware), there should not be any modification of the crestal point, the zone of cellulalgia, or the spontaneous pain.

RADIOLOGIC EXAMINATION

In most cases of low back pain of TL origin, the standard radiologic examination of the affected zone is unremarkable or demonstrates only minor degenerative changes. From time to time, sequelae of spinal apophysitis are observed. At that level, they are a cause of fragility for that overexerted zone and foster refractory or recurrent low back pain. In women over 60, some degree of disk degeneration can be seen, sometimes with retrolisthesis of L1 or L2 or a compression fracture of T11, T12, or L1 that was ignored is sometimes found. CT examination has shown us lesions that are not well revealed by conventional radiography, such as facet joint spondylosis, periarticular calcifications, and calcifications of the ligamentum flavum.

Malmivaara et al. studied 24 cadavers with degenerative lesions of the lumbar spine. They noted the relative frequency of degenerative changes at the TL junction, and they found T11-T12 to be the most frequent transitional segment. They noted that at that level, the degeneration is on the

- Whole segment (intervertebral disk, facet joints, costovertebral articulations)
- Anterior part (intervertebral disk) for the supra-adjacent segment (T10-T11)
- Posterior part (facet articulation) for the subjacent segment T12-L1

Radiologic examination can reveal uncommon pathology that may be the first signs of a spondyloarthropathy or of an infectious spondylodiscitis. Even a metastasis or multiple myeloma can, for some time, be manifested only by low back pain with mild discomfort. But we should emphasize that many patients with low back pain of TL origin show LS radiologic lesions such as discopathy, articular spondylosis, and spondylolisthesis that are asymptomatic, while the responsible TL region is radiologically normal or has only benign discrete lesions.

INCIDENCE

The incidence of low back pain of TL origin is 30% of all cases of common low back pain. The LS origin represents 40% of cases, and 30% are of mixed origin (personal statistical study of 500 cases). Our first statistics did not take enough notice of the mixed forms, in which the primary responsibility for the pain could sometimes alternate between one or the other origin, at an interval of a few weeks. A patient with low back pain of TL origin that was perfectly relieved by the specific treatment could very well consult us a few months later for a recurrence of what seemed to be the same pain, but whose origin this time was the LS spine. The following case is an excellent illustration.

Case History.   Mr. X., a 52-year-old patient had two successful operations for discogenic sciatica, 10 and 15 years previously. After the second operation, however, he developed a low back pain that became handicapping in a few years. After numerous treatments, he came to our department where the diagnosis of low back pain of T12-L1 origin was made. The treatment had a spectacular result, to the point that he could resume his athletic activities. During one of these, there was a recurrence, but this time it was a low back pain accompanied by acute sciatica. A diagnosis of recurrent disk herniation was made. Treatment of the new condition rendered a perfect result.

After a successful treatment of chronic severe low back pain of TL origin, often the patient, free from its inconvenience and pain, happy to feel at ease, undertakes activities that are not well tolerated by the LS spine with disk degeneration and completely lost or faulty coordination, which release LS low back pain or sciatica. Statistically, depending on when the patient is seen, it can be put in the LS or

TL category; but it is also common to see both categories simultaneously in the same patient.

Age plays also a role. TL low back pain can be seen in the young, but it is much more frequent in people over 45 years of age. The young subject with low back pain of LS origin will later show low back pain of mixed origin, LS and TL; with time, it will tend to have a TL origin.

ATYPICAL FORMS

Ectopic Referral Patterns

Some patients with low back pain of TL origin have referral patterns that appear to be sciatic and which disappear with treatment that is strictly localized to the TL zone. This referral pattern can be reproduced by injection of the facet joint at T12-L1 or L1-L2 or by injection of the crestal point. The two following cases are good examples.

Case History. D. G., a 50-year-old physician, while playing golf 2 years previously, felt a lumbogluteal pain radiating to the posterior aspect of the leg and the right testicle. The pain decreased in a few days. One year later, while lifting a child several times, he felt a low back pain that increased in the following days. The pain radiated up to the posterior aspect of the right thigh and occasionally as far as the heel. Bed rest and medical management improved it slightly. However, a wrong movement precipitated an acute attack that persisted, resulting in lumbogluteal pain referring to the posterior aspect of the right leg and under the heel. Pain was increased by prolonged standing and especially by sitting. There was no significant change after 20 days.

Treatment with anti-inflammatory medications, a reinforced LS corset, and injections did not help. The patient consulted a friend, a well-known rheumatologist who diagnosed "atypical sciatica" and prescribed epidural injections and different medical treatments. After numerous injections, rest, and traction, there was no change. The rheumatologist and two neurosurgeons advised radiologic studies. Then a neurologist advised a myelogram. At this point the low back pain was the dominant feature, with a mild S1 radicular component.

Before this examination, he sent the patient to us for our opinion. The spine was very stiff; anterior flexion was very limited (fingers to ground, 50 cm). The topography of pain was S1, but there was no Lasègue's sign. At 80°, a slight exaggeration of the gluteal pain occurred. This had already been noted by the different specialists who had been consulted. At the examination, the crestal point was very sharp, and pressure on it reproduced the lumbogluteal pain, and

curiously, referred it to the S1 region. There was a thick cellulalgic patch on the superior aspect of the right buttock and none on the other. Thoracic examination revealed the relative dysfunction of T12-L1, with tenderness to transverse pressure on the right side of the spinous process. Radiography showed a moderate discopathy at L5-S1 but nothing at the the TL junction. Injection of the facet point at T12-L1, which was very tender to palpation, resulted in immediate improvement (that no epidural injection ever gave) in flexion and resolution of the pain. After the third injection, the relief was complete, and the patient went back to his usual activities, which had been interrupted for 6 months. Manipulation of the T12-L1 segment completed this result, which was maintained for 3 years.

Case History. Mr. D., a 45-year-old patient, was operated on 6 months previously, unsuccessfully, for a persistent left S1 sciatica. At surgery, the surgeon found a disk protrusion that did not compress the nerve root. The pain was mostly lumbar, with some referral under the heel and to the posterior aspect of the thigh and calf. Pain at the heel was manifested especially when pressing on it and became very sharp when it was struck. The patient could not tap on the ground.

Local injections of the heel as well as epidural injections met with no success. When the patient came to our department for consultation, examination revealed a left low back pain of TL origin. A facet joint injection immediately relieved the low back pain, while his anterior flexion went from 50 to 10 cm distance, fingers to ground. Curiously, it also relieved the heel pain. After injection, he could tap and strike the ground.

This favorable result lasted a few days and disappeared. Several manipulations and injections were performed with the same momentary result. Two placebo injections that were performed two levels above, without the knowledge of the patient, brought no relief. A surgical capsulectomy was performed and produced an excellent result, with disappearance of low back and heel pain (capsulectomy T10-T11, T11-T12, T12-L1).

TREATMENT

Manipulation

If the state of the spine allows and the rule of no pain is respected, manipulation is the treatment of choice for this low back pain in young or average age persons; but it must be performed with impeccable technique. Ill performed or performed in the wrong direction, it aggravates, which is a true experimental test of the low back pain. Usually, the most helpful maneuvers are "astride technique" (Fig.

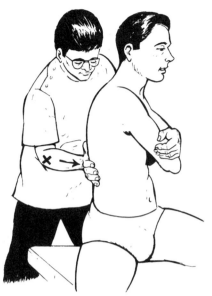

Figure 41.14. Technique for producing rotation with the patient sitting astride.

41.14), "epigastric technique," supine technique (Fig. 41.15, **right**), and "knee technique" (Fig. 41.15, **left**).

Facet Joint Injection

One mL of a long-acting corticosteroid derivative is injected at the affected facet joint.

It is a good idea to leave the needle in place after the lidocaine test has been performed. Just as the pain on pinch-rolling disappears, the corticosteroid derivative should be administered. Most often, two or three injections at 2-week intervals give an appreciable result, even disappearance of pain in chronic patients.

Depending on the case and the patient's age, it may be necessary to repeat a similar injection, two or three times per year. The result of the injection is particularly spectacular in the acute or subacute form, in which only one injection may bring immediate relief (Fig. 41.13, **left**).

Electrotherapy

Short wave diathermy applied to the TL junction can give good results in patients to whom the two preceding treatments cannot be applied.

Treatment of the Cellulalgic Lumbogluteal Region

Usually, the lumbogluteal cellulalgic zone will disappear with spinal treatment. Sometimes relief is total without having this zone completely eliminated, though it is decreased. When relief is incomplete and local treatment

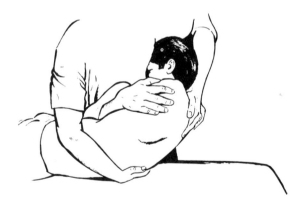

Figure 41.15. Left, Manipulation using both knees in extension. **Right,** In the supine position in flexion.

does not eliminate the zone, kneading maneuvers after injection with lidocaine over the crestal point or very progressive massage, with or without subcutaneous injection of diluted lidocaine, can also be of help.

Physiotherapy (iontophoresis, in particular) can be effective in refractory cases. Injection of the crestal point with lidocaine mixed with hydrocortisone can decrease or eliminate the pain in some patients, probably in cases in which the nerve is compressed and irritated in the fibro-osseous tunnel as described above (R. and J. Y. Maigne). This entrapment phenomena is added to the spinal irritation, as in a "double crush syndrome," but sometimes it seems to be the only cause, with no spinal component. The need for surgical release is exceptional; we have performed it twice.

Surgical Capsulectomy

In 1975, we tried surgical capsulectomy of the responsible articulation in very severe cases that were handicapping and relieved by manipulation or injection, but in which the result did not last. The capsulectomy was extended to the level above and the level below, which destroyed the posterior ramus of the spinal nerve that was attached to it. Henri Judet performed the surgery. We followed 16 patients who had been operated upon, from 4 to 10 years. Most operations had been done by Judet; the rest were done by other orthopedic surgeons who, after our publication, had diagnosed a low back pain of TL origin and had consulted us about the surgical indication. Results were excellent or good in 10 patients, fair in 3, and nil in 3. We should emphasize that these patients had refractory, chronic, and very incapacitating low back pain, usually due to work place injuries, and they had already been operated upon once or twice for sciatica.

The protocol was as follows. Notwithstanding the benign nature of the intervention, we were very restrictive. Only patients in whom only one level was responsible and in whom injection of lidocaine at the articular pillar resulted in clear relief of pain and temporary resolution of the crestal point and the sensitivity of the lumbogluteal subcutaneous tissues to pinch-rolling were operated on. The point of injection was marked, and the test was repeated three times. Unknown to the patient, a placebo injection was performed with saline injected 2 cm above and outside the facet joint point. No relief resulted.

Surgery was abandoned with the advent of percutaneous thermocoagulative rhizotomy. However, one of our patients, who was relieved just momentarily with two thermocoagulative rhizotomies, had a lasting result with surgical intervention.

Percutaneous Rhizotomy

The protocol is the same as that described above. One should be sure that the same segment is dysfunctional in different examinations at different times. Percutaneous rhizotomy is reserved for patients who are relieved by medical treatment, injection and possibly manipulation, but for whom the result does not last.

Practically, indication for thermocoagulative rhizotomy is infrequent, since most patients with low back pain of TL origin have good results with medical means. But when medical treatment yields only temporary results, rhizotomy may give a number of patients lasting results. After our publications describing this form of low back pain, Y. Lazorthes used thermocoagulative rhizotomy to denervate the facets at the TL levels in refractory cases of low back pain. According to him, it is the best indication for this technique, consistent with our own experience (70% of good results).

Corrective Actions

To avoid recurrences, patients should (a) avoid all trunk rotation and learn to turn with the feet, not the thorax; (b) avoid trunk twisting when sitting, as for instance, while speaking to somebody behind them or taking something from the back seat of the car when driving; (c) avoid seats that are too low or too soft; and (d) avoid cold in the lumbar region.

Therapeutic Exercise

In most cases, corrective actions are sufficient to prevent recurrences in a patient who has been relieved by medical treatment. But therapeutic exercise is necessary in patients with recurrences as well as in athletes (such as golfers) who stress their TL junction. Ledoux and Halmagrand studied the various therapeutic modalities in our department at the Hotel Dieu. The aims of the therapeutic exercise prescription are

- To increase the flexibility of the back, which often exhibits facet joint stiffness
- To normalize muscle balance by stretching the tight muscles and reconditioning the weak ones
- To restore normal proprioceptive balance

Increased flexibility helps to reduce articular stiffness (through mobilization and postural reeducation, so that the strains of rotation and lateroflexion do not adversely affect the TL junction) and to distribute these forces more widely. Muscular stiffness can also be alleviated by postural techniques or stretching of the spinal extensor muscles—latissimus dorsi, thoracolumbar, and hamstrings—and the hip flexor muscles—rectus femoris and psoas. Depending on the results of examination, muscle groups that tend to become deconditioned can be reinforced—abdominal, diaphragm transverse, psoas, and muscles of the thoracolumbar extensor group.

Proprioceptive reflexes are stimulated by teaching the patient to control movements on a very limited zone of the back and flank, which are best performed in sitting or quadruped position and completed by lumbopelvic adjustment exercises while sitting or standing. The patient is taught to use the legs to their best mechanical advantage in bending and turning by reinforcing the quadriceps and hip rotator muscles.

42

ACUTE LOW BACK PAIN

As in the case of chronic low back pain, it is common to attribute acute low back pain to the lumbosacral region (L4-L5 or L5-S1). But just like chronic low back pain, it can also be due to dysfunction of the thoracolumbar junction (Maigne). Furthermore, some may have a myofascial origin.

ACUTE LOW BACK PAIN OF LUMBOSACRAL ORIGIN

Clinical Picture

Acute low back pain of lumbosacral origin occurs most often after exertion, although it can occasionally occur spontaneously. The pain is usually described as sharp and is exacerbated by even the slightest movement. It is usually located in the low lumbar or sacroiliac region. During an acute episode, the patient remains stiff, even at rest, and is frequently unable to straighten up completely. Once patients are able to lie down and find a comfortable position, they prefer not to move anymore than is required because any attempt to move reproduces the pain.

In less acute cases, the patient moves en bloc, with great caution, and bent forward. The lumbar region is stiff, and the pelvis is often tilted to one side because of the antalgic attitude. The patient fears even the slightest movement, the least shaking, or coughing, for example. These low back pain syndromes come with an antalgic list that is generally quite pronounced, although it may sometimes be mild, revealed only when the patient bends the trunk slightly.

In 50% of cases, the patient can laterally flex freely away from the painful side but not toward it; the antalgic scoliosis is then convex to the side of pain (Fig. 42.1a). In 40% of cases, the patient can side bend freely toward the painful side, and the scoliosis is concave on the side of the pain (Fig. 42.1b). In 10% of cases, the antalgic list is in flexion (Fig. 42.1c).

The segmental examination performed on the patient supine across the table demonstrates dysfunction of a lumbosacral segment; L5-S1 or L4-L5, more rarely L3-L4.

The acute attack usually lasts 2–4 days and decreases progressively. It can last longer, especially when there is an antalgic attitude in flexion. Pain is usually relieved in supine, which is an often prescribed treatment. In some cases, a persistent low back pain can persist and propagate to involve the buttock and the leg, and sciatica develops.

Mechanism

Acute low back pain is produced by a posterior intradiscal blockage, according to de Sèze. A fragment of the nucleus, which has entered an annular fissure, distends the superficial fibers, which are the only ones that are innervated. This distention seems to be the principal cause of pain, which can also be due to the sudden pressure exerted by the bulging disk on the posterior longitudinal ligament.

Mac Nab thought that the facet joints were the most common source of acute low back pain. But it seems that both origins can be seen and even coexist. We can differentiate them with an epidural injection test performed via the sacrococcygeal hiatus. Assuming sound technique, the pain is immediately relieved if a discogenic mechanism is responsible and is not if the origin is facet joint. Conversely, injection of the lumbosacral facet found to be tender on examination, results in relief only if it is responsible for the lumbar pain.

320

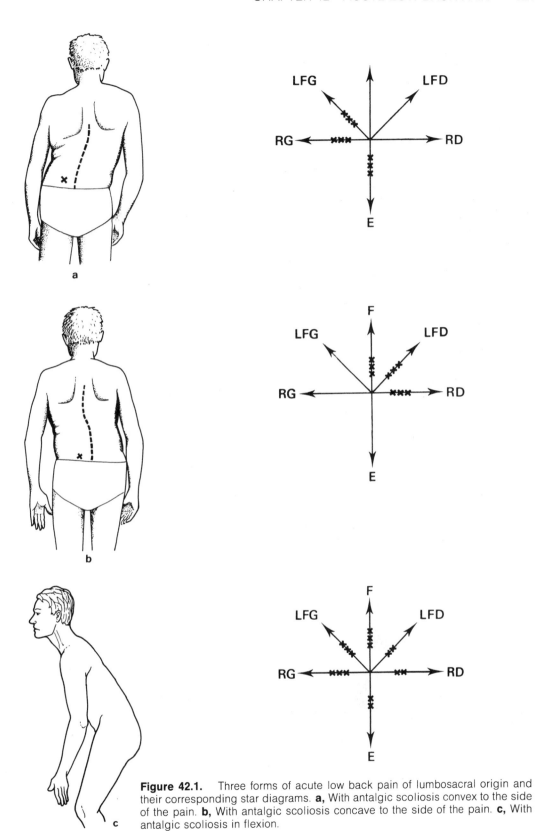

Figure 42.1.   Three forms of acute low back pain of lumbosacral origin and their corresponding star diagrams. **a,** With antalgic scoliosis convex to the side of the pain. **b,** With antalgic scoliosis concave to the side of the pain. **c,** With antalgic scoliosis in flexion.

Treatment

Periodic bed rest may relieve the spinal pain and shorten the acute episode; however, more rapid results can often be obtained by other means.

Manipulation

Acute low back pain has enhanced the reputation of manipulators and manipulations. Half of the patients are instantly relieved by the first manipulation. A second session performed 48 hours later relieves 25% more.

Not all forms of acute low back pain respond to the manipulative treatment in the same way. Forms with antalgic attitude in flexion are generally not a good indication. Most often, this treatment cannot be applied because the rule of no pain cannot be respected, since all directions are painful (Fig. 42.1c).

Low Back Pain with an Antalgic List, Convex to the Painful Side (Fig. 42.1a). This is the most common form seen. The patient lies on the painful side (side of the lumbar convexity), and the physician performs a lumbar manipulation in flexion (Fig. 42.2). Other techniques are possible including the "astride technique," with lateroflexion toward the pain-free side and a rotation in the same direction as the lateroflexion, or the "belt technique" if the patient can tolerate the prone position; the operator can be on the side of the free lateroflexion.

Low Back Pain with an Antalgic List, Concave to the Painful Side (Fig. 42.1b). The patient lies on the table on the pain-free side. The operator performs a manipulation in extension, thrusting on the iliac crest (Fig. 42.3). This technique allows the application of the rule of no pain and opposite movement in most cases. Occasionally, the opposite works well; that is, the patient lies on the concave side of the antalgic list (painful side) and is manipulated accordingly (i.e., either in extension, or in flexion).

Low Back Pain with an Antalgic Attitude in Flexion (Fig. 42.1c). This can be pure, the lateral flank concavity replaced by a convexity, with or without a scoliosis; they are always severe forms. Manipulation is rarely possible because all directions are painful. If two of them are free, repeated mobilizations in these directions should be tried to see if they free other movements; then proceed by successive approaches. Epidural injection is usually the only useful treatment (Fig. 42.4). Periodic bed rest is often necessary.

Relaxation Techniques in Acute Low Back Pain Syndromes

Whether manipulation is possible or not, mobilization can bring an appreciable relief.

- The patient is positioned in supine, on a firm base, with the hips and knees flexed (Fig. 42.5, left). Both knees are grasped under the operator's axilla, and gradually, the hip flexion upon the trunk is passively increased, bringing the knees toward the patient's head with a slow, insistent movement, with repetition if it is painless. The operator can also

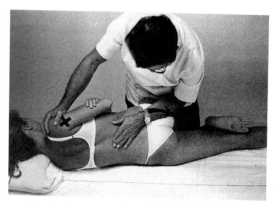

Figure 42.2.   (See Fig. 42.1**a**). Manipulation in flexion. The patient is lying on the left side for a manipulation and right rotation in flexion.

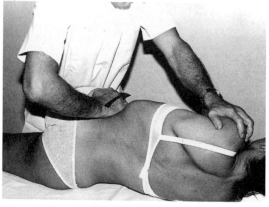

Figure 42.3.   (See Fig. 42.1**b**). Manipulation in extension. The patient is lying on the left side for a manipulation with left rotation and extension.

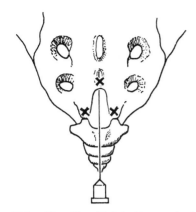

Figure 42.4. (See Fig. 42.1**c**). No manipulation is possible; the rule of no pain and opposite movement cannot be applied. Epidural injection is the best treatment if there is no contraindication.

pick the knees up on the shoulder (Fig. 42.5, right).

- The operator takes one knee in the hand and brings it slowly toward the ipsilateral shoulder (Fig. 42.6, left). This maneuver is performed several times, then the knee is directed toward the contralateral shoulder (Fig. 42.6, right), taking care that there is no pain with these maneuvers. The operator can thus obtain progressive mobilization. These maneuvers are usually painless on one side only; this is the one that is used.
- Another maneuver (described in Appendix 5) is useful in most cases of low back pain syndromes with antalgic attitude, direct or crossed (Fig. 42.7). The patient lies on the

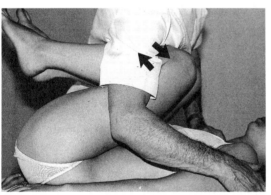
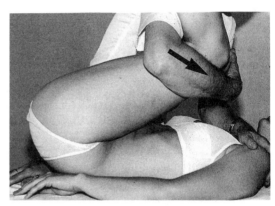

Figure 42.5. **Left.** Mobilization in lumbar flexion. **Right,** Mobilization with stretching of the lumbar musculature in flexion.

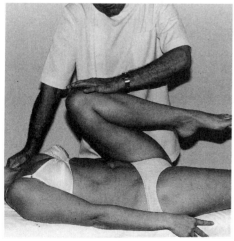
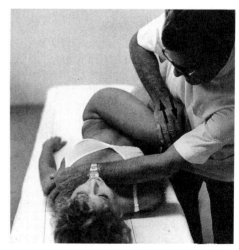

Figure 42.6. Mobilization in flexion with mild rotation. The knee is first flexed toward the shoulder, in a manner similar to that of the first mobilization, and then progressively toward the opposite shoulder.

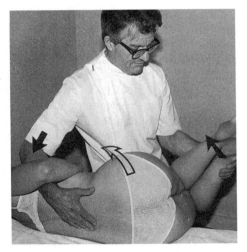

Figure 42.7. Mobilization in lateral flexion and rotation to the right.

most comfortable side, while the operator performs gentle progressive maneuvers in lateroflexion in the pain-free direction.

Injection

Epidural injection of corticosteroids can bring remarkable relief in acute low back pain of discogenic origin. In severe cases, an intrathecal injection of corticosteroids, using the technique of Luccherini, can give a spectacular result. The patient must remain in strict supine position for 24 hours.

Rigid Lumbar Orthosis

Rigid lumbar orthoses may obviate the need for bed rest and can sometimes replace it when the patient's activities cannot be interrupted. It is very useful in patients with a severe form that is relieved by manipulation or injection, who cannot rest or are required to travel.

Medication

From the beginning of the attack, anti-inflammatories should be prescribed if there is no contraindication, and they should be given for a few days. Muscle relaxants may be efficacious in certain cases. We find them to be more useful for the sequelae of an attack than for the attack itself. Analgesics are often useful.

Prevention (Prehabilitation) and Rehabilitation

A patient with acute recurrent low back pain has a good chance of progressing to a chronic stage. An appropriate therapeutic exercise program is the best way to avoid this, and it can limit the frequency and severity of recurrences as well as the risk of sciatica. Correcting poor postural habits and improving the ergonomics of the workplace are decisive elements in prevention.

ACUTE LOW BACK PAIN OF THORACOLUMBAR ORIGIN

This is the acute form of the low back pain of thoracolumbar origin of Maigne, described in Chapter 41. During a torsional movement (e.g., turning the shoulders, while sitting in a car, to take something from behind or on the side) and sometimes after an exertion or a chill, the patient often feels an acute pain in the low lumbar region, resulting in a generalized stiffness. Flexion is usually very limited and painful, and extension is difficult; the reverse can also happen. In addition, lateroflexion away from the painful side is limited. Unilateral trunk rotation is also painful, sometimes bilaterally. Protective paraspinal muscle guarding can be present, but the antalgic attitude is not as marked as it is in the acute low back pain syndromes of lumbosacral origin. This form of acute low back pain is more frequent in people over 40 years of age, but it can be seen in younger persons.

Clinical Signs

Clinical signs are the same as those in the chronic form described above (see "Clinical Signs" in Chapter 41).

At the Inferior Lumbar Level

Clinical signs include the crestal point produced by compression of the affected posterior ramus, against the lilac crest; pain on the pinch-roll test of the skin overlying the gluteal region that is adjacent to the crestal point, and a possible cellulalgic thickening of the subcutaneous tissues.

At the Thoracolumbar Junction

Segmental examination reveals pain of one and sometimes two segments (T12-L1 most often). If it is due to T11-T12, there is no crestal point, the cutaneous branch of T11 does not cross the iliac crest, and the zone that is painful on the pinch-roll test is located above the iliac crest.

Treatment

Manipulation

Manipulation is very useful if possible, according to the rules. Depending on the case, the most commonly used techniques are the "astride" technique in rotation (Fig. 41.14); the " epigastric" technique, the supine technique (Fig. 41.15, right), and the "knee" technique (Fig. 41.15, left). Facet joint injection replaces manipulation if the latter is impossible or complements it if it is insufficient. The following observation is characteristic of this form of acute lumbar pain.

Case History. Mrs. C. V., 60 years old, felt a left acute low back pain while taking a flower pot from the window. The pain was sharp. She was very stiff, very "blocked." The attack lasted 10 days and was persistent. Three epidural injections of cortisone were performed without improvement, but the pain was partially improved by anti-inflammatories, which she did not tolerate very well. She had had the same kind of attack 2 years previously; it dragged on for more than a month, leaving a kind of discomfort that finally disappeared. Radiography showed advanced degenerative changes of L4-L5 and L5-S1 that seemed responsible for the low back pain. In fact, these two levels were only slightly sensitive on the segmental examination, which revealed, however, sharp sensitivity of T12-L1, with a precisely localized pain on pressure over the right facet joint. Radiographs of that region were totally normal. An injection of 1 mL of a corticosteroid derivative with lidocaine was performed at the T12-L1 facet. There was nearly immediate relief, and the patient could bend. Manipulation was then possible, and one maneuver in left rotation relieved her completely.

ACUTE LOW BACK PAIN OF CALCIFYING DISCOPATHY

Isolated or integrated in the multiple tendinous calcifications, calcifying discopathy at the lumbar level, as at the thoracic level, can be responsible for a severe attack. Pain is induced rapidly. The slightest movement produces an extremely violent recurrence on a permanent basis, which is so painful that the patient cannot sleep. This pain is usually well localized and does not radiate very much. Fever of 38.5°C is present, and there is an elevated sedimentation rate. Examination is very difficult because the patient fears the slightest change of position; the abdomen is distended, the lumbar spine is stiff, and the paraspinal muscles are firm, with contracture.

Diagnosis is made by radiographs that demonstrate calcification of the intervertebral disk and the integrity of the vertebral end plates and the vertebral body. The attack lasts several days and decreases with nonsteroidal anti-inflammatories. Spontaneous resolution occurs in about 10 days. With such a picture, some other possibilities come to mind, especially an infectious discitis or an occult metastasis.

ACUTE LOW BACK PAIN OF MYOFASCIAL ORIGIN

Some chronic low back pain syndromes can originate at a trigger point, as described above. In some cases, pain can be acute and the attack can look like a low back pain of spinal origin. The painful muscular point is found on examination, when pressure reproduces the spontaneous pain. Trigger points can be found in the paraspinal muscles between L1 and the sacrum, in the lumbar iliocostal muscle, or in the longissimus. In these cases, the trigger point is localized over the lower ribs. Injection of a few milliliters of lidocaine or procaine produces relief.

43

SCIATICA

Common sciatica is the most frequent radicular pain syndrome of spinal origin. It is usually linked to irritation of a spinal nerve root associated with disk herniation at L4–L5 or L5–S1.

ONSET AND TOPOGRAPHY

The onset is often traumatic. Exertion or a forced movement results in acute low back pain, followed by referral to the leg. Often this is exacerbated by standing, sitting, exertion, coughing, and sneezing, and relieved by lying down. Its referral pattern follows that of the L5 or S1 territory: for L5, the buttock, anterior aspect of the thigh, lateral malleolus, dorsum of the foot, great toe or the three first toes (Fig. 43.1); for S1: the buttock, posterior aspect of the thigh, knee, leg and heel, to the sole or lateral side of the foot, up to the fifth toe (Fig. 43.3). In the distal limb, pain may be replaced by tingling or numbness.

CLINICAL EXAMINATION

There is usually an antalgic attitude with scoliosis, either convex (often L5) or concave (often S1), to the side of pain. If the patient tries to overcome the antalgic attitude by compensating for the lumbar shift, a relative blocking of spinal motion is encountered, manifested by a "break" in the normally smooth C-shaped curve formed by the line of the spinous processes. With antalgic kyphosis, if the patient tries to straighten up, the movement is also impaired. Forward flexion in standing, with the legs extended, is limited and often exacerbates the pain. The straight leg raise test,

performed either sitting (so that the pelvis is fixed) or supine (where the pelvis is free to move), often reproduces the referral pattern to the buttock and leg as a result of the dural irritation produced by the discogenic lesion. This is Lasegue's sign and is useful for following changes and assessing the efficiency of treatment. The neurologic examination is frequently negative or reduced to minor signs including

- Hypesthesia or hyperesthesia of the leg or the foot in the L5 or S1 distribution.
- Diminished or absent Achilles reflex in S1 sciatica.
- Occasionally, a subtle decrease in the motor power. For S1, the plantarflexors may be weak, and the patient may have difficulty performing heel raises (in subtle cases, it is only appreciable when the patient is asked to perform a series of heel raises, alternately on each side, to see whether the involved side fatigues sooner); for L5, the extensor of the great toe and, more rarely, the dorsiflexors.

Examination for Cellulotenoperiosteomyalgic Manifestations

It was with cases of sciatica that we first drew attention to the simultaneous presence of cellulalgic manifestations, trigger points, and tenoperiosteal tenderness located in the territory of the involved nerve root, and their role in certain persistent pain syndromes (Maigne, 1961). These cellulotenoperiosteomyalgic manifestations exist in all cases (Figs. 43.2 and 43.5), and include the following.

- Trigger points are constant in the gluteal

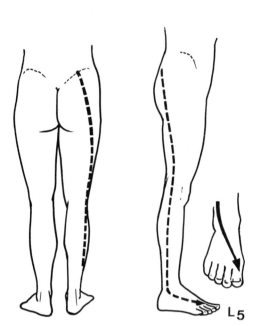

Figure 43.1.   Topography of pain in L5 sciatica.

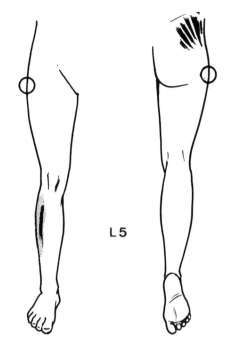

Figure 43.2.   Manifestations of the cellulotenoperiosteomyalgic syndrome in L5 sciatica.

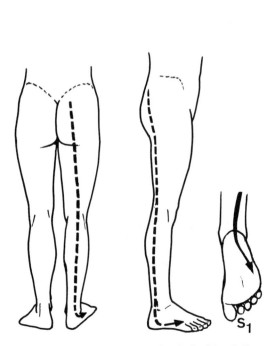

Figure 43.3.   Topography of pain in S1 sciatica.

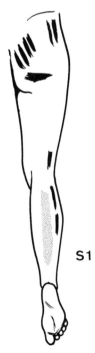

Figure 43.4.   Manifestations of the cellulotenoperiosteomyalgic syndrome in S1 sciatica.

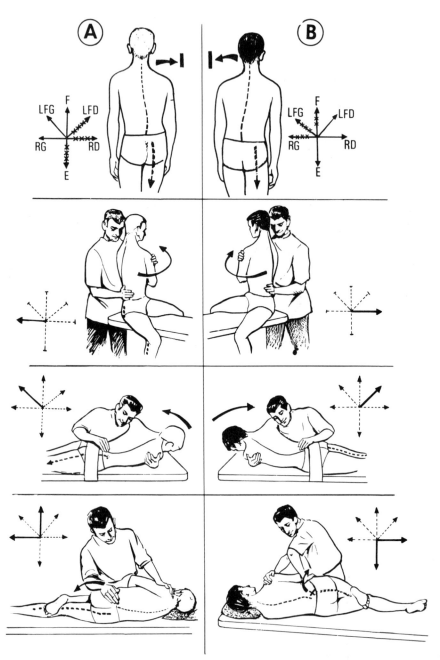

Figure 43.5. Examples of manipulations used in two cases of right sciatica with opposite antalgic scoliosis. **A,** The pain is convex to the side of the pain. **B,** The pain is concave to the side of the pain. The maneuvers performed are consistent with the rule of no pain and opposite movement and are thus performed in opposite directions in the two cases. (The star diagrams corresponding to **A** and **B** are shown).

From *upper* diagram to *lower* diagram: Manipulation in rotation to the left (subject on the *left*); manipulation in rotation to the right (subject on the *right*); manipulation in left lateral flexion (subject on the *left*); manipulation in right lateral flexion (subject on the *right*); manipulation in left rotation and flexion (subject on the *left*); manipulation in right rotation and extension (subject on the *right*).

muscles and often present in the inferior part of the biceps femoris, in S1 sciatica. They are much less common in L5 sciatica (extensor of the great toe).

- In 50% of cases, a cellulalgic zone is found overlying the posterior calf for S1 and at the superior anterolateral aspect of the leg for L5. It is usually more marked for S1 than for L5.
- Trochanteric tenderness to palpation is frequent in L5 sciatica. These manifestations may persist for years after the attack. They either become latent or responsible for residual and annoying pain. It is then possible to make a retrospective diagnosis of the involved segmental level.

Most often, trigger points are responsible for local or referred pain that persists and is reproduced by muscle fatigue or certain positions. For example, when compressed between the femur and the edge of a seat, the trigger point of the short head of the biceps femoris makes the sitting position painful; a trigger point of the lateral gastrocnemius (left leg) can be painful when the legs are crossed (left leg on right leg) as it can be compressed between the left shin and the right knee. They can also be a source of cramps during the night. Often the cellulalgic zone, which is usually latent, can be responsible for persistent moderate pain and, exceptionally, acute pain, as in the following case.

Case History. Mrs. Z., a 48-year-old patient, had L5 sciatica, not relieved by bed rest or by medical treatment. Myelographic studies confirmed the presence of a herniated disk at L4–L5. She was operated upon, and the surgeon found a large herniation that he removed easily. The antalgic attitude then disappeared, the spine became supple, and Lasegue's sign disappeared. However, the patient continued to complain that she had more pain than before, especially when in bed, which was not made worse by activity. She was rehospitalized, but no cause could be found for her refractory pain. She was given tricyclic antidepressant medication and anxiolytics, but was not relieved. We then decided to examine her, though the pain had lasted for 5 months. The clinical examination (spinal examination, Lasegue's sign) was unremarkable. There were only two trigger points of the gluteus medius, minimally painful on examination, and a cellulalgic zone of a few square centimeters on the lateral aspect of the leg, which was extremely painful to pinch-rolling. Injection of local anesthetic throughout this small zone, on two separated occasions, resolved the pain.

IMAGING

Radiography

The standard radiograph is useful to assess the state of the spine. But there is no relationship between the picture and the clinical state. The picture can be normal in a patient with acute severe sciatica and, in other subjects, can show significant degenerative lesions that have nothing to do with the sciatica. The other examinations are only indicated when a surgical intervention is being considered or when the diagnosis is difficult.

Computed Tomography

Computed tomography (CT) is a noninvasive modality that can readily demonstrate morphologic abnormalities relating to a herniated disk, including the relative impact on the adjacent soft tissues and whether there is any neuroforaminal or extraforaminal encroachment. CT is useful for demonstrating central and lateral recess stenosis, as well as lesions of the facet joints. In cases of recurrent disk herniation, and especially in those patients who have already undergone a surgical procedure, CT with intravenous contrast can be used to differentiate between a recurrent disk herniation and perineural fibrosis, because the former takes up contrast, while the latter does not.

Myelography

Myelography is excellent for assessing the entire subarachnoid space, from the cervical spinal cord to the sacral roots, and allows dynamic examination, which can reveal certain impingements that are only visible in standing position or in extension. It is also useful in the assessment of spinal stenosis. It has the same disadvantages as diagnostic lumbar puncture, including headaches, nausea, etc. (in approximately 35% of the cases). Problems of neurotoxicity of the contrast agent have now been eliminated thanks to modern products.

Myelography is insensitive to far lateral herniations, including both foraminal and extraforaminal encroachments. Epidural lesions are visualized only if they have left an impression on the dural sac. A central disk herniation at L5–S1, in a patient with a short thecal sac, with a thick epidural fat pad, will not be readily seen (Bard and Laredo).

Discography

Discography, an often neglected modality, is an excellent means of assessing disk pathology because of both its morphologic depiction and its provocative properties. Contrast injected into an intervertebral disk can demonstrate the following.

- Whether it is of normal morphology
- Whether there is evidence of annular or radial fissuring
- Protrusion within the confines of the posterior longitudinal ligament
- Extrusion beyond the confines of the posterior longitudinal ligament, with or without sequestration
- If the "end-feel" of the injection is firm or whether the disk accepts an abnormally large volume of contrast (e.g., when the annulus has ruptured)
- Whether the patient's typical pain is reproduced exactly

When followed immediately by CT, discography can provide an excellent three-dimensional morphologic analysis that is often indispensable in the preoperative evaluation.

Magnetic Resonance Imaging

MRI is the study of choice for a recurrence following discectomy, to differentiate recurrent herniation from perineural fibrosis. It can also detect other lesions such as a neuroma that is located higher than the supposed cause of the sciatica.

CLINICAL FORMS OF SCIATICA

Hyperalgic Sciatica

Hyperalgic sciatica is characterized by the severity of the pain. The patient prefers to remain in bed and is hesitant to move even slightly. These patients are often extremely difficult to examine. If the pain does not respond quickly to the treatment, sciatica can set in.

Of particular interest is a specific form of hyperalgic sciatica called myalgic sciatica. It is seen most commonly in disk herniations affecting the S1 nerve root, and the neuralgic pain is associated with intense and often continuous muscular pains and cramps affecting especially the biceps femoris, triceps surae, and, occasionally, the gluteal muscles. There is often a mild motor deficit. Fasciculations are usual.

Once the acute attack is over, moderate pain persists for months or years, with periodic cramps, often during the night or with certain positions. The segmental cellulotenoperiosteomyalgic syndrome is much accentuated; the trigger points of the gluteal muscles, biceps femoris, and triceps surae are very taut and very painful. They play an important role in the acute and chronic pain.

Paralytic Sciatica

On examination, a slight motor deficit can be detected. It is more frequent in L5 sciatica than in S1. In the latter case, however, the damage can be severe if the subject cannot perform a heel raise on the affected side. This deficit can be unmasked by applying pressure to the shoulders of a patient who is attempting to perform a heel raise against resistance.

Subtle motor deficits that always recover are not to be classified as paralytic sciatica. Only sciatica that has functional deficits (1% of cases, approximately) deserves that name. Most often, paralytic L5 sciatica leads to footdrop, which forces the patient to modify the gait pattern by increasing the amount of hip and knee flexion during the swing phase to avoid catching the toe on the ground at midswing. This deficit is readily detected by the examiner, because an audible foot "slap" is heard when the involved foot makes its initial contact with the ground as it begins a new stance phase.

There is a great difference between a motor deficit which has been graded as 0 or 1 compared to those graded as 3 or 4 (Held et al.). Motor deficits of paralytic sciatica often affect more than one nerve root, even when the painful topography affects only one.

Sciatica in the Young

Sciatica is rather rare in persons under 20 years of age. The antalgic attitude is generally quite marked, with a significant lumbar shift. Lasegue's sign is usually positive at 20° of leg elevation. If forward flexion of the trunk is tested with the legs extended, it is surprising to find that this flexion is quite impossible; only the superiormost portion of the spine goes into flexion; the lumbar spine remains as rigid as an iron bar. This contrasts with the possibilities of movement or of activities of the young patient, who manages to ''fake'' remarkably well.

In the child under 14 years of age, sciatica is rare. The antalgic scoliosis is marked in flexion, occasionally resulting in antalgic kyphoscoliosis. Most children with spontaneously painful scoliosis are seen by their physicians, and rarely is their presentation acute (Fauchet). Sciatica in these cases is generally due to large disk herniations. Spondylolisthesis is still the most frequent cause of sciatica in this age group.

Sciatica in the Elderly

Sciatica is uncommon in persons over 60 years old. If facet joint spondylosis and spinal stenosis often play a role, herniated disk is not exceptional. Interestingly, Lasegue's sign decreases in intensity with age. In the young, the sign at 10 or 20° is usual, and the patient has moderate pain and adapts well to it. The sign at 30° in a person of 40 years of age means a severe sciatica and confines the patient to bed. In an elderly patient, the signs of sciatica, although genuine, can be quite mild.

Sciatica and Spinal Stenosis

Verbiest pointed out the significance of congenital spinal stenosis in the development of compression of the cauda equina. Later, it was found that this condition, either acquired or congenital, could cause sciatica.

Two situations can occur:

1. When the spinal canal is narrow, especially at the the lateral recess, the slightest disk or articular alteration is capable of irritating the nerve root.
2. A spinal canal of normal dimensions can develop acquired narrowing by the simultaneous action of disk protrusions, hypertrophy of the ligamentum flavum, and facet joint spondylosis. This acquired narrowing can produce radicular pathology without necessarily causing a localized compression. The stenosis can be global or central, lateral or foraminal.

Central Spinal Stenosis

A chronic evolving sciatic pain can be present. It can sometimes be replaced by paresthesia. It can be monoradicular, often bilateral or alternating, or it can be polyradicular. Its physical signs are discrete. Symptoms of neurogenic claudication are pathognomonic but exist in only 50% of cases (Deburge, Lassale, et al.) and can have diverse clinical aspects including premature muscular fatigue that forces the patient to stop walking or sensory claudication with paresthesia and pain. Forward flexion of the trunk relieves this pain.

Sometimes, the picture is less typical. There is a persistent sciatic pain, generally of L5, worsening progressively, often in a solidly built man who bends slowly forward when walking to feel relieved. Hyperextension of the trunk increases the pain, which evolves progressively toward chronicity with improvement and aggravation phases, influenced by fatigue and relieved by rest.

Myelography reveals characteristic images, especially thinning of the epidural space; disappearance of the epidural fat pad; a festooned look like a string, of the intradural opacity in lateral view; and decreased contrast in the narrowed zones. CT/myelography is especially useful in demonstrating the morphology of the canal so that the stenosis is recognized.

Lateral Recess Stenosis

Lateral recess stenosis produces a monoradicular sciatica, most commonly L5, with a very strong mechanical component. Occasionally a degree of motor deficit occurs, usually in relation to the degree of facet hypertrophy, and occasionally there is an associated disk bulging.

Foraminal Stenosis

L5-S1 disk degeneration leads to a relative superior displacement of the articular process of S1, which narrows the intervertebral foramen without necessarily having spondylosis present.

DIFFERENTIAL DIAGNOSIS

Certain sciatic pains due to inflammatory, infectious, or tumoral causes can simulate common sciatica. In the young, there is the possibility of a spondyloarthropathy. Pain usually does not refer distal to the knee, is often bilateral or alternating occurring episodically, and is not modified by activity. Nocturnal pain is common, keeping the subject awake much of the night.

Diagnosis can be made by PA views of the pelvis or specialized Hibbs views of the sacroiliac joints as well as by an elevation in the sedimentation rate. It can be confirmed by rapid response to medication. The HLA B27 haplotype is commonly associated with this group of conditions and may be helpful diagnostically.

Intramedullary tumors, especially gliomas can produce a sciatica that does not quite follow a radicular topography. Nocturnal pain is common, and the patient will stand or walk to bring relief. Physical activity has no influence at all on the pain. The spine is sometimes very stiff. Radiographic studies are usually normal; it is rare to see the enlargement of the foramen intervertebralis, because of the thinning of the pedicle. Diagnosis is made by lumbar puncture and CT/myelography. Surgical intervention relieves the patient.

Metastatic lesions or a multiple myeloma can result in intense refractory sciatic pain. Infectious discitis and sacroiliitis can also be manifested by sciatic pain.

Pseudosciatic Syndromes

Some disorders can simulate sciatic pain, such as periarthritis of the hip (tendinitis of the gluteus medius), but are rarely confusing. On the other hand, dysfunction of the lateral perforating branch of the abdominal genital nerve or the subcostal nerve (ramus cutaneous lateralis and abdominalis) can sometimes appear to be a "mixed" or polyradicular sciatica (R. and J. Y. Maigne) (see Chapter 47, "Perforating Branch Syndrome of T12 and L1").

A trigger point of the gluteus minimus can cause a very misleading referred pain that refers distally to the foot. Pressure on this point reproduces the radiating pain, which disappears with an anesthetic injection. As we have seen above, certain low back pains of thoracolumbar origin can cause ectopic and pseudosciatic referral patterns (see "Ectopic Referral Patterns" in Chapter 41).

TREATMENT

Treatment of the Attack

Initial management of the acute episode should include back first-aid, of which a component is helping the patient to find a pain-free position. Intermittent bed rest, with movement for short periods in between, is probably the single most effective self-treatment the patient can implement. The patient should lie on a firm mattress, in the position that feels most comfortable: lying supine, with hips and knees flexed, most often alternating with lying on the side occasionally. In milder cases, a rigid lumbar orthosis can shorten the duration of, or obviate the need for, bed rest.

Medication

Pain relief is of paramount importance to the patient with sciatica. An epidural injection is often useful. In the hyperalgic forms, intrathecal injection of corticosteroids by Luccherini's technique can produce a remarkable reduction in pain. Anti-inflammatory medications and analgesics are the usual treatment.

Manipulation can decrease or shorten an acute attack, but it is usually performed in moderate or persistent forms, when the acute phase is over. It can produce an excellent result, sometimes even spectacular, if it is technically possible and well executed. Patients believe they are cured, although they are only relieved, with little or no pain; so they forget about caution . . . and there is a recurrence. For a patient who will not, or cannot, interrupt activities, a rigid lumbar orthosis is best.

In fact, the best treatment of acute sciatica is all of the above together, adjusted according to results and changes.

Surgery: Chemonucleolysis

For forms that are resistant to treatment and rest, additional examinations, such as CT or myelography, often reveal a herniated disk for which surgical interventions, including chemonucleolysis or percutaneous discectomy, may be considered. Sciatica caused by acute inflammatory arthritis of the facet joint can be successfully treated with one to three local injections of corticosteroids.

Treatment by Manipulation

The useful maneuvers (the same as those for the acute low back pain syndromes) are determined by the antalgic attitudes. However, even if the antalgic attitude is characteristic, careful study of muscle stretching during tests of free and painful movements (Fig. 43.5) is always best. It happens (rarely), especially in S1 sciatica, that there is not perfect coincidence between what is revealed by the antalgic attitude and the study of passive movements executed on the lower lumbar region.

Sciatica, whose star diagram has three free orientations, is a good indication for manipulation; this is the most frequent case. If there are only two free orientations, maneuvers of relaxation may be sufficient, and their result can be carefully monitored. In general, it is not a good indication. If there is no pain-free orientation, manipulation is contraindicated, as is the case in hyperalgic sciatica.

After each manipulation, the result should be retested: Lasegue's sign and pain of the gluteal trigger points on palpation; the subjective impression of the patient; and a functional activity (e.g., putting on a sock). No maneuver should be a setback. This cannot occur, of course, if the rule of no pain is applied, the maneuver is perfectly executed in the pain-free direction, the patient position is optimal, and the force used is adequate. In general, each maneuver has a positive effect; sometimes it produces nothing; but it should never cause aggravation.

The session should be well organized and well dosed: maneuvers of relaxation, then mobilization, and finally, the fewest manipulative maneuvers necessary (never more than three). Otherwise there may be further exacerbation. The patient should be forewarned, however, of the possibility of a temporary exacerbation that normally follows some manipulative sessions. After the reaction is over, there is generally an improvement, which is slight or significant, momentary or lasting. The second session is usually 3–4 days later. There is generally no flare-up after the second session. If the patient demonstrates good improvement after the first session, subsequent sessions can be spaced at longer intervals. Most patients are relieved after three sessions. In some difficult cases, two or three more might be necessary. However, if no partial or temporary improvement occurs during the first three sessions, the treatment should be stopped.

Treatment of Sequelae

In persistent sciatica, particular attention must be given to cellulotenoperiosteomyalgic manifestations, which are frequently responsible for refractory pain. They can be treated locally, but the responsible spinal segment should not have sufficient facet joint or ligamentous pain (interspinous ligament) to maintain them.

Trigger points should be treated by stretching and slow, deep, and progressive kneading massage. Acute trigger points can be injected with procaine or lidocaine, followed by stretching of the muscle; ultrasound often produces good results. Trochanteric pain (L5) will be relieved by the spinal treatment, but it occasionally requires local treatment. Cellulalgic manifestations are treated by anesthetic injection of the subcutaneous tissues followed by kneading. A stay at a spa for hydrotherapy can also have a very good effect in chronic cases.

Rehabilitation

Once the attack is over, therapeutic exercises can be introduced in cases involving a true low back pain after dysfunction of thoracolumbar origin has been ruled out or addressed.

Paralytic Sciatica

Certain authors (e.g., G. Lazorthes et al.) prefer an early surgical intervention, as soon as the first signs of neurologic deficit are noted. Others (e.g., Held et al.) attest that surgical intervention does not result in a more complete or more rapid recovery, especially when the original neurologic deficit is complete (as in such axonal lesions as axonotmesis or neurotmesis). Surgical interventions are usually reserved for patients without a total neurologic deficit, who seem to have the potential to recover normal neuromuscular function in the same manner and time course as nonoperated patients. Sany et al. believe that factors indicating a good prognosis are early treatment, the topography of pain, age of the patient (less than 40 years old), absence of any lumbalgic or sciatic antecedent and absence of any sensory or motor deficit. Therapeutic exercise will hasten recovery and should be continued long after the symptoms have resolved. Later-stage recovery, over 3 or 4 years, is not uncommon. The use of an ankle-foot orthosis can temporarily relieve the foot drop, as well as improve the lateral instability.

Sciatica in the Young Patient

Most authors prefer early intervention. The clinical signs and the duration of progression are deciding factors. Medical treatment is efficacious; there is no indication for manipulation. Cases in which the lumbar shift is moderate seem to us to be the most amenable to improvement. Treatment should be limited to the relief of the patient; dramatic improvements in spinal mobility or in Lasegue's sign are rarely an attainable goal. Sometimes young patients will declare that they feel better when the Lasegue's sign is still at 30° and anterior flexion of the trunk is still virtually impossible. If the relief is satisfactory and there is minimal lumbar shift, it is better to wait, because this stiffness will generally decrease progressively and disappear after several months without any other treatment. The best advice is to avoid overexertion and sports during that period.

However, if the pain is sharp and the lumbar shift is significant, these young patients should be operated upon as soon as possible, which means that, in general, surgery is more common in the young than in the adult.

Sciatica in the Elderly

Medical treatment is the same as that for the adult, except that manipulation is to be avoided in most cases. If this treatment is not efficacious and the patient is in great pain, then surgical treatment is necessary, whatever the age of the patient, if the diagnosis is disk herniation. In patients with spinal stenosis, the medical treatment is injections and complete rest in recumbent position for 2 weeks, followed by a rigid lumbar orthosis worn for 15–20 days, and then a reinforced lumbosacral corset and rehabilitation.

A flexion exercise program is usually prescribed, with particular attention to hip joint flexibility. The aim is to relieve the lumbosacral spine, which is often in hyperlordosis (Troisier, Rabourdin).

Surgical intervention is considered only after a well-planned medical treatment fails, as it is indicated only for sciatica associated with intermittent weakness and not for the associated low back pain. It consists of a laminectomy for central stenoses and a partial facetectomy in the lateral recess stenoses.

44

FEMORAL NEURALGIA

Femoral neuralgia is much less frequent than sciatica. It is most often due to irritation of the L3 or L4 nerve roots by a disk herniation. Facet joint spondylosis, narrowing the intervertebral foramina, can also be a source of aggravation. Femoral neuralgia is more often seen in men over 40 years of age. But besides "common femoral neuralgia," there are some symptomatic femoral neuralgias that are useful to understand.

INITIAL SYMPTOMS AND TOPOGRAPHY

Femoral neuralgia frequently starts with physical exertion. The pain is initially felt in the low back, followed by referral to the anterior thigh, toward the knee. If L3 is affected, pain is felt over the anteromedial thigh and stops at the patella. If L4 is affected, the pain may descend as far distally as the anteromedial leg to the ankle (Fig. 44.1, a and b). Mixed or overlapping topographies are common. Pain is internal, deep, and shooting, and nocturnal flare-ups are frequent.

CLINICAL EXAMINATION

On examination, the spine is stiff, but the possible antalgic attitude is less marked than it is in sciatica. The "sign of Léri," or the "inverse Lasègue sign," is characteristic of femoral neuralgias. This sign is elicited with the patient in the prone position. The physician, fixes the pelvis with one hand while hyperextending the thigh with the knee flexed. This maneuver stretches the femoral nerve and, when it is irritated, produces or increases the pain and the referral pattern. The following can be found.

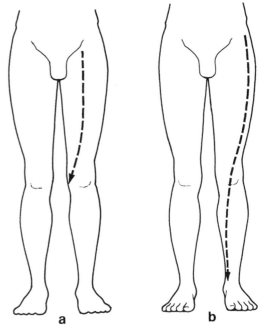

Figure 44.1. Topography of pain in L3 femoral neuralgia on the left (**a**), and L4 on the right (**b**).

- Hypesthesia or hyperesthesia in the L3 or L4 region (medial aspect of the knee, medial aspect of the leg)
- Blunting of the patellar reflex
- Decrease in the strength of the quadriceps, which become hypotonic and often amyotrophic

L3 contributes to the innervation of the psoas, adductor, and quadriceps muscles and, with its posterior ramus, the spinal muscles. The L4 root contributes to the innervation of the gluteal, adductor, quadriceps, tibialis anterior, and extensor digitorum and, with its posterior ramus, the spinal muscles. When the quadriceps is involved, the patient cannot raise the heel from the supine position. In a severe attack, the lower limb gives way, which leads to falls.

According to Godebout et al., sartorius weakness is a constant sign in femoral radiculopathy. They note the absence of the "band of sartorius," which can only be confirmed in lean or muscular persons.

Cellulotenoperiosteomyalgic Manifestations

The midpoint of the rectus femoris is often the site of one or two firm trigger points. They can be a source of chronic pain and even exacerbate it in the acute phase. Their injection often decreases the pain. They are less frequently seen in the vasti medialis and lateralis, but when present, they may be a source of pseudopatellofemoral pain and pseudoblockage.

Cellulalgia is practically constant. It is found at the thigh (L3, L4, over the medial knee, where it is often persistent) and in the region of the pes anserinus (L4). Pain with palpation in the superior medial aspect of the tibial periosteum (L4) is frequent (Fig. 44.2).

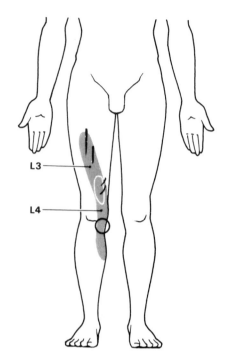

Figure 44.2.   Manifestation of the cellulotenoperiosteomyalgic syndrome of L3 and L4: cellulalgic zones (gray); trigger points (quadriceps and vastus medialis); tenoperiosteal pain (circle).

DIFFERENTIAL DIAGNOSIS

Nerve impingement due to disk herniation is not the only possible cause of femoral neuralgia. The nerve could be impaired along its path by sacroiliac arthritis or as a result of an appendicular or colitic disorder. There can also be infection, spinal metastases, or neuroma, which is always a possibility with any radicular pain. The nerve can be compressed at the hip by a truss or a large ganglion.

In some cases, a viral origin has been proposed. In hemophiliacs or in patients on anticoagulants, a retropsoas hematoma can result in motor deficits that are often significant. An antalgic posture in psoasitis is the rule. The femoral nerve might also be the victim of compression by the retractors during pelvic surgery. It can also be irritated by the cement of a hip prosthesis (methyl methacrylate).

TREATMENT

Treatment is the same as for true sciatica. Rest, injections, and anti-inflammatories are the essential modes of therapy. Manipulation, as in sciatica, can be very useful, especially in the moderate and chronic forms. The most used manipulations are those involving the lateral decubitus, astride, and knee techniques, which are, of course, tailored to each case according to the rule of no pain and opposite movement.

Treatment of the cellulalgic, tenoperiosteal, and myalgic manifestations can shorten the persistent pain. Once the attack is over, reconditioning of the quadriceps mechanism is necessary. Priority is given to isometric exercises, with particular attention to good stability during single support.

MERALGIA PARESTHETICA

Meralgia paresthetica was described by Roth, who observed it in 1895 in German riders wearing tight abdominal belts that compressed the emergence of the femorocutaneous nerve at the level of the ilioinguinal angle, below the anterior superior iliac spine. They complained of curious symptoms, characterized by bizarre feelings over the lateral thigh. Meralgia paresthetica is in fact characterized by paresthesia along the anterolateral side of the thigh, corresponding to the distribution of the femorocutaneous nerve (Fig. 45.1, left).

Exquisitely sensitive, this nerve comes from the anterior ramus of the second, and occasionally from the third, lumbar spinal nerve roots. It becomes superficial at a point located 2 cm anteromedial to the anterior iliac spine, then goes down along the anterolateral side of the thigh.

Meralgia paresthetica is almost always unilateral. The patient complains of a feeling of "dead skin" in that zone, with tingling (pins and needles) or prickling. The skin is hyperesthetic, and contact with clothes can be disagreeable. Most often, these feelings are triggered by walking or prolonged standing and are soothed by rest.

Sensory disorders are frequent but not constant: loss of pain and temperature sensation, hypesthesia, and pain on contact. In all cases, there is an unrecognized sign, a sharp pain of the skin (often thickened) on pinch-rolling (Maigne).

Meralgia paresthetica is perhaps not as rare

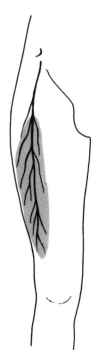

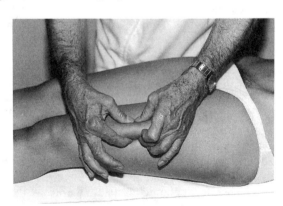

Figure 45.1. **Left,** Lateral femoral cutaneous nerve (gray). **Right,** Painful zone on the pinch-roll test in meralgia paresthetica.

337

as is thought, but when it is mild and intermittent, it is just a moderate inconvenience. The different therapeutic approaches tried at the onset of this disorder are often of little benefit, causing the patient to just accept this small annoyance and not always mention it to the physician. During a systematic examination of patients presenting with another painful disorder, it is not rare to find a zone of hyperesthesia and cellulalgia over the lateral side of the thigh, discovered by pinch-rolling (Fig. 45.1, right). When asked, the patient recognizes having had disagreeable feelings in that region for a long time, separated by long intervals of relative calm in which a prolonged walk does not produce any disagreeable feeling. With a more pronounced form, the daily discomfort motivates the patient to look for a solution and seek some opinions.

CANALICULAR ORIGIN

Meralgia can be due to the irritation of the femorocutaneous nerve at its emergence near the anterior superior iliac spine. There can be microtrauma (e.g., weight bearing on the thigh, hernial bandages). In some rare cases, meralgia is symptomatic (e.g., abscess, tumor). Most often, it is caused by a fibro-osseous entrapment mechanism. Between its abdominal path, which is horizontal, and its femoral path, which is vertical, the nerve undergoes angulation, putting it under particular stress. At that level, it can be compressed by the thickening of the fascia iliaca (Stookey, Dupont et al.). When decompressed surgically, there is a prestenotic swelling (Claustre et al.). This abnormality was also found at autopsy in subjects who never had any meralgia. In 60 autopsies, Nathan found 36 cases of enlargement of the nerve and 10 cases in which that nerve showed a fusiform "pseudoganglionic" aspect. If this anatomic factor predisposes, it is thus not sufficient; an additional factor, usually spinal, is necessary.

SPINAL ORIGIN

A spinal origin is sometimes considered when the segment L2–L3 demonstrates disk degeneration or spondylosis. This presumptive sign is of no more value than is a low lumbar discopathy seen in radiographic studies to a lumbar pain. In fact, systematic use of the segmental examination enabled us to find out that meralgia is very frequently of spinal origin, by revealing a pain in segment L2–L3, while this segment is most often radiologically normal. The patient sometimes complains of low back pain ipsilateral to the meralgic symptoms, but they are not necessarily concomitant, and they are usually left in the background.

The pinch-roll test is painful on all or part of the anterolateral side of the thigh and, in some cases, in the medial iliac crest region 7 or 8 cm lateral to the midline. This corresponds to the "crestal point," where the the posterior ramus of L2 can be compressed against the iliac crest. According to our anatomic findings, this ramus passes at this point in one-third of cases (in two-thirds it is L1) (J. Y. and R. Maigne) (see Chapter 41).

MIXED ORIGIN

As it is the case in many pains of spinal origin, meralgia paresthetica seems to have generally a dual origin.

• Dysfunction of the spinal segment L2–L3
• Irritation of the femorocutaneous nerve in its course along its abdominal path and its femoral path

These contributors are of variable importance, depending on the case. Suppression of one of the two factors usually suffices to suppress the symptom. Spinal treatment alone (manipulation and/or facet joint injection) yielded an excellent response in 30 of the 42 patients that we studied. Most of these patients had been suffering for several years (20 years for the oldest). Sometimes, an occasional manipulation (1 or 2 yearly) is necessary, because the causative PMID tends to recur.

N.B. As we shall see in Chapter 47, meralgia paresthetica can be simulated by irritation of a nearby nerve: the lateral cutaneous perforating branch of the abdominogenital and iliohypogastric nerve (L1) or the subcostal nerve (T12) (R. Maigne).

COCCYGODYNIA

Coccygodynia is a benign disorder, often refractory, and "wearisome for the patient and for the physician" (Louyot). It can be a simple inconvenience or a handicapping disorder with strong psychologic effects; it affects women slightly more than men. We propose here a technique that can give quick, sometimes immediate, relief in coccygodynia of mechanical origin.

The usual cause of traumatic coccygodynia is a fall on the buttocks, which occurs, according to authors, in 60–70% of the cases. The coccygeal pain is generally immediate, but in some cases, it may remain latent for 1 or 2 years between the fall and establishment of the coccygodynia. In the meantime, there is generally a slight pain with prolonged sitting or at contact.

Coccygodynia may occur on recovery after giving birth. Some seem to be linked to lumbosacral problems; they come after or with low back pain, and they can disappear after lumbosacral manipulation or epidural injection. Others result from anorectal infections and are seen especially by the proctologists. We observed a chordoma that was manifested for 2 years by coccygeal pain. Finally, some others are called essential, since no cause can be found. Psychologic causes are classic, with coccygodynia appearing, for example, after the loss of a loved one or a divorce.

DIAGNOSIS

Pain of the sacrococcygeal region is too easily called "coccygodynia." To arrive at this diagnosis, the characteristic sign of pain on pressure of the tip of coccyx should be found.

Occasionally, pressure on the sacrococcygeal articulation is painful.

In some cases, we have observed trigger points at the level of the sacrococcygeal insertions of the gluteus maximus or a trigger point of the pyriformis. Occasionally, one can detect a significant unilateral paracoccygeal cellulalgic zone. Most often, there is only pain on the tip of the coccyx. On rectal examination, there are taut bands in the levator ani and the pyriformis.

TREATMENT

In general, coccygodynias have the reputation of being refractory to treatments. Massages of the levatores and injections give only irregular success. Almost always, coccygodynia occurring after a fall or labor and delivery are immediately cured by the maneuver that we propose below. The others are cured much less often.

Massage of the Levatores

Thiele proposed this massage. Françon considered it a rather efficient maneuver, but its action is far from consistent; a certain number of sessions are generally necessary. We have abandoned this technique because the one we propose appears to be faster and more frequently efficacious, at least in our hands.

Osteopathic Technique

The manipulation (Fig. 46.1) involves mobilization of the coccyx by grasping it between the thumb (external) and the index finger (intrarectal) and applying flexion, extension, and

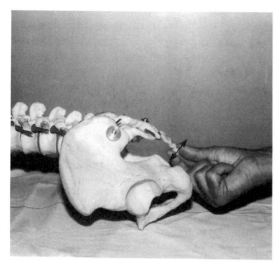

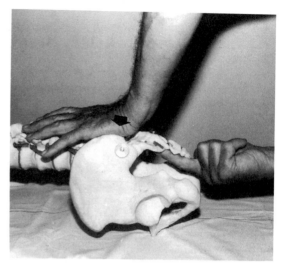

Figure 46.1.   Osteopathic technique. The operator introduces the index finger into the rectum and pinches the coccyx between the index finger and the thumb. The coccyx can then be mobilized in extension or in lateral flexion and rotation. This is the technique proposed by J. B. Mennell.

Figure 46.2.   Author's technique (see the description in the text).

rotation. Performed this way, we find the manipulation to be very unreliable.

The Author's Technique

The patient is in a prone position (Fig. 46.2). The physician introduces the right index finger in the rectum (with palmar side of the finger applied against the inferior aspect of the anterior sacral surface). The examiner maintains the coccyx in hyperextension, rather than pulling strongly on it.

Then the physician places the heel of the left hand on the superior aspect of the posterior sacral surface and applies firm and progressively increasing pressure. Pressure is maintained for 20–30 seconds while the right index finger maintains the coccyx in hyperextension.

Without ever pulling back, the operator, at a given moment, has the impression of a sudden release, which is probably from the levators. The maneuver is over. Pressure on the tip of the coccyx is usually asymptomatic, allowing the patient to sit without inconvenience. Sometimes, repeating the maneuver 2 or 3 times over several days is necessary for a lasting result.

This maneuver seems to stretch the levator, which relieves the spasm and the essential element of the coccygodynia. Indeed, the ''cord'' of the levatores disappears as soon as the maneuver is successful. For some, this maneuver acts on the sacroiliac, whose blocking in ''posterior sacrum,'' according to the osteopathic terminology (Renoult), could play a role in this disorder. An L5–S1 segmental dysfunction seems to be responsible for referred pain to the coccyx. Lumbosacral manipulation and epidural injection can then be useful.

47

PERFORATING BRANCH SYNDROME OF T12 AND L1

Irritability of the lateral perforating cutaneous branches of T12 and L1 is part of the "syndrome of the thoracolumbar junction" of Maigne (see Chapter 60). There is a spinal cause (T12–L1 or L1–L2) that requires spinal treatment. But these branches are also susceptible to entrapment as they traverse the iliac crest (R. and J. Y. Maigne). These two etiologies can be associated.

ANATOMY

Classic Studies

According to the classical notions, the iliohypogastric nerve (or abdominogenital nerve) (L1) gives off a branch near the midaxillary line. It courses downward, prior to crossing the obliquus muscles above the iliac crest, which it crosses. It then supplies the cutaneous surface of the buttock (according to Testut); it innervates the superiolateral part of the buttock and the thigh (according to G. Lazorthes it is the lateral cutaneous perforating branch) (Fig. 47.1).

Similarly, another perforating branch, the gluteal ramus, comes off laterally from the 12th intercostal nerve (T12). It traverses the iliac crest in front of the preceding branch and innervates the cutaneous surface of the lateral and superior buttock (Testut) (Fig. 47.1). In the anatomic drawings that show them, these nerves stop above the trochanter.

Maigne Study

Our anatomic study, done with J. Y. Maigne, had 20 subjects studied bilaterally (i.e., 40 dissections). It demonstrated that

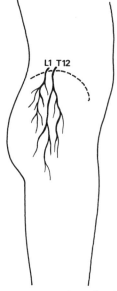

Figure 47.1. The lateral perforating cutaneous branches originate from the subcostal nerve (T12) and the iliohypogastric nerve (or abdominal-genital) (L1). These branches may vary in size.

- The perforating branch of the subcostal nerve (T12) becomes superficial 1–2 cm above the iliac crest in perforating the internal and external lateral oblique muscles of the abdomen, and it crosses the iliac crest 5–8 cm behind the anterior superior iliac spine (Fig. 47.5).
- The perforating branch of the iliohypogastric nerve (L1) becomes superficial slightly lower, 1–2 cm behind the preceding one. It often leaves the impression of a small bony gutter on the iliac crest, through which it passes. This gutter (which has not been described, as far as we know, but which is palpable in the living) is transformed into a fibro-osseous tunnel by the oblique muscles

of the abdomen and their aponeurosis (Fig. 47.6). This passage is relatively narrow and can sometimes compress the nerve along its course, as we saw in one dissection that demonstrated pre- and poststenotic swelling, which opens the possibility of an entrapment syndrome. (We made the same observations during some surgical decompressions to free the nerve.) The crossing point with the iliac crest is not a right angle; the two branches lie on it for 1–2 cm and then resume their vertical path.

After traversing the iliac crest, these nerves supply the skin overlying the lateral aspect of the hip. The iliohypogastric nerve (L1), which is usually the longer of the two, then passes 2–3 cm anterior to the greater trochanter. Three variations were noted: short (Fig. 47.2, left), medium (Fig. 47.2, middle), and long (Fig. 47.2, right). In the short variety (8 cases), it does not reach the trochanter. In the medium one, which is the most frequent (22 cases), it branches out at that level. In the long variety (6 cases), it can be dissected up to 7–9 cm distal to the greater trochanter and branches out below. In four cases, this nerve did not exist. Its homologue arises from the subcostal nerve, which occasionally anastomoses with it, and can present the same variations: short, 28 cases; medium, 8 cases; and long, 4 cases.

In summary, the results of our study show that

- The lateral perforating cutaneous branches, in many cases, terminate much more distally on the thigh than the classical descriptions mention.
- An entrapment syndrome is possible at the crossing point of the iliac crest.

CLINICAL EXAMINATION

Pressure over the iliac crest, on a line passing through the trochanter, reveals a very tender point, the "lateral crestal point." One is often able to palpate a small notch on the iliac crest, which corresponds to the bony "notch" noted in the cadaver (Fig. 47.3, left and right).

The skin overlying the trochanter, which corresponds to the territory of the lateral perforating branch, is painful to pinch-rolling and is often thickened. It can cover a narrow band which, especially for L1, can go down to midthigh and sometimes lower, following the path of the seam of the trousers (Figs. 47.2, right, and 47.4).

When the syndrome manifests with neuralgic pain or paresthesia, lateral stretching in forced adduction of the lower limb (with pa-

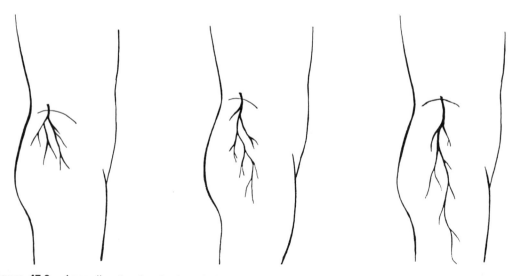

Figure 47.2. According to classic description the perforating cutaneous branches only go as far as the trochanter. In fact, we have been able to demonstrate three varieties (J. Y. Maigne): The short variety, which corresponds to the classic description (see Fig. 47.1); the median variety, which overlies the trochanter; and the long variety, which descends to midthigh.

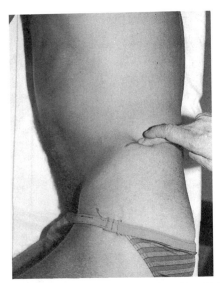

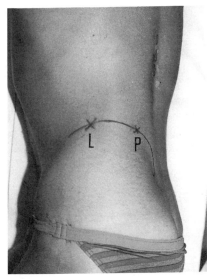

Figure 47.3. Left, Examination for the "lateral crestal point." The patient is lying on the right side and is seen from above. The finger is often able to feel a small notch over the iliac crest, in which one can find nerve branches. **Right,** The same position as noted in the prior patient. L, "lateral crestal point"; P, "posterior crestal point," the point where compression of the posterior ramus of T12 or L1 can occur.

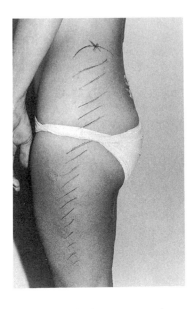

Figure 47.4. The topography of the cellulalgic zone is variably limited through the trochanteric and intratrochanteric region. It presents as a narrow straight vertical band following the lateral crease of the pants. In fact, it corresponds to the territory of the perforating branches (Fig. 47.2).

tient in supine) can sometimes reproduce the pain, analogous to a "lateral Lasegue's" sign. All examination signs and spontaneous discomfort disappear transiently with anesthetic injection at the level of the lateral crestal point.

CLINICAL PRESENTATION

We have seen three clinical presentations involving the dysfunction of these branches.

1. The first is associated with periarthritis of the hip and is by far the most frequent (90 of 103 cases).
2. The second is meralgia paresthetica (7 of 103).
3. The third is a truncated sciatica (6 of 103).

Pseudoperiarthritis of the Hip

Most often, pain simulates periarthritis of the hip, such as tendinitis of the gluteus me-

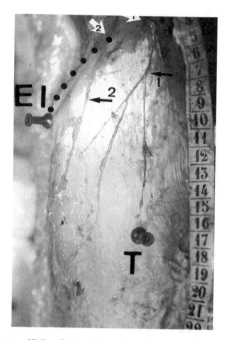

Figure 47.5. Perforating branches of the lateral thigh. This is a medium-length variety: the branches descend slightly below the trochanter (T). EI, Anterior superior iliac spine; the dark spot follows the iliac crest. Arrows show the crossing points of the branches in relation to the iliac crest: 1, perforating branch of the iliohypogastric nerve (L1); 2, perforating branch of the subcostal nerve (T12).

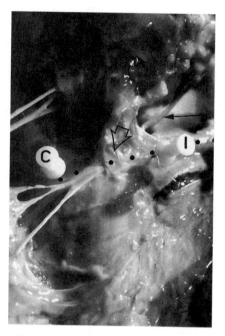

Figure 47.6. The perforating branch of the iliohypogastric nerve (L1) crosses over the iliac crest in a small bony notch, which is palpable and which passes through a fibro-osseous tunnel where it can sometimes be compressed in an entrapment syndrome (R. and J. Y. Maigne).

dius. The patient complains of pain along the lateral aspect of the hip, radiating sometimes toward the groin, and lateral thigh. Pressure on the trochanter is very painful, but local injection does not bring any relief. Indeed, pain is caused by compression of the cellulalgic subcutaneous tissues against the trochanter, which is painful to pinch-rolling. Anesthetic injection of the lateral crestal point relieves or decreases the pain to pinch-rolling as well as the spontaneous pain from pressure on the trochanter. This injection combined with a few milliliters of a corticosteroid derivative and repeated two or three times often results in lasting relief. The following case history is typical. It involves a patient believed to have an entrapment syndrome of this perforating branch, the first patient for whom we prescribed surgery to release the nerve; yet there was also a PMID at L1–L2 that was partially responsible.

Case History. Mrs. P. M., a 30-year-old athletic woman, suffered for years from pain over the right trochanter, radiating toward the anterolateral thigh. It re-

stricted her greatly. Pain started after a motocross race. The diagnosis of tendinobursitis of the gluteus medius was made. Several injections were performed without any success. Radiographs demonstrated two lacunas at the level of the right femoral neck. She was hospitalized in an orthopedics department, and a biopsy of the neck was performed. "Nonspecific bony lesions" were found but were not felt to be responsible for her pain. Other treatments yielded no results. She was followed for 2 years in a pain center. She wore a stimulator for a year with mediocre results.

When we saw her, she could not remain in a sitting position for more than a few minutes, especially if the seat was hard. Standing was also painful, extension of the trunk (position in lumbar hyperlordosis) was unbearable, as was left lateroflexion. Pinch-rolling was very painful on a narrow vertical zone, going from the supratrochanteric region to the inferior third of the lateral side of the thigh. A lateral crestal point was particularly clear in the trochanteric line. The spinal segmental examination revealed sensitivity of L1–L2, with right facet joint tenderness. Radiographic studies showed an old fracture of the superior endplate of L2 (result of a fall from a stool 10 years before) and lesions from sequelae of spinal apophysitis at T12–L1 and L1–L2. Thus, it was a traumatic PMID on a segment that had become fragile. The first session was a spinal manipulation and injection of the crestal point, which brought distinct relief for the first time since the start of her pain.

After a few more treatments on the spine and the local cellulalgia, she could resume a nearly normal life. However, prolonged sitting was still very difficult for her, and spinal treatments during a systematic examination no longer improved the situation. Because of our anatomic discoveries (i.e., the possibility of entrapment compression), we proposed surgical intervention. The surgeon, Dr. Touzard, discovered that the perforating branch was being compressed at the level of the iliac crest with a prestenotic dilation. Decompression completely relieved the patient; 5 years later, the result is maintained.

Pseudo–Meralgia Paresthetica

The patient has dysesthesia of the lateral thigh suggesting paresthetic meralgia paresthetica, but the topography is higher and more lateral than in meralgia paresthetica, which the painful zone on pinch-rolling reveals very well.

Pseudosciatica

Pain radiates toward the gluteal region, down the lateral thigh to the knee. It occurs in attacks that persist, like episodes of truncated sciatica. In one of our patients, the symptomatology was particularly painful; the origin was mixed, spinal and local simultaneously.

Case History. Mrs. S., a 50-year-old active woman, had had very painful episodes for the last 6 years, which required prolonged periods of bed rest, which did not completely relieve her pain. The pain was located over the lateral left buttock and radiated toward the lateral side of the knee.

She traveled a great deal and was hospitalized several times in different countries. The diagnosis of L5 sciatica was made, though Lasegue's sign was absent, but epidural and even intradural injections had no effect. The attacks lasted about 2 weeks and were recurring more frequently (six in the last year). Several CT scans were done at different times. All were normal for the inferior lumbar levels that were explored. An American orthopedist took out a large, calcified, gluteal hematoma, but this did not relieve the patient.

We saw her during an acute phase which, like the preceding ones, occurred suddenly during a very small movement. She suffered a great deal and held herself very stiffly. Any trunk movement exacerbated the pain radiating along the lateral side of the thigh.

The Lasegue sign was negative, and there were no cellulotenoperiosteomyalgic manifestations. A narrow cellulalgic band that was very painful to pinch-rolling went from the trochanter to the thigh. A lateral crestal point was particularly sharp. Its anesthetic injection brought appreciable relief, which made the examination easier and revealed the sharp pain of segment T12–L1. Radiographic studies performed immediately showed no lesions at that level. In the hours following the injection, pain reappeared, slightly diminished. The next day, a manipulation performed at T12–L1 resulted in rapid improvement, allowing her to move. A few other treatments, including manipulation, facet joint injection, and injection of the lateral crestal point, brought a total relief for 1 year. A recurrence was provoked by a forced rotation of the trunk. The same signs, though decreased, were again found; 1 year later, she had had no further attacks.

In this form, very sharp pain is rare; it is usually subacute.

N.B. During a systematic examination, it is common to find a cellulalgic band along the lateral thigh in patients who do not suffer spontaneously. Like all latent cellulotenoperiosteomyalgic manifestations, this can last a long time before pain occurs, for whatever reason, isolated or associated with lumbar or abdominal pain (see Chapter 60).

TREATMENT

Treatment can be spinal, local, or both, depending on the patient. With a spinal origin and thoracolumbar junction syndrome, treatment can consist of manipulation, articular injection, and electrotherapy. For an entrapment syndrome, an injection of the lateral crestal point with a mixture of a local anesthetic, 0.5% lidocaine, and a corticosteroid derivative can be tried. When relief is insufficient or only temporary, surgical decompression may be indicated (5 patients in our series of 103 cited above were operated upon). In mixed cases, local and spinal treatments can be used together.

In chronic cases, the cellulalgia should also be treated (tracing injections and massages with progressive kneading).

48

HEADACHE OF CERVICAL ORIGIN

In the presence of chronic headache, a cervical origin is generally considered only if the pain has a posterior topography and if the superior cervical spine demonstrates some signs of radiologic abnormalities (especially facet joint spondylosis). For most authors, the cervical spine does not play a major role in common headaches (1% for Nick). Muscular, cervical, static, or postural origins are sometimes alluded to. But in general, common headaches are attributed to a psychologic origin (80% for Wolf and Wolff) that manifests with protective guarding of the neck and shoulder girdle muscles, commonly referred to as the "tension headache."

The superior cervical spine seems to us to play a frequent role in common headaches. We have observed a faciocraniocervical semiology that makes it easy to recognize them and to find useful treatments. If psychologic factors are frequent in common headaches, they are perhaps sequelae, while the real cause of the headache is often cervical.

But, headache is a very nonspecific symptom with multiple causes. Statistics show that 2–3 of 1000 headaches are caused by a serious disorder (Nick). Therefore, before a headache is classified as "common," a detailed and thorough history and physical examination of the patient are necessary. If there is still any doubt, ancillary studies should be performed and advice from specialists sought.

COMMON CHARACTERISTICS OF CERVICAL HEADACHES

Cervical headaches have their own semiology (Maigne 1968, 1976, 1981). They are most often unilateral. In all cases, there is tenderness to palpation of the C2-3 articular pillars ipsilateral to the headache (Fig. 48.1, *left* and *right*). During the different acute episodes, their topography is fixed, always right or always left for a given patient. With time, it can become bilateral, as can the physical signs elicited.

For a given patient, the cause triggering the attack can always be the same or vary from one attack to the other: postural, psychologic, digestive, menstrual periods, etc. It is sometimes impossible to determine the exact nature of the trigger. The attacks may vary in frequency and intensity and may last a few hours to a few days.

It is important to note that the cervical and craniofacial signs of examination described below are constant and permanent and can be found even between acute attacks. Suitable cervical treatment is regularly useful. Attacks and clinical signs of the examination disappear, even if the usual triggering factors persist.

Cervical Semiology

For us, the only spinal sign showing the cervical origin of a headache is tenderness to palpation of the C2-3 facet joint on the affected side. In 20% of cases, that pain is bilateral. A possible decrease in active or passive mobility has no particular value; it certainly demonstrates the existence of a cervical problem, but it does not establish the cervical origin of the headache. It is unusual to provoke the headache by various cervical maneuvers. However, pressure maintained on the facet joint point can reproduce the usual referral pattern (Fig. 48.1, *left* and *right*).

In most cases, radiographic studies of the superior cervical spine are normal. The exis-

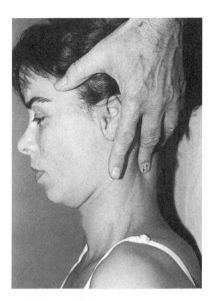
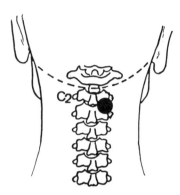

Figure 48.1.   Left, Cervical segmental examination. Examination for facet joint tenderness. **Right,** In all cervical headaches, the segmental examination demonstrates facet joint C2-C3 tenderness on the side where the headache usually presents. The C2-C3 facet joint is the highest that one can palpate. Stress on this facet joint translates to a dysfunction of C2-C3 and eventually to segments that are supra-adjacent, including C0-C1 and C1-C2.

tence of arthritic lesions does not automatically imply that they are responsible for the headaches. In a patient having repeated attacks, facet joint (C2-C3) palpation is tender ipsilateral to the headache and is found even between acute attacks. In general, it is the result of a PMID. Occasionally, it can be due to synovitis.

DIFFERENT ASPECTS OF HEADACHE OF CERVICAL ORIGIN

Three forms of cervical headaches can be distinguished, each with its own semiology.

1. Occipital (Fig. 48.2*a*)
2. Occipitotemporomaxillary (Fig. 48.2*b*)
3. Supraorbital, the most frequent, which corresponds to a projection of the cervical pain in the territory of the ophthalmic division of the trigeminal nerve (Fig. 48.2*c*)

Occipital Headache

Occipital headache is felt at the occiput and can radiate to the vertex. It corresponds to the territories of the posterior rami of C2 and C3 (Fig. 48.3). Isolated, it represents 20% of headaches of cervical origin, but it is often associated with other forms. The acute form is Arnold's neuralgia; it is rare, and its paroxysms are generally provoked by forceful or strenuous movements of the neck. The chronic form is frequent. It is responsible for episodic occipital headaches of variable duration and intensity. In both cases, the "friction sign of the scalp" (Maigne) can be found.

Friction Sign of the Scalp (Maigne)

Friction applied to the scalp replaces the pinch-roll test. It consists of pressing firmly with the pad of the fingers against the scalp and mobilizing it with small to-and-fro motions (Fig. 48.4). This maneuver is painless on a normal scalp, but it is very disagreeable and even painful in the case of an occipital headache of cervical origin. Ipsilateral to the C2-3 facet joint, tenderness is found.

The territory that is painful to friction can correspond to the posterior ramus of C3, which innervates the paramedian zone, or to the posterior ramus of C2, which innervates the lateral part of the occiput (Fig. 48.3). It can

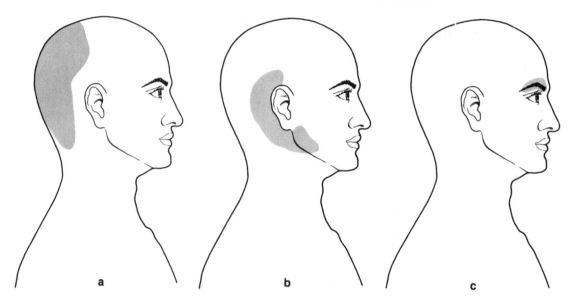

Figure 48.2.   Three types of cervical origin headache (Maigne). **a,** Occipital form. **b,** Occipital temporal maxillary form. **c,** Supraorbital form (the most frequent). These forms can exist as mixed types.

be more diffuse, but it does not go beyond the biauricular line. The periauricular region also receives innervation from C2 or C3, but it comes from their anterior rami.

Occipitotemporomaxillary Headache

The occipitotemporomaxillary headache is located in the retroauricular, mastoid, and parietal region and radiates toward the inferior maxilla. Pain is found ipsilateral to the facet joint tenderness at C2-3, with a positive friction sign over the painful scalp in the retroauricular territory that is innervated by branches arising from the superficial cervical plexus (an-

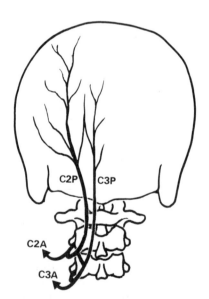

Figure 48.3.   Posterior primary rami of C2 and C3 (*C2P* and *C3P*) and anterior primary rami of C2 and C3 (*C2A* and *C3A*) (according to G. Lazorthes).

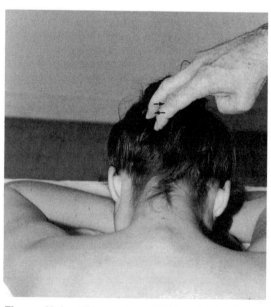

Figure 48.4.   "Friction sign" (Maigne). The fingers rub the scalp against the skull. This maneuver is painful in territories that are irritated. This test replaces the pinch-roll test in this area.

terior ramus of C2, sometimes of C3) (Fig. 48.5).

Pain with pinch-rolling at the angle of the jaw is seen (Fig. 48.6). A fold of the skin is pinched firmly between the thumb and index finger and rolled between these two fingers. The maneuver should be controlled and be compared with the opposite side. It requires

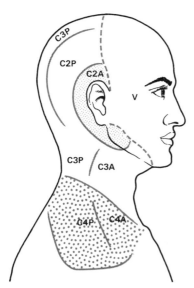

Figure 48.5.   Topographies of innervation. *C2P*, Posterior ramus of C2; *C2A*, anterior ramus of C2; *C3A* and *C3P*, anterior (*A*) and (*P*) posterior rami of C3.

practice, as do all the maneuvers that we propose here. The sign is positive if the maneuver is painful (the fold can be thickened). It is painless on the contralateral side if the impairment is unilateral.

The discomfort elicited at the angle of the jaw is referred to as ''the angle of the jaw sign'' (Maigne). This skin region at the angle of the jaw is innervated by the anterior ramus of C2 and not by the trigeminal nerve. Isolated, this form makes up about 5% of headaches of cervical origin, but it is often associated with another form of headache, presenting with mild features.

Supraorbital Headache

Supraorbital headache is the most frequent headache of cervical origin (67% of cases in our statistics). The topography of the pain is usually supraorbital, sometimes occipitosupraorbital, and in a few cases, retro-orbital. It always carries with it the ''eyebrow sign.''

''Eyebrow Sign'' (Maigne)

The eyebrow is pinched between thumb and index finger and kneaded and rolled like a cigarette. It is explored from one end to the other, going over the skin of the forehead (Fig. 48.7). When the sign is positive, the fold is painful and often thickened throughout all or part of

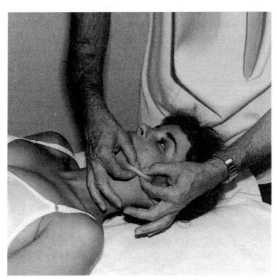

Figure 48.6.   Pinch-roll sign of skin overlying the angle of the jaw (Maigne).

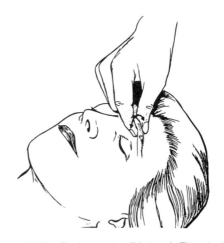

Figure 48.7.   Eyebrow sign (Maigne). The pinch-roll eyebrow sign is painful, and the skin is thickened on the side of the cervical-origin headache. This is essentially the sign of supraorbital headache of cervical origin. This sign disappears with anesthetic injection of the C2-C3 facet.

the length of the brow. This sign is found only on the side of the usual headache, which is generally the side of the C2-3 articular pain. The maneuver is painless on the other eyebrow, except in cases of bilateral headache.

The link between this sign and an origin in the cervical spine is shown by the response to injection of local anesthetic at the C2-3 facet joint. A few moments after the injection, the eyebrow is no longer painful to pinch-rolling (Fig. 48.8). The fold becomes supple and thin. The same result can be obtained with any manual therapy maneuver that renders the C2-C3 articulation painless (Fig. 48.9). Conversely, a poorly performed manipulation that increases C2-C3 tenderness also increases the sensitivity of the eyebrow and usually results in headache.

We did not find this sign in the true migraines, even when they had a dominant radiation toward the eye, nor in the other forms of headaches (sinusitis, psychologic headaches, etc.). On the other hand, the supraorbital cervical headache can have a migrainous character (see Chapter 49, "Cervical Migraines").

Cheek Sign (Maigne)

Some patients with the eyebrow sign also have some tenderness to pinch-rolling the skin of the cheek, located below the maxilla (cheek sign). This maneuver is particularly painful in some facial pain syndromes that are relieved by cervical treatment.

Different Aspects of the Supraorbital Headache of Cervical Origin. This headache repre-

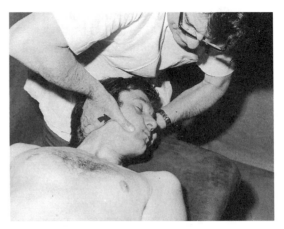

Figure 48.9. Example of the manipulation of the superior cervical spine in the treatment of cervical-origin headache.

sents 67% of headaches of cervical origin. It can have three clinical presentations: simple form (85% of cases), vascular form (10% of cases), and the migrainous form (5% of cases). These are personal statistics from 162 cases of cervical headache. They probably vary depending on the recruitment. For all these forms, frequency, intensity, and duration of the episodes of headache are extremely variable from case to case, spanning a spectrum from mild low-frequency headache to the intense, daily, incapacitating headache.

Simple Form. The most common form, it has a supraorbital or occipitosupraorbital pain. It is always located on the same side for a given subject. It can migrate to the other side if the episode is severe, but its examination signs remain unilateral. It can be truly bilateral in some cases. Some patients describe it as the pain of a frontal sinusitis. It is sometimes felt as a retro-orbital pain; the patient has the impression that his eye is "pulled backwards."

Vascular Form. In this less frequent form with supraorbital pain, there is also nasal congestion (the nostril is clogged with or without rhinorrhea) and occasionally a unilateral tearing. These manifestations are always ipsilateral to the C2-3 facet joint tenderness, and the eyebrow sign is always positive on the same side during successive attacks. The efficacy of medications for the headache is generally poor, whether antiserotonin or an ergotamine derivative. The cervical treatment is the only one that is useful. The following case is typical.

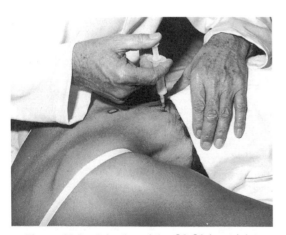

Figure 48.8. Injection of the C2-C3 facet joint.

Case History. A 42-year-old woman suffered from headaches for the last 13 years. They had become progressively worse during this time, with increasing frequency and duration, without any precipitating cause. When she consulted a physician, the attacks occurred three to four times a month, lasting 2–3 days. Topography was supra- and retro-orbital, always on the left, with swelling of the left nostril, then rhinorrhea and watering of the left eye. She was followed in two departments of neurology, and their diagnosis was vascular headache. She was not relieved by ergotamine tartrate, dihydroergotamine, or antimigrainous medication but was well relieved with amidopyrine (6 tablets/day of Optalidon). On examination, the left eyebrow was thickened and very painful to pinch-rolling, and there was a sharp pain at the left C2-3 facet joint. Cervical radiographs were normal. Four manipulative treatments and two injections relieved her.

She did not have any more attacks for the next 12 months. This form of headache represents 8.5% of cases of cervical headaches in our statistics (14 cases of 162).

Migrainous Form. In some cases, the migrainous form has the characteristics of true migraine. It is a nonalternating migraine, localized always on the same side in a given patient during the successive attacks. It often responds poorly to antimigrainous medications, but cervical treatment is very useful (see Chapter 49, "Cervical Migraines").

TRIGGERING FACTORS

Whatever its variety, headache of cervical origin can be episodic, with variable intervals between attacks. It can be mild or severe, but as stated above, the examination signs that we describe persist beyond the attacks.

The triggering factor can be cervical. It is often postural, such as improper neck positioning on the pillow (sleeping prone) or improper work place ergonomics that place patients in a strained position. These headaches can also be provoked by cold drafts on the neck. They can also be triggered by gynecologic, dietary, or psychologic factors. Often the headache is fallaciously attributed to these factors without considering a cervical etiology, despite the fact that cervical treatment is the only one that is efficacious and long lasting.

These headaches can also be triggered by minor factors in persons whose tolerance threshold is very low. The slightest articular dysfunction is then felt even while the physical

or psychologic state is good. This is considered to be the mechanism in slightly depressed or anxious individuals and "spasmophiles" (M. Duc, M. Janel), etc. In these people, the psychologic factor is often, wrongly, the only one tended to.

FREQUENCY OF CERVICAL HEADACHES

Cervical headaches are frequent. The frequency found in various studies depends on the recruiting; in our statistics, they represent 80% of unscreened headaches (162 cases on a known sampling of 200 cases). J. L. Garcia (1977) used our semiology and diversified its recruiting; he obtained identical figures on 110 cases. His studies demonstrated the efficiency of the cervical treatment that we propose. He studied three groups of patients with common headaches.

1. The first group was recruited from patients referred for neurologic consultation.
2. The second group was recruited from patients referred for rheumatologic consultation.
3. The third group was recruited among patients in general medicine selected in a population group that was easy to follow (military and their families). A total of 110 patients was recruited, and of these, 87 met the criteria for cervical headache as we have defined them; 78 were followed up and seen regularly. Treatment by manipulation and sometimes by articular injection brought 90% good results with 1 year of follow-up.

Frequency of the Different Forms

All the forms described above can be seen in isolated or mixed forms. However, a painful topography is most often dominant. In the 162 cases of our study, the dominant pain was

- Frontosupraorbital or supraorbital in 110 cases
- Occipital in 35 cases
- Occipitomaxillary in 7 cases
- Diffuse in 10 cases

There was always a correlation with the examination signs. But the signs can be present without the pain of the attack occupying all the painful territories at examination. For example, the eyebrow sign can be positive in a cervical headache that is painful only in the occipital region, but in this case, the friction sign is always positive.

Remark

Persons showing C2-3 facet joint tenderness on examination do not all have headache. But those who present some other signs of the craniofacial semiology that we propose are rarely without any episodes of headache, at least mild and of low frequency.

PATHOPHYSIOLOGIC MECHANISM

There are two questions about the mechanism of these headaches: the first is about the cause of the C2-3 facet joint tenderness, the second about the supraorbital projection of pain and the eyebrow sign.

C2-3 Facet Joint Tenderness

Facet joint tenderness is a constant sign of PMIDs at all levels of the spine. C2-3 facet joint tenderness is found on palpation in all cases of cervical headache. Does it express only the dysfunction of the segment C2-C3? Probably not. C2-C3 is the highest cervical facet joint that is palpable. It is at the junction of the two functional units of the cervical spine:

- Inferior part, with the last five vertebrae, whose biomechanical characteristics are the same and which function in a synchronous manner
- Superior part, with atlas and axis, whose great mobility allows precise adjustment of the finest and most varied movements of the head

The possible isolated dysfunctions of the occiput-atlas-axis cannot be clearly shown. Some signs of palpation or radiologic examination have been proposed; they seem to us to be only presumptive signs.

But, any isolated dysfunction eventually affecting C0-C1 or C1-C2 also perturbs all of the superior cervical spine, which functions as a unit. This perturbation is reflected at the junction of the latter with the inferior cervical spine, which has different biomechanical characteristics than C2-C3. And so, tenderness to palpation at C2-C3 seems to us to reflect all mechanical perturbations of the superior cervical spine.

Disappearance of this tenderness after treatment means the return to normal of the musculoskeletal functions of the whole. The small suboccipital muscles, which are stretched on palpation, are probably essential to maintain these dysfunctions. They also play a role in the production of pain, through the formation of taut bands that persist sometimes in spite of the spinal treatment; a local treatment then becomes necessary.

Craniofacial Signs

Some signs that we describe correspond anatomically to the territory of the anterior and posterior rami of C2 and C3 (Fig. 48.5). This is the case with the friction sign, which reveals the hypersensitivity of the scalp in the C2-C3 region. It is also the case with the angle of the jaw sign, which corresponds to the cutaneous region of the anterior ramus of C2 (masseter notch).

On the other hand, the supraorbital projection and especially the eyebrow sign are more unexpected. The zone of the eyebrow is innervated by a branch of the trigeminal nerve (ophthalmic division) and seems to have no anatomic connection with the cervical spine. However, their clinical link is easy to demonstrate.

In a previous study (1981), we had 50 patients with unilateral supraorbital headaches for more than 2 years and C2-3 facet joint tenderness and the eyebrow sign on the same side. In 47, we were able to eliminate the tenderness to pinch-rolling of the eyebrow by injection of 0.5% lidocaine in the tender C2-3 facet joint. Not only did the fold become painless, but it was supple after a few minutes, although it was thickened prior to injection.

Hypotheses about the Mechanism

The observations outlined can be explained by some connections between the nucleus of the trigeminal nerve and the cervical spinal cord. The gelatinous nucleus of the trigeminal nerve descends very low and becomes continuous with the posterior column of the spinal cord. Anastomoses of branches from C1, C2, and even C3 probably unite with the ophthalmic division of the trigeminal nerve, as Kerr has demonstrated. It is generally accepted that the fibers carrying nociceptive information have a more inferior location in the inferior part of the gelatinous nucleus, descending as far distally as the second or third cervical segment of the spinal cord. The ophthalmic fibers project to the inferior and anterior part of the trigeminal nucleus (Lazorthes). These common anastomoses explain the painful supraorbital projection that we have noted.

Another mechanism might also be at work here. Sympathetic fibers are carried by branches of the trigeminal nerve and go to the cutaneous regions along with the sensory nerves. These fibers come from the periarterial sympathetic nerves of the internal carotid. After a relay in the superior cervical ganglion, they arrive at the ganglion of Gasser through the internal pericarotid plexus. But this classic cervicogasserian anastomosis was never really shown by anatomists.

On the other hand, numerous peripheral anastomoses unite the trigeminal branches and the vascular plexus of the collateral of the external carotid (Lazorthes). In its intracranial segment, the internal carotid receives, from the superior pole of the superior cervical ganglion, two nerves that anastomose in the plexus and are distributed to the collaterals and the terminals of this artery and, therefore, to the supraorbital artery, which goes out by the supraorbital foramen. The superior (C1, C2, C3) cervical ganglion is bound to the spinal nerves by communicating branches.

Whatever the actual cause of the eyebrow sign, it is a common sign of the dysfunction of the first three cervical segments, as appears to be the case with the C2-3 facet joint tenderness.

TREATMENT OF HEADACHE OF CERVICAL ORIGIN

Treatment confirms the cervical origin of the headache because the examination signs disappear and the patient is relieved.

Manipulation

The basic treatment is manipulation if it is not contraindicated because of the vascular or spinal state (postural tests) and when it is technically possible, respecting the rules of application. It should be very precise and perfectly executed. If it is performed correctly, it relieves or cures; performed incorrectly, it aggravates and can create a local perturbation that could make any other treatment difficult. Application of the rule of no pain and opposite movement is sometimes difficult at the superior cervical spine. To determine the directions of the maneuver to be performed, it is often better to perform repeated stretching in the different orientations. Performed in favorable directions, they definitely decrease the facet joint tenderness on palpation and relax the suboccipital muscles (Fig. 48.9).

Depending on the patient, two to five sessions are necessary. Soon after the first maneuvers, the result on the friction sign or the eyebrow sign allows the diagnosis to be made. A reaction occurring during the night following the first session is not rare, and the patient should expect it.

Facet Joint Injection (C2-C3)

If manipulation is contraindicated or insufficient, facet joint injection is useful. For the injection, the patient is seated on a stool, with the forehead resting on a table. The point of injection is at the painful facet joint point, C2-C3, about 1 cm lateral to the spinous process of C2, which is easily found (Fig. 48.8).

A corticosteroid derivative, 0.25 mL is injected strictly on contact with the bone, after checking by aspiration that there is neither blood nor spinal fluid. To avoid any accident, it is better to use a corticosteroid derivative that is safe for intrathecal use without producing any disturbance, and no local anesthetics should be used.

Other Treatments

Massage can be a very useful adjunct (even if the patient has been relieved of the headache), when applied to the subcutaneous tissues of the neck if they are cellulalgic or to suboccipital trigger points.

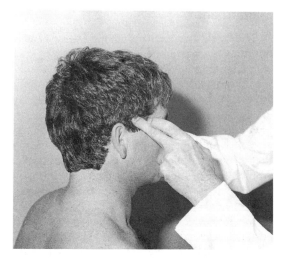
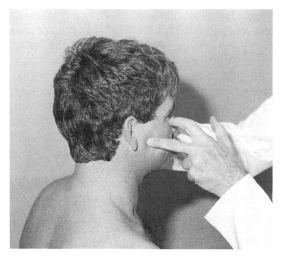

Figure 48.10. Trigger points either involving the temporalis (**left**) or the masseter (**right**) can be responsible for persistent cervical headaches. They are often due to problems with the temporomaxillary joint (due to poor dental articulation).

The patient should learn to avoid extreme rotation of the neck (prolonged backing up in a car, for example). Patients with morning headaches should remove or modify the pillow, depending on the case. Sleeping in prone places the neck in extreme rotation, which can be harmful and cause morning headaches. Patients should not sleep in that position.

CERVICAL MUSCLES AND HEADACHES

Some headaches seem to be provoked by trigger points, which can have several origins.

- They can be postural.
- They may result from articular dysfunctions. The masseter or temporal muscle (Fig. 48.10, *left* and *right*) is disturbed in the syndrome of temporomandibular joint dysfunction. The trigger points provoke pains that radiate to the supraorbital and temporal regions, and to the teeth (dental pseudopain) (J. Travell, D. Simons).
- Some of these "trigger points" can be localized to a taut band that is part of a cellulotenoperiosteomyalgic syndrome of cervical origin (Maigne). They affect especially the suboccipital muscles, the trapezius and the sternocleidomastoid (Fig. 48.11). Some can

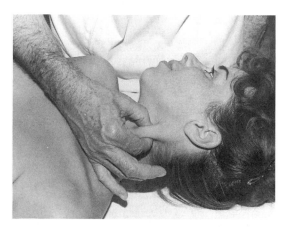

Figure 48.11. Sometimes the sternocleidomastoid muscle has a taut band that plays a role in cervical-origin headache. It is often attenuated by cervical treatment. However, local treatment may be necessary.

cause headaches. When they are linked to a cervical PMID, they disappear or become inactive after treatment of the PMID; but they can persist if they also have a postural origin, and a local treatment is necessary.

The trapezius and the sternocleidomastoid are innervated by the cranial accessory nerve, which receives a contribution from C2 and C3 as the spinal accessory nerve. The latter participates to a variable degree with the motor fibers of this nerve and assures the propriocep-tive innervation of the muscle (Winckler). That explains the possibility of having taut bands with a segmental C2 or C3 syndrome. For the sternocleidomastoid, the trigger point usually is located at the junction of the superior one-third and the inferior two-thirds, but it can be higher or lower. The pain is projected toward the mastoid or the orbital region. It can be pro-voked by compression of the trigger point be-tween thumb and index finger and maintained for about 15 seconds (Fig. 48.11).

With the trapezius, the upper fibers are gen-erally affected along its superior border. Pain referral is in the temporal region. The trigger points of the suboccipital muscles (rectus and obliquus posterior) have occipitotemporal pro-jections (J. Travell, D. Simons).

The treatment consists of two to three trig-ger point injections of 0.5% lidocaine.

49

CERVICAL MIGRAINE

TRUE MIGRAINE

Far too many headaches are categorized as migraine. True migraine is frequent and affects women more than men. It occurs by paroxysmal attacks that last a few hours and is usually preceded by signs that are well known to the patient. Symptoms include unilateral pain, photophobia, pallor, nausea, and vomiting. Most often, it goes from right to left or vice versa from one attack to the other (80% of cases). The first attack often occurs in the very young, before the age of 10. A familial or genetic pattern is usual.

Although a vascular origin has been proposed, the etiology of migraine has not yet been clearly delineated. It can present in various clinical forms such as ophthalmic migraine, mixed migraine, and migrainous equivalents.

Classic migraine has nothing to do with the cervical spine. However a patient with a definitive diagnosis of migraine can also have headaches of cervical origin. The patient can usually distinguish the two types of "headache." However, there are headaches with migrainous characteristics, with a cervical component or a cervical origin.

The first type of cervical migraine has been described by Bartschi-Rochaix. Below, we describe a second one, based on our semiology of cervical headaches.

CERVICAL MIGRAINE

Bartschi-Rochaix has described a migrainous syndrome of cervical origin. Cervical osteophytes and episodic synovitis of cervical elements, according to the author result in vertebral artery vasospasm. According to Taptas, Ricard, Girard, and Dupasquier, cervical discopathies act essentially on the preganglionic fibers of the white rami communicants, which join the cervical sympathetic chain to the cerebrospinal axis while following the path of the last five cervical roots. Irritation of these elements seems to cause vasomotor problems in the whole carotid system, both extracranial and intracranial.

MIGRAINE AND THE SUPERIOR CERVICAL SPINE

There is another form of cervical migraine whose origin is in the superior cervical spine (Maigne). Supraorbital headaches of cervical origin can, as we have seen above (see "Different Aspects of the Supraorbital Headache of Cervical Origin" in Chapter 48), have a clear vasomotor character, associated with nausea in some patients. In others, the migrainous character is clearly so prominent that most of the patients we examined had consulted in other departments or in specialized centers and been given the diagnosis of "migraine." But their response to the treatment was suboptimal or nonexistent, even with treatments that usually help those suffering from migraine. These cervical migraines that we isolate have many other characteristics.

- They do not alternate; they are located always on the same side, right or left.
- They show the usual signs of cervical headaches that we have described; the eyebrow sign is always present, as is tenderness of the C2-3 articulation on the side of the usual attack.

• Their response to the treatment is good (manipulation and possible posterior articular injection).

The following observation is typical.

Case History. A 41-year-old woman, storekeeper, had unresponsive migrainelike headaches for 10 years. Eight years earlier, she received minor cervical trauma in a motor vehicle accident. She subsequently developed temporary frontal headaches, which were progressively decreasing after 1 year. Ten years ago, without any apparent cause, attacks of frontal headaches occurred, always on the left, with a feeling of a retro-orbital stretching. These headaches were accompanied by nasal obstruction on the same side and, when the pain was severe, with an abundant rhinorrhea and watering of the left eye. She looked for calm darkness and sometimes vomited. Attacks quickly increased in frequency and became daily.

Different sedatives were tried to no avail. After some ophthalmologic and ENT examinations were negative, a first consultant physician prescribed Niamid for a year, without success. An orthodontist then extracted a wisdom tooth on the left, with no effect on the headaches. She was seen by a neurologist, and the diagnosis of true migraine was made. Different medications, such as dihydroergotamine, caffeinated Gynergen, and dimetiotazine, were tried but had no effect. Only amidopyrine in high dosage had a mildly positive effect. Finally, she was hospitalized in a neurology department where (among other examinations) she underwent an arteriogram, which was normal. Dihydroergotamine was tried without effect. Attacks became more severe and handicapped her at work. She was then hospitalized in a second department of neurology. A pneumoencephalogram was performed and was normal. A third neurologist, a well-known headache specialist, ordered an allergy panel. Tests were positive to dust and mildew. After 1 year of desensitization, she noted no effect, and the migraine remained unchanged. She then saw a faith healer who prescribed hand baths with plants and sitz baths, without result. She consulted in another department of neurology, where the diagnosis of migraine was made. She was treated with methysergide, which produced a slight improvement. Every 6 months, an intravenous pyelogram was performed. The third one revealed the beginnings of retroperitoneal fibrosis, and the treatment was stopped. Pyramidon was then tried in high dosage, and to some extent, it relieved her. Upon her return, she consulted in the same department of neurology, and after all these failures, she was told that all of her problems were probably of psychologic origin. She was told that perhaps it was having her mother live with her; however, she thought this was not a major problem. For some reason her mother had to leave, but this did not change the headaches.

Then a physician that she saw in the Southwest sent her to us: "it is about a woman who cannot stop her work (she works in a store alone) and who is very handicapped by quasi-daily attacks." The fixed topography was always on the left. Her negative extensive workup allowed us to concentrate on examining the cervical spine. X-rays had already been performed, and since they were normal, a cervical origin was not considered. With the patient in supine position, palpation of the suboccipital region revealed marked tenderness of the left C2-3 facet joint. Pressure even reproduced the retro-orbital radiation that she felt during the attacks.

The remaining cervical segments—above, below, and on the right—were unremarkable. On palpation, the left suboccipital subcutaneous tissues were thickened, infiltrated, and very sensitive to pinch-rolling. Pinch-roll of the right eyebrow was painless, but the left was thickened, infiltrated, and very painful. A diagnostic injection of the left C2-3 facet joint was performed, and in a few minutes, both the sensitivity to pinch-rolling and the left eyebrow sign decreased. Manipulation was performed, combined with a left C2-3 corticosteroid injection. After the third treatment, attacks were less frequent and severe, and the pinch-roll test was much less sensitive. After the fifth treatment, the "migraines" and the positive clinical findings disappeared. A recurrence occurred 4 months later, after she carried a suitcase. The left pinch-roll tenderness and the left C2-3 sensitivity returned.

One treatment was enough to put everything in order! Two years have passed without an attack.

This is an example of a cervical headache with a typically migrainous aspect. In summary, this women suffered from severe migraines for 10 years. She was hospitalized three times and underwent an angiogram, a pneumoencephalogram, and multiple investigations repeated many times. Treatment with methysergide resulted in the beginning of retroperitoneal fibrosis. No medical treatment improved her, except Pyramidon. She was relieved by a few manipulations and cervical injection.

The following case is similar.

Case History. Mrs. C. L., a 39-year-old bookkeeper, had migraines since the age of 16. In the beginning, they were linked to her menstrual periods. Then they occurred outside the cycle, with increased frequency for the last 5 years, following a motor vehicle accident. Pain was always on the right, never the left.

She was hospitalized twice in a department of neurology. All investigations were negative (including angiography and pneumoencephalography). Specialized examinations (e.g., ENT, orthodontic, ophthalmology, allergy) were all negative. She consulted many specialists, and the diagnosis of true migraine was always made because the clinical picture was typical. Treatment with antimigraine medications provided no results. She had partial relief with Optalidon (30–40 suppositories a month, usually), the only treatment that allowed her to continue her work.

When we saw her, on referral by her physician, we noticed marked tenderness over the right C2-C3 articular pillar, with a clear eyebrow sign. On radiologic evaluations, the cervical spine was normal except for a slight loss of cervical lordosis. After three treatments consisting of two facet corticosteroid injections and a manipulation, there was clear relief, which was definitive after three manipulations done 15 days apart. In 1 year after the treatment, she had only two mild attacks of short duration after a long trip.

CERVICAL SYNDROME

In 1925, Barre and his student Lieou (thesis in 1928) brought attention to the cervical origin of a certain number of headache syndromes, vertigo, tinnitus, etc. They thought the mechanism was irritation of the "sympathetic system by a cervical rheumatism," and therefore they described the "posterior cervical sympathetic syndrome."

The existence of this syndrome is at present very controversial. Most authors attribute its manifestations to circulatory disorders of the vertebrobasilar system due to insufficiency or psychologic problems. But knowledge of the vertebrobasilar insufficiency brought many clarifications to these problems, though it did not explain everything. In a preceding chapter, we noted the frequency of cervical headaches and showed that they have their own clinical signs. They are relieved by cervical treatments. These patients often present also with vertiginous sensations or true vertigoes, visual problems, difficulties in concentration, and memory loss, which usually disappear (like the headaches) after a cervical treatment or, on the contrary, are aggravated or worsened by ill-performed manipulations.

If one thinks that the essential merit of Barre was to affirm the cervical origin of the manifestations of his syndrome, these results confirm his opinion. But those who do not agree with the Barre thesis of a "sympathetic mechanism," disputed by most authors, can say that the syndrome of Barre and Lieou does not exist. To avoid confusion, we use the term *cervical syndrome*, after others (Toussaint), to refer to all the manifestations in which the cervical spine plays a dominant role. We should emphsize the complexity of the problem and remember that multiple causes—some benign, some serious—can create symptoms whose frequency and benign nature constitute the essential trap.

ELEMENTS OF THE CERVICAL SYNDROME

The elements of this syndrome include headache, disequilibrium, visual and auditory dysfunction, laryngopharyngeal problems, vasomotor problems, and psychologic problems.

Headaches

Headache is by far the most common manifestation of this cervical syndrome. It is treated in Chapter 48, "Headaches of Cervical Origin."

Vestibular Symptoms

Some patients complain of poor balance and are afraid to cross the street. Others have the impression of being drunk. Most often, these patients have vertiginous symptoms, usually triggered by rotation of the head to one side or cervical extension. Sometimes, these are true rotary vertigoes. Vestibular symptoms show only minor abnormalities in most cases, with hypoexcitability of the labyrinth. Spontaneous nystagmus is very rare, but electronystagmography can give interesting results (Waghemacker).

Auditory Symptoms

Tinnitus, ringing, whistling in the ear, and hyperacusis constitute the auditory symptoms.

Visual Symptoms

Some patients complain of visual fatigue, floating specks, tingling, or a feeling of dust in the eyes.

Pharyngolaryngeal Symptoms

Symptoms include pharyngeal paresthesia (feeling a foreign body) and for singers, difficulties with high notes.

Vasomotor and Secretory Symptoms

Symptoms include rhinorrhea and watery eyes, generally affecting only one nostril or eye.

Psychologic Symptoms

Patients often complain of intellectual fatigue, difficulty concentrating, and memory loss. They have a tendency toward depression and anxiety. A history of mental illness can perpetuate the problem. Often, symptoms occur in patients without any antecedent history. Because these symptoms frequently manifest after cervical trauma and disappear after cervical treatment, they are considered an integral part of the syndrome, rather than a psychologic reaction to the accident.

All these symptoms are rarely seen together. Occurrence, expression, and intensity vary. They are not always the consequence of a minor cervical trauma. They are also seen in patients over 50 years old who have some neck stiffness due to spondylosis and who present with a PMID of the superior cervical spine provoked by spondylosis or synovitis. Often, the symptoms are transitory, but they are persistent in a few cases, with little tendency to spontaneous regression.

External perpetuating factors include cold drafts, postural factors (e.g., poor posture during sleep or work, driving the car for too long), and especially psychologic factors. The psychologic factors are manifest by a feeling that one's cognitive function (memory, concentration) is declining and not improving after treatment. Patients often have medicolegal issues and become very vulnerable. A personal problem or a professional setback is taken very badly at this point, and the depressive reaction becomes the essential therapeutic problem.

DIAGNOSIS

The diagnosis is sometimes difficult to make, because the symptoms seen in patients with the cervical syndrome can be very similar to those seen in psychiatric patients. In the anxious, depressed patients, one should differentiate a true cervical pain and hypochondriacal neck pain.

Vertebrobasilar insufficiency (VBI) should be evaluated by Doppler studies of the carotid arteries. Rancurel's maneuver is an excellent means of uncovering a hemodynamic VBI that may be present (see "Vertebrobasilar Insufficiency" in Chapter 22).

EXAMINATION OF THE CERVICAL SPINE

Examination of the cervical spine does not differ from that described in Chapter 48, "Headaches of Cervical Origin." The important thing to look for is tenderness of the C2-3 facet joint ipsilateral to the supposed problems. This sensitivity is generally the result of a PMID, although occasionally, posterior element inflammation can be the causative factor. Other common physical signs ipsilateral to the symptoms include the eyebrow sign, friction sign over the scalp, and tenderness to pinch-rolling at the angle of the jaw. The sternocleidomastoid and trapezius muscles should be examined very thoroughly to determine whether there are trigger points that can be treated. They can play a role in the painful manifestations (headaches, pseudovertigo).

MECHANISM

Chapter 48, "Headaches of Cervical Origin," discusses a mechanism for the headaches. Disorders of equilibrium in the absence of any other lesion can be explained by perturbation of articular and muscular receptors, which are very numerous at the superior cervical level. They play an important role in the control of equilibrium and posture. When there are lesions, afferent misinformation can be relayed to the central nervous system. This is well known in cases that involve the superior cervical segments. However, irritation of certain taut cervical muscles can also produce the same sympathetic phenomenon with visual and vestibular dysfunction (J. Travell).

Trigger points can have a postural origin; however, we have frequently found them associated with a PMID of the superior cervical spine and have frequently seen them disappear after treatment of the cervical spine. The sternocleidomastoid is innervated by the cranial accessory nerve as well as by branches of C2 and C3 (Winckler) or the spinal accessory nerve. Thus nociceptive information arriving from the muscles can induce the disturbances that are commonly seen with the cervical spine syndrome.

TREATMENT

Manipulation can be performed with the usual precautions, and it is often effective. At each session, one should evaluate the results of the manipulation and reexamine the spine for pain and associated signs (see Chapter 48, "Headaches of Cervical Origin") such as eyebrow pain, if it is present. If one can make these various signs disappear without the patient feeling better, then one should assume that there is no relationship between the cervical spine and the patient's complaints. Usually the response to treatment is positive and rapid, especially in those who have headaches and vertigo.

If manipulation is contraindicated or if the results are poor, one can try injecting corticosteroid at the painful C2-C3 articulation. Three to four injections should be sufficient. One can also try soft tissue release techniques for the neck, without any mobilization. Petrissage of the subcutaneous tissues, if they are injected subcutaneously, can also be useful. Trigger point injection is a complementary treatment that is often very effective. Electrotherapy can be of use in those whose conditions are the sequelae of old trauma and especially in those with arthritic spines.

Cervical treatment usually gives excellent results in those with cervical headaches and those with vertigo. It is somewhat less useful in those who complain of difficulty with hearing or tinnitus (less than 10%). It can be good for complaints of visual fatigue and pharyngolaryngeal complaints. We have seen many singers with acute difficulty after a cervical trauma who regain their normal voices after several manipulations.

Some patients require a cervical collar during the night, particularly if they sleep in prone and produce extreme torsion because of their nocturnal posture. This extreme torsion can result in facet joint irritation. Such individuals should be counseled about neck movement and taught to avoid extreme torsion.

Physical Modalities

Physical modalities are rarely useful in the cervical syndrome, especially when it is of traumatic origin. Sometimes they may further irritate the articular discomfort. In addition, the repetitive sessions can condition the patient psychologically. This is particularly seen in posttraumatic syndromes that involve medicolegal issues.

When improvement in the condition is noted, one should lengthen the time between treatments and reassure the patient. The patients should also be taught how to prevent future trauma to the cervical spine.

Remarks
R. Waghemacker made interesting observations regarding victims of minor cervical trauma, their complaints, and the efficacy of their treatment. Decroix and he performed electronystagmography before and after cervical treatment. In 40 patients with cervical syndromes, usually of posttraumatic origin, they noted that manipulative treatments tended to normalize the abnormalities, while subjective improvement tended to follow objective graphic improvement in complaints such as vertigo and headaches. Their work helped to identify the complaints of the patients, show the role of the cervical spine, and document the efficacy of manipulative therapeutic approaches and the good results that could be obtained with them.

51

LEVATOR SCAPULAE SYNDROME

The levator scapulae is attached distally at the superior-medial angle of the scapula and to the superior part of the spine of the scapula, and proximally to the transverse processes of cervical vertebrae 1–5 (Fig. 51.1). It has a dual action: when the cervical spine is fixed, it elevates the scapula; if the scapula is fixed, it produces ipsilateral rotation and a lateral bending of the cervical spine. Tenderness to palpation of its scapular attachment is found very frequently on systematic examination. It is sometimes sufficiently sharp to cause spontaneous pain (Fig. 51.2).

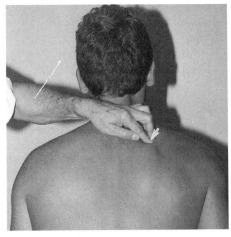

Figure 51.2. Palpation of the scapular attachment of the levator scapulae.

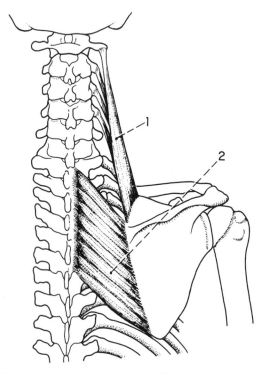

Figure 51.1. Levator scapulae (*1*) and rhomboideus (*2*).

CLINICAL PICTURE

Different Aspects of Pain

Dysfunction of the levator is expressed as

- Upper thoracic or periscapular pain
- Chronic low cervical pain with limitation of movement to the opposite side or an acute pain like a torticollis (wryneck)
- Pain radiating, in some cases, to the arm; it can be dull and poorly localized or acute, mimicking cervicobrachial neuralgia

In all cases, anesthetic injection of the scapular attachment of the muscle immediately suppresses the pain and relieves the limitation of movement.

Mechanism

Tenderness of the levator attachment can be due to a local cause, a vertebral cause, or both.

Local Cause

Muscle fatigue can be due to overworked muscles or strenuous postures (e.g., turning the head for a prolonged time while backing a car, speaking to somebody seated on the side, typing while reading text on the side, holding a telephone receiver between shoulder and neck, using too long a cane as a support). Prolonged or repeated fatigue of the muscle produces taut bands at its inferior part.

Cervical Cause

As we have seen, tenoperiosteal hypersensitivity of the superior-medial angle of the scapula is usually found in the cellulotenoperiosteomyalgic syndrome of C4, sometimes of C5. The segmental examination reveals dysfunction of C3-C4 or C4-C5, with ipsilateral facet joint tenderness and often cellulalgia of the ipsilateral supraspinous fossa.

Mixed Causes

Local and cervical factors are often found in combination. Generally superimposed on this background is recent muscle fatigue, postural stress, or another irritant, which then provokes a cervical or thoracic PMID.

TREATMENT

If there is a cervical element, such as a C3-C4 or C4-C5 PMID or synovitis, it can be treated, depending on the case, by facet joint injection or manipulation. Usually this will suppress the spontaneous pain. Sometimes an injection of the scapular attachment, followed by physiotherapy may be necessary. Trigger points should be looked for, one or two fingerbreadths above the scapular insertion. If found, an injection of Xylocaine should be tried.

52

ACROPARESTHESIAS OF THE UPPER LIMBS AND THE CERVICAL SPINE

Acroparesthesias of the arms are characterized by feelings of pins and needles, tingling, numbness, and pinching, which can affect all fingers or be localized to only some of them. They can be unilateral or bilateral. Depending on their topography and character, one can distinguish

- Global acroparesthesias, affecting the whole hand and occurring usually during the night
- Acroparesthesias with radicular topography
- Acroparesthesias with entrapment topography

They may originate from lesions in the spinal cord (syringomyelia) or the cerebrum. Multiple causes can provoke the feeling of numbness, of a swollen hand, or of a dead finger, which characterizes this syndrome. The leading pathologic cause of this syndrome by far is carpal tunnel syndrome.

ACROPARESTHESIAS WITH RADICULAR TOPOGRAPHY

A form of cervicobrachial neuralgia, acroparesthesias with radicular topography are linked to irritation of a cervical root, producing paraesthesia in the thumb (C6), middle finger (C7), or ring and little fingers (C8) (Fig. 52.1).

NOCTURNAL GLOBAL ACROPARESTHESIAS

Especially frequent in women during menopause, nocturnal global acroparesthesias occur between 2 and 4 o'clock in the morning, awakening the patient with a feeling of numbness, the impression that the hands are dead

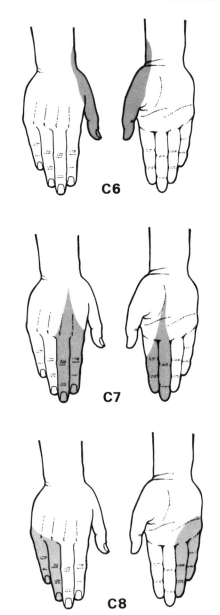

Figure 52.1. Radicular topography of C6, C7, and C8.

364

or swollen, and intense prickling in the whole hand. The patient wakes, shakes her hands, rubs them, and sometimes gets up, hoping that these disagreeable feelings will disappear. It is usually bilateral, but it can be unilateral.

First, one should ascertain that the hand and all fingers are affected. For example, upon awakening, when the patient feels the symptoms coming, she should softly rub the affected hand with a clothes brush. This will determine whether the fifth finger is involved or not. Usually it is not, which may be consistent with a carpal tunnel. If all the fingers are affected, the diagnosis of a bicanalar syndrome can be made (carpal tunnel syndrome with the syndrome of Guyon's tunnel). But as we shall see below, participation of the cervical spine should not be excluded.

ACROPARESTHESIAS WITH ENTRAPMENT

Acroparesthesias with entrapment are the most frequent and the consequence of an entrapment syndrome (Figs. 52.2–52.4). Entrapment of the palmar branch of the median nerve as it traverses the carpal tunnel is the most common entrapment syndrome. Although less common, the ulnar palmar branch can also become entrapped at the wrist in Guyon's canal. Nerve conduction studies and needle electrode examination are the fundamental examinations. They can localize the site of the entrapment, measure the degree of conduction block, assess the amplitude of the evoked response, and measure the velocity of the motor and sensory fibers that comprise the nerve.

The median nerve can also be compressed between the two heads of the pronator teres or at the fibrous edge of the flexor digitorum superficialis. Compression of the anterior or posterior interosseus nerves in the midforearm is less common. The ulnar nerve can be compressed in the cubital tunnel. When the proximal nerve fibers at the level of the brachial plexus are (occasionally) compressed at the thoracic outlet, the term *thoracic outlet syndrome* is applied. In this case, the origin is often postural, located in the C8-T1 or lower trunk territory, and is rarely isolated.

Carpal Tunnel Syndrome

Compression of the median nerve at the wrist as it traverses the carpal tunnel is the most frequent cause of acroparesthesia. The symptoms are classically nocturnal but may occur during the day. Their topography is that of the median nerve; that is, it involves the first three fingers and the medial half of the fourth finger. In some cases, it may only involve one or two fingers. Tapping over the wrist (Tinel's sign) and sustained passive wrist flexion (Phalen's test) can trigger the usual pain. In severe cases, there is hypesthesia over the tips of the involved digits and wasting of the thenar eminence with weakness of the muscles innervated by the median nerve, including the opponens pollicis and the abductor pollicis brevis.

Electrodiagnosis may reveal decreased sensory nerve conduction velocity across the wrist compared with the median nerve on the opposite side or with the ipsilateral ulnar and radial nerves over equidistant segments. There

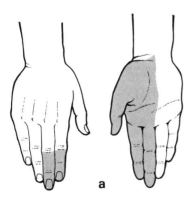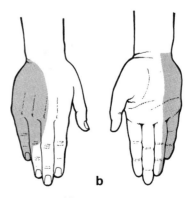

Figure 52.2.   Sensory territories. **a,** Radial nerve. **b,** Ulnar nerve.

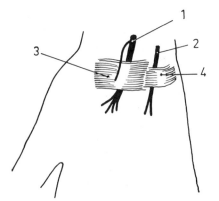

Figure 52.3. Anterior view of the median nerve in the carpal tunnel and of the ulnar nerve in the Guyon's canal. *1,* Median nerve; *2,* ulnar nerve; *3,* annular ligament; *4,* anterior ulnar expansion.

may be evidence of either conduction block across the wrist or, in severe cases, axonal loss manifested by decreased amplitude of the evoked response. Motor studies may show a prolonged wrist latency; the needle electrode examination is abnormal only in severe cases.

The diagnosis is confirmed by injection of the carpal tunnel with anesthetic and corticosteroid and treated with surgical release in refractory cases. A hypertrophic synovitis of the tendons is usually responsible for the compression. The cause can also be also traumatic: a Colles fracture with an imperfect callus, intracarpal fractures and dislocations, contusions or sprains of the wrist, or retractable scars of the anterior side of the wrist. Muscular abnormalities can also play a role and, rarely, lipomas of the carpal tunnel.

Treatment

In the purely sensory forms, injections are usually sufficient, but one should not resort to them frequently. If the disorders persist, only surgical intervention can avoid motor lesions and sensory problems. Jesel has shown that if the injections relieve low back pain of thoracolumbar origin, the objective electrical signs of nerve compression can remain unchanged.

Guyon's Canal Syndrome

The ulnar nerve can sometimes be affected by an entrapment syndrome at Guyon's canal. It is really rather rare, and its causes are variable: vascular, muscular, or tendinous abnormalities; synovial cysts of the carpus; fractures of the pisiform bone or the hook of the hamate bone, etc.

The clinical picture is characterized by paresthesia in the small and ring fingers. Atrophy of the first dorsal interosseous space is usually the first clinical sign of a motor damage.

CERVICAL SPINE AND ACROPARESTHESIAS

If the role of the cervical spine seems evident in the acroparesthesias with radicular topography, it seems that no such role exists if the acroparesthesias are global or in the case

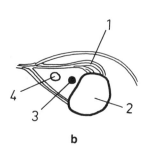

Figure 52.4. **a,** Section of the wrist at the second carpal row. *1,* Median nerve; *2,* palmaris longus tendon; *3,* flexor digitorum superficialis; *4,* flexor digitorum profundus; *5,* hamate; *6,* capitate; *7,* trapezoid; *8,* trapezium; *9,* flexor retinaculum. **b,** Section through the canal of Guyon. *1,* Tendon of the flexor carpi ulnaris; *2,* pisiform; *3,* ulnar nerve; *4,* ulnar artery.

of carpal tunnel syndrome. Howev
cases, if cervical manipulation is p(
justified by an inferior cervical PM
often bring appreciable relief or ever
pearance of all symptoms.

The explanation for this is not
though this observation is frequent enough to
be more than mere coincidence. Thus, unless
contraindicated, when a patient demonstrates
acroparesthesias and an inferior cervical
PMID with facet joint tenderness on the side
of the paresthesia, a trial cervical treatment is
justified. If successful, the local treatment may
be unnecessary or more efficacious.

To determine whether there is cervical participation and thus a role for manipulative
treatment, we use the "arm elevation test" or
the "arms up test" (Maigne).

Arm Elevation Test

Patients are asked to keep their arms up for
1 minute. Often, not always, after 20–30 seconds, this elicits the usual numbness and paresthesias.

- The time it takes to happen is noted.
- The exact topography of the numbness and
  paresthesias is checked by rubbing the fingers softly with a small dry brush to better
  detect sensory problems.
- If the examination reveals cervical signs,
  (PMID at C5-C6 or C6-C7), manipulation can
  be performed according to the usual rules.

? acropares-
; up. If the
atment will
es even the
is, in two to
obtained in
the global forms and in some moderate forms
of the carpal tunnel syndrome in which the
nerve conduction velocity is only slightly impaired. If there is an inferior cervical segmental dysfunction, the cervical treatment
can suppress the symptomatology.

All this indicates that the painful phenomena was due to a local and a cervical factor
together. If one or the other is decreased, the
paresthesias can disappear.

DOUBLE CRUSH SYNDROME

Cases in which a favorable result can be obtained by either a local treatment or a vertebral
treatment (if there is a PMID) represent the
"double crush syndrome" described by Upton
and Mac Comas; the combination of the two
factors creates the syndrome. This phenomenon is found in many painful disorders with a
vertebral component that we describe in this
book (e.g., syndrome of the perforating
branches, of the twelfth intercostal nerve and
of the first lumbar nerve; pain in the knee; and
some low back pain of thoracolumbar origin).

SHOULDER PAIN AND THE CERVICAL SPINE

The most frequent common presentation of shoulder pain is tenderness at the tendinous insertion. It is frequently linked to degenerative lesions, whose frequency is well known.

However, a few painful shoulders are remarkably relieved by cervical treatment only. They are the result of the cellulotenoperiosteomyalgic manifestations of a segmental dysfunction at C4-C5 or C5-C6 (by PMID or synovitis), which may simulate tendinitis or exacerbate it. These totally or partially "cervical" shoulders should be recognized so they can be treated efficiently.

GENERALITIES ON TENDINOUS AND CAPSULAR LESIONS

Common shoulder tenosynovitis has been well studied, which permits study and classification of lesions that were not usually held responsible.

S. de Sèze et al. (1964) classified these conditions as follows:

"Scapulothoracic periarthritis"
(a) "Simple painful shoulder" linked to a tendinitis affecting most often the long biceps and the supraspinatus
(b) "Frozen shoulder" due to adhesive capsulitis
(c) "Acute hyperalgic shoulder," part of the evolution of a calcific tendinitis, a microcrystalline acute attack
(d) "Pseudoparalytic shoulder" due to rupture of the rotator cuff tendon

In 1972, Neer highlighted the role of impingement between the rotator cuff tendon and the coracoacromial arch, known as the *subacromial impingement syndrome*.

Subacromial Impingement (Neer)

The subacromial impingement syndrome is a term used to describe compression of the soft tissues between the greater tuberosity of the humerus and the undersurface of the acromion and the coracoacromial ligament, especially during shoulder abduction and flexion. The subacromial impingement syndrome has three phases, which reveals the progression of the lesions.

1. Stage 1: edema, hemorrhage, and acute tendinitis due to excessive physical exertion: patients are usually young
2. Stage 2: tendinitis and fibrosis; patients are older, but under 40; overworking the shoulder produces pain; the shoulder is not painful in mild activities
3. Stage 3: tendinous ruptures of the rotator cuff and bony modifications; patients are over 40; the supraspinatus is most often affected; radiologic lesions appear

On examination, the characteristic sign is the painful arc produced by passive shoulder abduction. Between 60° and 90°, this movement produces a sharp pain, increased by the least resistance. This pain disappears with injection of local anesthetic into the subacromial bursa at the zone of impingement. This sign cannot be considered specific.

Neer's concept, which is based on anatomic and clinical findings, is very interesting. It is useful in refractory cases, in medical treatments in which physical therapy has an essential role, and when the patient will not or cannot undergo corrective surgery.

More recently, the "impingement" has been shown to be more a dynamic dysfunction of shoulder mechanics than a static problem reflecting unfavorable anatomy. Dynamic impingement is the result of abnormal energy and force distribution across the rotator cuff and labrum, which can account for the pathoanatomic findings described in this condition. The existence of structural injury does not necessarily imply that a decompressive procedure (which attempts to modify a structural lesion, without adequately identifying the dysfunctional elements that are producing the impingement) is a valid approach. The source of the dysfunction is the muscle imbalance altering the various force couples that control shoulder motion, including the rotator cuff and scapular rotator muscles, and, to some extent, the cervicothoracic muscles as well. Treatment of this dysfunction is necessary to avoid recurrent attacks.

Asymptomatic Lesions

Codman has shown the frequency of degenerative lesions in the supraspinatus tendon (focus of fibrillar necrosis, calcifications, microruptures, etc.), but there is no correlation between the severity of these lesions and the pain and dysfunction felt by the patient. Many of them are asymptomatic.

Subcoracoid Impingement Syndrome

In addition to the anteroposterior and subacromial impingement, there can be impingement of the anterolateral subcoracoid (subcoracoid impingement syndrome), evidenced by pain on internal rotation of the shoulder when the arm is in horizontal abduction (Gerber's sign).

EXAMINATION OF THE SHOULDER

Each painful shoulder should be thoroughly examined, both clinically and radiologically. Ultrasonography may be useful (especially in posttraumatic shoulders) and, if necessary, arthrography with or without CT.

A systematic examination of the cervical spine should always accompany the examination of the shoulder. This should be performed as follows:

- Assessment of active range of motion
- Assessment of passive range of motion
- Assessment of resisted range of motion
- Assessment of tender sites
- Palpation of the subcutaneous tissues, muscles, and tendons
- Examination of the acromioclavicular and sternoclavicular joints
- Assessment of scapular mobility
- Assessment of the glenohumeral joint and the signs that could reveal a lesion of the glenoid labrum

Assessment of Active Range of Motion

Active range of motion assessment allows better evaluation of the mobility of the shoulder and the discomfort of the patient. The patient is asked to do the following movements:

- Vertical elevation of the arm: in the sagittal, frontal, and scapular planes.
- Hand behind the back (combined adduction and internal rotation)
- Hand behind the head (combined abduction and external rotation)

Assessment of Passive Range of Motion

The same movements are used, but they are pushed to a maximum by the physician.

Muscles of the Shoulder Girdle

A complex coordination of prime movers, stabilizers, agonists, synergists, and antagonists is required for optimal shoulder function. It can be schematized in the following way:

- Abduction: deltoid (C5, C6) supraspinatus (C5-C6)
- Adduction: teres major (C5, C6), latissimus dorsi (C6, C7, C8), pectoralis major (C5 to T1)
- External rotation: infraspinatus (C5, C6) teres minor (C5, C6)
- Internal rotation: subscapularis (C5, C6, C7)
- Accessory internal rotators: teres major, latissimus dorsi, pectoralis major
- Vertical flexion: anterior head of the deltoid, clavicular head of the pectoralis major and the coracobrachialis (C6)
- Extension: posterior head of the deltoid, teres major, latissimus dorsi

Assessment of Resisted Range of Motion

In this phase of the examination, the patient is directed to perform a specific active movement with maximal force while the physician simultaneously applies an equal and opposite resistance. Contraction of a muscle-tendon unit against resistance increases the pain of tendinitis because of the increased tensile load imposed upon the inflamed tissue. Each specific maneuver can detect the muscle or muscles that are affected.

Supraspinatus (Abduction)

The arm is positioned in about 30° of horizontal abduction and full internal rotation and raised vertically in the plane of the scapula. The physician applies a downward torque on the outstretched arm, while instructing the patient to resist isometrically (Fig. 53.1).

Infraspinatus (External Rotation)

Maneuver 1. The arm is kept against the body in slight internal rotation, the elbow flexed at a right angle. The examiner opposes the external rotation performed in slight abduction (Fig. 53.2).

Maneuver 2. The arm is kept horizontal, the forearm is vertical at 90°, and the examiner opposes the external rotation with the hand at the wrist.

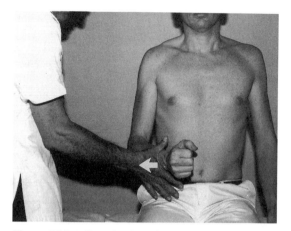

Figure 53.2. Examination of shoulder: external rotation against resistance.

Subscapularis (Internal Rotation)

The arm is kept against the body, forearm flexed at a right angle, and a slight internal rotation is started. The patient tries to bring his hand toward the abdominal wall while the examiner opposes the movement. This maneuver can also be performed with the arm horizontal and the forearm at a right angle.

Biceps

When the long head of the biceps is affected, it is rare to evoke pain with resisted elbow flexion, with or without associated resisted forearm supination. In this case, direct palpation renders the best information.

Pectoralis Major, Latissimus Dorsi, Teres Major

These are adductors and tested by resisted adduction.

The Painful Arc

On occasion, the shoulder may not be painful when certain selective maneuvers are performed against resistance. However, a painful arc of motion may detected during active or passive range of motion assessment. For example, in some supraspinatus tendinopathies located in an hypovascular zone (Codman) within 1 cm of its insertion, pain can be evoked at a precise point during active motion at end range in flexion, abduction, or horizontal ad-

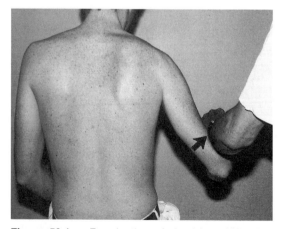

Figure 53.1. Examination of shoulder: abduction against resistance.

duction (Cyriax). Sometimes, a painful arc is noted with abduction of the arm to about 80°, especially if the arm is in internal rotation. This painful arc means that there is impingement of the affected tendon between two obstacles.

Neer proposed provocative testing of this impingement by passively flexing the arm in internal rotation, in an attempt to impinge the the rotator cuff attachment between the greater tuberosity beneath and the coracoacromial arch. Hawkins proposed a similar test, with the arm passively flexed at the shoulder and elbow at 90° (the 90/90/90 position). In this position, the examiner increases the amount of internal rotation at the shoulder, attempting to impinge the the rotator cuff attachment to the greater tuberosity beneath the coracoacromial arch. Both of these provocative maneuvers produce pain in shoulders with rotator cuff tendinopathy due to impingement.

Palpation

Subcutaneous Tissues

Some falsely localized shoulder pain syndromes are linked to tenderness of the subcutaneous tissues of the supraspinous fossa and lateral shoulder. A very painful cellulalgic zone is often found at the deltoid insertion. This zone can have a local or a cervical reflex origin (C5). Local treatment is sometimes necessary.

Muscles

Palpation of the muscles, particularly the infraspinatus, often reveals very painful trigger points even when manual muscle testing against resistance is painless. These trigger points can play a role in the painful shoulder. They can have cervical or local origin (overuse) (Fig. 53.3). The deltoid can also be affected.

Tendons

There are some limitations to examination against resistance. In some painful shoulders, movements performed against maximal resistance are painless, while direct palpation reveals pain of the tendon involved. This is particularly true for the biceps.

Indeed, a movement against resistance per-

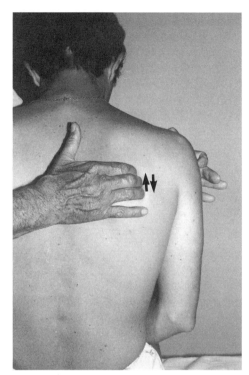

Figure 53.3. Palpation of the supraspinatus for trigger points.

formed to test the biceps (flexion of the forearm plus supination) is rarely painful although its tendon is very tender to palpation. Yet, injection of local anesthesic around the tendon temporarily relieves the habitual shoulder pain, demonstrating its involvement in the pain syndrome.

To palpate the tendon of the supraspinatus, the arm is internally rotated (back scratch test), which brings the tendon into a subacromial position under the anteromedial edge of the acromion. The arm should be in external rotation to palpate the tendon of the infraspinatus. It is better to have the elbow held by the examiner's other hand (or resting on a table of the correct height) and placed in slight adduction and flexion. The tendon is then palpable under the edge posterior to the acromion.

The tendon of the long head of the biceps is easily palpated at the deltopectoral groove in the deltopectoral sulcus (Fig. 53.4) It is first palpated statically, and then while subjecting the arm to small repeated movements of rotation with the hand holding the elbow. The best position for palpating the biceps tendon is with

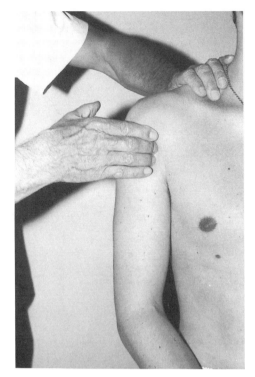

Figure 53.4. Palpation of the biceps tendon.

the shoulder and elbow in extension. The tendon is then pulled on the humeral pulley. So sensitized, its dysfunction is clearer.

The tendon of the subscapularis muscle is palpated in the deltopectoral groove, just lateral to the coracoid process. The patient is positioned in supine, with the arm in slight external rotation. The coracoacromial ligament can be palpated just below the coracoid, with the patient in supine and the arm in external rotation.

All these maneuvers should be compared with maneuvers on the healthy side.

Assessment of the Clavicular Joints

Acromioclavicular Joint

Dysfunction of the acromioclavicular joint often results in shoulder pain, poorly localized by the patient, and felt during flexion and abduction to 120° and internal rotation (back scratch test). Horizontal adduction is limited and sometimes painful against resistance. The diagnosis is made by the pain felt on palpation and confirmed by an anesthetic injection that relieves it.

The joint line is palpated while the scapula is mobilized by grasping it between thumb and index finger, laterally, like a piano key. Normally painless, these maneuvers are painful if the joint is injured (Fig. 53.5).

This joint has a small meniscus that can be torn or subluxed during rapid and violent movements or even during simple forced movements; it undergoes degenerative changes in 9 of 10 patients over the age of 50. Acute joint blockage is rare, but there is often a chronic dysfunction of the joint.

Radiography sometimes demonstrates joint space narrowing with sclerosis, osteophytes and in some cases, remodeling and deformations of the involved bony extremities. Initially, widening of the superior part of the joint space is noted. This degenerative arthropathy is often "silent"; it can become painful after forceful physical movements.

Particular Cases

Overhand athletes (e.g., pitchers or tennis players) can develop a microtraumatic arthropathy seen on radiographs as a subchondral cyst in the lateral third of the clavicle. Resting the joint is the best treatment. In a few cases, Wenders observed osteonecrosis of the distal clavicle several months after trauma.

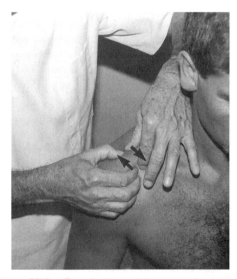

Figure 53.5. Examination of the acromioclavicular joint.

Sternoclavicular Joint

Whatever the nature of the injury, it is generally revealed by swelling and always by tenderness on palpation (Fig. 53.6). Pain from the sternoclavicular joint is rarely felt at its level; it is often referred toward the shoulder, the supraspinous fossa, or the neck. This joint also has a small meniscus that (rarely) can produce a mechanical pathology characterized by painful swelling.

Manipulation can be useful, with or without corticosteroid injections. Degenerative arthropathy of the sternoclavicular joint occurs later than acromioclavicular degeneration, but it is practically constant at 60 years of age. Radiographs demonstrate narrowing of the joint space, with subchondral sclerosis and osteophytosis. These lesions can cause acute inflammation, but they also foster painful dysfunction that can be treated successfully by manipulation. They are usually asymptomatic. Generally the acromioclavicular joint is spared in inflammatory and rheumatic conditions; the sternoclavicular joint, in contrast, is frequently affected.

Assessment of Scapular Mobility (Scapulothoracic Joint)

Free mobility of the scapula upon the rib cage is essential for normal glenohumeral range of motion. The mobility of the joint is

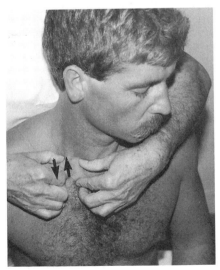

Figure 53.6. Examination of the sternoclavicular joint.

examined with the patient lying on the side opposite the one to be examined. The examiner grasps the shoulder tip in both hands, pulling it backward while simultaneously taking hold of the medial edge of the scapula with the fingers of both hands (Fig. 53.13); in this way the examiner can mobilize the scapula in all directions and evaluate any limitation of glenohumeral mobility.

Glenohumeral Mobility and Assessment of the Glenoid Fossa

Various maneuvers are used to test the anteroposterior joint play of the humeral head on the glenoid fossa. The patient is sitting or lying down.

Testing Joint Play

The "pylon" or hammerhead technique allows one to test the separation of the humeral head from the glenoid cavity and at the same time move it in all directions. When pain or limitation precludes maintaining the humerus at an elevation of 90° as shown in Figure 53.7, the maneuver can be adapted by maintaining the humerus at 30–40° of abduction. Thus the two shoulders can be compared with respect to joint play and pain. Joint play is absent in capsulitis. It is very limited in the rare glenohumeral spondylosis, and there is painful crepitus. Joint play is increased in lesions of the glenoid fossa.

Glenohumeral play can also be tested with the patient completely relaxed in supine. The examiner grasps the humeral head with the hand contralateral to the side being assessed, with four fingers posteriorly and the thumb anteriorly, while the opposite hand applies pressure to the clavicle.

Humeral head mobility can also be tested with the patient seated and bending slightly forward (Fig. 53.8, *left* and *right*). With one hand, the examiner fixates the shoulder, while the other hand grasps the upper part of the arm and applies slow anteroposterior movements (Rodineau).

Glenohumeral arthropathies are characterized by shoulder pain, with restrictions in both active and passive motion. Diagnosis is completed by appropriate radiographic views to rule out other entities such as spondylosis, ne-

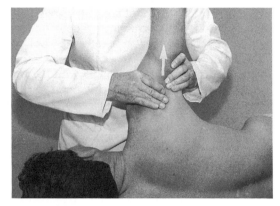

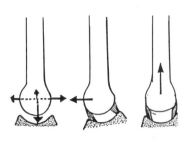

Figure 53.7. Left and **right.** This maneuver, the "pylon," permits the examiner to assess the mobility between the humeral head and the glenoid fossa. It can also be used to mobilize the shoulder, allowing separation. If the patient is unable to abduct beyond 90°, this maneuver can be modified by placing the patient's arm in less adduction.

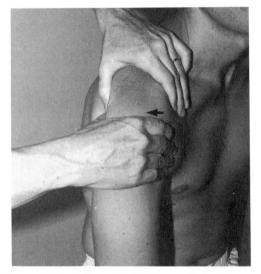

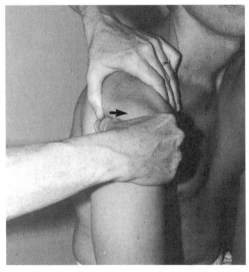

Figure 53.8. Left and **right.** Examination of the anteroposterior mobility and glenohumeral joint. This movement is often increased in lesions of the glenoid labrum. The patient should be relaxed and bent forward slightly.

crosis, arthritis, benign tumors (chondromas, osteomas, osteoid, osteochondromatosis), or malignant tumors (primary or secondary).

Glenoid Fossa

Some shoulder tenderness may be due to a lesion of the glenoid fossa and labrum from athletic trauma or without clear cause. These lesions can become progressively more painful and lead to shoulder instability. These lesions are especially seen in overhand athletes, whose shoulders are submitted to violent and repetitive anteroposterior shear forces associated with internal and external rotation. Injury to the anterior labrum, the most common site of injury, is improved by local warm compresses. The patient sometimes senses an abrupt alteration in joint mobility or transient locking of the shoulder.

Manual muscle testing against isometric resistance is normal. The back scratch test (adduction plus internal rotation) is limited by pain. Palpation of the glenohumeral fossa cavity at its anterior border is painful. If the patient is asked to simulate the motion of "throwing a javelin," it is noted that the range of motion is greater on the affected side than on the normal side. At maximal external rotation, in this position, the examiner exaggerates the movement by applying a posteroanterior shear to the humeral head with one hand and pulling the patient's wrist backward with the other. This maneuver, similar to the dislocation-relocation test performed in the supine position, reproduces the usual pain.

Radiographic studies can show a fracture of the inferior glenoid labrum, a flattening of the glenoid cavity, or a blunted aspect of the rim. Lateral views performed with Sernageau's technique are a useful way to demonstrate glenoid lesions. In difficult cases, CT arthrography, MRI, and possibly arthroscopy complete the examination.

If pain is improved by medical management, the patient should be rehabilitated by working the internal rotators (subscapularis) in a program similar to that used in patients with recurrent dislocations of the shoulder. If there is any failure, then surgery is indicated if the instability is not well tolerated. The techniques used are the same as those used for recurrent dislocations.

Examination of the Cervical Spine

After a thorough shoulder examination, the origin of the shoulder pain can be diagnosed, and the treatment can be tailored to the diagnosis. However, sometimes a thorough examination will find no lesion to explain the shoulder pain. Often examination of the cervical spine will then reveal the answer, as the pain can be due to the cellulotenoperiosteomyalgic syndrome, C5 or C6 (tendinalgias, trigger points, periosteal tenderness).

The "cervical shoulder" can present with symptoms consistent with tendinitis, including pain on movement against resistance, and motion restriction. Often the cervical and local factors are additive; thus lesions that would be latent in isolation become painful.

CERVICAL SHOULDER

Often, a patient with a painful shoulder, with or without motion restriction, where a diagnosis of "tendinitis" might be made, will obtain immediate relief from manipulation of the cervical spine, which may restore pain-free movement as well (Fig. 53.10). Here it is important to demonstrate the segmental dysfunction of the midcervical segments (C4-C5 and C5-C6), with facet joint tenderness ipsilateral to the painful shoulder. This segmental dysfunction is almost always the result of a PMID and occasionally is due to synovitis (Fig. 53.9, a and b).

Radiologic examination of the cervical spine and shoulder is indispensable for diagnosis. However, radiographic examinations have a high incidence of both false-positive and false-negative findings. The presence of spondylosis at C4-C5 or C5-C6 or the existence multilevel disk degeneration is only presumptive. They neither affirm nor invalidate the

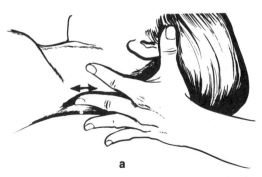

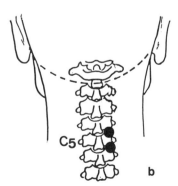

Figure 53.9. **a.** The cervical segmental examination. Examination for facet joint tenderness in the lower cervical spine. **b.** C4-C5 and C5-C6 segments can produce pain in the shoulder through intermediary cellulalgic, tenoperiosteal, or myalgic manifestations.

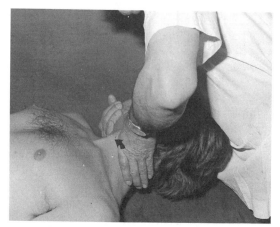

Figure 53.10. Immediate reduction in pain and increase in shoulder mobility with cervical manipulation supports the participation of the cervical segment as the origin and cause of this dysfunction. Here the manipulation in right rotation is demonstrated on C5-C6.

possible cervical origin of the painful shoulder. The following case is typical of "cervical shoulders."

Case History. Mr. P., a 56-year-old athletic male was an accomplished tennis player who played regularly. After a fall down some stairs, he began complaining of right shoulder pain with limitation of movement into abduction and behind the head. The diagnosis of rotator cuff "tendinitis" was made, and a few subacromial injections resulted in partial improvement. His condition remained unchanged in spite of anti-inflammatory treatments, more injections, and physical therapy trials. This lasted for 4 months, with persistent painful motion restriction. Abduction and rotation against resistance were impossible, as they produced a very sharp pain. Both the infra- and supraspinatus muscles as well as the tendon of the right biceps were tender to palpation.

Examination of the cervical spine did not reveal any limitation of movement. Radiographic studies showed only minor spondylosis. But, palpation revealed marked tenderness over the right C4-C5 facet joint (on the side of the affected shoulder). Soon after, a manipulation in left rotation, followed by a manipulation in left lateroflexion was performed. After the manipulation, the patient was able to lift his arm freely without the least discomfort, and the tests against resistance in abduction and external rotation were much improved. Two more sessions of manipulation, at weekly intervals, were performed. Every time, there was an improvement of the tests against resistance. After the third session, the movements were free, and contraction against maximal resistance was painless. The patient took up tennis without the least inconvenience.

In summary, in this case, the diagnosis of tendinitis was considered; however, on closer examination the pain turned out to be of cervical origin. Even when the pain seems to be undeniably linked to a lesion of the biceps tendon or the rotator cuff, the cervical factor, if it exists, can play a determinant or facilitating role.

Diagnosis of the Cervical Shoulder

In the patient presenting with shoulder pain accompanied by features of tendinitis such as pain, with or without motion restriction, two diagnostic possibilities may be considered.

1. Cervical facet joint tenderness at C4-C5 or C5-C6 is not found on palpation. In this case, the cervical factor may be eliminated.
2. There is facet joint tenderness C4-C5 or C5-C6 ipsilateral to the painful shoulder. It is then possible, but not certain, that the cervical spine may be totally or partially responsible for the shoulder pain. To make this determination, the following therapeutic test should be performed.
   —If it is an acute synovitis, injection of corticosteroid can be performed, without manipulation.
   —If it is due to a PMID and manipulation is possible, a test of manipulative treatment can yield an instant answer.

The first manipulation should be performed (e.g., in rotation). Soon after, testing of the painful movements should be repeated. If the cervical spine is involved, as is frequently the case, a well-performed manipulation should result in appreciable improvement in the patient's condition; for example, a patient who was unable to abduct his arm can do it soon after and without pain, even against increased resistance.

After the first manipulation, one or two more manipulations may be performed; for example, in lateroflexion and then in chin pivot. The examination should be repeated after each of these maneuvers. Thus, from the first session on, when manipulation can be done without any difficulty, one knows whether there is a link between the cervical spine and the painful tendon or tendons.

If the result obtained with manipulation is not satisfactory with respect to facet joint sensitivity, an injection with corticosteroid can be tried. If the shoulder pain is not improved after the first treatment, there is little chance that further cervical treatment will be useful.

In some cases, the patient may come back a few days later reporting a painful 24 hours associated with a temporary or persistent improvement in the condition. This result helps to confirm that the pain syndrome originated in the cervical spine. Two or three more sessions of cervical treatment will often bring complete and lasting relief.

Sometimes it is necessary to inject a residual trigger point. Depending on which segment is involved, C5 or C6, the corresponding cellulotenoperiosteomyalgic syndrome can be seen involving the infraspinatus (Fig. 48.11), the supraspinatus, or the teres minor.

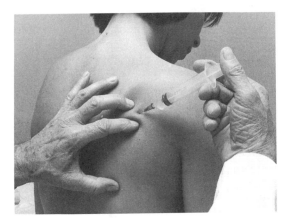

Figure 53.11.   Injection of an infraspinatus trigger point.

MIXED SHOULDER PAIN SYNDROMES

In some cases, local treatment produces incomplete improvement. Cervical treatment produces total relief or, on the contrary, it clearly improves the pain and the tests against resistance, but relief is incomplete and injection of the tendon results in complete relief. In these "mixed shoulders," the contributions to the painful syndrome made by its two components can vary from case to case and over time in individuals.

Taut Bands, Trigger Points, and Atypical Shoulder Pain

We have already emphasized the role in shoulder tenderness of some "active" trigger points belonging to a cellulotenoperiosteomyalgic C5 or C6 syndrome. But at the shoulder especially, certain trigger points can have a local origin. They can result from excessive exertion: carrying too heavy a suitcase in the case of the supraspinatus; repeated maneuvers in a car without power steering for the teres major; working with the arms held horizontally for the deltoid, etc. A forceful, strenuous, or overly wide movement can also be responsible, as can prolonged, sustained, stressful postures.

Taut bands often harbor "trigger points" that are often the source of referred shoulder tip tenderness and refer in a consistent pattern: to the anterior shoulder for infraspinatus, the lateral shoulder for supraspinatus, and the posterior shoulder for teres minor.

One often finds trigger points along the lateral border of the subscapularis. They can be palpated along the lateral border of the scapula with the patient supine. Severe cases can limit shoulder movement and mimic adhesive capsulitis.

The trigger points of the coracobrachialis interfere with the ability to reach behind the back. Trigger points of the deltoid are frequent, easy to find, and are more often linked to nonvertebral causes (trauma, exertion). They cause discomfort with abduction. The trigger points of the triceps prevent complete arm flexion. The treatment is injection of xylocaine followed by stretching of the affected muscle (Fig. 53.11).

MANUAL THERAPY FOR THE PAINFUL SHOULDER

Theoretically, manual therapy does not have a dominant place in the treatment of shoulder tenderness linked to rotator cuff pathology. Rotator cuff tendinitis needs specific treatment (essentially medical), including injections in acute cases, provided they are used judiciously. Electrotherapy and ultrasound can be recommended.

A therapeutic exercise prescription is the best treatment in total or partial ruptures of the rotator cuff as well as in tendinitis caused by subacromial impingement. The basic principle of the program is to teach the patient to depress the humeral head during abduction, thereby decreasing the subacromial impingement. Physical therapy can start with passive mobilization of the humeral head into a depressed position that will free external rotation. This humeral head depression is performed first with the help of the physiotherapist, then performed actively and repeated frequently so that the patient can automatically depress the humeral head at all times with flexion or abduction of the arm. It is also necessary to strengthen the adductor muscles, pectoralis major and latissimus dorsi, because they also participate in humeral head depression. There are also cases in which some manual techniques have their indication.

Mobilization of the Glenohumeral Joint

The technique shown in Figure 53.7 allows glenohumeral mobilization and separation of the articular surfaces. The technique shown in Figure 53.12 also permits efficient glenohumeral distraction.

Mobilization of the Scapulothoracic Joint

Full mobility of the scapulothoracic joint can help to compensate for inadequate mobility of the glenohumeral joint in adhesive capsulitis or in spondylosis. Mobilizations shown in Figure 53.13 (see also Fig. 54.13) are very useful. They also allow for good stretching and relaxation of the muscles of the scapula.

Manipulation of the Acromioclavicular Joint

The acromioclavicular joint is often affected in shoulder tenderness associated with other conditions. Injection can prove its involvement and often relieve it, but it is not always sufficient, and manual techniques can be of help. Figures 53.14 and 53.15 show two usual techniques.

Lesage uses a slightly different technique from the one shown in Figure 53.15. For a right acromioclavicular joint: the patient sits on a stool, right hand on the hip and thumb forward. This point can be the pivot point. The examiner stands behind with the left foot slightly forward and right foot back, legs bent. The examiner's left side flank is against the lumbar

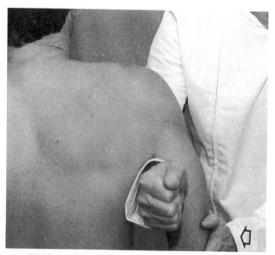 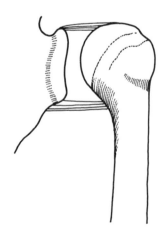

Figure 53.12.   Left and **right.** Demonstration of glenohumeral distraction. The examiner, standing in front of the patient, places the arm under the patient's axilla with the patient's arm dangling at the side. With the left hand, pressure is applied rhythmically to the lateral inferior aspect of the arm, using it as a lever to produce progressive glenoid humeral distraction. This maneuver stretches the lateral joint capsule to permit distraction.

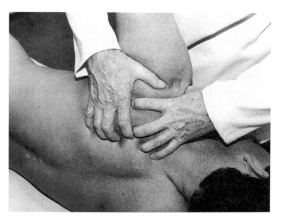

Figure 53.13. Mobilization of the scapulothoracic joint with stretching of the scapular rotators.

region of the patient. The examiner's left arm rests on the right clavicle of the patient; the right hand grasps the patient's right shoulder. The examiner's right forearm rests on the lateral side of the patient's arm. Manipulation is performed by suddenly bending the two legs with an elbow motion that brings the shoulders into retraction.

Manipulation of the Sternoclavicular Joint

The sternoclavicular joint is manipulated with the technique shown on Figure 53.16. The technique shown in Figure 53.17 simultane-

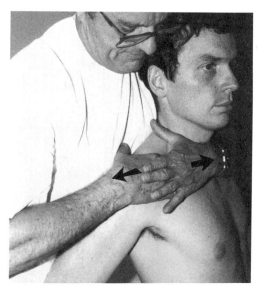

Figure 53.15. Acromioclavicular manipulation (second technique). The patient is sitting on a table with the right arm hanging slightly posteriorly and the hand in supination. The doctor, standing behind, presses with the left hand over the medial surface of the clavicle and places the right hand over the acromion. Then while firmly maintaining pressure with the sternum and left hand, the examiner progressively applies posterior lateral traction with the right hand to "take up the slack" and then applies a manipulative thrust.

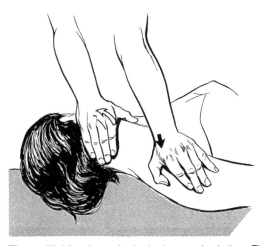

Figure 53.14. Acromioclavicular manipulation. The left hand fixes the lateral surface of the clavicle, while the right hand places pressure at the base of the neck, applying lateral tension to the axis of the clavicle to "take up the slack." A brief thrust is then applied with the left hand on the acromioclavicular joint.

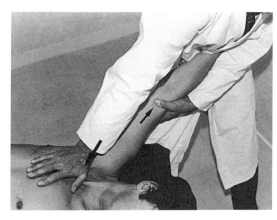

Figure 53.16. Sternoclavicular manipulation. The patient is supine. The examiner takes the left arm of the patient and pulls it outward and in abduction, slowly applying pressure on the axis of the clavicle so that the heel of the right hand applies pressure to the median clavicle. The examiner "takes up the slack" while applying pressure to the medial aspect of the clavicle. Repeated mobilizations are performed.

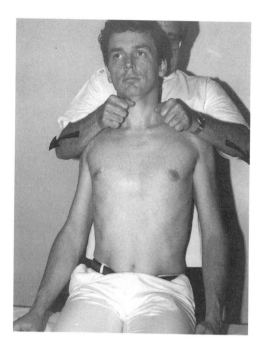

Figure 53.17. The examiner stands behind the seated patient, with the forearms flexed and placed over the anterior aspects of both humeral heads. Counterpressure is then applied with the sternum against the patient's back. Posterior lateral tension is progressively increased rhythmically or with a thrust to mobilize or manipulate the glenohumeral, acromioclavicular, and sternoclavicular joints.

ously mobilizes the three joints of the shoulder: sternoclavicular, acromioclavicular, and glenohumeral. A direct manipulation is possible. The patient is supine, arms along the body. For a right sternoclavicular manipulation, the examiner stands on the right side of the patient and presses on the medial part of the right clavicular head with the heel of the right hand and applies a counterpressure with the left hand on the left clavicle. The examiner takes up the slack by pressing downward and laterally (in the direction of the acromioclavicular joints)

then applies a thrust of the right hand in the same direction.

In some cases, the sternoclavicular and acromioclavicular joints are painful at the same time (syndrome of both ends of the clavicle [Troisier]). This is often a posttraumatic sequela, but in these cases, there is never a local pain, but rather, radiating tenderness (e.g., supraspinatus fossa, ear). The usual treatment is the injection of the two joints, but manipulative treatment (Fig. 53.17) can be useful in some cases.

54

LATERAL EPICONDYLAR PAIN

Lateral epicondylar pain or epicondylitis refers to pain localized to the lateral epicondyle in which some movements (e.g., turning a doorknob or pouring a drink) are very painful or even impossible if the disorder is severe. It is often called "tennis elbow," since it is frequent among tennis players. But workers whose jobs require repetitive pronation and supination (e.g., using a screw driver) are often affected, as are people who are neither athletes nor manual laborers.

Pain is generally attributed to tenoperiosteal irritation of mechanical origin caused by overwork of the long wrist and finger extensors, which have a common origin on the lateral epicondyle (hence the name, lateral epicondylitis). However, the efficiency of treatment by cervical manipulation demonstrates that "insertion tendinitis" is not the only process involved in the lateral epicondylar pain.

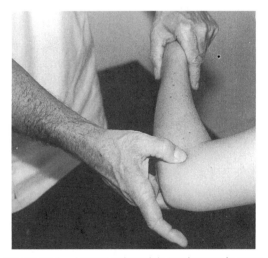

Figure 54.1. Lateral epicondyle tenderness is an essential sign of this disorder.

Six muscles have their proximal attachment on the lateral epicondyle including:

- Supinator
- Extensor carpi radialis longus and brevis (ECRL, ECRB)
- Extensor digitorum communis (EDC)
- Extensor digiti minimi
- Extensor carpi ulnaris,

Among those muscles originating from the epicondyle, the surface of attachment of the extensor carpi radialis brevis represents half of the total surface of attachment of all the epicondylar muscles.

CLINICAL EXAMINATION

Elbow

Palpation

Tenderness to palpation over the lateral epicondyle is the characteristic sign of the condition (Fig. 54.1). It is performed with the elbow flexed at a right angle. The common extensor tendon, the radiohumeral joint line, the circumference of the radial head, and the point of emergence of the posterior interosseous branch of the radial nerve are also palpated. One or two trigger points in the supinator or in the radialis muscles are often palpated also. Sometimes, a cellulalgic zone painful to pinch-rolling is found at the lateral side of the elbow.

Manual Muscle Testing against Resistance

Pain produced by resisted isometric contraction of the epicondylar muscles is a quasi-constant sign. This should be assessed by first having the patient extend the wrist against resistance, with fingers clenched, and then extend the fingers against resistance, usually directed at the middle finger.

Examination of Active and Passive Range of Motion

Mobility is normal in general, but extension may be limited on occasion. More rarely, the limitation involves both flexion and extension. Passive mobility is tested in flexion-extension, then in pronation-supination. It can sometimes give the impression of "hooking" in cases of radiohumeral subluxation; but as we have already emphasized, the lateral joint play should be studied.

Lateral Joint Play of the Elbow

The elbow is extended. With the physician facing the patient, the affected forearm is held under the examiner's axilla, in supination. The lateral elbow is then grasped with both hands. Then, while firmly grasping the patient's forearm, the examiner applies gradual varus and valgus stresses to the elbow to assess the passive range and end feel. The joint play varies from one patient to another but is readily appreciated in the intact patient. The physician compares both sides, knowing that the lateral play is always a little less free in the dominant elbow (Fig. 54.2). In some lateral epicondylar pain syndromes, this play is globally decreased, and elbow mobilization is painful; it is painless in the normal state. Sometimes, this maneuver is very painful in abduction or in adduction, giving the impression of joint blockage.

Joint Play of the Distal Radioulnar Joint

In some persistent lateral epicondylar pain syndromes, there is a decrease in the passive mobility of the distal radioulnar joint together with a decrease of the lateral mobility of the elbow. The examiner grasps the distal radius with the thumb and index finger of one hand and grasps the distal ulna with the thumb and index finger of the other. Gliding mobilizations can be performed to assess joint play. Mobility of both sides is compared. This test can be disagreeable for the patient.

Radiography

Radiography can reveal small periarticular calcifications that indicate joint overuse and are usually not the cause of the pain.

Cervical Spine

The patient is in supine position and the physician examines for tenderness over the C5-6 or C6-7 facet joints ipsilateral to the lateral epicondylar pain. Tenderness suggests that there may be a cervical component to the elbow pain, and the cervical spine should be carefully examined with the usual techniques. Radiographic studies will be necessary.

EVALUATION OF LATERAL EPICONDYLAR PAIN

It is important to be able to evaluate lateral epicondylar pain, not so much to compare the lateral epicondylar pain of a patient with the one of another patient, but to appreciate, in a given patient, the evolution of the condition and the efficiency of a therapeutic treatment. In 1975, we proposed a series of maneuvers performed with the physician applying isometric resistance in two different elbow positions.

1. Extension of hand and fingers with
   —The elbow flexed at a right angle and the arm adducted at the side (Fig. 54.3, *left*)
   —Elbow extended (Fig. 54.3, *right*).
2. Pronation: the physician grasps the patient's hand and instructs the patient to

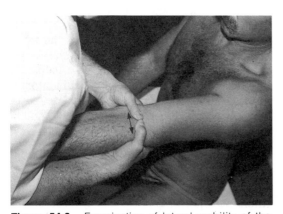

Figure 54.2. Examination of lateral mobility of the lateral epicondylar joint.

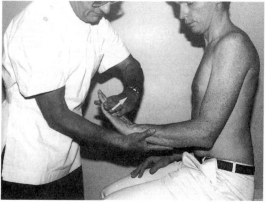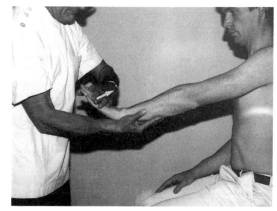

Figure 54.3. Wrist extension against resistance. **Left.** With the forearm flexed to 90° **Right.** With the forearm extended.

"turn the palm to the floor" (pronate) against isometric resistance supplied by the examiner
— Elbow flexed at a right angle (Fig. 54.4, *left*)
— Elbow extended (Fig. 54.4, *right*).

3. Supination: same maneuver as above, except the patient is asked to "turn the palm up" (supinate) against isometric resistance
— Elbow flexed at a right angle (Fig. 54.5, *left*)
— Elbow extended (Fig. 54.5, *right*).

Each maneuver is rated as follows:

- 0–no pain
- 1–some resistance, but painful
- 2–some weak resistance, with marked pain
- 3–resistance impossible, pain too severe

If there is pain at rest, it is rated from 0 to 2. Thus the total range is between 0 and 20 (3 for each of the 6 maneuvers, and 2 for pain at rest), but it is not absolute. One cannot conclude that a patient with a score of 14 is more affected than a patient with a score of 10. But this scoring system allows one to reliably judge the evolution of pain in a given patient and the response to treatment. It is particularly useful in lateral epicondylar pain syndromes with cervical involvement, in which a suitable cervical maneuver can, for example, improve and sometimes even render the tests negative.

Classification

The examination allows the examiner to classify the pain syndrome with respect to the

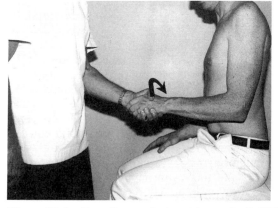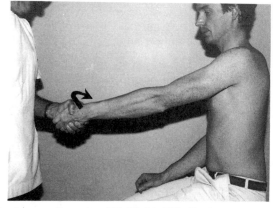

Figure 54.4. Pronation against resistance. **Left.** With the forearm flexed to 90° **Right.** With the forearm extended.

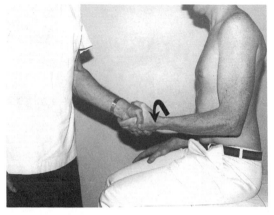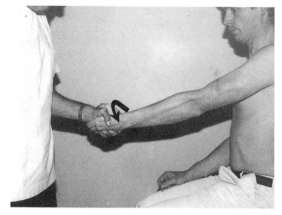

Figure 54.5.   Supination against resistance. **Left.** With the forearm flexed to 90° **Right.** With the forearm extended.

underlying pathophysiologic mechanism. It may be

- Lateral epicondylar pain of local origin
- Lateral epicondylar pain of tenoperiosteal, muscular, articular, or neurogenic (due to compression of the posterior interosseous branch of the radial nerve) origin.
- Lateral epicondylar pain of cervical origin
- Lateral epicondylar pain of mixed origin

Periarthritis of the elbow and sometimes also a decrease in the range of motion of the distal radioulnar articulation can be associated with each of these forms.

Lateral Epicondylar Pain of Local Origin

Lateral Epicondylar Pain due to Tenoperiosteal Irritation.   Most authors believe that lateral epicondylar pain is due to irritation of the tendinous attachment to the periosteum, caused by overuse of the epicondylar muscles. This seems to be confirmed by the often favorable results of only local treatment. The diagnosis is made on:

- Pain on palpation of the common extensor tendon
- Pain on resisted contraction of the epicondylar muscles (ECRB, EDC)
- Pain caused by forced varus and hyperextension

In our experience, a purely local origin accounts for only a fraction of the cases, because the pain of tendinous insertion is often facilitated, or even caused, by a cervical factor that

responds to cervical treatment. If the cervical factor is moderate or transient, local treatment can be sufficient. If not, the result can be temporary or insufficient (see "Lateral Epicondylar Pain and the Cervical Spine," below).

Treatment.   Treatment consists of injection of the painful site on palpation, using a corticosteroid derivative, with or without a local anesthetic. Physiotherapeutic modalities, including electrical stimulation and ultrasound, can also be most useful.

In refractory cases of tendinitis, deep transverse massage has been recommended by Cyriax. Transverse friction massage of the tendon is a painful treatment, demanding three to six sessions of about 15 minutes each. It does not seem very logical, if the tendon is thought to have inflammatory or necrotic lesions, but it is useful in some cases.

In "very refractory" cases, Troisier, after Cyriax, advocated the technique of subcutaneous tenotomy of the common extensor tendon, followed 6 weeks later by one or two injections of corticosteroid. It is after that injection that the patient is relieved. Troisier reported 34 good results out of 39 with this technique.

The technique is as follows: using sterile technique, the operator inserts a short-blade scalpel under the skin and detaches the common extensor tendon from the lateral epicondyle. The tenotomy is followed by a Mill's manipulation: the operator maintains the patient's hand and fingers in maximal extension, with the forearm in abduction, and then forces extension of the elbow. Six weeks later, the patient, who generally is still in pain, is reexamined and receives one or two injections of corticosteroid, which usually brings relief.

Epicondylalgia of Muscular Origin. During epicondylitis, it is common to palpate a few trigger points in the body of the epicondylar muscles (Fig. 54.6). They can belong to a cellulotenoperiosteomyalgic segmental vertebral C6 or C7 syndrome. They can have a local origin, such as muscular fatigue or articular pain or they can be of mixed origin.

Treatment. If a cervical origin is suspected, spinal treatment should be performed first; often it is sufficient. The result is immediately noted on the rating tests.

If the origin is local or mixed, local treatment is indispensable. The trigger points are usually found in the supinator muscle and occasionally in the extensor carpi radialis longus and brevis muscles. The trigger points should be injected with 1 mL of Xylocaine or 0.5% lidocaine. Pressure should be maintained for 90 seconds on the trigger points, and repeated several times. Ultrasound is often useful in these forms.

Radiohumeral Articular Blockage (Locking). Sometimes, testing the lateral joint play of the elbow reveals that it is impaired and very painful in some directions while free in others. This usually corresponds to a mechanical pain of the articulation; it is related to either adduction, abduction, or hyperextension. The opposite movement is usually free and painless. Most often, there is exquisite pain on palpation of the radiohumeral joint line. This lateral epicondylar pain often starts rapidly during a certain movement.

Frequently, an appropriate manipulation or a series of mobilizations performed in the pain-free direction, sometimes with intra-articular

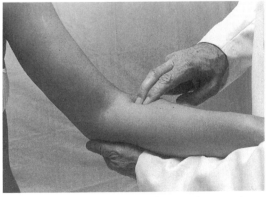

Figure 54.6.   Palpation of supinator trigger points.

injection, relieves the patient. Does this "radiohumeral disturbance" (Maigne, 1959) correspond to the impingement of a synovial fringe or a fragment of the radiohumeral pseudomeniscus? Both have been found in surgical interventions. In 1959, De Goes opted for the pseudomeniscus, and Benassy had operative findings suggesting the same thing. In other cases, chondromalacia lesions of the radial head have been found.

A test that we trust seems to confirm the existence of an intra-articular factor: the transient disappearance of pain after the intra-articular injection of local anesthetic. In chronic cases, there is an associated periarticular reaction, resulting in restricted elbow range of motion with pain increasing markedly in a given direction. This can be tested by oscillating the joint at end range in all directions. In our experience, a radiohumeral origin accounts for 8% of all the lateral epicondylalgias.

Treatment. In acute cases, manipulation of the elbow is often useful. The technique to be used depends on the type of blockage. The rule of no pain always determines which manipulation can or should be used. In chronic cases, it has to be performed progressively and, in some cases, may require an intra-articular injection of corticosteroid and anesthetics prior to manipulation.

MANIPULATION IN ADDUCTION. These techniques are used when there is a blockage in abduction, which is the most frequent (Fig. 54.7).

First technique. The patient's forearm is positioned in extension and full supination. The operator grasps the patient's wrist with the opposite hand (operator's left hand for the patient's right and vice versa) and grasps the medial elbow with the other hand, keeping the forearm perpendicular to the patient's arm. Manipulation consists of a brief thrust that exaggerates elbow adduction, following several maneuvers that take up the slack.

Second technique. The operator is on the right side of the patient (for a right elbow). The elbow is extended, with the forearm in supination. The examiner's left arm is flexed around the patient's elbow with the fist tightened to make that position rigid. The operator's forearm is in contact with the medial side of the patient's elbow. The operator's right hand grasps the wrist, maintained in supination. This hand will give the manipulative thrust in forced adduction (Fig. 54.8).

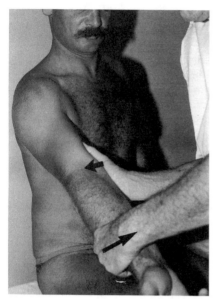

Figure 54.7. Manipulation of the elbow in adduction (first technique).

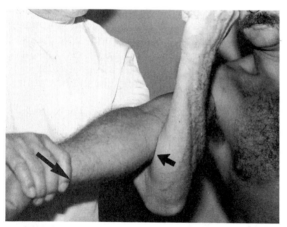

Figure 54.8. Manipulation of the elbow in adduction (second technique).

MANIPULATION IN ABDUCTION. This manipulation is the opposite of the above.

First technique. Here the right hand takes the right wrist of the patient, while the left hand grasps the lateral elbow, with the left forearm of the operator kept perpendicular to the patient's arm (Fig. 54.9).

Second technique. The operator blocks the patient's extended right elbow in the V formed by the operator's flexed right arm. The forearm is in contact with the lateral aspect of the patient's elbow. The left hand grasps the wrist,

which is maintained in supination. It gives the manipulative thrust in abduction after several maneuvers to take up the slack (Fig. 54.10).

MANIPULATION IN EXTENSION. This manipulation is performed in anterior or anterolateral blockage of the radiohumeral joint (Fig. 54.11). The forearm of the patient is extended and su-

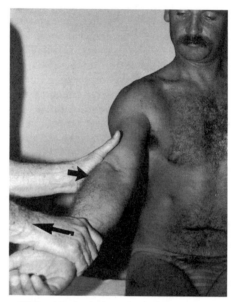

Figure 54.9. Manipulation of the elbow in abduction (first technique).

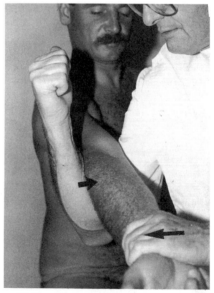

Figure 54.10. Manipulation of the elbow in abduction (second technique).

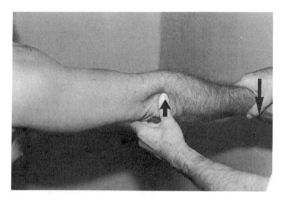

Figure 54.11. Manipulation of the elbow in extension.

pinated; the thumb applies pressure to the posterior radial head, while the operator exaggerates the extension of the elbow with a brief push on the wrist.

MANIPULATION IN PRONATION (FIG. 54.12). The patient's arm is extended. The physician's right hand grasps the right wrist of the patient

in forced pronation. The elbow is held by the operator's left hand, with the thumb against the posterior radial head. The maneuver consists of inducing a hyperextension and forced pronation of the patient's elbow while the thumb keeps the pressure against the radial head. Then, while maintaining this pressure, the elbow is brought back slowly to the starting position. This maneuver is performed several times, progressively.

MANIPULATION IN FLEXION-SUPINATION (FIG. 54.13). This maneuver is used in the "pediatric pulled elbow child," but it can also be applied to certain epicondylalgias of the adult. The pediatric pulled elbow is generally caused when the child is lifted up by pulling the hand to go up a sidewalk or stairway. The operator supports the patient's elbow with the right hand and presses with the right thumb on the anterior part of the radial head. The operator grasps the patient's wrist with the left hand, the thumb pressing on the back of the patient's hand. A strong traction is then applied on the forearm, and while maintaining the wrist in su-

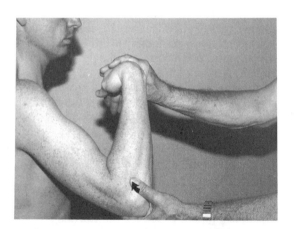

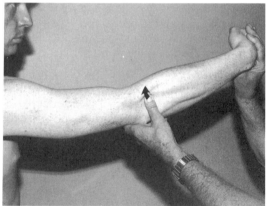

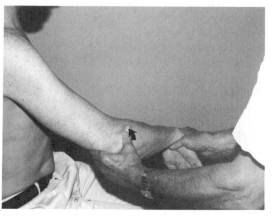

Figure 54.12. Three phases of the manipulation of the elbow in pronation. This is actually more of a mobilization, because the movement performed is repeated several times.

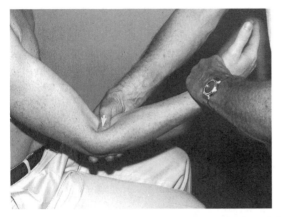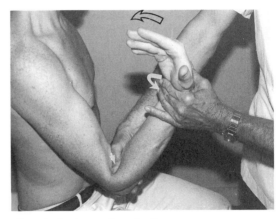

Figure 54.13.   Manipulation of the elbow in flexion and supination.

pination, the elbow is brought in forced supination and in complete flexion. This maneuver, which is simple in the child because traction is not necessary, should usually be repeated in the adult to be useful. Its indication is rarer than that for the maneuver in pronation.

N.B. The operator can also apply pressure on the radial head with the pad of the fingers of the right hand while the left hand encloses the patient's wrist. The execution of the maneuver is the same.

Periarthritis of the Elbow. A certain number of epicondylalgias of local origin or with a cervical factor present with a global decrease in the lateral joint play of the elbow when tested by the above technique (Maigne) (Fig. 54.2). The test is a little painful, but it is perfectly free and painless on the other elbow. This seems to correspond to a periarticular reaction, which can be responsible for the persistence of pain. Indeed, in some cases, the lateral epicondylar pain is decreased by either local treatment or cervical treatment, but it disappears completely only when the lateral joint play of the elbow is reestablished.

TREATMENT. To free lateral play, we use the same maneuvers used for assessment. They are repeated progressively and insistently, 10–20 times. The periarticular reaction seems to be the consequence of an articular dysfunction caused by the lateral epicondylar pain.

Lateral Epicondylar Pain due to Compression of the Radial Nerve. Irritation of the posterior interosseous branch of the radial nerve as it passes through the two heads of the supinator into the radial tunnel can cause lateral epicondylar pain (Kopell and Thompson, 1963). It is refractory to local treatment, is often increased during the night, and can radiate toward the anterior forearm. According to Roles, the characteristic sign is the increased pain with contraction against resistance of the ECRB (resisted extension of the 3rd ray). This sign lacks specificity. Electromyography confirms the diagnosis (Roles, Bence, and Commandré).

If local injections do not bring any improvement, a surgical decompression should be considered. At surgery, a fibrous arcade is often seen (arcade of Frohse) that increases the irritation of the nerve. In pronation, the supinator is stretched and compresses the posterior interosseous branch of the radial nerve (80 of 90 cases, [Werner]). In chronic cases, lesions of the nerve are noted. Moreover, the roof of the radial tunnel is formed by the fibrous edge of the ECRB, which can be a source of irritation. In their examination of 36 cases of chronic lateral epicondylar pain, Jesel et al. showed a compression of the posterior interosseous branch of the radial nerve in 5 cases.

Local injections are the best treatment. When they fail, the patients should be considered for surgery.

Remark
In most epicondylalgias, whatever the mechanism, palpation of the epicondylar muscles reveals the presence of painful taut bands, which may have a cervical origin (cellulotenoperiosteomyalgic syndrome C6 or C7) or

which could be the result of a radiohumeral articular dysfunction or a muscular strain. Under favorable anatomic conditions, these trigger points might be able to cause a functional entrapment syndrome that could be another factor in the development of lateral epicondylar pain.

DISTAL RADIOULNAR DYSFUNCTION

Certain patients with persistent lateral epicondylar pain also have decreased passive mobility of the distal radioulnar joint. To test for this, the distal end of the radius is grasped between the examiner's thumb and index finger and the distal ulna is grasped between the thumb and index finger of the other hand while applying opposite movements from front to back, like playing the piano. Mobility is compared with that of the opposite side. This maneuver can be disagreeable on the affected side.

Treatment consists of repeating this maneuver several times and trying progressively to free the movement.

This distal radioulnar block can perpetuate a persistent lateral epicondylar pain (Fig. 54.14). In several cases, we have been able to eradicate chronic refractory epicondylalgia. The patients had no pain at the wrist, but passive movements of forced supination were painful.

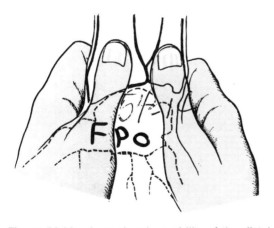

Figure 54.14.   Assessing the mobility of the distal radioulnar joint.

LATERAL EPICONDYLAR PAIN AND THE CERVICAL SPINE

Most authors agree that common lateral epicondylar pain is caused by an insertional tendinitis due to overuse of the epicondylar muscles. This opinion seems to be confirmed by the favorable results of local treatment (injections).

But in many cases, there is a cervical factor (C5-C6, C6-C7) whose treatment can also ease the lateral epicondylar pain, often immediately. This factor may precipitate and perpetuate the lateral epicondylar pain. The more prominent the cervical factor is, the more likely it is that lateral epicondylar pain will result with minimal effort or routine movements.

J. Lacapére (1950) first considered the cervical origin of lateral epicondylar pain. Renoult (1955) and Maigne (1955) found that cervical manipulation produced favorable results. A semiologic and statistical study of 150 cases (Maigne 1959) indicated that two of three cases of epicondylitis showed a variable degree of cervical participation. The mechanism can be understood in terms of a PMID and segmental vertebral cellulotenoperiosteomyalgic syndrome (Maigne). Hypersensitivity of the lateral epicondyle to palpation is common in dysfunction of the C5-C6 and C6-C7 segments. The slightest overuse can cause lateral epicondylar pain (Figs. 54.15 and 54.16).

The origin or facilitation of lateral epicondylar pain by cervical factors should be considered when the examination demonstrates ipsilateral tenderness to palpation of the C5-6 or 6-7 facet joints. Of course, it is definite if treatment produces amelioration, which is usually rapid with a manipulation. The result of each treatment can be shown by evaluation tests; it can be shown immediately with manipulation.

We drew attention a long time ago (1959) to the frequent hypersensitivity of the lateral epicondyle in patients with a segmental dysfunction of C5-C6 or C6-C7 due to a PMID or facet joint spondylosis. Recently, with J. C. Goussard, we examined patients with minor cervical pain in whom the segmental examination revealed the contribution of C5-C6 or C6-C7. None of them complained about the lateral epicondyle.

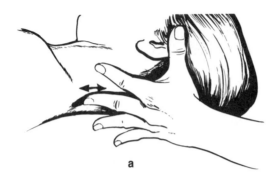
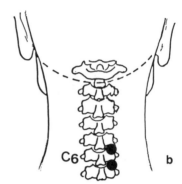

Figure 54.15. **a.** Cervical segmental examination: palpation of the facet joints. **b.** Lateral epicondylar pain can be related to dysfunction of the C5-6 or 6-7 segments, found ipsilateral to the facet joint tenderness.

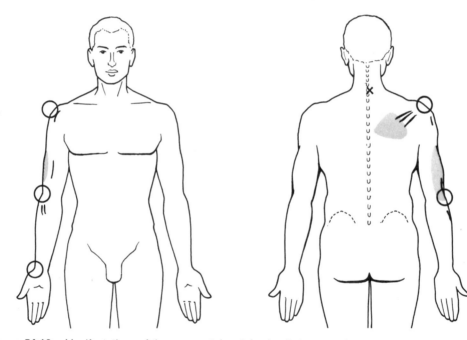

Figure 54.16. Manifestations of the segmental vertebral cellulotenoperiosteomyalgic syndrome of C6.

In 80 selected patients, the lateral epicondyle was found to be tender to palpation, and in 53 cases, it was ipsilateral to the facet joint tenderness and painless on the other side. In a control group of 40 patients with no cervical signs on examination, the lateral epicondyle was painful in only 3.

In patients with cervical signs, the examination frequently showed some manifestations of the segmental C6 or C7 cellulotenoperiosteomyalgic syndrome. In an unpublished study, we found the same results in patients with no cervical pain but whose routine examination also showed a latent PMID at C5-C6 or C6-C7. American osteopaths have studied the origin of some lateral epicondylar pains. However, Steiner (1976), in an article published in the *Journal of the American Osteopathic Association*, wrote about all the pathogeneses that have been proposed for lateral epicondylar pain without mentioning the cervical causes.

Certain authors, with the help of electromyographic examination, have looked for evidence of neural dysfunction in the C6 or C7 territory to invalidate or confirm the cervical thesis of diverse epicondylalgias: Illouz and

Limon (1974) and Bence et al. (1978). In 40% of cases, the latter found a narrow relationship between lateral epicondylar pain and cervical radiculopathy.

The Canadians Gunn and Milbrandt suggest a cervical origin in 42 patients with lateral epicondylar pains that were resistant to local treatment (1976). In an electromyographic study involving 36 patients with refractory epicondylalgias, Jesel et al. (1986) found that 8 showed evidence of nerve dysfunction from C5 to C7. A cervical spine origin is generally considered only when there are radiologic lesions of spondylosis, which prove nothing, or when there are electromyographic signs, which are very conclusive, but can only be applied to a portion of the cases. Indeed, given the present state of affairs, we cannot expect to find objective signs of neural irritation in all patients with only a PMID and reflex cellulotenoperiosteomyalgic manifestations. The following case is typical.

Case History 1. A 35-year-old woman had pain for 2 years and had to stop playing tennis (a ranked player). She had 36 consecutive local injections. She was relieved for a while in the beginning, but later the injections had no effect. Then she showed a PMID at C5-C6 on examination. After the third session of cervical manipulation, she was clearly improved and was relieved after the sixth. She then resumed her normal competition.

The following case is more interesting because the patient, after the failure of the medical treatments, had been unsuccessfully operated on and then relieved by cervical treatment:

Case History 2. A 45-year-old male manual laborer had lateral epicondylar pain for 2 years prior to being seen, which, after having been partially relieved, was refractory to medical treatments. He was operated on (lengthening of the ECRB), but the intervention did not relieve him. A few months later, he was examined in our department at Hotel Dieu. The cervical examination demonstrated a PMID at C6-C7. Three sessions of cervical manipulation relieved him completely, and he was able to resume his work.

In chronic cases, if the improvement brought by the cervical treatment is clear but incomplete, a local treatment generally acts very quickly, even if it had been ineffective before. It consists in injection of the lateral epicondyle or the trigger points and/or electrotherapy.

Treatment. The proof of the cervical origin is the success of the treatment. C5-C6 or C6-C7 facet dysfunction is usually the consequence of a PMID, but it can be due to acute synovitis. In the first case, manipulation can be used for treatment (Fig. 54.17) if there is no contraindication and if it is technically possible. In favorable cases, cervical maneuvers can result in clear improvement in the evaluation tests, sometimes even the disappearance of any pain against resistance. In persistent cases, 2–3 sessions and sometimes 5–6 sessions may be necessary.

When the articular pain does not disappear after a well-performed manipulative treatment, injection of the cervical articulation with a corticosteroid derivative is useful. This can be the first treatment if manipulation is contraindicated or in cases of synovitis. To be effective, the manipulation should be technically possible, precise, and rather forceful. Cervical electrotherapy (shortwave diathermy, ultrasound) can be useful when the above treatments cannot be used.

In chronic cases, patients often show limitation in the lateral joint play of the elbow. This should be treated by the above described mobilizations.

Surgery is reserved for cases refractory to medical treatment. They are relatively rare. Most lateral epicondylar pain resistant to classical treatment (injections) shows a cervical or articular factor, and suitable treatment relieves

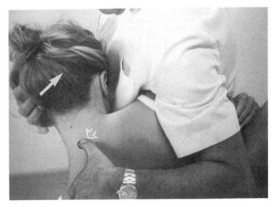

Figure 54.17. Example of a cervical manipulation in lateral flexion useful for treating an inferior cervical PMID. When the C-spine plays a role in lateral epicondylar pain, amelioration of the pain (Figs. 54.3–54.5) is often immediate after a properly performed cervical manipulation.

them. Nevertheless, in some resistant cases, relief is impossible with medical treatment, and there is no great need to defer action, especially if a simple extra-articular intervention considered. The proposed interventions are numerous. Some authors (Narakas) classify them according to the type of pain present. The principal interventions are

- Denervation of the lateral epicondyle (Kaplan, Wilhem)
- Excision of the inflamed tendinous tissue
- Tenotomy with debridement of the lateral epicondyle (Hohmann) together with an annular ligament release (Bosworth)
- Lengthening of the ECRB (Garden)

- Excision (ablation) of the pseudomeniscus or the synovial fringes (de Goes, Benassy)
- Release of the posterior interosseous branch of the radial nerve (Roles and Maudsley)

According to Saillant et al., most of the proposed techniques have a common denominator, principally the lateral epicondylar muscles. They propose systematic and complete detachment of all epicondylar muscle with (possibly, and only if clinically warranted) a radiohumeral arthrotomy. Results are good when a true entrapment syndrome of the posterior interosseous branch of the radial nerve exists (87% for Narakas) and a little poorer in other cases.

55

MEDIAL EPICONDYLAR PAIN

Medial epicondylar pain is much less frequent than lateral epicondylar pain. In fact, on examination, palpation often demonstrates a particular sensitivity of the medial epicondyle, while the patient has no spontaneous pain. It is generally caused by repetitive activity of the forearm in flexion and in pronation. It is frequent in manual therapists.

Often, it is noticed only when the patient leans on a table with the elbows apart; the medial epicondyles are then directly in contact with the table and become very painful. At the next level of activity, the patient complains of pain over the medial elbow, increased with exertion, especially by movements such as the forceful shaking of hands in flexion and pronation of the forearm.

A cervical element may exist, which facilitates it (a PMID C7-T1). In those cases, the neck should then be treated. Local injection is performed in the same manner as for lateral epicondylalgias. Frequently, injection of trigger points found in the body of some epitrochlear muscles is more useful if it is combined with the stretching of these muscles.

Rest is necessary in difficult cases. Patients at risk for developing this condition should be instructed in stretching techniques for the common flexor muscles that originate from the medial epicondyle: with the elbow extended, the wrist and fingers are extended with the palm and fingertips pressed on a table, for example, to increase the stretching.

PUBIC PAIN AND SPINAL FACTORS

Pubic pain, or pubalgia, is currently common because it frequently strikes athletes, especially tennis and soccer players. This pain is due to mechanical stresses peculiar to these sports, which affect the pubis. They are promoted by some morphologies (hyperlordosis and anteversion of the pelvis) associated with abdominal insufficiency. Some authors (Durey) think that overtraining can also be a cause. Pain in the pubis is generally attributed to

- Arthropathy of the symphysis (osteitis pubis)
- Tendinitis of the adductors
- Tendinitis of the abdominal muscles

Arthropathy of the symphysis is associated with lesions that progressively worsen and are classified in four stages (Luschnitz). After the initial period, there is a period of a progressive healing that lasts several years. The painful period lasts only a few months and responds well to rest and anti-inflammatory medications. However, similar radiologic abnormalities can be found in individuals who do not complain of pain.

THEORIES

Nesovic Theory

According to Nesovic, the essential cause of pubalgia is a musculoaponeurotic disequilibrium between weak abdominal muscles and hypertonic adductors. It is common, particularly in pubalgic soccer players, to see a dehiscence of the obliquus superior in a prehernial state and pain in the internal opening of the inguinal tunnel.

The Nesovic procedure consists of putting the large muscles of the abdomen in tension.

It is indicated in patients who are not relieved by medical treatment that usually consists of rest, injection, physiotherapy, and therapeutic exercise.

Spinal Factor (Maigne)

Nesovic's theory describes well the local conditions that can promote and result in the decompensation that maintains the pubic pain. But our observations indicate that another factor affects the pubalgia and is probably the first to appear—the spinal factor. Thus we would add to Nesovic's theory a "reflex spinal" origin of pubalgia (Maigne, 1981).

We had noticed that pain on palpation of the hemipubis is found in one-third of patients with a PMID of the thoracolumbar junction (T11-T12, T12-L1) (Fig. 56.1). The affected hemipubis is ipsilateral to the articular pain of the PMID. In chronic cases, the condition may become bilateral (see Chapter 60, "Thoracolumbar Junction Syndrome"). These patients are usually unaware of having pubic sensitivity, and they are very surprised when it is discovered at the insertion of the rectus abdominis muscle or on the whole surface of the bone (Fig. 56.2). Frequently, a cellulalgic zone painful to pinch-rolling is detected on examination, overlying the ipsilateral groin and superomedial thigh. Sometimes, one or two small trigger points are found in the inferior aspect of the rectus abdominis, which are very painful to palpation (Fig. 56.3).

Most of these patients will never experience pain in the pubis. They usually complain of low back pain or abdominal pain, which are the most frequent manifestations of the thoracolumbar junction syndrome. But if the patient with a "sensitized" pubis subjects the muscles

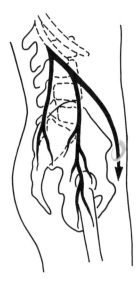

Figure 56.1. Sketch of the territory of the posterior and anterior rami of T12 and L1, including the lateral cutaneous branch that arises from the anterior ramus.

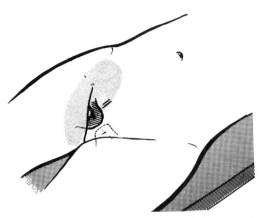

Figure 56.3. The anterior cellulotenoperiosteomyalgic manifestations are related to segmental dysfunction of the thoracolumbar junction: zone of cellulalgia, trigger points of the rectus abdominis, and hemipubic tenderness to palpation (seen in one-third of cases).

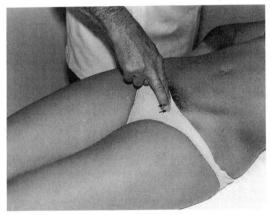

Figure 56.2. The hemipubis is tender to friction-rubbing in one-third of cases of thoracolumbar junction syndrome (PMID at T11-12, T12-L1). This is a facilitating factor for pubalgia.

that are inserted on it to excessive use, they will reproduce the pubic pain and periosteal tenderness during a sudden movement or physical effort.

Soccer players frequently strike the ball with the trunk in extension. This imparts a strong rotatory torque to the thoracolumbar junction. Indeed, rotation at the lumbar spine, which is minimal under normal circumstances in neutral position, becomes impossible in ex-

tension because of the locking of the facet joints.

At the onset of this condition, spinal treatment suffices to bring relief. In our first publication, we successfully treated a number of diverse patients with pubalgia, including a few soccer players. After that, Zimmermann, one of our students, conducted a study on soccer players.

Zimmermann, himself a soccer player, had followed several soccer teams regularly for many years as a consulting physician, including teams of young players. His findings confirmed our hypothesis; he even found a spinal factor at the thoracolumbar junction in all pubalgic patients. For the last 6 years, no player on the teams he took care of had to be operated on for pubalgia, thanks to prevention based on systematic spinal and pubic examination and to the spinal treatment used as soon as the first signs of thoracolumbar PMID were noted.

This very interesting experiment should be developed. But it demands a high quality segmental examination—which is not as simple as it seems if one is not used to that type of examination—and extensive experience in manipulative treatment. If it is done inexpertly, the results can be very poor. A. Gourjon noticed the same things and relates the following amusing observation (personal communication).

Case History. X., a 24-year-old rugby player, had head trauma and loss of memory following a motor vehicle accident. After hospitalization for a few days, he left the hospital complaining of pain in the groin. Radiographs revealed a pubic diastasis. He was treated with six local injections, bed rest, and electrotherapy but was not relieved. Two months later, radiographs were repeated, and osteophytes were noted on the symphysis pubis. Pain continued to increase, and surgery was proposed. The patient then consulted Dr. A. G., who noticed a typical thoracolumbar junction syndrome on the side of the pubalgia, with a PMID at T12-L1. A facet joint injection was performed at this level, and the patient was able to spread his thigh without pain. Three manipulations at the thoracolumbar junction brought total relief, and the patient was able to resume rugby. Seen again 1 year later, he did not suffer anymore, and the radiologic image was unchanged. This does not imply that all pubalgias are of spinal origin. However, the spinal factor should be considered in the diagnosis and treatment of pubic pain.

CLINICAL STAGES OF PUBIC PAIN WITH SPINAL FACILITATION

Zimmermann has classified the clinical stages of pubic pain with spinal facilitation into four stages.

Stage I

In the subclinical stage, there is no spontaneous pain, but palpation reveals hypersensitivity of the pubis on one side. There is often a discrete, intermittent, well-tolerated low back pain. In all cases, thoracolumbar examination reveals dysfunction of the thoracolumbar junction, in the form of a PMID affecting one or two segments. The affected hemipubis is on the side of the facet joint tenderness.

Stage II

The patient complains of unilateral pubic pain that occurs after prolonged physical exertion, usually not severe enough to restrict the activities. Low back pain is constant but often unrecognized, mildly inconvenient, and considered by the patient to be a minor problem.

Stage III

Pubic pain is confirmed and is diffuse and bilateral. Pain on exertion is increased and

may bring a temporary halt to competition. There is a specific sign: the patient finds that sitting while resting on both hands is particularly painful, if not impossible. Low back pain is more pronounced, with pains projected to the muscles of the legs (quadriceps, hamstrings, calves).

Stage IV

The pain is sufficiently severe to make participation in athletic activities impossible. All tests are painful, and there is always weakness of the abdominal obliquus muscles, with pain and widening of the inguinal ring, sign of Malgaigne, etc.

Zimmerman also noted that at stages I and II, spinal perturbations are occasionally located at the thoracolumbar junction and on one or two intervertebral segments, generally T11-T12 or T12-L1. The cellulotenoperiosteomyalgic syndrome is usually well represented and localized to the territory of the posterior or anterior rami of the corresponding spinal nerve root.

During stages III and IV, the spinal dysfunction reaches the subjacent lumbar and intervertebral segments, resulting in dysfunction in the region of L3-L4. This explains the pain referral to the anteromedial thighs that is frequently observed. At the back, a cellulalgic zone of the entire lumbosacral region is seen, but the mobility of the spine remains normal.

TREATMENT

Stage I

In most cases, it is sufficient to treat the thoracolumbar PMID or PMIDs and the related possible cellulalgic manifestations. Activities that involve significant spinal rotation must be limited, and the abdominal muscle balance must be restored.

Stage II

Spinal treatment is by manipulation, combined if necessary with thoracolumbar facet injections and local treatment of the cellulomyalgic manifestations that persist after the spinal treatment. Abstinence from competition or sport is not compulsory. The player is relieved in less than 6 weeks.

Stage III

Same treatment as above, but competition must stop for 2 months.

Stage IV

Surgical intervention is required. This stage should be seen rarely. Nesovic's technique is used most commonly. It strengthens and short-ens the obliquus muscles to rebalance the forces that act on the pubis; but it may also denervate the pubic region.

N.B. Pubic pain or tendinitis of the rectus abdominis muscle can be caused or precipitated by a spinal factor (PMID of the thoracolumbar junction) (Maigne). This concept is of therapeutic interest because spinal treatment at the first stage can suffice to relieve the patient, and at a more advanced stage, it can contribute to the cure. It also has a preventive effect. Supervision of the spine should help to avoid a certain number of pubalgias.

FALSE HIP PAIN OF SPINAL ORIGIN

Certain pain syndromes of spinal origin can mimic hip pain. The pain is felt over the lateral aspect of the hip, sometimes with pain in the groin and in the buttocks. Mobility of the hip is normal; extreme movements are sometimes slightly limited and painful. This picture resembles periarthritis of the hip, especially when the palpation of the trochanter is painful (Fig. 57.1), but local injections have no effect or (sometimes) act only briefly.

This false pain of the hip can have *two origins*. Examination shows a different picture in each of these cases.

- Tendinitis of the gluteus medius with periosteal sensitivity of the trochanter in relation to an L5 cellulotenoperiosteomyalgic syndrome

- Cellulalgia (producing pain that feels deep) related to the thoracolumbar junction syndrome, with involvement of the iliohypogastric nerve (L1) or subcostal nerve (T12) lateral perforating branches; the nerves are usually found to be subject to entrapment as they cross over the iliac crest (R. and J. Y. Maigne).

TROCHANTERIC PAIN AND THE L5 SEGMENTAL VERTEBRAL SYNDROME (Fig. 57.2)

Pain on palpation of the greater trochanter and trigger points in the gluteus medius is regular when the L4-5 segment pain is due to a PMID, a herniated disk, or facet joint synovi-

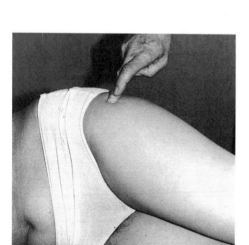

Figure 57.1. Pressure over the greater trochanter is painful. This can be due to a painful trochanter or a tendinobursitis of the gluteus medius. It can also represent pain due to a painful cellulalgic zone compressed between the examiner's finger and the trochanter.

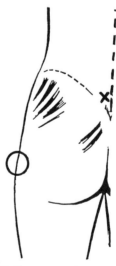

Figure 57.2. Cellulotenoperiosteomyalgic L5 syndrome consists of taut bands in the gluteus medius and hypersensitivity of the trochanter to palpation.

tis. Generally, the picture is that of hip periarthritis. Injection of the trochanter or the trigger points of the gluteus medius can relieve the patient if the spinal factor that is responsible is sufficiently decreased, but there is recurrence. If segmental spinal pain persists, only spinal treatment can bring lasting relief.

FALSE HIP PAIN AND THE T12-L1 SEGMENTAL VERTEBRAL SYNDROME

False hip pain can be caused by irritation of the lateral perforating branches coming from the subcostal (T12) or iliohypogastric nerve (L1) (Fig. 57.3a). Irritation of the latter can be part of the thoracolumbar junction syndrome (see Chapter 60), be due to entrapment at the iliac crest, or be of mixed origin.

In the thoracolumbar junction syndrome, the picture may include pain in the buttock and the groin.

Generally, periarthritis of the hip is diagnosed. The trochanter seems tender to palpation, but injections have no effect, even temporarily. In fact, the trochanter is not painful, but the subcutaneous tissues pressed against it at the hip are (Fig. 57.3b). External rotation of the hip can be impaired in severe cases, but it disappears quickly after a spinal treatment.

ENTRAPMENT SYNDROMES OF THE PERFORATING CUTANEOUS BRANCHES OF T12 AND L1

The picture is the same as above, but there is no spinal factor. Branches of the subcostal or iliohypogastric nerve can be entrapped at the iliac crest and show the same symptomatology (R. and J. Y. Maigne) (see Chapter 47). It is common to find some mixed pictures in which the spinal factor is associated with a local factor.

TOTAL HIP ARTHROPLASTY AND FALSE HIP PAIN

These falsely localizing pains are seen particularly in patients with a total hip arthro-

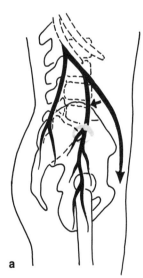

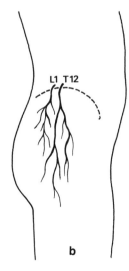

Figure 57.3. **a.** Diagram of the posterior and anterior branches of T12 and L1 with the perforating branches (*circled* in one, and on the other in *gray*). **b.** Lateral cutaneous perforating branches of the subcostal nerve (T12) and of the iliohypogastric nerve (L1). The pain can be projected toward territory beyond the thoracolumbar junction (R. Maigne). It can also be involved in an entrapment syndrome at the iliac crest (R. and J. Y. Maigne).

plasty. Chronic pain often occurs, even when the technical result of the operation is good and there is no infection or technical problem with the joint. When they recover mobility of the hip, these patients modify their usual postures and gestures because of the pain. Generally, in older patients, the spine does not adapt well to the new constraints; thus, dysfunction of the thoracolumbar junction is frequently seen together with pain referred to the trochanter and groin simulating pain arising from the joint (see Chapter 60).

KNEE PAIN OF SPINAL ORIGIN

Certain pain syndromes of the knee seem to be due to tendinitis, cruciate ligament sprains, or meniscal blockage or be atypical, which can originate at the T12 level of the lumbar spine. These pains are related to the cellulotenoperiosteomyalgic manifestations of L3 or L4 origin (Fig. 58.1).

EXAMINATION

The segmental examination reveals pain at the L2-L3 or L3-L4 level. Some patients report having had a femoral neuralgia in the past, but usually no previous history is noted. Often, there is cellulalgia over the medial aspect of

the knee (L4) (Fig. 58.2), tenoperiosteal tenderness of the superior medial aspect of the tibia (Fig. 58.3), and trigger points of the vastus

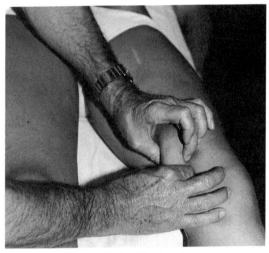

Figure 58.2. Pinch-roll test.

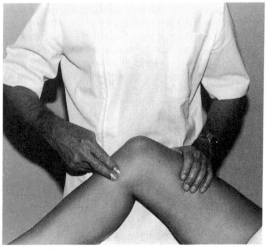

Figure 58.3. Palpation for tenoperiosteal tenderness.

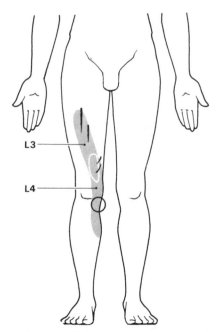

L3

L4

Figure 58.1. Cellulotenoperiosteomyalgic syndrome of L3 and L4.

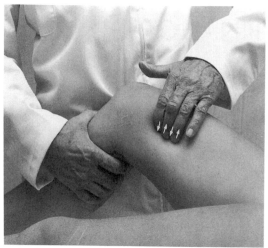

Figure 58.4. Palpation of trigger points of the vastus medialis.

medialis (L3, L4) (Fig. 58.4). A minimal entrapment syndrome affecting the saphenous nerve seems to occasionally exacerbate the cellulalgic manifestations.

CLINICAL PICTURE

Cellulalgia of L3 or L4

The observation of this young classical dancer is typical.

Case History. A. C., 24 years old, had been complaining of pain in the right knee for the previous 3 months. She was able to do all the dancing exercises, but especially when she was tired or stretching, she felt a diffuse, poorly localized pain at the anteromedial region of the knee. She was examined several times by different specialists. A sensitivity of the pes anserinus tendon was found; two injections did not result in any change. On the other hand, the knee was strictly normal. When we examined her, we found the same thing. We performed the pinch-roll test of the skin and noticed that the pes anserinus ligament was not sensitive, but a sensitive cellulalgic zone overlying the ligament covered an area as large as the palm of the hand. The pinch-roll test was very painful at that level and painless on the other knee. The skin was thickened and lumpy.

The segmental examination demonstrated L3-4 segmental dysfunction; spinal radiographs were normal. Three lumbar manipulations were performed on the affected segment, and the pain disappeared. The cellulalgia decreased. After two local injections with dilute local anesthetic, followed immediately by a brief kneading massage on the affected tissues, the pain completely disappeared. She complained only of a few episodes of low back pain, causing little inconvenience, which disappeared after the spinal treatment.

Tenoperiosteal Tenderness (L4)

Tenoperiosteal tenderness is easily confused with pes anserinus bursitis, but it does not respond well to local injection. On the other hand, it is generally relieved by spinal treatment (L4). It can be associated with cellulalgia.

Trigger Points of the Vastus Medialis and Pseudoblockage of the Knee

The patient complains of pain localized to the medial knee, which increases with walking and prevents running. Sometimes a real blockage limits the total extension of the leg, simulating a blockage of the meniscus, which (amazingly) can yield immediately after a lumbar manipulation. Injection of local anesthetic into the trigger point of the vastus medialis can have the same effect, but is often transient.

Case History. L., 24 years old, while running 6 months prior, felt pain on the medial side of the left knee and limped for a few days. It recurred several times during diverse activities until the day 2 months prior when the pain became sharper, making stretching the knee impossible. A meniscal lesion was suspected, but arthroscopy was normal. Injections, electrotherapy, and massages did not result in any relief. When examined, an extension lag was noticed, and any attempt to force it was very painful. There was no joint line tenderness, and a negative Apply's grind test. Palpation of the vastus medialis was painful and revealed a hypersensitive trigger point. Spinal examination revealed segmental pain at L3-L4; the radiograph was normal. A referred pain of spinal origin was suspected and was confirmed by a lumbar manipulation that brought rapid clear relief. After the second session, the patient could jump, run, and extend the knee against resistance without pain. One year later, there had been no recurrence.

Such cases are not rare. Recurrence can occur following exertion or a false lumbar movement. This is not too frequent in our experience.

Entrapment Syndrome of the Saphenous Nerve

The saphenous nerve can be entrapped in its course where it crosses Hunter's canal. The patient feels a diffuse pain in the medial region of the knee. Initially some discomfort while running may be felt, then walking becomes very difficult. To decrease pain, the patient starts to walk with the knee partially flexed and with the foot equinus. Pain increases with hyperextension of the hip. It is exacerbated with pressure over the nerve at about four fingerbreadths above the medial condyle, at the anterior edge of the sartorius muscle. Treatment can consist of injection of the point with local anesthetic mixed with corticosteroids. In severe cases, the nerve must be "released" surgically.

The nerve can also be entrapped at the medial aspect of the leg by the saphenous vein, usually in women with a history of thrombophlebitis. In certain cases, there can be two origins: an entrapment syndrome and a spinal problem at L3-L4, each one contributing in variable proportion.

Case History.   M. C., 25 years old, complained of pain in the medial knee for about a year. She was able to run and even to walk quickly. The knee was examined several times. Arthroscopy was normal, and nothing could explain her discomfort. When examined in the department, there was significant cellulalgia of the medial knee and L3-4 segmental tenderness with normal radiographs. A few lumbar manipulations brought enough relief to enable her to resume playing tennis; but 8 months later, the identical pain reappeared, with the same cellulitic infiltrate. This time, neither pain nor infiltrate yielded to spinal treatment. However, injection of the saphenous nerve resulted in temporary relief. The diagnosis of an entrapment syndrome was made. The patient was completely relieved by surgical release of the entrapment in Hunter's canal.

This observation shows that certain false knee pains can have a dual origin, spinal and local entrapment. When the entrapment is mild, the spinal treatment suffices. At the next stage, a few injections can be added, performed at the point of entrapment. At a more severe stage of compression, surgical intervention is indicated.

KNEE PAIN AND THE PROXIMAL TIBIOFIBULAR JOINT

The proximal tibiofibular joint only moves in relation to the subtalar joint. The presence of cartilage proves the existence of the movement. Flexion-extension at the ankle is transmitted automatically to the two tibiofibular joints. The talus is wider anteriorly than posteriorly. It is inserted like a coin in the tibiofibular notch, which it widens during dorsiflexion of the foot.

When the tibiofibular joint diverges or converges, there is a simultaneous associated axial rotation. The amplitude of movement is 30°. Simultaneously, the fibula pistons up and down, because when it diverges from the tibia, the interosseous membrane draws it upward. Conversely, it is drawn downward during ankle plantar flexion. These movements have repercussions on the proximal tibiofibular joint. During ankle dorsiflexion, the fibula slides upward; it slides downward with plantar flexion.

The joint also glides anteroposteriorly because of its orientation. Gliding backward is easier than gliding forward because the articular facet is at the back of the tibia, and its obliquity outside and backward does not facilitate gliding forward.

In the normal state, joint play is palpable. It is tested with the patient supine. The knee to be examined is flexed to 90°. The physician grasps the head of the fibula between the thumb and index finger (left hand for the right knee and vice versa) and slowly performs to-and-fro movements. It is a good idea to sit on the patient's foot to stabilize it on the table. Joint play should be compared with that of the knee on the other side (Fig. 58.5).

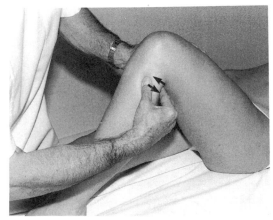

Figure 58.5.   Examination of the proximal tibiofibular joint.

Isolated dislocation or fracture-dislocation of the tibia is seen in children and adolescents (Sirbrandij). They complain that the knee hurts and that it seems to give way or that there is a "click" in the knee with a vague pain that seems to come from the knee. Since this lesion is not found in adults, it seems to improve spontaneously.

On the other hand, one can see cases in which mobility is difficult and painful in the tibiofibular joint. The pain does not occur spontaneously, but it can happen after flexion or extension. Sometimes it looks like a joint periarthritis. Pain with mobilization is often seen as a manifestation or sequela of sciatica.

Proximal Tibiofibular (PTF) Blockages

A minor mechanical dysfunction of the PTF joint can exist without radiographic abnormality, which can be considered a blockage of the fibula. It results in knee pain or, more surprisingly, pain along the instep; on examination, there is a precise tender point on the talus at the talar insertion of the anterior talofibular ligament (Maigne) (Fig. 58.6).

This pseudoblockage occurs most often after prolonged squatting, but it can also be seen in subjects who have stood on tiptoes for a long time or did series of jumps without having been trained to do so (e.g., volleyball on the beach) or after a long drive in the car, with the legs overly bent or a seat that is too soft

or too low. It is as if the joint being used in its maximal course in elevation or in lowering the head of the fibula has been blocked in that position. But the anteroposterior joint play, which is the only one that can be tested, decreases or disappears. The therapeutic maneuver should attempt to restore the anteroposterior mobility.

Proximal Tibiofibular Arthritis and Sciatica

Dysfunction of the PTF joint sometimes follows an episode of sciatica. The patient complains of lateral leg pain and instep pain, which is sometimes sharp. In some cases, the instep pain can exist alone.

Anteroposterior mobilization of the PTF joint is used to assess whether the joint play is limited or painful. Manual therapy using mobilization treatments usually produces good results, in some cases immediately. If a periarticular pain is present, one must consider the possibility that it could be part of the segmental cellulotenoperiosteomyalgic syndrome or the mechanical consequence of a gait that is altered by sciatic pain.

Treatment

Mobilization is performed exactly as in the examination. The knee is flexed to 90° and the head of the fibula is grasped between the thumb and index finger and mobilized from front to back progressively. If mobilization is

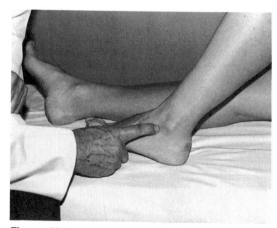

Figure 58.6. In cases of blockage of the proximal tibiofibular joint, there is often marked tenderness to palpation at the insertion of the anterior talofibular ligament.

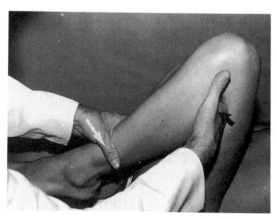

Figure 58.7. Manipulation of the proximal tibiofibular joint.

insufficient, manipulation can be performed. Depending on the case, it can be performed by pushing the fibula toward the front or the back (according to the rule of no pain and opposite movement).

First Technique (Left Leg): Leg at 90°

The right hand is placed on the popliteal surface so that the metacarpophalangeal joint of the index finger is on the head of the fibula. The left hand grasps the inferior part of the leg and progressively flexes the knee until the hand is well wedged, the support against the fibular head is firm, and there is some tension.

The manipulation is then performed with a sharp exaggeration of the left hand, which exaggerates the flexion of the knee. The head of the fibula is pushed forward with a cracking sound (Fig. 58.7).

Second Technique

The patient is supine with legs extended. The operator pushes on the fibular head with the heel of the hand applying a progressive downward pressure that is suddenly exaggerated. When these maneuvers are insufficient (which is rare), injection or electrotherapy can be used.

59

PSEUDOVISCERAL PAIN OF SPINAL ORIGIN

Certain types of pain originating in bony structures can simulate visceral pain. They often have a spinal origin, which is confirmed by the effectiveness of the spinal treatment. However, finding objective spinal manifestations does not eliminate the subjacent viscera as the painful source, because there is often an association between certain visceral conditions and a reflex cellulalgia that is painful to the pinch-roll test.

ORIGIN OF PAIN

Role of Cellulalgia

It has been known for a long time that pseudoanginal pain can be linked to cellulalgia overlying the chest wall. Laroche, Debray, and May have drawn attention to the diagnostic errors brought about by a cellulalgia of the abdominal wall.

On the other hand, the spinal origin of these cellulalgic zones is rarely considered. However, these zones are found rather frequently during systematic examinations of the chest wall. They are not always the cause of the painful symptoms, but they could become so. Nearly all belong to the cellulotenoperiosteomyalgic syndrome (Maigne), and the responsible spinal segment is demonstrated with regularity. Usually it is a PMID, but all possibilities can occur.

Frequently, a second cellulalgic zone is found in the region of the corresponding posterior ramus. These cellulalgic zones, unknown by the patient, are very painful to pinch-rolling. The pain that is elicited is curiously felt as deep pain or burnlike. Pain is generally chronic and sometimes sharp. Anesthetic injection of the affected cutaneous zone relieves them mo-

mentarily and confirms that it is not the viscera that is painful on palpation.

Trigger Points

In certain cases, small trigger points are responsible for the pseudovisceral pain. They are rather rare in the abdominal muscles but more frequent in the muscles of the thorax (pectoralis major). They can have a local origin or belong to a segmental cellulotenoperiosteomyalgic syndrome. These misleading pains can be found at all levels, but they are particularly frequent at the inferior abdominal region in the territory corresponding to the thoracolumbar junction.

THORACIC PAIN

Pseudocardiac Pain

Pseudocardiac pains are the most common pseudovisceral pain. Precordial cellulalgia, which can mimic anginal pain, can have a cervical (C4) or thoracic (T2–T5) origin (Fig. 59.1). Trigger points of the left pectoralis minor or major can also be implicated (C6–C7).

False Breast Pain

Certain pain syndromes felt as breast pain can have a spinal origin. They can be due to a cellulalgic zone but, generally, are due to trigger points of the pectoralis major or minor, which can be of spinal or local origin (overwork of the muscle) (Fig. 59.2).

Pseudopleuropulmonary Pain

Pseudopulmonary pain can be simulated by interscapular pain of cervical origin (see Chap-

generally due to a very localized cellulalgia, which can be misleading because during the abdominal palpation, the cellulalgic skin is compressed between the hand of the operator and the subjacent viscera, so that the pain seems to come from those viscera (Figs. 59.3 and 59.4).

Abdominal pain can be minor, intermittent, barely noticeable, or blamed for minor gastrointestinal or gynecologic problems. It can also be chronic and tenacious as well as distressing and alarming because no cause is found during the multiple necessary examinations. In some cases, the presentation is acute, simulating a surgical emergency.

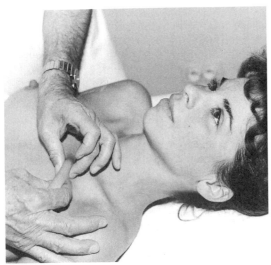

Figure 59.1. Precordial cellulalgia (which is often of spinal origin) can mimic pain of cardiac origin.

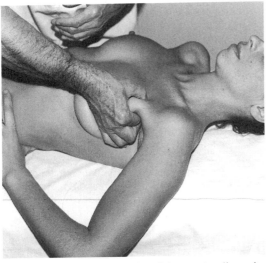

Figure 59.2. A trigger point of the pectoralis major can be responsible for falsely localized chest pain.

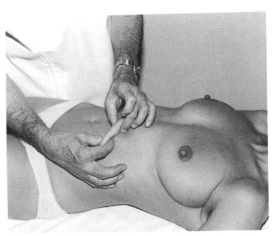

Figure 59.3. Abdominal cellulalgia of spinal origin can produce a sense of profound pseudovisceral pain, which can be misleading.

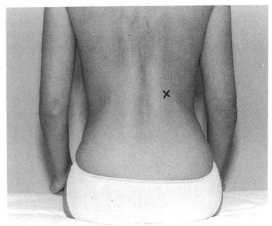

Figure 59.4. A myalgic pain along the border of the erector spinae can produce abdominal or low back pain.

ter 36, "Chronic Thoracic Pain"), which is sometimes felt as an intrathoracic pain and is increased by deep breathing or by trigger points of the iliocostalis muscle.

ABDOMINAL PAIN

Cellulalgia, usually of spinal origin, can simulate gastrointestinal, urologic, testicular, and (especially) gynecologic pain. At the abdominal level, these pseudovisceral pains are

These abdominal pains can be seen at all levels of the abdomen, but they are particularly frequent in the lower quadrants supplied by T12 and L1. They are then part of the thoracolumbar junction syndrome of Maigne (see Chapter 60). The observations below will show more clearly what we mean.

Pseudogastrointestinal Pain

The following case is a good example of a pseudogastrointestinal pain syndrome.

Case History. A 67-year-old man had suffered for the past 35 years from refractory epigastric pain occurring without any cause. During certain particularly painful attacks, he had to interrupt any activity and lie down. He had found that using hot water bottles shortened and notably decreased these attacks. The many investigations done over these years had always been negative. In fact, he had right epigastric cellulalgia linked to a PMID T7. Several spinal treatments brought total relief.

Cellulalgic zones linked to PMIDs can simulate pain of the entire digestive system. They are common in the epigastric region and subcostal zones, but they are more frequent at the inferior part of the abdomen (thoracolumbar junction syndrome).

Pain Can Be Moderate and Episodic. In these cases, they do not result in anxiety or in visits to physicians looking for a diagnosis.

Pain Can Be More Severe and More Tenacious. These pains can lead to distressing situations for the patient and difficulty for the physician, as can be seen in the following observation.

Case History. M. X., 50 years old, complained of a left-sided abdominal pain, which was low, dull, continuous, and soothed by bed rest. The intensity of this pain (which lasted for a year) led to several hospitalizations in such specialized departments as urology, gastroenterology, and rheumatology; all investigations were negative.

This persisted until, during a new hospitalization, gastrointestinal radiologic examinations led to the suspicion that there was a carcinoid tumor of the small intestine. After a mesenteric arteriography and other intestinal imaging studies, this diagnosis was discarded. He was transferred to the department of neurology, where he underwent the usual examinations, including myelography, which was normal. A lymphangiogram and a laparoscopy were also negative. The psychiatrist found the patient somewhat depressed (!) and prescribed a treatment that was not well tolerated and was quickly stopped.

All this lasted a year; then his own physician, suspecting a spinal origin, sent him to us. Examination of the abdominal subcutaneous tissues revealed a very painful zone of cellulalgia in the region of the iliac fossa and the left groin. The ipsilateral pubis was painful to palpation. The lumbar examination revealed a "crestal point" on the left and gluteal cellulalgia. The patient also complained of low back pain, but he believed it was radiating abdominal pain. Segmental examination showed pain at T12-L1. The radiographic examination was unremarkable. A PMID at T12-L1 was diagnosed.

After the first manipulation, he was relieved. After the second, palpation of the cellulalgic zone was less painful. After the third, he had no further pain. After a few sessions of massage the residual cellulalgia disappeared. Seen 2 years later because of moderate recurrence of the low back pain, he declared that he had no more abdominal pain.

Acute Pain

Acute pain can lead to useless interventions.

Case History. M. C., 38 years old, was an avid cyclist, who would frequently take long rides during his leisure time. One day, during a strenuous workout, he felt a very sharp pain in the right inferior abdominal region and had to stop. With difficulty, he arrived at a neighboring town and went directly to the hospital emergency department. The diagnosis of acute appendicitis was made. He underwent a laparotomy, but the appendix was normal. Pain decreased over the following days. From time to time afterward, he felt a disagreeable sensation. Then he had another acute attack, which disappeared spontaneously. This happened several times.

Right-sided low back pain brought him for examination in our department, where the diagnosis of low back pain of T12-L1 origin was made. A cellulalgic zone sensitive to palpation, yet previously asymptomatic, was discovered over the right lower quadrant of the abdomen, which was responsible for the false appendicitis. Spinal treatment completely relieved this patient; on follow-up after 6 months, he had no further abdominal pain.

In most cases, intermittent abdominal pain is thought to be due to "irritable bowel syndrome," because these patients have flatulence with periods of constipation that also respond to spinal treatment.

Pseudogynecologic Pain

In the gynecologic domain, pain of spinal origin is particularly misleading and frequent. During the examination, the painful subcutaneous tissues are compressed between the intravaginal fingers and the adnexa. The pain that is elicited reproduces the usual pain; to both patient and physician, it seems to come from the organ that is palpated.

This pain is especially frequent at the inferior abdominal region, which is innervated by the anterior rami of T12 and L1, or the thoracolumbar junction, a zone that is subject to overuse and which is a frequent site of PMID. We have observed numerous patients who were operated upon because of sharp pain attributed to PMIDs (some histories are collected in the thesis of J. C. Goussard). Endometriosis was suspected and verified at OR, but no relief resulted from it. The pain was coming through the wall from the spine and was relieved by spinal treatment.

Case History.   Mrs. Z., 40 years old, had severe right-sided abdominal pain with each menstrual period, which increased on the second day. This started at first menstruation at the age of 14. Failure of medical treatment led to surgical intervention when she was 17. Endometriosis of the right broad ligament was detected and it was resected, but the pain was unchanged. For 10 years, other medical treatments failed. One day, exertion resulted in acute low back pain of thoracolumbar origin and abdominal pain. We examined her at that time. Her examination confirmed low back pain of thoracolumbar origin without any radiologic lesion. Her pain complaints disappeared after the first manipulation.

We saw her again 12 years later. She came to ask for pain relief "as in the past" for her "endometriosis." The pain that was attributed to this disorder had totally disappeared with the low back pain. They had reappeared acutely a few months later, after she had engaged in physical activities. First she had severe low back pain; later, the abdominal pain had reappeared with menstruation.

A manipulation done by an orthopedist had aggravated both pains. Examination revealed sensitivity to pinch-rolling over the inferior right iliac fossa, tenderness of the right hemipubis, and pain at T12 to transverse pressure from right to left. Radiographs of the spine were normal. Three manipulations again relieved the abdominal pain and the low back pain.

The point in this case history is that the abdominal pain occurred only during menstruation. The findings were similar in other patients with abdominal pain of spinal origin. Generally, the pain is more constant, with episodic attacks having no clear precipitating cause.

When the gynecologic examination is normal, it limits the value of other investigations and surgical procedures and often leads to a diagnosis of psychosomatic origin. Occasionally, the investigations discover abnormalities that mislead the gynecologist to falsely attribute causation to them, particularly if the pain is severe.

More rarely, the pain is strictly vulvovaginal, usually unilateral. The skin of the groin and the labia majora is painful to pinch-rolling, and the hemipubis is tender to palpation. It is usually due to a PMID at T12-L1 or L1-L2.

Pseudourologic Pain

Pseudourologic pains lead to fewer interventions than do the gynecologic ones, as the examinations are usually normal. They are rather frequent and may mimic renal colic and testicular pain.

Case History.   Mr. C., 42 years old, had right low back pain chronically for 15 years, with occasional periods of exacerbation. An orthopedist prescribed physical therapy, which was done for a long time with no noticeable result. Since then, he had several painful attacks of the right lumbar fossa, radiating to the right testicle. The first attack was considered to be renal colic, but the patient always pretended that it was the result of exertion in rotation. The second acute episode happened a few months later. Hospitalized in the department of urology, he had three intravenous pyelograms (IVPs), which were all normal. He was then referred to orthopedics and rheumatology.

Nothing abnormal was found that could explain these attacks. After 12 years, a particularly severe attack brought him to the urology department as an emergency. Again, the IVP was normal. He was then hospitalized under rheumatology, where two spinal injections of corticosteroid failed to relieve either the low back pain or the right testicular pain, which had persisted since the attack. A myelogram was done and was normal. The attack gradually subsided.

At the end of another acute attack, he came to us from another department of urology for his refractory right-sided low back pain and the unexplained testicular pain. On examination, he showed right low back pain of typical thoracolumbar origin, with a "crestal point," gluteal cellulalgia, and a PMID of the T12-L1 segment. There was also a cellulalgic zone above the right groin and medial side of the thigh. Pressure on the right hemipubis was painful. Radiographs showed a completely normal thoracolumbar junction.

After three manipulations, he was considerably improved. The low back and testicular pain were less intense and episodic rather than constant. A T12 facet joint injection along with an anesthetic injection of the residual cellulalgic zone ended the treatment.

These pains of spinal origin are generally unilateral, but they can be bilateral, as in the following case.

Case History.   M. T., 65 years old, was operated upon for a prostatic adenoma 2 years previously with excellent results. Since that time, he complained of bilateral testicular pain that increased with any pressure, for example, thigh adduction or crossing his legs. The urologic examination was unremarkable. His surgeon sent him to our department. He also had bilateral low back pain that had appeared soon after surgery, just as testicular pain had. The T11-T12 segment was painful with transverse pressure in both directions, and the two facet joints were painful. Palpation revealed bilateral cellulalgic bands over the inferior part of the iliac fossa, and the pubis was painful on both sides. Several radiologic examinations were normal. The result of the spinal treatment was excellent.

Sprain of the false ribs can also simulate renal pain, because it is felt in the lumbar fossa and sometimes radiates toward the groin. One of our patients was hospitalized three times and underwent five IVPs (all negative) for attacks that were attributed to renal colic. He had an unrecognized sprain of the twelfth rib.

A CASE EXAMPLE

Abdominal Pain and Lumbar Herniated Disks

Inguinal pain is often seen in sciatica. It is rarely significant, and the patient has to be questioned to have him notice it.

In certain cases, the inguinal pain can be more severe, isolated (i.e., without low back pain), or associated with sciatica, making the diagnosis difficult (Fernstrom). Halmagrand and Seror have reported a case of lumboabdominal pain, occurring with acute attacks, associated with an anterior L5-S1 herniated disk revealed by discography and cured by chemonucleolysis. An identical observation was reported by Lelong et al. These authors emphasize the importance of discography, which reproduces the usual abdominal pain.

TREATMENT

Treating the responsible PMID usually removes the pseudovisceral pain, and the cellulalgic zone disappears or decreases considerably. In certain chronic cases, the improvement obtained by spinal treatment is only partial, and an additional local treatment of the cellulalgia is necessary, such as massage or possibly local injections.

60

THORACOLUMBAR JUNCTION SYNDROME

The term *thoracolumbar junction syndrome* (TLJS) (1981) was coined to refer to all the painful manifestations, combined or isolated, that are the consequences of dysfunction of segments of the thoracolumbar junction: T12-L1 and, more rarely, T11-T12 or L1-L2 (Fig. 60.1a). The TLJS includes:

• Low back pain, the most frequent manifestation

• Lower abdominal, pseudovisceral pain

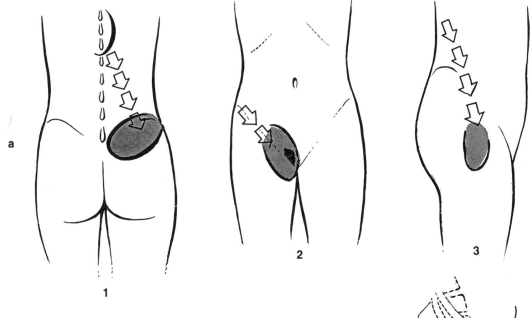

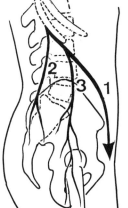

Figure 60.1. **a.** Three pain referral patterns of the thoracolumbar junction syndrome (Maigne). *1,* Posteriorly—low back pain; *2,* anteriorly—pseudovisceral pain, pubic tenderness; *3,* laterally—pseudotrochanteric pain, false meralgia paresthetica. Patients with these syndromes often do not complain of pain at the level of the thoracolumbar junction. **b.** Three branches of the divisions of the T12 and L1 spinal nerve (diagram). *1,* Anterior ramus; *2,* posterior ramus; *3,* lateral perforating branch.

- False hip pain
- Pubic tenderness
- Irritable bowel symptomatology

Pain distribution and the clinical signs found on examination correspond to the branches of the T12 and L1 spinal nerve roots (Fig. 60.1*b*). Their posterior rami innervate the superior gluteal and inferior lumbar subcutaneous tissues. Their anterior ramus innervates the inferior part of the abdomen and the groin region. A perforating lateral cutaneous branch arising from the anterior ramus innervates the trochanteric region.

Low back pain, the most frequent manifestation of the syndrome, is often the patient's only complaint. It is the topic of a special chapter (see Chapter 41) and is described with the other low back pain syndromes. When we first isolated low back pain of thoracolumbar origin (1974), we brought attention to its frequent association with abdominal pain on the same side.

TLJ ANATOMY AND PHYSIOLOGY

The lumbar spine has only a limited amount of rotation available, especially when it is in extension. On the other hand, the thoracic spine is very free in rotation. T12 (and sometimes T11) is a transitional vertebra. The TLJ is thus a zone that is particularly used in all efforts of everyday life and sports.

PHYSICAL SIGNS

Dysfunction of one or more segments of the TLJ is revealed by segmental examination. Usually, it concerns T12-L1, sometimes T11-T12 or L1-L2. Among the referred signs are

- The cellulotenoperiosteomyalgic manifestations located in the regions corresponding to one of the posterior or anterior rami or one of the lateral perforating cutaneous branches.
- Tender points palpable on the iliac crest, including, "the posterior crestal point," and the "lateral crestal point." They correspond to the site of compression of an irritated nerve branch—the posterior ramus and/or lateral perforating cutaneous branch.

Examination of the Thoracolumbar Junction

The segmental examination reveals dysfunction of only one segment in 6 of 10 cases, of two in 3 of 10 cases, and of three in 1 of 10 cases. For this examination, it is best to have the patient prone, across the table or at the end of the table (Fig. 60.2).

Segmental dysfunction is generally related to a PMID, sometimes to an episode of facet joint arthritis, and very exceptionally to discogenic pathology. Radiographic examination is usually unremarkable, but sometimes an old and unrecognized compression fracture of T12 or L1 is found. It is quite unusual for the patient to complain of pain at the level of the TLJ.

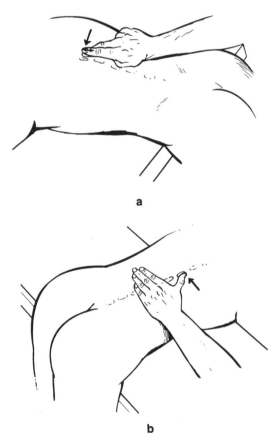

Figure 60.2. Two maneuvers that are essential in the segmental examination of the thoracolumbar region. **a.** Examination for facet joint tenderness. Generally it is unilateral, involving one or two segments. The painful manifestations are always on the painful side. **b.** Transverse pressure against the spinous process.

Cellulotenoperiosteomyalgic Manifestations

Cellulotenoperiosteomyalgic manifestations are unilateral, located ipsilateral to the facet joint tenderness. If the pain is bilateral, the manifestations are also bilateral. Cellulalgic zones are a constant finding, whereas the tenoperiosteal tenderness to palpation of the pubis is rather frequent.

Zones of cellulalgia are found uniformly in the cutaneous region of the three terminal branches of T12 and L1. The cellulalgia manifests the cutaneous territory of a single nerve or region common to two levels. This can be due to the presence of numerous anastomoses but also to the physiopathologic mechanism of the cellulalgia itself. In practice, there is usually concordance with what we know of the cutaneous distribution of these nerves.

The TLJS has two characteristics that are frequently seen in cellulotenoperiosteomyalgic manifestations:

- The spontaneous pain linked to the cellulalgia is felt by the patient as a deep intense pain, and (very exceptionally) as a superficial burnlike pain.
- These manifestations can also be found on the systematic examination when they do not cause any pain (they are then called *latent*).

In the TLJS, one can find, for example, cellulalgia simultaneously in the anterior, posterior, and lateral regions, while the patient complains only of low back or abdominal pain.

Cellulalgia

1. The posterior region corresponds to the territory of the posterior ramus, inferior lumbar and superior gluteal (Fig. 60.3), and is practically constant (97%). Only in 3 cases out of 100 was it missing.
2. The anterior region corresponds to the territory of the anterior ramus; it was found in 60% of cases: inferior abdominal region (Fig. 60.4, *top left* and *top right*) and the superomedial part of the thigh (Fig. 60.4, *top left* and *bottom right*), forming a triangle with an inferior apex with very clear limits.
3. The lateral region covers the trochanter and sometimes extends as a narrow band following the "seam of the trousers" up to the PMID thigh and even beyond (Fig. 60.5) (56% of cases). This territory corresponds to the lateral perforating cutaneous branch coming from the anterior rami of T12 and L1.

Trigger Points

Trigger points are infrequent and small. They can be found along the inferior border of the rectus abdominis muscle and occasionally in the quadratus lumborum muscle (Fig. 60.4, *top left*).

Tenoperiosteal Tenderness

Tenoperiosteal tenderness to friction-rubbing is found on the ipsilateral hemipubis,

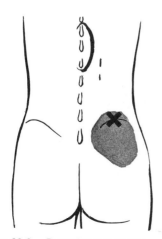 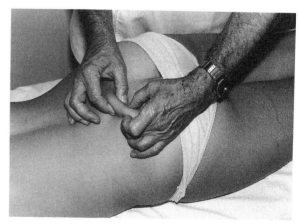

Figure 60.3. Posterior cellulalgic zone (**left**) and its examination (**right**). X, Posterior crestal point.

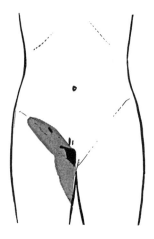

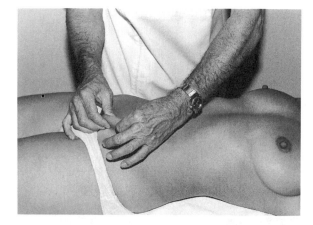

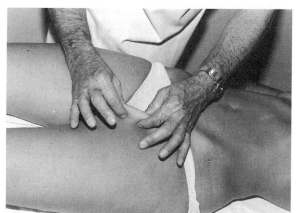

Figure 60.4. Top left. Anterior cellulalgic zone. **Top right.** Abdominal examination. **Bottom right.** Medial examination. **Top left.** Hypersensitivity of the hemi-pubis examined by friction-rubbing.

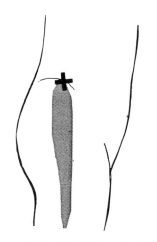

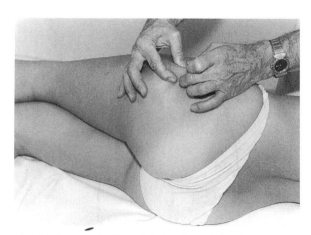

Figure 60.5. Left. Lateral cellulalgic zone. **Right.** Its examination. *X,* Lateral crestal point.

compared with the opposite side (32% of cases) (Figs. 60.4, *top left,* and 60.6).

"Crestal Points"

Painful points can be noticed on palpation of the iliac crest.

- A posterior crestal point is detected at the site of pressure by the physician's finger over the traversing posterior ramus of T12 or L1 (Fig. 60.7, *left*). It is generally located 7–8 cm lateral to the midline (see "Clinical Signs" in Chapter 41).
- A lateral crestal point, on a line passing through the trochanter, corresponds to the pressure over the lateral perforating branch of the iliohypogastric nerve (L1) or the sub-

costal nerve (T12) (Fig. 60.7, *right*). The iliac crest often has a small notch in which the first of these two rami goes (J. Y. Maigne), and which can be palpated during the clinical examination (see Chapter 47).

CLINICAL SYMPTOMS

Clinical symptoms may appear in isolation or in multiple combinations.

Low Back Pain

Low back pain of thoracolumbar origin of Maigne can be acute or chronic and is by far the most frequent manifestation (Table 60.1). It is felt in the sacroiliac or gluteal region and is often isolated or dominant. When the other symptoms (e.g., previous pains or pains of the external side of the hip) are moderate, they are generally not mentioned right away by the patient. (A detailed description of this lumbar pain is given in Chapter 41.)

Pseudovisceral Pains

Pseudovisceral pains are located at the inferior part of the abdomen and simulate gynecologic pains or low gastroenterologic, urologic, or even testicular pains. When they are the dominant pain, the patient does not report the associated moderate low back pain, which is less handicapping. These pains are misleading and often lead to consultation with a general physician, internist, or gynecologist rather

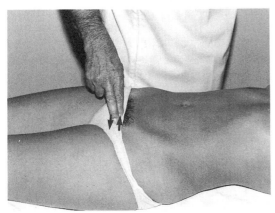

Figure 60.6. Hemipubic tenderness to friction-rub examination is found in one-third of cases.

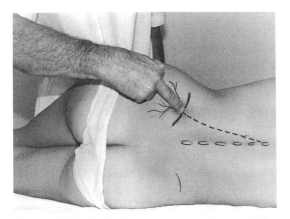

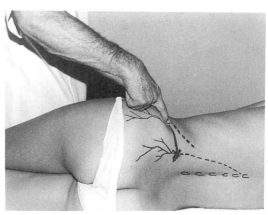

Figure 60.7. Left. Examination of the posterior crestal point where the posterior ramus crosses the iliac crest. **Right.** Examination of the lateral crestal point where the lateral perforating branch crosses over the iliac crest.

than a specialist in musculoskeletal conditions. If the pains are discrete and moderate, they are attributed to a colitis or a minor gynecologic disorder. If they are sharp and severe, diagnostic errors can be made. (They are described in Chapter 59, "Pseudovisceral Pain of Spinal Origin," where they are well demonstrated by our observations.)

False Hip Pain

Pain is localized to the lateral side of the thigh, sometimes the groin. It feels deep and is sometimes accompanied by sudden sharp stabs toward the groin during certain movements or with a sudden increase in pace while walking. It can mimic periarthritis of the hip but also can resemble a truncated sciatica or even meralgia paraesthetica. It often is exacerbated by wearing a belt or clothing that is too tight. A detailed description can be found in Chapter 47, "Perforating Branch Syndrome of T12 and L1" and Chapter 57, "False Hip Pain of Spinal Origin."

Pubic Tenderness

Pubic tenderness to palpation is frequently found in the thoracolumbar junction syndrome—up to 32% of cases. It is most often unilateral and is found only on examination. Sometimes it is only inconvenient, but it can be of prime importance, especially if the subject uses the adductor muscles or the rectus abdominis (e.g., in soccer), as both are inserted on the sensitized pubis. When the TLJ is affected, it presents a form of pubic tenderness that readily responds to treatment (see Chapter 56, "Pubic Pain and Spinal Factors").

Functional Disorders

Functional disorders show the participation of the visceral sympathetic system, but they do not have the same systematic clinical character as the manifestations discussed above. Nevertheless, in certain patients, they are sufficiently pronounced and stereotypic to be noticed, especially since they disappear with the spinal treatment. There are feelings of bloating, of abdominal meteorism, and sometimes constipation. Certain patients complain of a strong need to urinate, without any evidence of other organic lesions.

Table 60.1

	Present on Examination	Presenting Complaint
Lumbogluteal cellulgia	97	89 Lowback pain
Abdominal cellulalgia	60	16 Pseudovisceral pain
Lateral hip cellulalgia	56	14 Pseudo–hip pain
Pubic tenderness	32	4 Pubic pain

Table 60.1, based on 100 cases of TLJS that we have studied, gives the frequency of these different signs and their correlation with the patient's entrance complaint. The figures may vary depending on the patient sample. There were only 4 complaints of pubic pain among the 100 cases, probably due to the fact that the study included a number of athletes.

N.B. On examination, a patient having only low back pain may very well have a very painful abdominal cellulalgia that does not cause abdominal pain.

TREATMENT

The first treatment is spinal and is generally sufficient. Sometimes it is necessary to treat the cellulotenoperiosteomyalgic manifestations.

1. In most cases, the spinal treatment consists of mobilization and manipulation of the affected segment. Sometimes manipulation can be replaced by a facet joint injection (with corticosteroids) after the joint or joints involved are accurately located. For patients who are clearly relieved but not cured, a *percutaneous rhizotomy* should be considered. When manipulation and injection are contraindicated, electrotherapy (e.g., pulsed short wave diathermy) is very beneficial. Global treatments (e.g., anti-inflammatories, analgesics) are sometimes effective for limited periods.

2. In certain cases, local cellulomyalgic

manifestations can be treated by injections of the cellulalgic zones followed by progressive maneuvers of kneading of the cutaneous surface by pinch-rolling. Injection of anesthetic plus corticosteroids into the posterior or lateral crestal points is useful, especially when an en-trapment syndrome is present. Intervention is rarely necessary to free a later perforating branch involved in an entrapment syndrome or, rarely, a posterior ramus.

3. Therapeutic exercise is prescribed for recurrent cases. This is discussed in Chapter 41.

61

TRANSITIONAL ZONE SYNDROME

The "spinal transitional zones" are located at the junction of two adjacent spinal regions with various differences in posterior element orientation and differing degrees of mobility. There are five transitional zones (TZs), top to bottom: cervico-occipital (CO), cervicothoracic (CT), thoracolumbar (TL), and lumbosacral (LS) (Fig. 61.1). While they may differ significantly, vertebrae of the same region (cervical, thoracic, or lumbar) have common characteristics. Vertebrae of a junction or TZ have intermediate characteristics.

The cervico-occipital junction is interposed between the cervical spine, which has a very great mobility, and the occiput that it supports. The cervicothoracic junction is located between the superior thoracic spine, which has limited mobility because of the thoracic cage, and the cervical spine, which is free in all directions. The thoracolumbar junction links the lumbar spine, which has limited capacity for rotation, and the thoracic spine, where this motion is easy. The lumbosacral junction articulates the spine with the pelvis; there are considerable constraints to mobility in this zone, which explains the frequency of its mechanical pathology.

A PMID (painful minor intervertebral dysfunction) can be the source of simultaneous and diverse symptoms. The thoracolumbar junction syndrome, the topic of the preceding chapter, is a good example.

Another kind of association of symptoms and pain of spinal origin can exist. Located at different levels, but all on the same side, right or left, they are the consequence of the simultaneous presence of PMIDs localized to the transitional zones and the cellulotenoperiosteomyalgic manifestations that they develop: these are the transitional zone syndromes (Maigne). The result is a distinct clinical picture, with a curious interdependence between these PMIDs that reflects on the way they have to be treated (Fig. 61.2).

CHARACTERISTICS OF THE TRANSITIONAL ZONE SYNDROME

The TZ syndrome has distinct semiologic, clinical, and therapeutic characteristics.

Semiologic Characteristics

There is a PMID on each of the transitional zones (initially, 2 of 3). On examination, these PMIDs reveal themselves with ipsilateral facet joint tenderness, right or left. The cellulotenoperiosteomyalgic manifestations caused by these segmental dysfunctions are also unilateral and on the same side. They can be "active" (i.e., responsible for pain complaints), or they can be "latent."

Clinical Characteristics

The patient complains of pain at one or several levels: lumbar, cervical, or cephalic; usually unilateral and always on the same side. Occasionally, the pain is described as diffuse and even as bilateral although the clinical signs are unilateral. The patient may complain of only one region. Examination reveals the involvement of the other transitional zones with PMIDs and latent cellulotenoperiosteomyalgic manifestations.

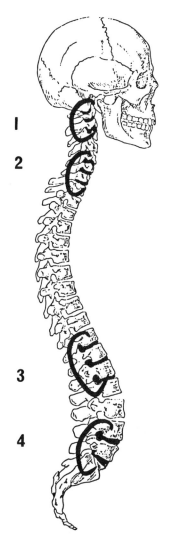

Figure 61.1.   Transitional zone. *1,* Cervico-occipital (*CO*); *2,* cervicothoracic (*CT*); *3,* thoracolumbar (*TL*); *4,* lumbosacral (*LS*).

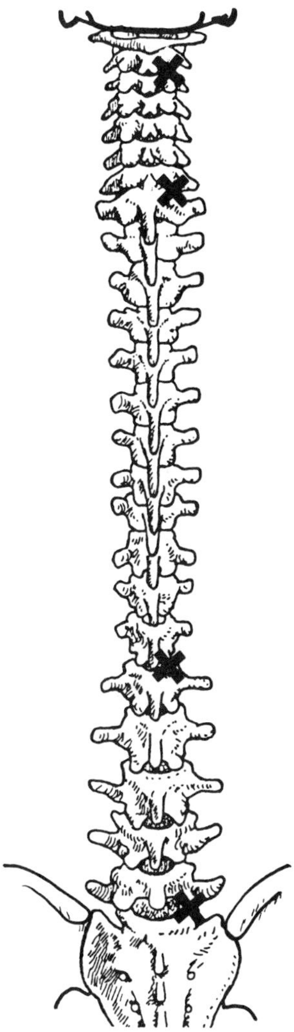

Figure 61.2. The transitional zone syndrome (Maigne) is characterized by the presence of a PMID at each level. The facet tenderness in patients with a PMID is always located on the same side.

Treatment

There seems to be true interdependence between the PMIDs of the different transitional zones. Sometimes, treating the most irritable of them causes the others to disappear as well. But, often all the PMIDs of the different transitional zones, even the latent ones, must be treated to obtain a lasting result on the one that is most inconvenient for the patient and which is often the only reason for consultation. In certain cases, it is good to treat the residual cellulotenoperiosteomyalgic manifestations locally, as well.

The patient's general condition has an important role in the expression of these common pains. Pain will persist in a subject with a low tolerance threshold, who is anxious, tired, or "spasmophilic." In such cases, the slightest perturbation may result in "acute diffuse pain," especially in a depressed patient. In these instances, psychologic treatment is necessary. Finally, when the PMIDs have been treated, and the causative factors have been recognized and corrected, therapeutic exercise will stabilize the result, and recurrences will be avoided.

PERPETUATING AND PRECIPITATING FACTORS

In refractory or recurrent cases, the perpetuating or precipitating factors must be sought. They are sometimes quite evident—compensatory postures, repetitive rotation, etc. Occasionally, none are found.

Compensatory Postures

There is a possible interrelationship between the different TZs: a static disequilibrium results in repercussions from the base to the top, and any functional perturbation of one of them has its repercussion on the others, be they super- or subjacent. The antalgic attitude of sciatica demands a compensatory adjustment from the thoracolumbar, cervicothoracic, and cervico-occipital TZs. This compensatory adjustment can be well tolerated without creating PMIDs if the junctional zones are supple and tolerant. If not, they can foster them and aggravate preexisting PMIDs.

Daily experience shows that a marked antalgic attitude is not necessary for a lumbar mechanical problem to have repercussions at a distance. A chronic low back pain can lead to functional adaptations that can persist beyond the resolution of symptoms. A patient needs horizontal vision, and any postural deviation of the trunk is compensated at the cervical or cervico-occipital level to maintain the eyes at the same level. The modifications imposed on the spine by a change in a given region, readily result in PMIDs in the transitional zones; it is different with the static problems that have existed since childhood or adolescence.

Repetitive rotation from a seated position (car, office, etc.) is an example of a typical movement expected of the cervico-occipital, cervicothoracic, and thoracolumbar junctions. In repetitive activities, the dominant side of the subject (right or left) seems sometimes to play a role. Right-handed persons who must rotate frequently to the left do it in a less coordinated manner and more awkwardly than if they were doing them from the right side and therefore more easily produce some PMIDs in the involved zones.

Postural habits play a frequent role. Sleeping on the abdomen creates excessive stress on the cervico-occipital and cervicothoracic TZs. A seat that's too low or too soft results in lumbar kyphosis and a cervical hyperlordosis.

CLINICAL PICTURE

Typical Clinical Picture

The most typical and currently the most commonly seen clinical picture of the transitional zone syndrome has the following clinical presentation:

- Supraorbital headache (cervico-occipital TZ)
- Interscapular pain (thoracocervical TZ)
- Low back pain, which can be of thoracolumbar origin (thoracolumbar TZ), lumbosacral origin (lumbosacral TZ), or both (Fig. 61.3).

These pains are all localized on the same side, right or left. Sometimes the patient notices the consistent laterality, sometimes not. Symptoms that the patient cannot analyze very well can seem confusing, ''I have the impression I am aching all over.'' But the facet joint tenderness of the responsible PMIDs and pain of the subcutaneous tissues to pinch-rolling show the usual unilaterality and the clear systematization of the symptomatology.

In certain cases, the patient complains only about one of the three symptoms: headache, thoracic pain, or lumbar pain. But a systematic examination reveals, on the other transitional zones, some latent PMIDs with the usual cellulotenoperiosteomyalgic manifestations. With excessive fatigue or for any other cause, the latent PMID and the cellulotenoperiosteomyalgic manifestations can become active.

Other Clinical Features

The association between headache and thoracic or lumbar pain on the same side is by far the most usual, as each of these manifestations is the most frequent combination for each of the corresponding TZs. Other associations are possible. There can be several symptoms for the same transitional zone; for example, low back pain and abdominal pain for the thoracolumbar junction and cervical pain and shoulder pain for the cervicothoracic junction.

During the systematic examination, it is common to see tenoperiosteal or tendinous hy-

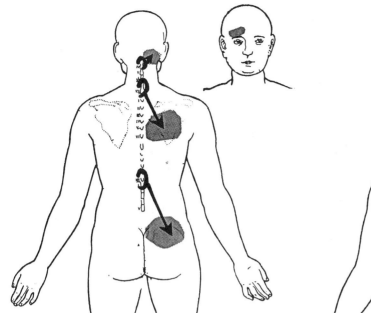

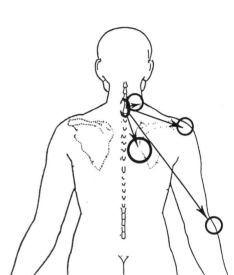

Figure 61.3. The most common form of the transitional zone syndrome is associated with a low back pain overlying the iliac crest (of thoracolumbar origin (*TL*)); interscapular pain (of cervicothoracic origin (*CT*)); and headache, usually occipitosupraorbital (of cervical occipital origin (*CO*)). They are unilateral and always located on the same side.

Figure 61.4. A C5-C6 or C6-C7 PMID is often characterized by interscapular pain. It can also produce cervical pain or pseudotendinous pain of the shoulder or elbow.

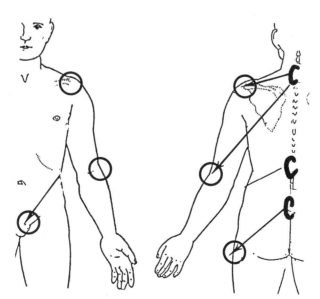

Figure 61.5. A transitional zone syndrome can present as tenoperiosteal insertional tenderness. The transitional zone PMID syndrome, be it CT, TL, or LS, is often associated with tenoperiosteal tenderness to palpation, noted at the shoulder and elbow (C6-C7), pubic region (L1, T12), and the trochanter (L5). They can be latent (not noted by the patient) but become active because of the stress of repetitive activities.

persensitivity as a consequence of a PMID localized to the TZs. With the cervicothoracic TZ, one sees pseudotendinous pain of the shoulder or hypersensitivity of the lateral epicondyle, which is found in 6 of 10 cases if the segments C5-C6 or C6-C7 are affected (Fig. 61.4). With the thoracolumbar TZ, tenderness to palpation of the hemipubis is found in one case out of three. When the lumbosacral junction is affected, the trochanter can be painful on examination if the segment L4-L5 is affected.

Usually, the subject does not get any pain spontaneously; only palpation reveals the hypersensitivity of these zones of insertion. But if repeated violent movements stress the tendons too much, the patient can easily cause a refractory pain. The simultaneous damage of the TZ in a patient who exercises excessively favors the association of these insertional pains (Fig. 61.5).

The thoracolumbar junction syndrome and the transitional zone syndrome demonstrate well the multiplicity of clinical manifestations that benign spinal dysfunction or PMIDs can produce. These syndromes also show the interrelations between the PMIDs and the cellulotenoperiosteomyalgic manifestations they produce, and they emphasize the interdependence between PMIDs located at different levels of the spine, particularly if they are at the spinal TZs.

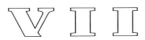

VII

MANUAL
TECHNIQUES

A1° Introduction

EQUIPMENT

For the practice of manual therapy, certain basic equipment is necessary:

- Examining/treatment table (Figs. A1.1 and A1.3).
- Stool with crossbars (Fig. A1.2)
- Firm pillow, for patient comfort
- Two or three small firm bolsters, which can be replaced by terry towels that can be folded or rolled if necessary
- For certain techniques, a wide belt of 5 × 200 cm, with Velcro closure (see Fig. A5.47).

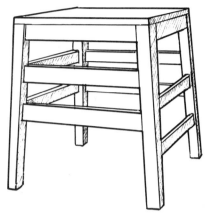

Figure A1.2. A stool is necessary for certain techniques. The stool should have bars at three levels, which can serve as support for the examiner's feet in certain maneuvers.

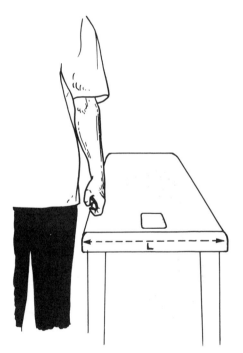

Figure A1.1. The best height for the treatment table is that which just reaches the fingers of the examiner's hands while resting at the side. It is best to have a table that can adjust to different heights to best accommodate the morphology of the patient and all techniques. It should not be too wide (about 60 cm) and should taper in width to the foot of the table, allowing the patient to sit astride without difficulty for the performance of certain techniques.

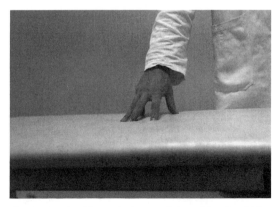

Figure A1.3. The upholstery of the table should be comfortable, but firm, with rounded edges. A hole should be provided for the patient's face (15 × 7 cm), so that the patient can lie comfortably in the prone position.

In the following chapters, we describe in detail, region by region, the techniques for soft tissue mobilization, stretching (when possible), and manipulation. Since numerous manipulative techniques are possible, we concentrate only on the indispensable techniques, which include seven basic techniques and seven accessory techniques.

BASIC MANIPULATIVE TECHNIQUES

Seven Basic Techniques

One should first learn and master the seven basic techniques of manipulation. The study of manipulation should not be started until mobilization is understood. With their variations, mobilizations can be adjusted to a great number of circumstances. All manipulative techniques make use of mobilization to "take up the slack." These seven techniques include two cervical, two thoracic, one thoracolumbar, and two lumbar.

Cervical Spine: Techniques 1 and 2

The "chin free" technique can be used at all levels of the cervical spine by varying the point of application. It is mostly a technique of rotation, but it can accommodate all combinations with lateroflexion, flexion, or extension (Fig. A1.4) (see description in Appendix A2).

The second technique is a maneuver performed in lateroflexion (Fig. A1.5). It is most often used at the cervicothoracic junction. While it can be mastered quite well in its simplest form, (pure lateroflexion), it can be combined quite easily with all the available degrees of freedom, including lateroflexion, rotation, flexion, or extension, to impart a triplanar manipulative thrust (see description in Appendix A3).

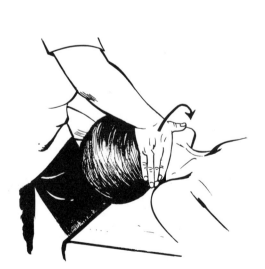

Figure A1.4. Technique 1.

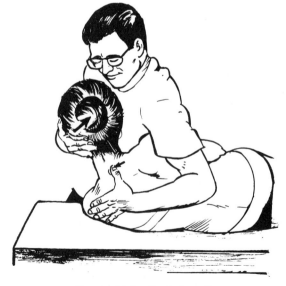

Figure A1.5. Technique 2.

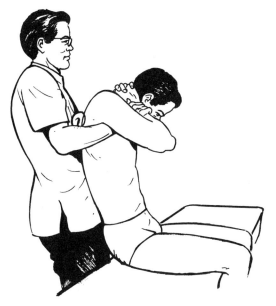

Figure A1.6. Technique 3.

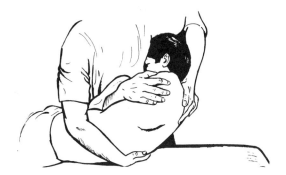

Figure A1.7. Technique 4.

Thoracic Spine: Techniques 3 and 4

The "epigastric" (Fig. A1.6) and "supine" (Fig. A1.7) techniques are the classic techniques used for the middle and inferior regions (see description in Appendix A4). Technique is performed with the patient seated, using a rolled towel or bolster as the contact point; the latter is performed in prone, with the point of contact made by the examiner's hand.

Thoracolumbar Junction: Technique 5

The "astride" technique is ideal for rotational manipulation of this region (Fig. A1.8). It allows numerous combinations with flexion, extension, and lateroflexion.

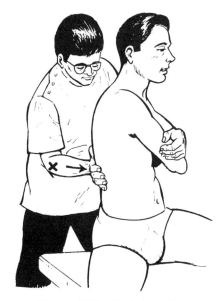

Figure A1.8. Technique 5.

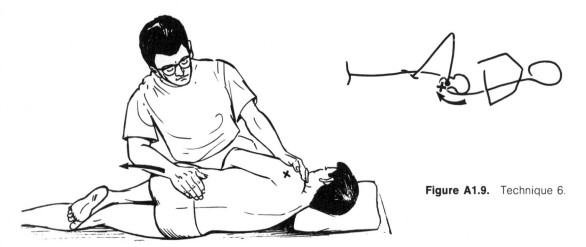

Figure A1.9.   Technique 6.

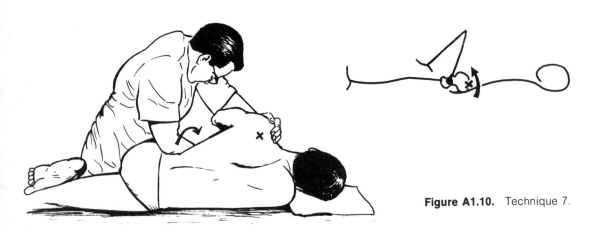

Figure A1.10.   Technique 7.

Lumbar Spine: Techniques 6 and 7

The "lateral decubitus" techniques impart rotation to the lumbosacral spine, either in flexion (Fig. A1.9) or in extension (Fig. A1.10) (see description in Appendix A5). In both variations, the examiner fixates or blocks the patient's shoulder while applying the manipulative thrust to the pelvis.

The basic maneuvers, like all manipulative techniques, are routinely effective only if they are executed perfectly. These techniques have the advantage of permitting some imperfection in technique, which makes them somewhat less effective, without rendering them systematically dangerous. This is not true for the accessory techniques, described below. They require more technical expertise, may be painful if performed incorrectly, and carry a degree of risk if they are not executed correctly.

These basic and accessory techniques are the ones that are routinely used. There are many other interesting techniques, and the principal ones are described. They can be adapted to an examiner's own capabilities, and the examiner can even "invent" a new technique that is personally more comfortable or efficient. The most important point is to be certain of the indication for the technique and to act on the appropriate segment in the pain-free direction, gently and with precision.

We insist on the use of mobilization and stretching techniques that are gentle and progress gradually, yet firmly, in all phases of treatment. These techniques, which are imperative in older patients, are to be used initially in most cases. They can often produce very good results by themselves and possibly also indicate the best way to execute the manipulative thrust if it is necessary.

Manipulation, like all complex manual acts, needs a lengthy apprenticeship to be well executed. The practitioner may be more or less gifted to succeed. One does not learn to play tennis or golf in a few weeks, and in each of these activities, they are obvious differences between amateurs and professionals. The same can be said for manipulation.

Manipulation, as a form of treatment, is only useful in the context of a sound understanding of all the clinical conditions that bring patients for consultation. Each application must be carefully planned, must be tailored to the particular patient, and must respect the various indications and contraindications particular to the patient. The entire spectrum of manipulative techniques represents a whole armamentarium of tools from which the physician may draw, and with experience, these techniques prove to be invaluable. Even though the novice may initially meet with success, it is the experienced manipulator who regularly finds these techniques to be efficacious, while at the same time avoiding the many possible adverse effects.

Seven Accessory Techniques

In general, the accessory techniques require greater precision to execute correctly than the basic techniques do, and most have less tolerance for error.

Cervical Spine: Technique I

The "chin grasp" technique allows very precise maneuvers, but it is powerful and must be done with the tips of the fingers (Fig. A1.11) (see detailed description in Appendix A2).

Cervicothoracic Junction: Techniques II and III

The "transverse thrust" (Fig. A1.12) and "chin pivot" (Fig. A1.13) are two excellent techniques that also require great precision (see description in Appendix A3).

Thoracic Spine: Technique IV

The "knee" technique is a very precise technique (Fig. A1.14) but may be quite painful if performed incorrectly.

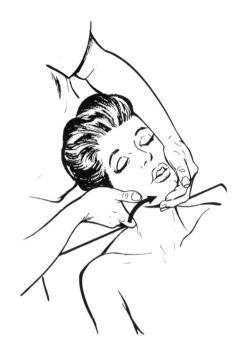

Figure A1.11.   Technique I.

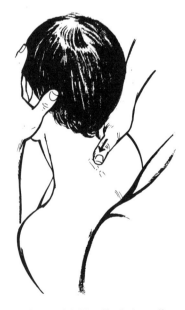

Figure A1.12.   Technique II.

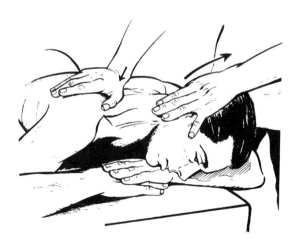

Figure A1.13.   Technique III.

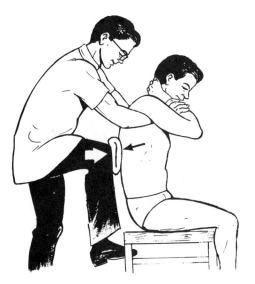

Figure A1.14.   Technique IV.

False Ribs: Technique V

The manipulation shown in Figure A1.15 is the most frequent indication for costal manipulations (see Appendix A6).

Lower Thoracic and Lumbar Levels: Techniques VI and VII

The "double knee" technique uses both knees as the contact point (Fig. A1.16) and is an excellent maneuver for extension manipulation of the lower thoracic and lumbar spine (see Appendix A5). The "belt" technique is a very precise (Fig. A1.17) but powerful maneuver (see Appendix A5).

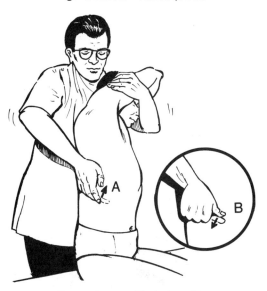

Figure A1.15.   Technique V.

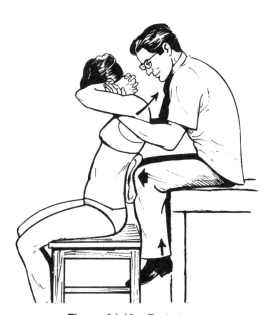

Figure A1.16.   Technique VI.

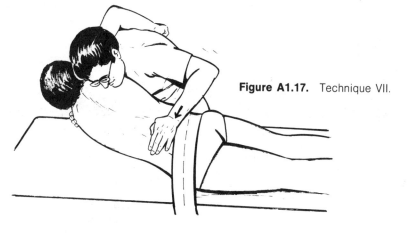

Figure A1.17.   Technique VII.

A2· Cervical Techniques

MASSAGE

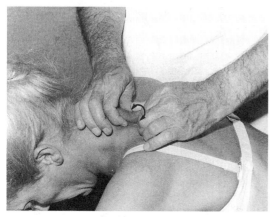

Figure A2.1. The pinch-roll test that we use for examination can also be used as a therapeutic maneuver in the treatment of cellulalgic zones. It should be performed in a measured and progressive manner, with the patient sitting on a stool, arms crossed and resting on a table, and the head rested on the arms.

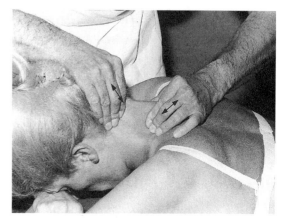

Figure A2.2. Stretching and distraction of the subcutaneous tissues and skinfolds. Same position as the preceding one.

RELAXATIONAL MANEUVERS

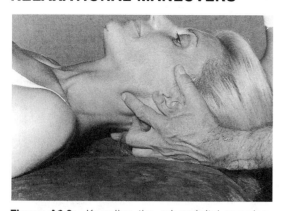

Figure A2.3. Kneading the suboccipital muscles. The examiner stands or sits at the head of the supine patient. Deep kneading of the suboccipital muscles is executed with the fingertips of both hands. This maneuver is very relaxing.

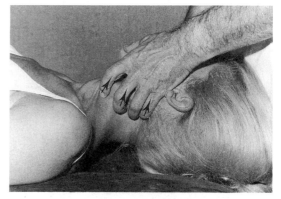

Figure A2.4. Stretching of the lateral cervical paraspinal muscles. The patient is supine. The examiner stands at the head, grasps the neck with the fingertips along each side of the paraspinal muscles, and stretches them alternately from one side to the other, pulling them toward him or her as if trying to detach them slowly from the spine and then releasing them rhythmically from one side and then the other.

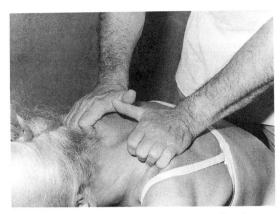

Figure A2.5. Kneading the suprascapular fossa. The same position as for Figure A2.1.

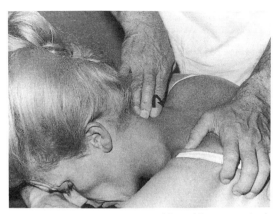

Figure A2.6. Transverse stretching of the paraspinal muscles. The fingertips grasp the taut muscular bands and stretch them to the other side of the spinous process. Same position as for Figure A2.1.

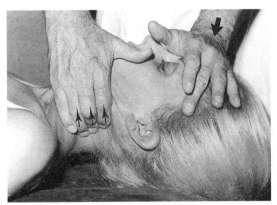

Figure A2.7. Kneading-stretching. The patient is supine. The examiner grasps the left paracervical muscles with the right hand and pulls them toward him or her, while the heel of the left hand prevents the head from turning to the right. These movements are to be performed slowly and rhythmically.

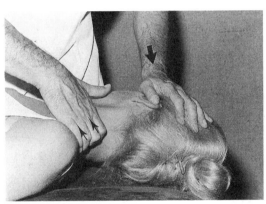

Figure A2.8. Kneading-stretching of the suprascapular fossa. Same principal as for the preceding figure. The left hand fixates the lateral side of the head of the patient while the right hand stretches the muscles, with the fingers in a "hook" position.

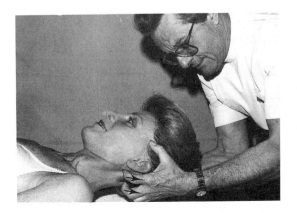

Figure A2.9. Suboccipital stretching. The patient is lying supine. The backs of the examiner's hands and the wrists rest on the table, with the fingers strongly maintained in a hook grasp—like position along the inferior edge of the occiput. The wrists pushing firmly on the table allow the hands to act like a lever in stretching the occiput and the suboccipital muscles.

MOBILIZATION AND MANUAL TRACTION

Among these techniques are mobilizations in rotation, lateroflexion, flexion, and extension. These maneuvers are useful for muscular stretching.

Mobilization

Rotation

Patient is in supine position.

First Technique.   This example is in right rotation. The physician supports the head of the patient with the right hand over the right occipitomaxillary region. The left hand, with the fingers flat against the neck, brings the spine into right rotation until end range is reached. At this point, the pressure is maintained for a few seconds, then the examiner releases and starts again with slow, rhythmic, and oscillating movements. Depending on the position of the left hand, the action will be applied to the middle, superior, or inferior cervical spine (Fig. A2.10).

Second Technique.   For right rotation, the examiner fixates the patient's left shoulder with the right hand while imparting right rotation to the cervical spine with the left hand applied to the patient's occiput and superior cervical segments (Fig. A2.11).

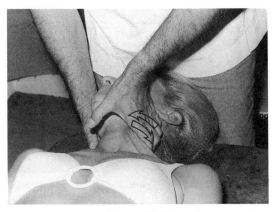

Figure A2.10.

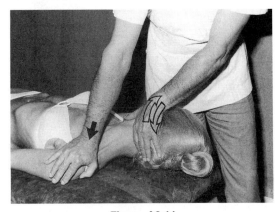

Figure A2.11.

In Lateroflexion

Patient is in supine position.

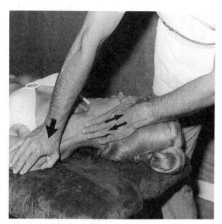

Figure A2.12.   The patient and the physician are positioned as in the preceding techniques. However, the physician's left hand makes contact with the parietal region and stretches the cervical spine in lateral flexion.

Patient is in lateral decubitus position.

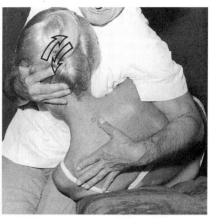

Figure A2.13.   Mobilizations in right lateral flexion. The patient lies on the left side, firmly maintained in that position with the right shoulder under the physician's axilla. The movement is repeated slowly in stretching and in an "elastic" manner in an upward direction and then letting go.

In Flexion

Patient is supine. The operator's forearms are crossed behind the patient's neck, blocking the patient's shoulders with the hands (Fig. A2.14). By gently alternating between flexion and extension of the wrists, the operator acts as a lever and pushes (Fig. A2.15) the neck into flexion, then releases. It is a powerful maneuver, to be done very slowly, with great caution. It has to be repeated several times.

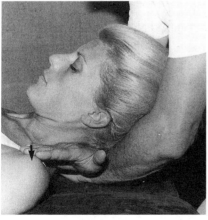

Figure A2.14.   Start.

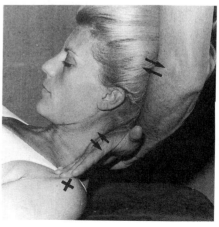

Figure A2.15.   Finish.

Superior Cervical Spine.   This maneuver is for the superior cervical segments, especially the atlanto-occipital joint. The patient is supine. The physician, standing at the head, grasps the base of the occiput with the thumb and tips of the 3rd, 4th, and 5th fingers of one hand, while the other hand pushes on the fore-head (Fig. A2.16). With the occipital hand, the physician applies traction while the frontal hand applies simultaneous downward pressure, which results in hyperflexion on the upper neck. The movement, as always, is slow, rhythmic, and repetitive (Fig. A2.17).

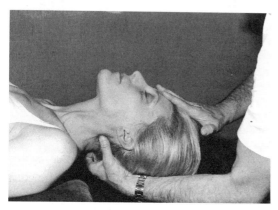

Figure A2.16.   Start.

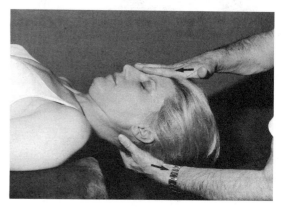

Figure A2.17.   Finish.

Manual Traction

Several methods can be used for cervical traction, a maneuver of stretching and relaxation that is often useful. It is also a necessary test before deciding on treatment with mechanical cervical traction. The head is supported in one of three ways. In the first technique, the examiner grasps the base of the occiput with both hands placed on each side (Fig. A2.18). In the second technique, the examiner simulates a Sayre's collar by grasping the chin with one hand and the occiput with the other (Fig. A2.19). In the third technique, the examiner holds the occiput and the forehead. The occipital hand applies traction, while the other hand maintains the forehead (Fig. A2.20).

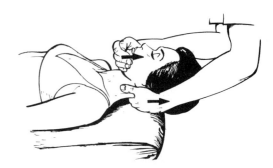

Figure A2.19.   Second method.

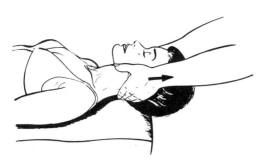

Figure A2.18.   First method.

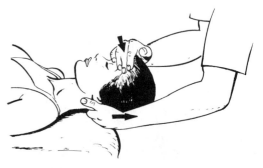

Figure A2.20.   Third method.

The first method is an easier means of applying manual traction in extension. With the second technique, traction in flexion can also be performed. The third method avoids the possibility of discomfort with mandibular contact, which occurs with certain patients with a dental apparatus. This principle has been applied in our apparatus for cervical traction (see Chapter 23, "Traction"). The operator pulls slowly, regularly, progressively and firmly toward himself, maintains the traction for about ten seconds, then releases and starts again. This is repeated about ten times. In doing so, the examiner should lean backward with arms outstretched, because it is better to use the weight of the body than to rely on the strength of his arms.

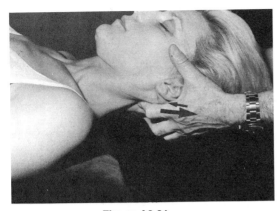

Figure A2.21.

Suboccipital Traction (Fig. A2.21)

With the fingertips, the operator grasps the occiput, maintains it in traction for several seconds, releases it, and starts again. This is a soft, relaxing maneuver of the suboccipital muscles.

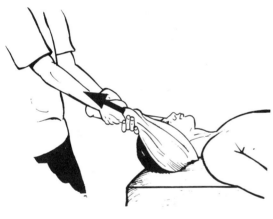

Figure A2.22.

Traction with a Towel (Fig. A2.22)

A very good system for maintaining traction of the cervical spine is as follows: the examiner places the patient's head in a folded towel that is passed like a sling under the occiput.

Traction with a Belt (Fig. A2.23)

The patient is supine. A belt, 5-cm wide, is passed under the patient's occiput, forming a long loop passing behind the physician's back. By leaning backward, the examiner applies tension to the belt and produces cervical traction that is easy to measure and to control and much less fatiguing for the examiner. The examiner can either simply maintain the traction while maintaining the position of the head with the hand or perform a manipulation in rotation under traction or simply mobilizations. With a step to the left or to the right, the examiner can apply right or left lateroflexion.

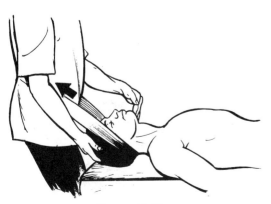

Figure A2.23.

MANIPULATION

Basic Technique: Chin Free

The example chosen is a manipulation of the middle cervical spine in pure rotation. In this example left rotation is used. The chin free technique is used more frequently than the "chin grasp" technique described later.

Example

Manipulation into left rotation (Fig. A2.24) is performed with the patient supine. The physician is standing at the end of the table and slightly to the right. The patient's head, placed in left rotation, is supported with the left hand, while the physician applies pressure with the radial edge of the right index finger to the lateral aspect of the target vertebra. The physician then brings the cervical spine to end range in left rotation to take up the slack. With end range well assured, a brief and brisk thrust of the right index finger exaggerates the left rotation result in a *manipulation*, accompanied by the usual "cracking."

Note that

- The right forearm is maintained in a vertical plane perpendicular to the plane of the table throughout the entire movement. This implies that the examiner's shoulders play an important role in the execution of the manipulative thrust. In this example, the right shoulder goes up while the left one goes down (Fig. A2.25, *left*).
- The left hand supports and maintains the head throughout the movement and assists the right hand to take up the slack and apply the terminal phases of the manipulation. The

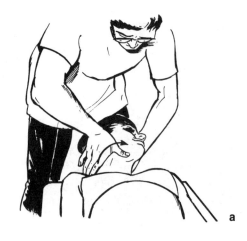

a

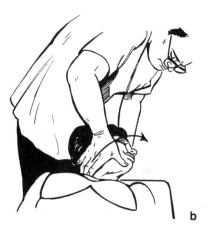

b

Figure A2.24.   **a.** Start. **b.** Finish.

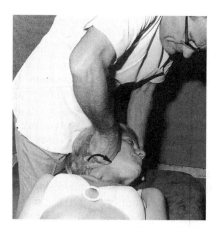

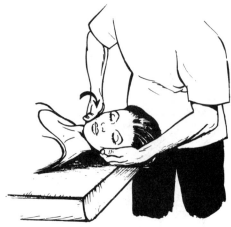

Figure A2.25. Position of the examiner's arms.

left forearm is nearly horizontal (Fig. A2.25, *right*), the right forearm remains perpendicular to the patient's neck (Fig. A2.25, *left* and *right*). The thumb of the right hand does not play a role and should not apply pressure to the patient's cheek (Fig. A2.25, *left*).

The part of the index finger that contacts the vertebral segment is the fleshy part located between the lateral edge and the palmar surface of the finger (*full stroke* in Fig. A2.26) rather than the bony edge of the phalanx (*hatched* in Fig. A2.26). The fingers should not be tightly adducted as in Figure A2.27a. The active index finger overlaps the dorsal aspect

of the middle finger (Fig. A2.27b). The index finger plays the role of shock absorber. Even though the manipulative thrust is brisk, it is painless. However, if the fingers are held too firmly, the pressure of the soft tissues against the vertebra is very painful.

To properly position the fingers, the hand must first be placed flat on the neck (Fig. A2.28, *top*); then, while the contact is main-

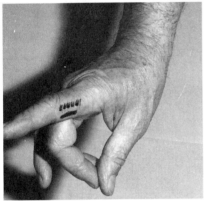

Figure A2.26.

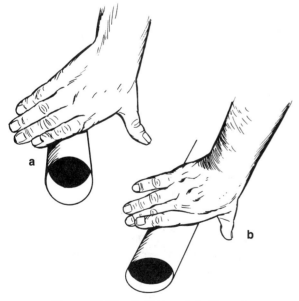

Figure A2.27.   a. Incorrect. **b.** Correct.

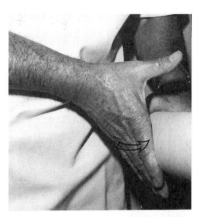

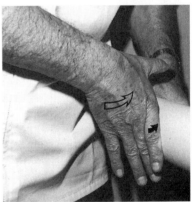

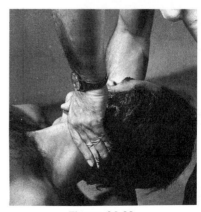

Figure A2.28.

tained with the index finger, pronation of the wrist is performed (Fig. A2.28, *middle* and *bottom*).

With a few minor adjustments in position, this manipulation can be executed at all levels of the cervical spine. The active index finger is placed at the level of the segment to be manipulated as seen in Figures A2.29–A2.31:

- Superior cervical spine (Fig. A2.29)
- Middle cervical spine (Fig. A2.30)
- Inferior cervical spine (Fig. A2.31)

These maneuvers can be executed on the spine

- In neutral position (without flexion or extension)
- With flexion or extension
- With or without associated lateroflexion (Fig. A2.26–A2.27)

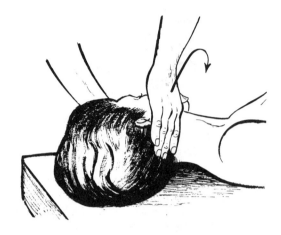

Figure A2.29. Manipulation in left rotation of the superior cervical spine.

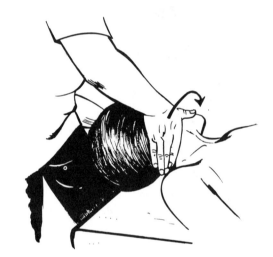

Figure A2.30. Manipulation in left rotation on a midcervical segment.

Remarks

We have chosen to describe the technique in which the examiner keeps the forearm (here the right one) perpendicular to the axis of the patient's neck. We consider this best for a precise and well-measured maneuver, but the technique can also be done with the forearms parallel to the ground, in the axis of the neck of the patient. Movement is then essentially at the forearms, wrists, and hands.

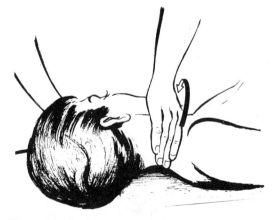

Figure A2.31. Manipulation in left rotation on a segment of the inferior cervical spine.

Pure Rotation (with or without Flexion or Extension)

Superior Cervical Spine

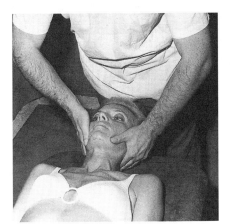

Figure A2.32. Starting position for a manipulation in left rotation in neutral position (neither in flexion or extension).

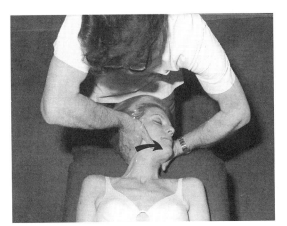

Figure A2.33. Final position.

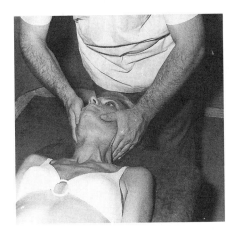

Figure A2.34. Starting position for a manipulation in left rotation on the superior cervical spine placed in extension.

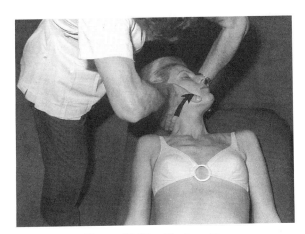

Figure A2.35. Final position.

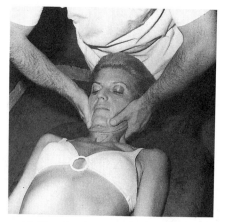

Figure A2.36. Starting position for a manipulation in left rotation on a spine in flexion.

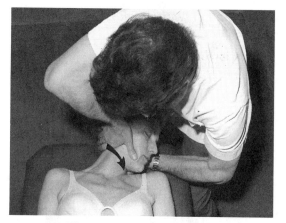

Figure A2.37. Final position.

Middle Cervical Spine

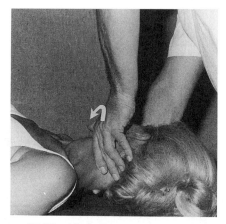

Figure A2.38. Manipulation in right rotation on a spine in neutral position of a midcervical segment.

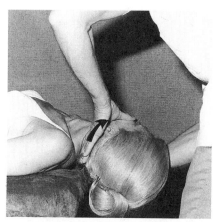

Figure A2.39. Manipulation in right rotation on a spine in extension (with the head of the patient maintained over the end of the table).

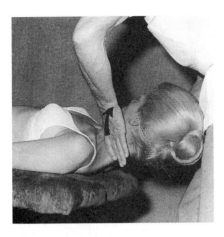

◄
Figure A2.40.   Manipulation in right rotation of the midcervical spine in flexion.

Inferior Cervical Spine

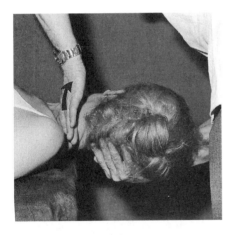

◄
Figure A2.41.   Manipulation in right rotation on a segment of the inferior cervical spine in neutral position.

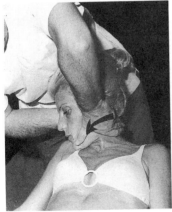

Figure A2.42.   Manipulation in right rotation on the inferior cervical spine in flexion.

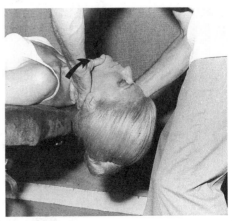

Figure A2.43.   Manipulation in right rotation on the inferior cervical spine (starting position).

Accessory Technique (Chin Grasp)

Manipulation with Combined Rotation and Lateroflexion.

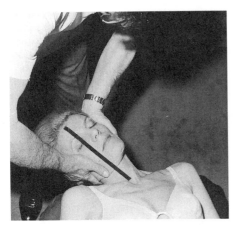

Figure A2.44. Right lateral flexion on the inferior cervical spine.

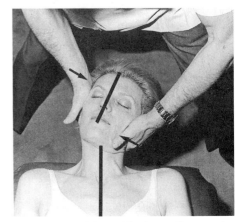

Figure A2.45. Left lateral flexion on the superior cervical spine.

Superior Cervical Spine

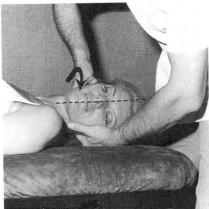

Figure A2.46.

Both hands combine to impart lateroflexion to the spine. The apex of the lateroflexion is the site where the manipulation is performed.

Figure A2.46. Left rotation without lateral flexion.

Figure A2.47. Left rotation with right lateral flexion. The right lateral flexion is produced by simultaneous action of the hand and left forearm of the examiner and the countersupport of the right hand.

Figure A2.48. Left rotation with left lateral flexion. Here the action of the two hands is opposite. Their simultaneous actions put the head in left lateral flexion.

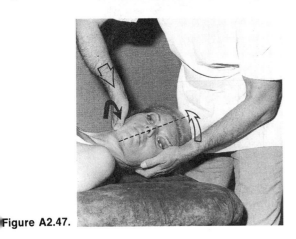

Figure A2.47.

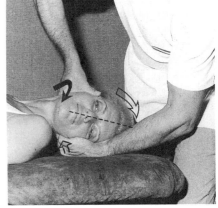

Figure A2.48.

Middle and Inferior Cervical Spine

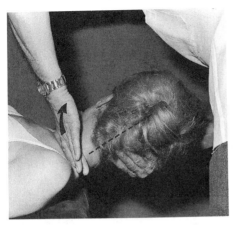

Figure A2.49.   Right rotation and left lateral flexion.

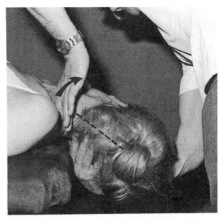

Figure A2.50.   Right rotation and right lateral flexion.

Chin Grasp Technique

The chin grasp technique can be very powerful by using the head as a lever and must be extremely precise and perfectly controlled from beginning to end (Fig. A2.51). This technique allows manipulation of the superior, middle, and inferior cervical spine with all the desired combinations.

The patient lies supine. For left rotation, the examiner grasps the chin of the patient with the left hand. The top of the patient's head is supported against the arm or the thorax of the examiner, similar to carrying a football. This hand assures the desired degree of flexion or extension. The other hand contacts the target vertebra. Both hands must move in perfect synchrony to properly take up the slack and then perform the manipulative thrust.

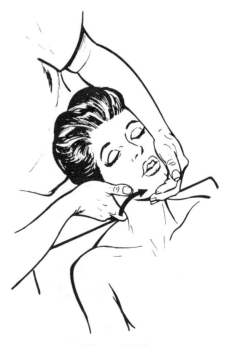

Figure A2.51.

Manipulation in Rotation with or without Flexion/Extension

Superior Cervical Spine

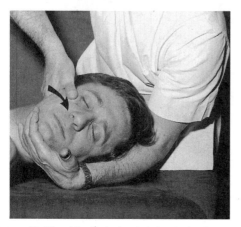

Figure A2.52. Manipulation in left rotation in neutral position.

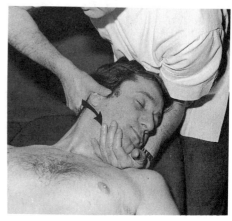

Figure A2.53. Manipulation in left rotation on the spine in flexion.

Figure A2.54. Manipulation in left rotation on the superior cervical spine in extension.

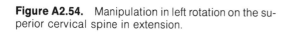

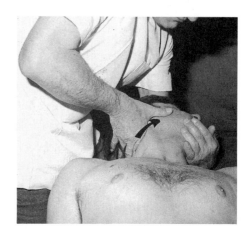

Middle and Inferior Cervical Spine

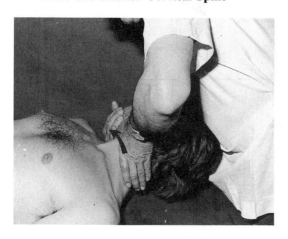

Figure A2.55. Manipulation in right rotation in neutral position of the midcervical spine.

Variation

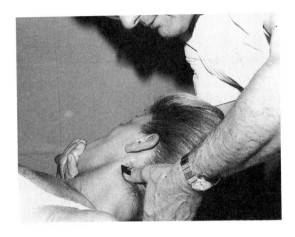

Figure A2.56. Manipulation in right rotation of the superior cervical spine in neutral position. Instead of providing the manipulative thrust with the radial edge of the index finger, it is provided by the thumb.

Manipulation in Rotation and Lateroflexion

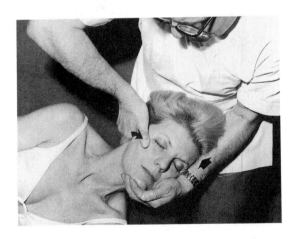

Figure A2.57. Manipulation of the superior cervical spine in left rotation and right lateral flexion. Lateral flexion is being applied by the left forearm of the examiner. The patient lies on the left side. The pressure of the right index finger is directed on the occiput. The "chin" hand performs the right lateral flexion. The manipulative thrust is performed downward and forward.

Anterior Hand Technique

Manipulation in Left Rotation

Middle Cervical Spine

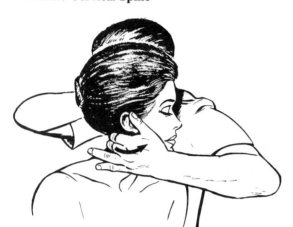

◄

Figure A2.58.

The patient is seated, with legs dangling over the edge of the table. The physician, standing beside the patient (on the side of the rotation), places the middle finger in contact with the right transverse process of the vertebra on which the maneuver will be executed, while the right hand pushes on the left fronto-parietal region and brings the neck to end left rotation. Once the slack has been taken up, the physician pulls toward the left and anteriorly with the middle and index fingers as they "hook" the vertebrae and exaggerate the left rotation to execute the manipulation.

➤

Figure A2.59. Rotation with neutral flexion/extension performed on the middle cervical spine.

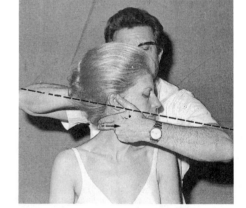

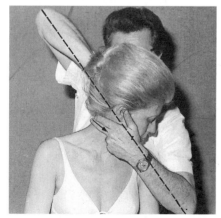

Figure A2.60. Manipulation in rotation with flexion. Note the direction of the forearms of the examiner.

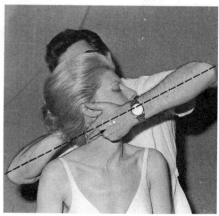

Figure A2.61. Manipulation in rotation with extension. Note the direction of the forearms of the examiner.

Superior Cervical Spine

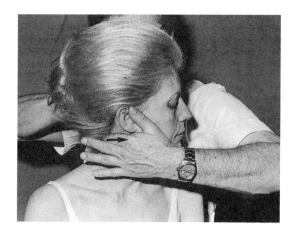

◄

Figure A2.62. Manipulation in pure left rotation performed on C2. The active finger is the index, which contacts the occiput.

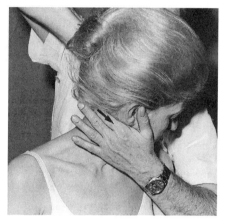

Figure A2.63. Manipulation in left rotation and flexion on C2.

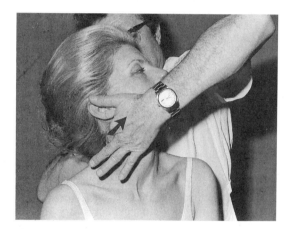

Figure A2.64. Manipulation in left rotation and extension on C2.

Inferior Cervical Spine

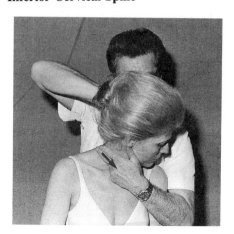

◄

Figure A2.65. Here, the inferior cervical spine is subjected to a left rotation, and it is always the left hand that puts the cervical spine in position. The middle finger is active. To effect a manipulative thrust at C7, it is generally more comfortable to use the 4th or 5th finger as the active finger, with the hand flattened against the neck. Shown is a left rotation on a spine in flexion.

N.B. This technique can include a component of lateroflexion.

Posterior Hand Technique

This personal technique is closely related to the preceding one. The patient is seated. The physician does not put the active hand in front of the patient's neck, but in the back, with the active finger (usually the index or middle finger) applied at the level of the vertebra to be manipulated (here the right middle finger for left rotation) to assist the manipulation. The other hand places the patient's head and neck in position by contact with the temporal region (Fig. A2.66) or the inferior maxilla (Fig. A2.68).

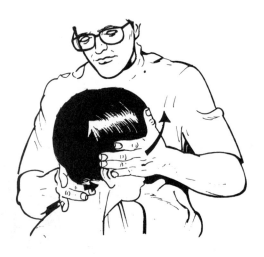

◄

Figure A2.66. For a left rotation, the left hand of the examiner grasps the right side of the patient's forehead or chin. With this hand, the physician positions and then takes up the slack. To give the manipulative thrust, the physician suddenly exaggerates the rotation, helped by a synchronized pressure with the right middle finger. This technique allows all maneuvers of lateroflexion, flexion, and extension, all combined.

There is choice of movement because only one finger guides the rotation, and the maneuver is well localized to a specific segmental level. Moreover, as the slack is taken up, the head and neck are positioned very precisely by the combined action of the two hands (Figs. A2.67 and A2.68).

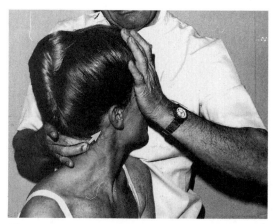

Figure A2.67. Manipulation of the superior cervical spine in left rotation. Note the position of the examiner's hands.

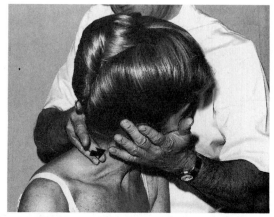

Figure A2.68. Manipulation of the inferior cervical spine in left rotation. Note the position of the examiner's hands.

MASSAGE OF THE SUBCUTANEOUS TISSUES

The pinch-roll (Fig. A3.1) or skinfold (Fig. A3.2) maneuvers are used for petrissage of the cellulalgic skin and subcutaneous tissues. They must be very progressive.

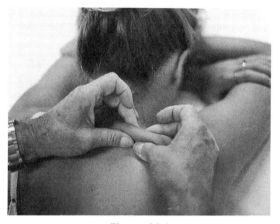

Figure A3.1.

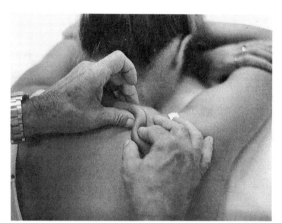

Figure A3.2.

RELAXATIONAL MANEUVERS

Patient Seated

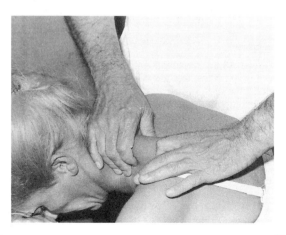

◄

Figure A3.3. The patient is seated on a stool, arms crossed in front and resting over a table and the head resting on the arms. This position is also excellent for relaxational maneuvers. They are performed with the thumbs, which form a deep petrissage of the muscles and apply traction to them going from the midline and directly, obliquely, superiorly, and laterally. The same maneuver can be performed with the patient supine.

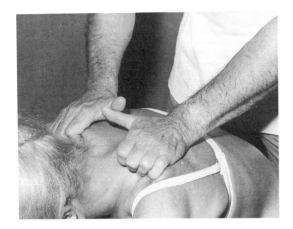

Figure A3.4. Same patient position. The examiner's fingers, in a hook position, grasp the muscles of the supraspinous fossa and pull them backward and inward, maintaining them, then releasing them and starting again in a slow rhythmic pattern.

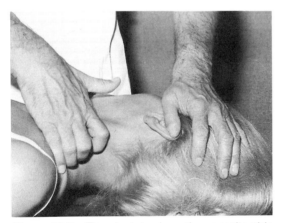

Figure A3.5. The physician is on the opposite side of the one to be treated. The right hand grasps the mass of the lateral muscles of the neck at their inferior attachment and pulls them toward the physician, releasing them in a slow repeated rhythmic fashion. The other hand applies counterpressure to the shoulder.

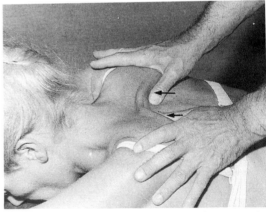

Figure A3.6. Massage and deep "gliding" is performed with the thumbs of each side of each hand along the side of the line of the spinous processes. The examiner glides parallel to that line, slowly, progressively modifying the pressure applied.

MOBILIZATION

In Extension

Patient Seated

The patient is seated, with the head resting on the crossed forearms. The physician, standing in front, places the forearms under the patient's forearms and the hands over the thoracic region on each side. By lifting the arms slowly and pulling toward himself or herself, the physician is able to mobilize the superior thoracic spine in extension.

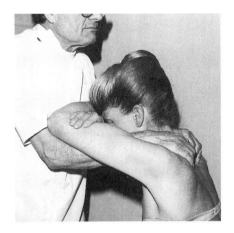
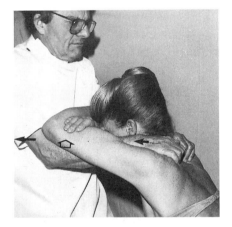

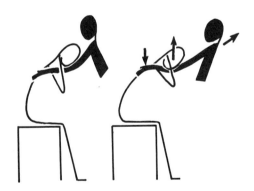

Figure A3.7.

In Flexion

Patient Supine

With the patient lying supine, the examiner's forearms are crossed behind the patient's neck, with the hands on the patient's shoulders to block them. With light, alternating flexion and extension movements of the wrist, the examiner can act as a lever and bring the neck into flexion and release it. It is a powerful maneuver, to be performed slowly with great caution. It must, of course, be repeated several times (Fig. A3.8).

For a lateroflexion maneuver, the hand is placed on the parietal region as support, while the other hand fixates the shoulder. Movement is slow, rhythmic, and tailored to the needs of the patient. The maximum time that stretching should be maintained is 2–3 seconds (Fig. A3.8).

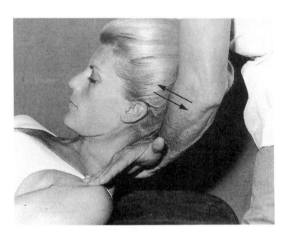

Figure A3.8.

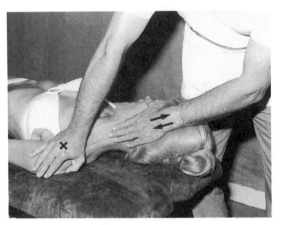

Figure A3.9.

In Rotation

Patient Supine

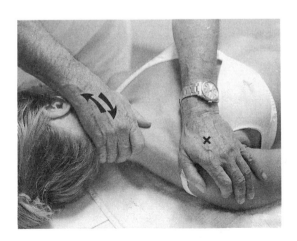

Figure A3.10.

MANIPULATION: BASIC TECHNIQUES

Cervicothoracic Technique in Lateral Decubitus Position

Pure Lateroflexion (without Rotation)
Preparation.   The patient is lying in lateral decubitus, with both legs and thighs slightly flexed. Manipulation into right lateroflexion is pictured, so the patient is lying on the left side (Fig. A3.11, *left*).

Execution.   Manipulation in right lateroflexion in neutral flexion/extension.
Placing in Position.   The examiner is standing, semiupright, with the left thigh resting against the table. The upper part of the patient's body is slowly brought over the edge of the table (Fig. A3.11, *right*) until the patient's head and neck are practically perpendicular to the axis of the table (Fig. A3.12, *left*). The physician's right hand supports the patient's head at the ear, taking care not to compress it, which would be uncomfortable for the patient. The fingertips have contact with the skull (Fig. A3.12, *right*).

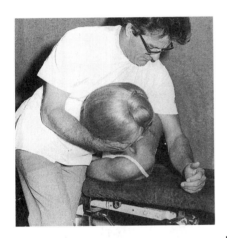
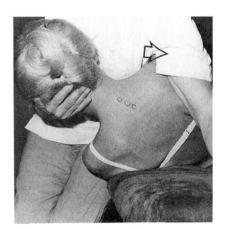

Figure A3.11.

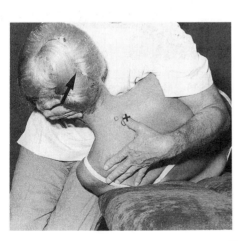
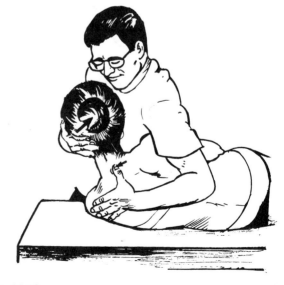

Figure A3.12.

The patient's superior shoulder must be fixated firmly under the examiner's axilla. The examiner pushes it posteriorly and, by so doing, verifies that the scapula is pulled upward and outward, not pushed back toward the spine (Fig. A3.12, *right*).

The examiner presses the left thumb against the right edge of the spinous process of the subjacent vertebra of the segment that is to be manipulated (Fig. A3.12, *left*). In this position, the examiner is nearly lying on the patient. The patient should not be crushed but must be firmly fixated. Only the neck remains mobile.

Taking up the slack.   The right hand of the physician, which supports the head, brings the neck into lateroflexion toward the physician's left. Taking up the slack, assured when the physician feels the "break" (which depends on the given lateroflexion), is done at the height of the segment to be manipulated; it locks the subjacent segments.

Thrust.   From the point of taking up the slack, the manipulative thrust is delivered by a brief ascent of the examiner's right hand (Fig. A3.12, *right*).

This manipulation can be done on the thoracolumbar junction in neutral position (no flexion, no extension) as in Figure A3.12. It can also be done in the spine positioned in extension (Fig. A3.13) or in flexion (Fig. A3.14).

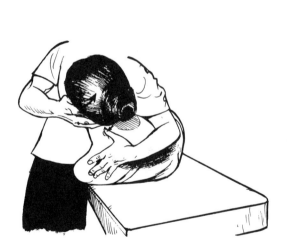

Figure A3.13.   Manipulation in lateral flexion on the spine in extension.

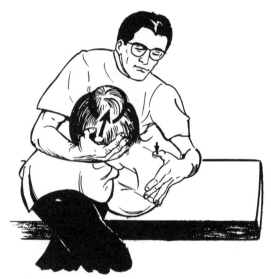

Figure A3.14.   Manipulation in right lateral flexion on the spine in flexion.

In Lateroflexion Associated with Rotation

This manipulation in lateroflexion can be associated with

• Rotation in the same direction as the lateroflexion

    —Right lateroflexion with right rotation (homologous lateroflexion) (Fig. A3.15).

• Rotation in the opposite direction

    —Right lateroflexion with left rotation (heterologous lateroflexion) (Fig. A3.16).

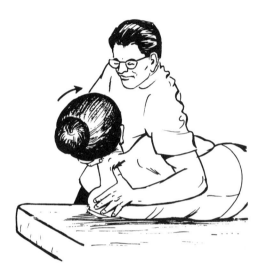

Figure A3.15.   Manipulation in right lateral flexion and right rotation.

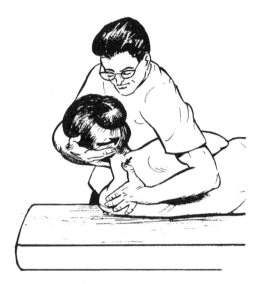

Figure A3.16.   Manipulation in right lateral flexion and left rotation.

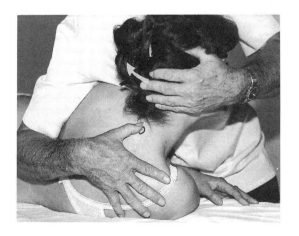

All of these maneuvers can be performed on segments of the cervicothoracic junction in neutral position, in extension, or in flexion. Figure A3.17 shows left lateral flexion combined with right rotation of the C6-C7 segment (note support of the thumb on the spinous process of C7) in the spine in extension.

◄

Figure A3.17.   Manipulation in left lateral flexion, extension, and right rotation.

Chin Pivot (Accessory Technique)

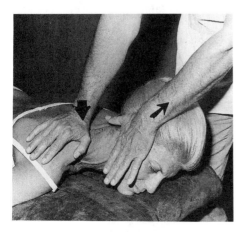

Figure A3.18.

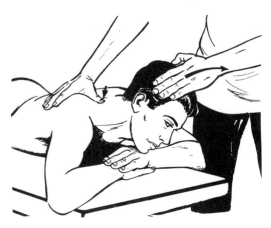

Figure A3.19.

Patient in Prone

The patient is prone, with arms apart, hanging on each side of the table (Figs. A3.18 and A3.20). The chin rests on the table. It is often more comfortable for the patient to rest the chin on the hands resting flat on the table (Fig. A3.19). This position puts the spine in slight extension.

The physician stands (here on the left side of the patient) at the corner of the table and places the thenar eminence over the right transverse process of the first, second, or third thoracic vertebra (Figs. A3.19 and A3.20). The

hand grasps the patient's right temporomaxillary region, taking care not to compress the ear. The patient's neck is brought into right rotation with stretching toward the left (Fig. A3.21).

When the taking up the slack is assured, the manipulative thrust is given by accentuating the action of the hand taking support on the head, while the counterpressure is firmly maintained on the transverse process by the thenar eminence of the other hand, which remains fixed.

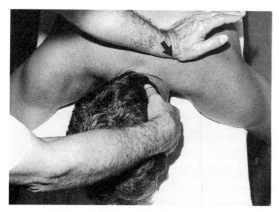

Figure A3.20. Placing in position.

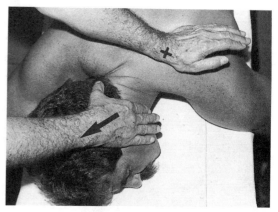

Figure A3.21. Taking up the slack.

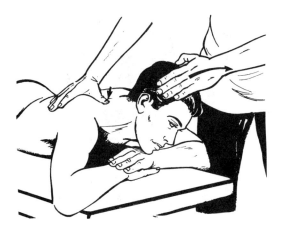

◄

Figure A3.22. Same maneuver as Figure A3.19, but here the thumb is used by the examiner to assure counterpressure.

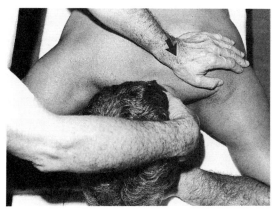
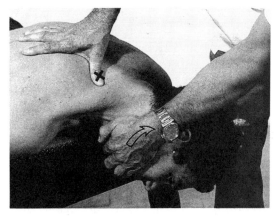

Figure A3.23. Variation of the basic technique. The manipulative thrust is performed by the dorsal hand (*thick arrow*). **Left.** Start. **Right.** Taking up the slack. Thrust.

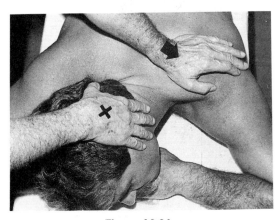

Figure A3.24.

Variant. The maneuver can be done by taking up the slack in the same manner as above (Fig. A3.23, *left*), but at the terminal thrust, pressure on the head is the fixed point. The thrust is given by the sudden increase in pressure on the transverse process of the thoracic vertebra (Fig. A3.23, *right*).

Same Maneuver on the Spine in Flexion. The maneuver can be done on the spine in flexion. The head of the patient must be over the edge of the table. It is supported by the examiner's knee (Fig. A3.24); the counterpressure is supplied by the thumb against the transverse process of the vertebra subjacent to the segment to be manipulated. This delicate and powerful maneuver has only rare indications.

Same Maneuver Associated with Lateroflexion. The left hand takes a slightly different support. It is placed in front of the patient's ear, on the temporomaxillary region. The examiner brings the neck into right lateroflexion, while the counterpressure on the thenar eminence (or the thumb) of the left hand is applied to the left transverse process of the first, second, or third thoracic vertebra, depending on which segment will bear the maximum effect. The neck is then in strong right lateroflexion with slight left rotation (Fig. A3.25). The manipulative thrust is given by sudden and limited accentuation of the examiner's right hand on the transverse process. Its direction is slightly caudal.

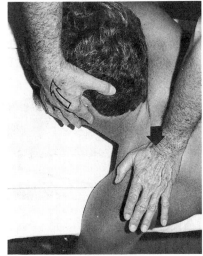

Figure A3.25. The patient is prone, with the arms on either side of the table.

Lateral Pressure Against the Spinous Process (Accessory Technique)

Patient Seated

The physician stands behind the patient. In this example, the physician places the left hand over the patient's left parietal region and brings the neck into right lateroflexion. The right thumb applies pressure against the right lateral part of the vertebra subjacent to the joint to be manipulated (Fig. A3.26). The physician gradually increases the right lateroflexion of the neck, until the left thumb senses that the flexion has reached end range (i.e., the point at which the peak of the lateroflexion reaches the vertebra on which it rests). The manipulative thrust is given by increasing the pressure of the thumb with a small brief movement directed downward and to the left, in the direction of the line that bisects the angle formed by the neck and the shoulder of the patient. The examiner's wrist and forearm are maintained firmly throughout the maneuver.

To execute this maneuver and have it strictly painless for the patient, both patient and physician should be perfectly positioned, with lateral inclination of the trunk of the patient. Two techniques can be used.

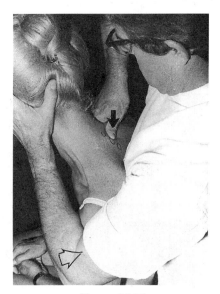

Figure A3.26.

Technique A (Fig. A3.27)

The patient's body is maintained slightly to the left. The physician's elbow grasps the patient's left shoulder, like a pair of pliers. The physician's chest is flat against the back of the subject, forming a kind of block. The patient's trunk is brought into slight left inclination, and the cervicothoracic junction into slight right inclination. The right thumb applies pressure against the spinous process; the right forearm is oriented obliquely, with the elbow raised superiorly.

When the examiner senses that end range has been reached, the terminal thrust is applied; the direction is given by the obliquity of the forearms, which practically bisect the neck-shoulder angle.

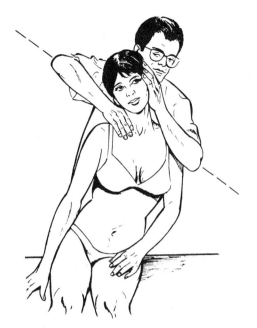

Figure A3.27.

Technique B (Fig. A3.28)

The physician's foot is placed on the table, against the left hip of the patient. The patient's left axilla rests on the physician's left knee. The inclination of the knee gives the inclination of the patient's trunk.

N.B. Note in all cases the strict parallelism of the two forearms of the operator.

When the manipulation is applied on the 6th cervical vertebra, the active pressure is not provided by the thumb against the spinous process (as it is too small) but with the thumb and the index finger which are half-folded, forming pliers. The so-formed pliers take the lateral part of the spinous process and the posterolateral part of the affected vertebra.

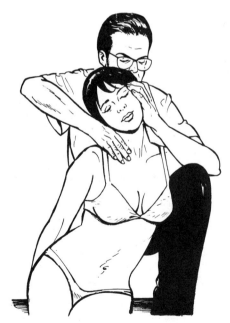

Figure A3.28.

A 4. Thoracic Techniques

MASSAGE

Techniques for this region are identical to those of the cervicothoracic junction (see Appendix 3).

RELAXATIONAL MANEUVERS

The patient is prone.

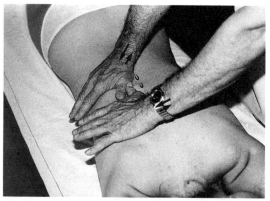

Figure A4.1. The patient is prone with the head turned to the direction opposite to the side being treated. The examiner stands at the side opposite to the one to be treated and applies the hands, with the fingers spread apart, to the paraspinal region. The thumbs are together at their extremity, forming a line parallel to the line of the spinous processes.

With the "bar" formed by the thenar eminences and thumbs, the examiner pushes the paraspinal muscles slowly, as if trying to pull them away from the spinous process and detach them from the deep planes. When maximal tension is reached, the examiner pauses, increases the pressure slightly, and then releases it. This should be done in a rhythmic well-controlled way, without losing any contact, even during the release.

In many conditions, this is a relaxing and useful maneuver, particularly in the treatment of acute and chronic thoracic pain. At the start of the massage, the elbows of the examiner are partially flexed, and during the maneuver, they are extended. The examiner finishes with the elbows fully extended, permitting a strong tangential pressure to be transmitted to the thorax and allowing good stretching of the paraspinal muscles.

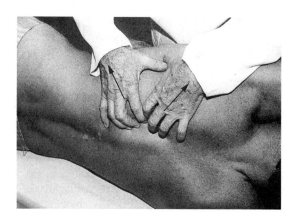

Figure A4.2. The patient is in lateral decubitus (here on the right side) the arm resting on the head. The examiner stands facing the patient. The examiner's two hands are side by side, and the fingers in a claw-like position can grasp the paraspinal muscles at the spinous process. The examiner pulls the muscles, with hands slightly apart, and then releases them in a slow and rhythmic fashion, allowing an elastic movement that is firm at the moment of maximal stretching. At that moment, there is a brief pause.

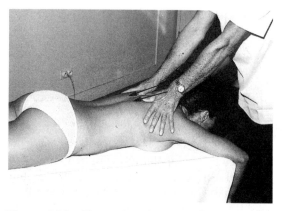

Figure A4.3. The patient is prone. The examiner stands at the head, and places the hands flat on each side of the spine near the midline over the superior thoracic vertebrae. The forearms are partially flexed. The examiner slides the hands along the spine, downward in a parallel fashion, stretching the forearms. The maneuver should be performed slowly and rhythmically, applying pressure in a constant manner according to the results that are desired.

Scapular Muscle Stretching

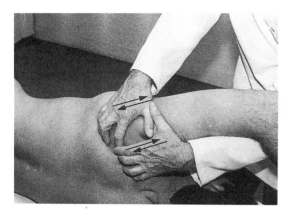

Figure A4.4.

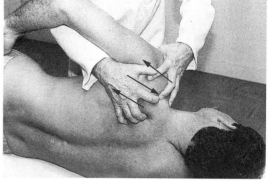

Figure A4.5.

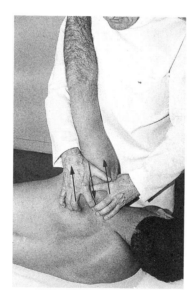

Figure A4.6.

The patient is positioned in side lying. The examiner faces the patient and grasps the medial scapular edge with the fingertips. The scapula is circumducted slowly, stretching the soft tissues in the different directions while kneading the muscles laterally (Fig. A4.4); inferiorly (Fig. A4.5); and superiorly (Fig. A4.6).

Note the variations in the position of the patient's upper limb. The different maneuvers are performed slowly and rhythmically, stretching to end range and pausing as maximal tension is reached. These maneuvers are also an excellent way to mobilize the scapulothoracic joint.

MOBILIZATION

Mobilization can be performed in extension, lateroflexion, rotation, and occasionally flexion.

In Extension

The patient is seated. Upper thoracic spine is shown in Figs. A4.7 and A4.8. Midthoracic spine shown in Figs. A4.9–A4.13.

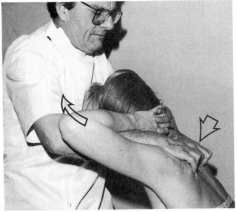

Figure A4.7.   The patient is sitting on the table with hands folded behind the neck. The examiner, in front, passes the forearms between the forearms and the shoulders of the patient and applies the hands at each side of the line of the spinous process at the first thoracic vertebrae. The examiner pulls the arms back, bending slightly backward, while the forearms act as a lever on the patient's forearms. The hands act on the back of the patient while supporting the patient's forearms (pressing them upward) to bring the affected region into extension.

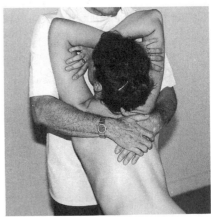

Figure A4.8.   The patient, with arms crossed over the forehead, rests on the physician's chest in front. The physician's hands are placed on each side of the region to obtain mobilization in extension and pulls, while going back slightly. The physician then releases the pressure, going a little forward, and starts again gently.

N.B.   Because the patient has a tendency to slide forward, with these maneuvers, the examiner uses his knees to block the patient and prevent them from sliding (Figs. A4.8–A4.13).

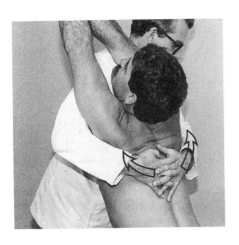

◄

Figure A4.9.   This variant is also useful for the inferior thoracic spine. The patient's two stretched arms are rested vertically on the examiner's right shoulder. The examiner, in front, crosses the hands over the segment to be treated and presses on it, while pushing the shoulder forward. With backward and forward movement of the trunk, the examiner can execute repeated mobilizations in extension.

Figures A4.10–A4.12. The patient is seated on the table with the feet on the bar of the stool and the arms stretched forward. The examiner is at the side, with the outer foot on the stool and the forearm holding the stretched arms of the patient. The physician rests the forearm on the knee and, with the other hand, presses the thoracic region that has to be mobilized. While increasing the pressure, the examiner bends the knee outward, thus lengthening the thoracic spine in extension. The examiner then releases, puts the foot back at the starting position, and does a series of alternating slow, rhythmic, and elastic movements.

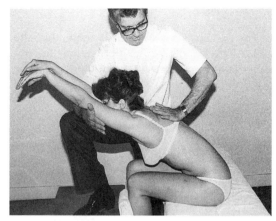

Figure A4.10.

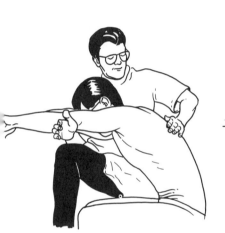

Figure A4.11. Positioning.

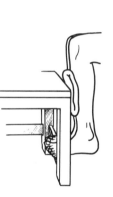

Figure A4.12. Taking up the slack.

Figure A4.13. The patient is sitting with arms crossed behind the head. The physician, from behind, passes the left forearm in front of the chest and grasps the patient's right arm. The physician, with right elbow on the right hip, presses with the right hand on the zone to be mobilized in extension. By rotating the pelvis and advancing the hip, the physician transmits increased pressure through the right forearm to the spine while applying counterpressure with the left forearm as it pulls the upper thorax into extension.

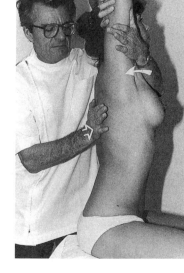

In Lateroflexion

The patient is seated astride the end of the table. This maneuver is performed slowly, with counterpressure well maintained by the operator's right hand by placing the right elbow against the iliac crest. At maximum tension, the pressure is gradually released and reapplied several times.

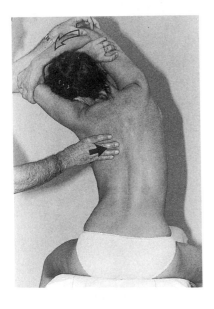

Figure A4.14. Left lateral flexion. The subject is seated astride at the end of the table, arms crossed over the head. The examiner stands to the left and grasps the patient's right elbow. The examiner's left forearm rests on the patient's right forearm. The examiner then applies the right hand to the patient's left lateral thorax and bends patient's thoracic spine to the left by pulling back with the left hand. The examiner can vary the degree of bending by changing the position of the right hand. The maneuver is performed slowly, with counterpressure from the right hand as the examiner's right elbow rests on the iliac spine. At the point of maximal tension, the pressure is relaxed. The movement is performed several times.

In Rotation

The patient is seated astride the end of the table in rotation.

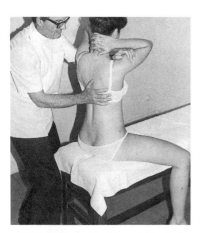

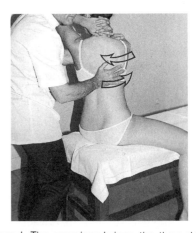

Figure A4.15. The patient is astride the end of the table, back to the examiner, and hands crossed behind the neck. The examiner grasps the patient's right arm with the left hand. The right hand grasps the region to be mobilized, with the heel of his hand overlying the right transverse process. The examiner's right elbow is at a 90° angle, and the forearm is parallel to the ground. The examiner brings the thoracic spine into left rotation with the left hand, while the right hand applies pressure on the transverse process in a synchronous manner, which increases the rotation on the affected vertebrae. The examiner takes up the slack, maintains it for a moment, and then returns to the starting point. This maneuver is repeated several times.

MANIPULATION

(Basic) Epigastric Technique

Two patient hand positions are utilized: hands folded behind the neck (hands-on-neck) and hands placed anteriorly across the thorax (hands-front).

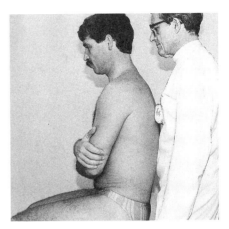

Figure A4.16. Positioning.

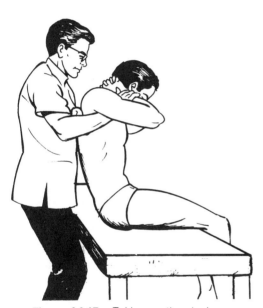

Figure A4.17. Taking up the slack.

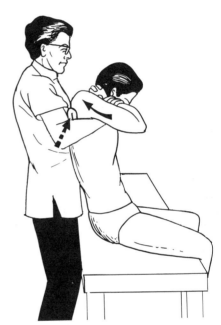

Figure A4.18. Taking up the slack. Manipulative thrust.

Hands-on-Neck Position (Figs. A4.17 and A4.18)

Positioning. The patient is seated on the table, with legs dangling over the edge and hands folded behind the neck. The physician, standing behind, passes the forearms under the patient's axilla and grasps the wrists. The physician's sternum is applied to the patient's midthoracic region, with a tightly rolled towel (or bolster) interposed between examiner and patient (Fig. A4.16).

Taking up the Slack. The examiner takes a deep breath while elevating the patient by the axillae, taking care that no downward pres-

sure is applied to the wrists (this would produce neck hyperflexion). Simultaneously, the sternal pressure against the patient's spine is increased by elevation of the examiner's chest at end inspiration with a Valsalva maneuver. Sternal pressure is further augmented by compressing the patient's thorax between the two forearms (Fig. A4.17).

Manipulative Thrust. The examiner briefly exaggerates the forward and upward sternal movement, without applying tension to the patient's neck, while the examiner's forearms elevate the patient's thorax posteriorly (Fig. A4.18).

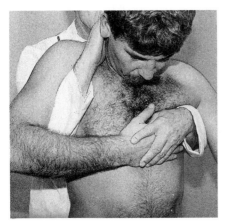

Figure A4.19.

variable height adjustment should be used or the examiner must adjust to the patient by bending the knees and keeping the chest straight (though the examiner always keeps the legs bent).

The examiner's right arm is passed under the patient's right axilla, with the hand on the patient's neck. This hand determines and maintains the degree of neck and back flexion. Its pressure must not vary because it maintains the chosen position throughout the maneuver, even during the terminal manipulative thrust.

With the left hand, the examiner then grasps the patient's right wrist (or hand) and firmly places it against the patient's chest immediately in front of the thoracic point of contact. The left arm of the patient remains free at the side (Fig. A4.19).

Placement is now completed (Fig. A4.20); subject and examiner must move together, en bloc, as the examiner firmly maintains the pressure against the sternum.

Taking up the Slack. The examiner simultaneously increases the sternal pressure against the patient's spine by elevating the chest at end inspiration with a Valsalva maneuver. Sternal pressure is further augmented by increasing the traction on the patient's forward arm, pulling the patient posteriorly.

Manipulative Thrust. As in the preceding technique, the manipulative thrust originates from the sternal pressure (Fig. A4.21) while the patient's upper thorax is elevated upward and backward.

Hands-Front Position (Figs. A4.20–A4.22).

This position is generally more efficacious than the hands-on-neck position, especially for the middle and inferior thoracic spine. It is also more comfortable for the patient.

Positioning. The patient is seated. A tightly rolled towel or bolster is placed between the examiner's lower sternum and the segment to be manipulated. To adjust to the various vertebral levels, either a table with a

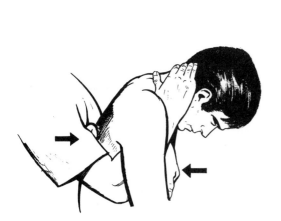

Figure A4.20.

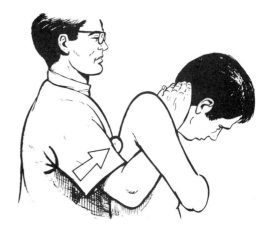

Figure A4.21.

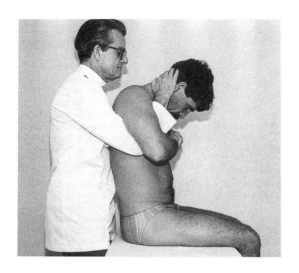

Localizing the Manipulation to a Specific Spinal Segment

Depending of the level chosen, the position of the patient is modified by varying the degree of posterior inclination, so that the segment to be manipulated is situated at the apex of the curve formed.

Hands-Front Position

For the midthoracic region, the patient sits normally on the table, with the chest vertical (Fig. A4.22, *top*).

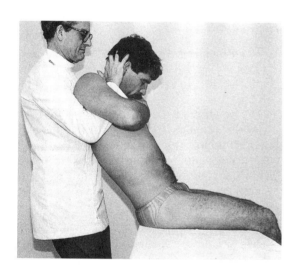

For the upper segments, the examiner must pull the patient backward so that the plane of the shoulders falls behind the table (Fig. A4.22, *middle*).

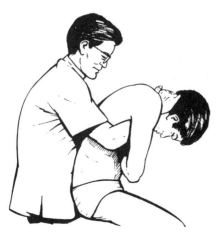

For the lower segments, the examiner positions the patient in slight forward bending, rounding the patient's back (Fig. A4.22, *bottom*).

Figure A4.22.

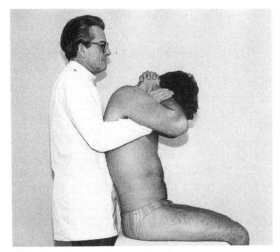

Figure A4.23.

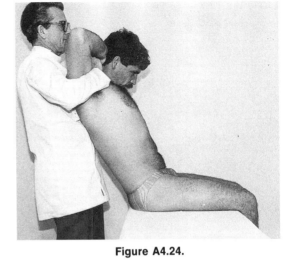

Figure A4.24.

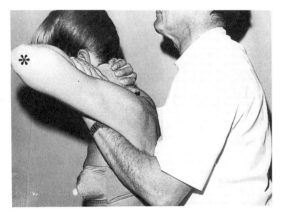

Figure A4.25.

Hands-on-Neck Position

The principle is the same as above: midthoracic spine (Fig. A4.23); superior thoracic spine (Fig. A4.24); inferior thoracic spine (Fig. A4.27).

The position of the patient's arms and the examiner's hands is important for the successful execution of the maneuver. The positions can vary depending on the patient's or physician's size, but in general, the following techniques can accommodate:

- The midthoracic spine (Figs. A4.23 and A4.25). The patient's arms are positioned horizontally or slightly lower. The examiner's hands are applied to the patient's wrists.

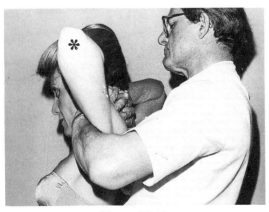

Figure A4.26.

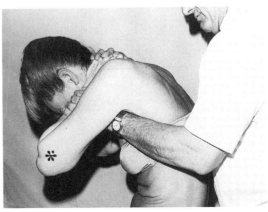

Figure A4.27.

- The superior thoracic spine (Fig. A4.24 and A4.26). The patient's arms are positioned more vertically and are abducted and externally rotated. The examiner's hands overlap those of the patient.
- The inferior thoracic spine (Fig. A4.27). The patient's arms rest below the horizontal. The examiner's hands grasp the patient's forearms, proximal to the wrists.

Variations in the Terminal Manipulative Thrust. An alternative technique of administering the manipulative thrust modifies the manner in which the examiner elevates the patient. This modification involves the sudden extension of the semiflexed knees or rising up on the toes while the examiner's trunk and lower limbs are maintained rigidly.

First Method
POSITIONING. The patient is positioned as above. The physician's knees are *partially flexed* because the muscles of the thighs and the legs are contracted.

TAKING UP THE SLACK. There is no change from above. The physician's chest is inflated at end inspiration and the sternum is pushed forward and upward while firmly maintaining the patient. Physician and patient move *en bloc*.

MANIPULATIVE THRUST. The physician begins by briefly externally rotating the hips and spreading the partially flexed knees, which suddenly stretches them a few degrees. This results in a sudden elevation of the examiner's upper body (which remains stiff throughout) including the thorax and sternal pressure. Contrary to what one might think, when performed with precision, this maneuver, is not traumatic.

Second Method. This method is quite similar to the first.

POSITIONING. As above.

TAKING UP THE SLACK. As above.

MANIPULATIVE THRUST. Although the principle is the same, the examiner's technique is modified slightly. The examiner's entire body becomes blocked and stiff, holding the subject firmly against it, while firmly maintaining the pressure of the hands on the patient's neck and sternum. The examiner's feet are flat on the floor and the knees are slightly flexed. The manipulative thrust is executed by suddenly raising the heels from the floor while maintaining the knees in their semiflexed position. This movement must be very rapid. The cervicothoracic segment must be perfectly fixated, without any loosening, throughout the maneuver.

(Basic) Sitting Astride Technique

Designed for manipulation in rotation, this technique is applicable at all levels, from the midthoracic to the low lumbar spine, in neutral position, flexion or extension. The rotation can be pure or combined with lateroflexion (Fig. A4.28)

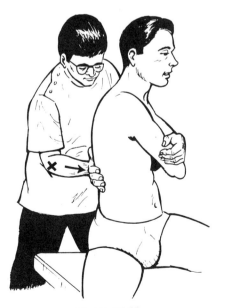

Figure A4.28.

In Pure Rotation (Fig. A4.29).

The technique is performed according to the usual three phases: placing in position, taking up the slack, and terminal thrust.

Example

Manipulation in Left Rotation.

Positioning. The patient is seated astride the end of the table with the physician standing behind. The patient's arms are crossed in front of the chest, with each hand grasping the opposite arm (Fig. A4.29, *left*). The physician's left arm passes in front of the patient's thorax and grasps the patient's right arm to bring the trunk into left rotation. The physician's right thenar eminence (or hypothenar eminence) is placed over the transverse process of the target vertebra (Fig. A4.29, *right*).

Taking up the slack. This is assured by the action of the physician's left arm as it brings the patient's trunk to end range. This movement is assisted by the palm of the right hand.

Manipulative thrust. The physician uses a brief simultaneous action of both hands.

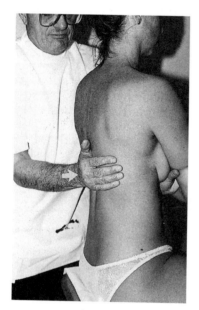 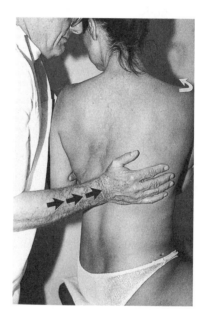

Figure A4.29. **Left.** Start of the maneuver (taking up the slack). **Right.** End of the maneuver (taking up the slack and manipulative thrust).

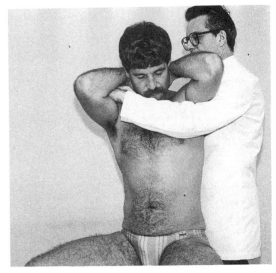

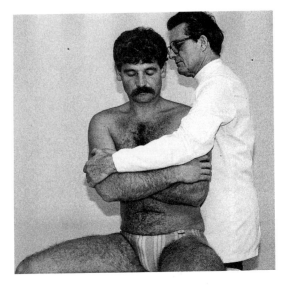

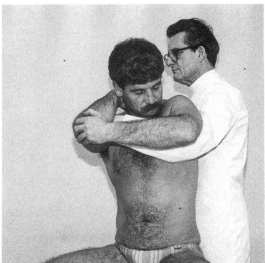

Figure A4.30.

Variations of the Patient's Arm Position

Several arm positions can be assumed by the patient. The choice depends on the size of both the examiner and the patient and especially on the level to be treated: hands-on-neck (Fig. A4.30, *top left*); arms crossed (Fig. A4.30, *top right*); mixed position, one hand behind the neck, the other grasps the elbow (Fig. A4.30, *bottom left*).

Positions of the Examiner's Arms and Feet

Arm Position (Fig. A4.30). Independent of the position chosen for the patient's arms, the examiner's right forearm must remain perpendicular to the spine during the manipulation (Figs. A4.31 and A4.32). The height of the table must be adjusted if possible to accommodate this. When using a table without a variable height, the physician varies the degree of knee flexion to adjust the position of the arms. The left forearm must also be horizontal.

The technique is more efficient if the examiner's elbow is against the iliac crest (for the lower and midthoracic segments) (Fig. A4.32). The thoracic pressure is then applied by a pelvic thrust anteriorly. The manipulation is therefore due to a vast rotation of the examiner's entire body to the left, while the forearms are maintained parallel to the floor and each other, subtending a horizontal arc (Figs. A4.31–A4.35).

Position of the Feet.   To perform the horizontal circle with the arms, the examiner must turn around the patient, in small steps. As the slack is taken up, the physician plants the foot ipsilateral to the contact hand and shifts the weight to that side. The pelvic rotation is thus transmitted to the elbow and contributes to the manipulative thrust of the forearm.

Example

For a manipulation in left rotation, the examiner's weight is shifted somewhat to the left, with the right foot positioned slightly behind the left (Figs. A4.32 and A4.35, *left*, starting position; Figs. A4.34 and A4.35, *right*, finishing position).

The movement of the feet (*white asterisk*) and the pelvis (*black asterisk*) is shown in the figures by the *arrows*.

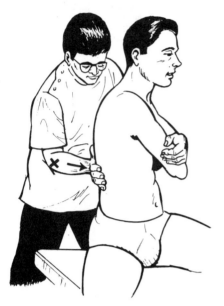

Figure A4.31. Starting position of the arm.

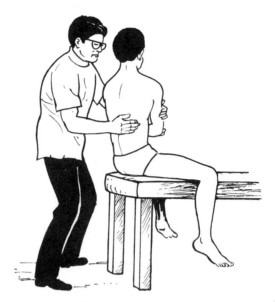

Figure A4.32. Positioning.

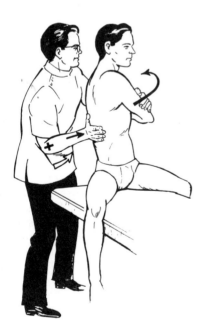

Figure A4.33. Intermediate phase.

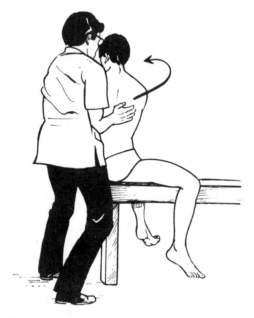

Figure A4.34. Taking up the slack. Manipulative thrust.

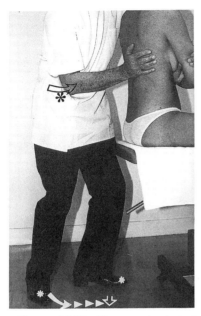

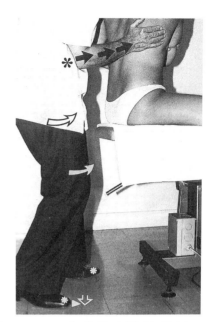

Figure A4.35. The examiner's foot position during the maneuver. **Left.** Start. **Right.** Finish.

In Rotation, Combined with Other Directions. The neutral position technique (pure rotation) described above can be combined with flexion, extension, or lateroflexion (Figs. A4.36–A4.40).

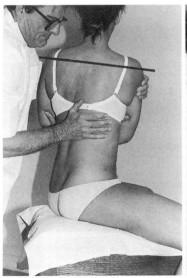

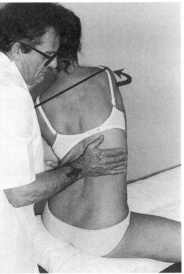

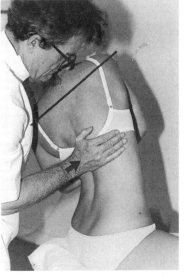

Figure A4.36 (left). Manipulation in left rotation of the inferior thoracic spine in neutral position, without flexion or extension (crossed arms position). The plane of the shoulders is horizontal.

Figure A4.37 (middle). Manipulation in left rotation of the inferior thoracic spine with left lateral flexion (crossed arms position), without flexion or extension. The plane of the shoulders is inclined toward the left.

Figure A4.38 (right). Manipulation in left rotation of the middle of the inferior midthoracic spine in left lateral flexion and in extension (crossed arms position).

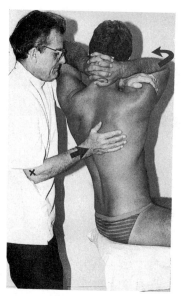

Figure A4.39. Manipulation of the midthoracic spine in left rotation in the neutral position (hands-on-neck position). Compare with Figure A4.40.

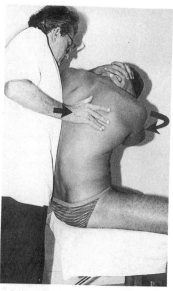

Figure A4.40. Manipulation of the midthoracic spine in left rotation and in flexion without lateral flexion (hands-on-neck position).

Resisted Manipulation. The previously described techniques are assisted manipulations, in which the manipulative thrust of the right hand is in the same direction as the trunk and the left hand.

In the assisted technique, pressure is applied to the transverse process of the supra-adjacent vertebra of the segment to be manipulated (see Fig. A4.34). In certain cases, the resisted maneuver may be used (Fig. A4.41).

For example, to produce left rotation of T11, the examiner can apply counterpressure to the left transverse process of T12 with the heel of the right hand, while the left hand takes up the slack in left rotation and applies the manipulative thrust. The examiner's right elbow is firmly in contact with the right iliac crest.

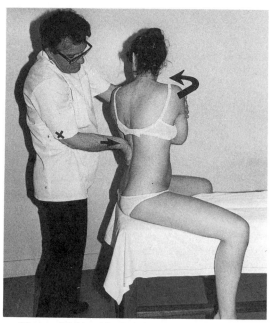

Figure A4.41. Manipulation in counterrotation.

(Accessory) Knee Technique

This is an extremely precise technique for manipulation of the thoracic spine.

Positioning (Fig. A4.42)

The patient is seated on a stool, with hands folded behind the neck. The examiner stands behind, with a foot on the bar of the stool, whose height is adjusted to the thoracic level to be manipulated. The examiner then grasps the patient's wrists with both hands, after having passing the forearms under the patient's axillae. The knee is then placed in contact with the spinous or transverse process (the latter introduces a rotational component to the thrust) of the vertebra on which the manipulation will be performed. The contact point is padded by a folded thick towel or bolster.

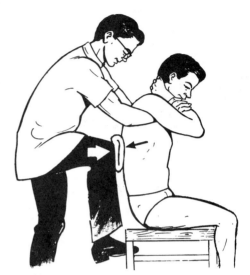

Figure A4.42. Positioning.

Manipulative Thrust

With the knee well fixed, the physician takes up the slack by elevating the patient's axillae upward and toward the physician, without applying downward leverage on the patient's wrists. The manipulative thrust consists of exaggeration of this traction slightly, without the least effort.

This maneuver can be performed at all levels of the thoracic spine, but it is technically more difficult at the superior thoracic level. Notwithstanding its appearance, this maneuver is not uncomfortable for the patient at all. It must be executed with the fingertips and with well-trained hands, so that it is soft and precise. Depending on the spinal level (mid-thoracic, Fig. A4.44; upper, Fig. A4.45; or lower, Fig. A4.46), the examiner positions the patient's trunk in neutral, flexion, or extension, so that the apex of the curve formed is over the segment to be manipulated (Figs. A4.44–A4.47).

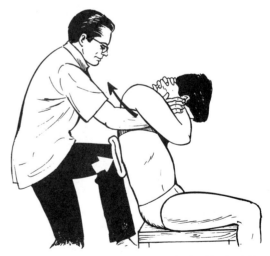

Figure A4.43. Taking up the slack. Manipulative thrust.

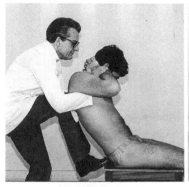

Figure A4.44.

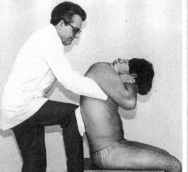

Figure A4.45.

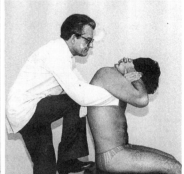

Figure A4.46.

Localizing the Manipulation to a Specific Spinal Segment

- Midthoracic spine (Figs. A4.44 and A4.47*A*).
- Superior thoracic spine (Figs. A4.45 and A4.47*B*).
- Inferior thoracic spine (Figs. A4.46 and A4.47*C*).

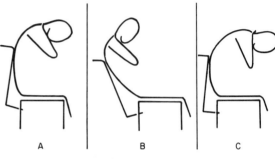

A   B   C

Figure A4.47.

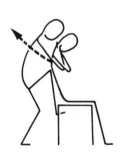

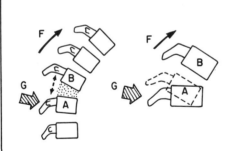

Figures A4.48 and A4.49. Mechanism of action of the maneuver on the spine.

Figure A4.48. The contact point of the knee (*G*) is applied to the spinous process of *A*. The global movement imparted by the examiner's arms results in flexion (*F*). This movement is maximal between *A* and *B* because of the position of the knee.

Figure A4.49. If the spine was initially in extension (which is not possible with all patients), the pressure applied here on *B* would facilitate the extension of *B* on the subjacent vertebrae (*A*). It should be considered an assisted maneuver. The segment *AB* would be manipulated in extension and no longer in flexion.

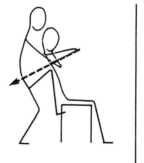

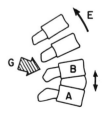

Supine (Basic Technique)

Hands-on-Neck Position (Figs. A4.50–A4.53)

The patient is supine, with the hands folded tightly behind the neck, elbows adducted forward, and the forearms resting under the chin. The physician stands to the right and grasps the patient's elbows with the left hand. The physician will act as a lever on them.

The patient places a hand in the "gutter" (here the right one) over the segment to be manipulated, while the left hand applies pressure to the elbows, to vary the degree of flexion necessary to place the segment to be treated under maximal tension. Once the slack has been taken up, a brief manipulative thrust of the left arm will suffice to obtain the manipulation, as it directs force toward the right hand (counter support).

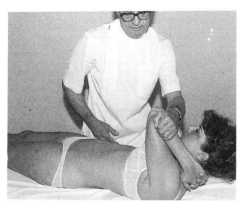

Figure A4.50. Preparation.

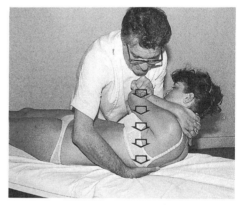

Figure A4.51. Execution.

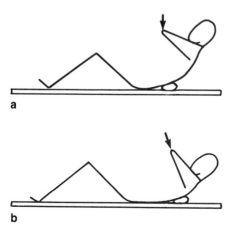

Figure A4.52. Diagram showing how to obtain a manipulation of the upper (a), mid-, or lower (b) thoracic spine, according to the position of the thoracic hand and the degree of flexion imposed on the spine.

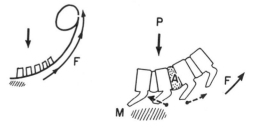

Figure A4.53. Diagram demonstrating the action of the manipulation on the spine. M, the counterpressure of the hand; P, the pressure provided by the weight of the physician; A, the segment on which the action is performed; F, the force of flexion imposed by the elbow pressure.

Crossed Arms Position (Figs. A4.54–A4.58)

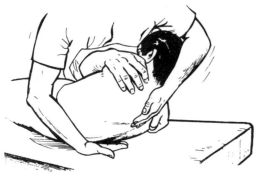

Figure A4.54. Preparation.

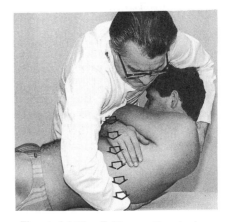

Figure A4.55. Taking up the slack.

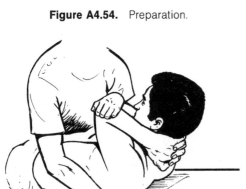

Figure A4.56.

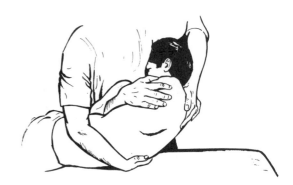

Figure A4.57.

The patient's arms are crossed in front of the chest (Fig. A4.54) while the examiner's thoracic spine applies pressure (which is performed in a protected manner, using a cushion). The examiner's left forearm and hand

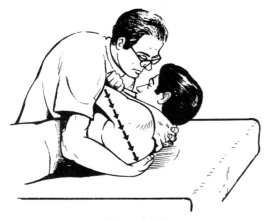

Figure A4.58.

maintain the thoracic spine in the necessary position of flexion. The fixed point of contact is provided (as in the above technique) by the right hand placed flat in the gutter on the table.

Note the position of the examiner's left arm (Fig. A4.55), which envelops the head in line with the axis of the body. This technique is especially useful for mid- and inferior thoracic spine problems. The manipulative thrust is given by sudden, but measured, accentuation of the thoracic pressure.

Figure A4.56 shows a manipulation performed on a midthoracic spine (patient: hands on neck); start of the maneuver.

Figure A4.57 shows a manipulation performed on the inferior thoracic spine (patient: crossed arms); start of the maneuver.

Figure A4.58 shows a manipulation of the superior thoracic spine (patient: hands on neck); end of maneuver, moment of manipulative thrust.

Direct Technique

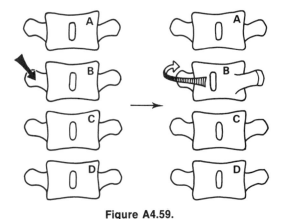

Figure A4.59.

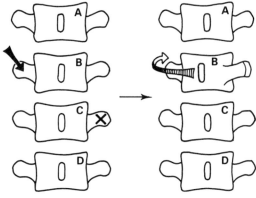

Figure A4.60.

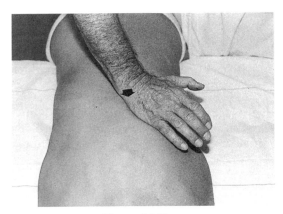

Figure A4.61.

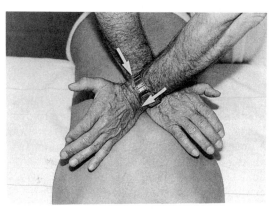

Figure A4.62.

This apparently easy technique readily produces the familiar ''cracking'' sound. In reality, it is difficult to measure it well.

In Figure A4.59, pressure on the left transverse process of *B* gives the vertebra *B* a rotation to the right in relation to *C*. Counterpressure on the right transverse process of *C* will add precision to the movement (Fig. A4.60). Pressure is applied with the pisiform of each hand (Figs. A4.61 and A4.62).

An analogous technique, done in a particular way, was one of the essential chiropractic maneuvers: the ''recoil'' of Palmer. The principle is shown in Figure A4.63. Pressure is maintained by the examiner's hand contact, with arms slightly flexed. The manipulative thrust is performed by the rapid contraction of the triceps, which relax immediately. This type

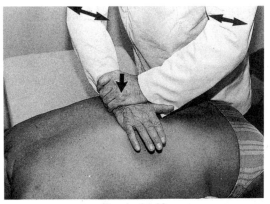

Figure A4.63.

of maneuver demands that patient's body and head rest on a support that absorbs a part of the manipulative force and offers a counterresistance to the segment that is treated.

MASSAGE

Superficial petrissage is used in the treatment of cellulalgic subcutaneous tissues. The maneuver is adjusted according to the severity and degree of induration. There are two typical cases.

The first type is a global cellulalgia of the lumbar region. The thickened subcutaneous tissues are sometimes difficult to mobilize on the deep fascial planes and difficult to pleat. In these patients, the superficial fascial planes must be mobilized on the deep planes. This is followed by maneuvers of progressive pleating (or folding?) of the skin and superficial soft tissues. The skinfolds are very thick at first, but they become more pliable as the treatment progresses.

The second type is a localized cellulalgia, often unilateral, usually corresponding to dysfunction of the thoracolumbar junction (Maigne's low back pain). It is the most frequent possibility (Fig. A5.1). Variable techniques can be used: pinch-rolling, Wetterwald's maneuvers, broken fold, etc.

The maneuvers are always somewhat uncomfortable. They must be well measured so that they are not painful; otherwise, the pain must stop at the same time as the maneuver.

RELAXATIONAL MANEUVERS AND MUSCLE STRETCHING

Relaxational Maneuvers

Buttock and Lower Limb Muscles

These techniques are used in the treatment of trigger points, often associated with segmental cellulotenoperiosteomyalgic syndrome of low lumbar origin.

Petrissage (Fig. A5.2). The treatment of gluteal trigger points associated with a lower lumbar PMID or to a discogenic problem is important in the treatment of the low back pain and the sequelae of sciatica. Slow deep petrissage of muscles with taut bands is generally effective. It must be performed in a rhythmic and progressive fashion.

When muscle involvement is very severe, petrissage can be contraindicated. This is often the case when the spine is the origin of the problem. Attention must be given first to that problem.

Slow pressure, maintained for 30–60 seconds on the most sensitive trigger points can also be effective.

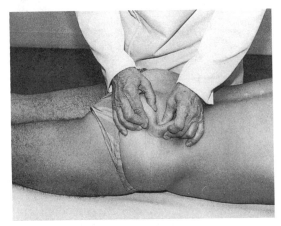

Figure A5.1.

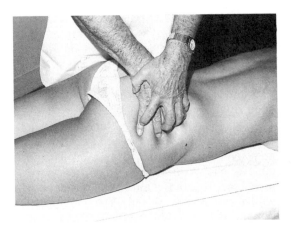

Figure A5.2.

Paraspinal Muscles

The patient is prone (head turned away from the side being treated) (Fig. A5.3).

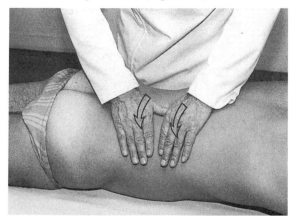

Figure A5.3. The examiner stands opposite the side to be treated, hands applied to the paraspinal region, with the fingers apart and the thumbs touching each other, in a line parallel to the line of the spinous processes. With the "bar" formed by the thenar eminence of the thumbs, the examiner slowly pushes the paraspinal muscles, as if trying to push them away from the spinous process and detach them from the deeper fascial plane. When maximum tension is reached, the examiner pauses, slowly exaggerates the pressure, and then releases it. This gesture is performed in a rhythmic and controlled manner, without losing contact, even during the period of relaxation.

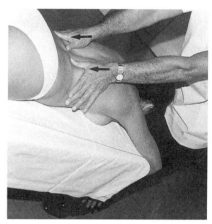

Figure A5.4. The examiner's thumbs are placed on each side of the line of the spinous process and perform slow, deep, gliding maneuvers. They are very relaxing and should be performed slowly and rhythmically.

N.B. These maneuvers are often an indispensable start to the spinal mobilization and manipulation.

Patient Supine.   (Figs. A5.4–A5.6.)

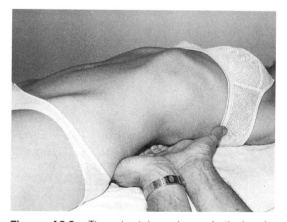

Figure A5.5. The physician places both hands under the patient's flank, with the fingertips nearly in contact with the transverse processes. The physician then pulls back on the closest lumbar muscles while the wrists act as a lever pushing the fingers upward. The pressure-traction is maintained for a while, relaxed, and then the movement is repeated. The maneuver is very sedating and is performed for acute low back pain.

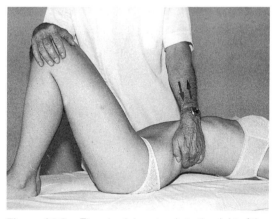

Figure A5.6. The physician stands to the right of the patient, whose legs are flexed. With the right hand, the physician takes the patient's knees while the left hand grasps the patient's left lumbar muscles. The knees are maintained in position, while the examiner pushes them back and pulls the erector spinae mass upward. This is performed slowly and rhythmically.

Patient in Side Lying: Fanning Maneuver (Fig. A5.7). The patient lies on the right side, with knees and hips flexed. The physician stands in front and rests the right forearm on the iliac crest, while the left forearm rests against the patient's axilla. The hands are placed side by side over the patient's flank. Using the fingertips in a clawlike fashion, the examiner grasps the left erector spinae mass. The examiner pulls the mass upward and back, while pulling the forearms apart, like a fan, which distracts the shoulder girdle away from the pelvic girdle.

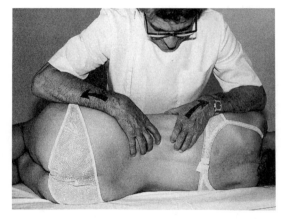

Figure A5.7. The fanning technique is used.

Stretching

These techniques constitute an efficacious means of treating trigger points.

Gluteus Medius and Tensor Fascia Lata

The patient is prone.

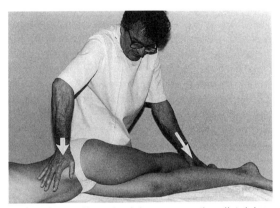

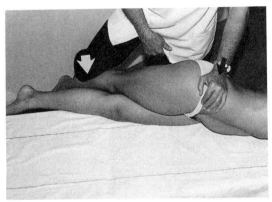

Figure A5.8. The physician grasps the distal leg above the knee and crosses it over the other leg, while applying counterpressure on the iliac crest with the other hand. This position is maintained for a few seconds, with stretching progressing a little more for each maneuver.

Figure A5.9. The examiner's knee can be used for this maneuver. The flexed knee rests on the superior part of the leg of the patient near the knee, and by pressing downward, stretches the gluteus medius and the tensor fascia lata.

External Rotators of the Hip

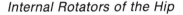

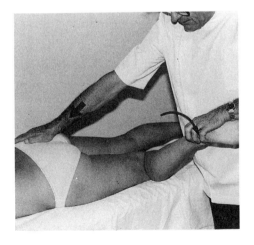

Figure A5.10. The patient is prone with the leg flexed 90° on the thigh (to the left). The examiner stands opposite the side being treated. The right hand blocks the pelvis, while the left hand pushes the sacrum and pushes the left foot of the patient outward, which causes internal rotation of the hip and stretches the external rotator muscles. This maneuver is performed progressively and interspersed with stretching in a slow, rhythmic pattern tailored to the reaction of the muscle (usually the pyriformis). A maneuver with the same effect can be performed with the patient supine, thighs and legs flexed at 90°.

Internal Rotators of the Hip

This maneuver, the opposite of the preceding one, can act especially on the gluteus minimus. A component of adduction incorporated into the technique increases the effectiveness of this maneuver on this muscle, which acts as an internal hip rotator as well as an abductor.

Extensors of the Hip and Spine

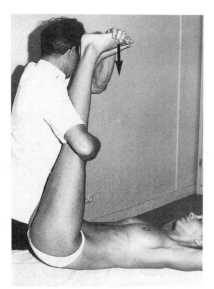

Figure A5.11. This maneuver stretches the triceps surae, hamstrings, and gluteus maximus. If the only aim of the maneuver is to stretch these muscles, the patient's hands can be crossed behind the neck (as shown). If the intent is to act on the paraspinal muscles as well, then the patient's arms should be kept along the body, with the shoulders down in a caudal direction and the chin in to eliminate the cervical lordosis.

At the start, the patient is supine, with the lower limbs extended. The physician squats and places both of the patient's legs on the shoulder. With the right hand, the physician dorsiflexes the feet. The dorsiflexion is maintained and slightly increased during the maneuver. With the left hand, the physician locks the knees in extension, and progressively stands up. In doing so, the physician slowly raises the patient's lower limbs until pain is reported (i.e., to the limit of what is bearable), then stops, lessens the tension slightly, and maintains this new position for 15–30 seconds (sometimes more). The tension is gradually increased in a stepwise fashion and interspersed with periods of relaxation, until the maximum length possible is reached. With each step, the initial painful feeling must dissipate gradually while the tension is maintained. Throughout the maneuver, the patient is encouraged to breathe regularly and deeply (Fig. A5.11).

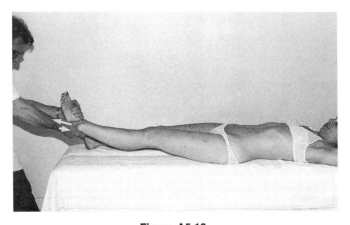

Figure A5.12.

Axial Traction of the Leg

This maneuver must be executed in three phases: (*a*) the examiner firmly grasps the patient's foot; (*b*) with the lower limb completely relaxed, the slack is taken up progressively; and finally (*c*) a sudden traction. The examiner's feet must be well under control.

This maneuver is contraindicated in sciatica, which could become serious. It can also produce good relaxation of the gluteal muscles (Fig. A5.12).

MOBILIZATION

These maneuvers act on the spine by mobilizing to end range and including the affected segments in the chosen direction. They also gradually lengthen the muscles. The movements must be applied slowly, repeatedly, and progressively. When muscular stretching is desired, they are maintained in tension for several seconds.

In Flexion

Contact on Both Knees

The patient is supine, with both knees and hips flexed (Fig. A5.13). The physician applies the hand and forearm to the patient's flexed knees and exaggerates pressure in the direction of the patient's head, bringing the lower limbs into hyperflexion. This maneuver must be repeated slowly, insisting a little more each time.

Variation. The examiner's shoulder holds the patient's legs. The examiner then bends forward and increases the lumbar flexion to take up the slack and then releases and starts again, slowly (Fig. A5.14).

Contact on One Knee (Fig. A5.15)

The physician stands beside the table (e.g., at right) and faces the head of the table. The examiner's left hand is applied to the patient's right shoulder while the right hand grasps the flexed knee. The degree of hip and knee flexion is then exaggerated, pushing the lower limb to-

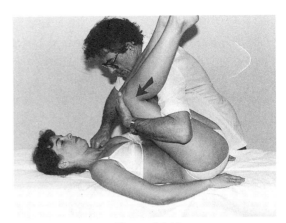

Figure A5.14.

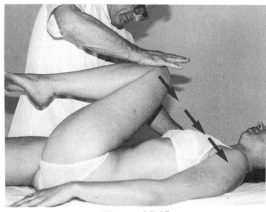

Figure A5.15.

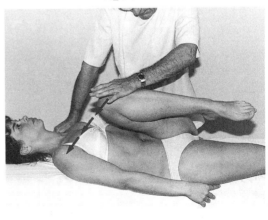

Figure A5.16.

ward the ipsilateral shoulder (Fig. A5.15). This maneuver is gradually released and repeated. This is a mobilization in pure flexion. However, if the physician pushes the thigh toward the contralateral shoulder, flexion and slight rotation result (Fig. A5.16).

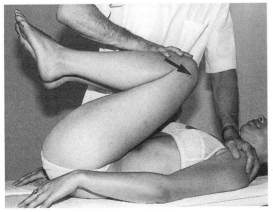

Figure A5.13.

In Lateroflexion

The patient is lying on the side. This maneuver is excellent, but powerful; it must be done with great care, progressively, and must be repeated slowly (Figs. A5.17 and A5.18).

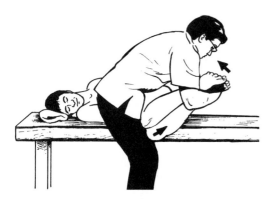

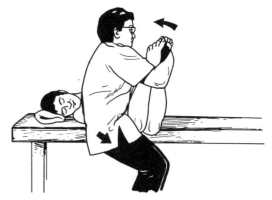

Figure A5.17. This maneuver mobilizes the patient into left lateral flexion. The patient lies on the right side, with legs and hips flexed 90°. The physician stands, hips and knees partially flexed, facing the patient. The physician's left elbow blocks the patient's left shoulder, and the right hand grasps the patient's ankles and places the knees on the physician's thighs.

The physician then pulls the patient's ankles upward while pushing anteriorly with the abdomen. This produces left lateral flexion of the patient's lumbar segments. The pressure is then released and returned to the starting position. **Left.** Positioning. **Right.** Taking up the slack.

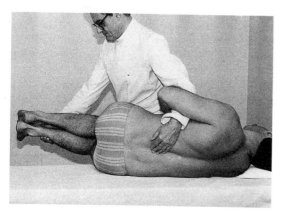

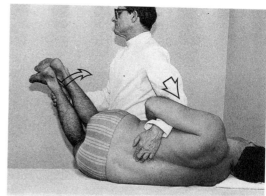

Figure A5.18. The same maneuver from another angle shows the position of the examiner's left arm. **Left.** Positioning. **Right.** Taking up the slack.

In Extension

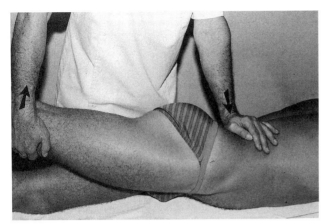

Figure A5.19.

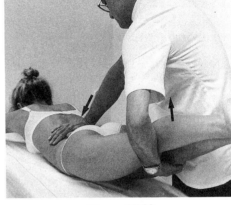

Figure A5.20.

The patient is prone. The physician stands beside the table and grasps the patient's farther thigh just proximal to the knee, while the other hand is applied to the lumbar region. The examiner then rhythmically extends the hip with counterpressure applied to the lumbar region (Fig. A5.19). With this technique, a certain degree of lateroflexion can be combined with the extension by combining hip adduction with the hip extension.

A similar maneuver can be done by simultaneously extending both of the patient's thighs (Fig. A5.20).

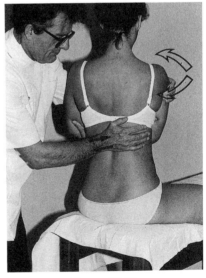

Figure A5.21.

In Rotation

The patient is seated astride the end of the table, arms crossed on the chest. The physician, stands behind and grasps the patient's right forearm with the left hand, while the right hand is applied to the paraspinal region. The examiner then gradually increases the degree of lumbar rotation imparted by the left arm. As in the thoracic techniques, the examiner's right elbow is held firmly against the iliac crest to transmit the force of pelvic rotation to the patient's lumbar spine. Mobilization is applied primarily by rotation of the examiner's pelvis, while the left arm acts in synchrony to bring the patient's trunk into left rotation (Fig. A5.21).

This maneuver is identical to that already described for the thoracic spine.

N.B.   From the astride position at the end of the table, all accessory orientations are possible (flexion or extension, ipsilateral or contralateral lateroflexion). It is the position that we use for examining the mobility of the lumbar spine as well as for certain manipulations.

MANIPULATION

(Basic) Lateral Decubitus Technique in Flexion (Fig. A5.22)

Positioning. The patient lies on the right side, with the head resting on a pillow, and the top lower limb flexed at the hip and knee (in this example, the left one). The examiner faces the patient and pulls the patient's lower arm (here, the right one) so that the plane of the shoulders is 45° to the plane of the table. The lower leg is extended at the knee, with the thigh in very slight flexion. The foot is positioned off the edge of the table at the corner and facing downward (Fig. A5.23).

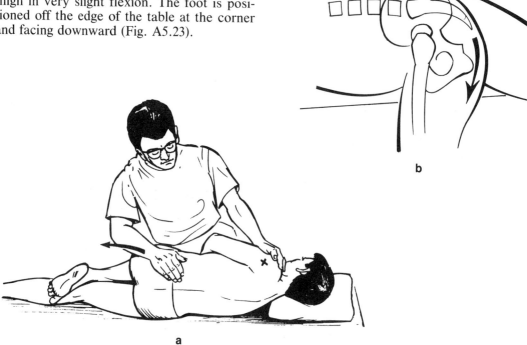

b

a

Figure A5.22. This maneuver imparts left rotation (**a**) to the lumbosacral segments by exaggerating the flexion (**b**).

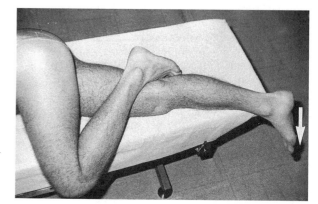

Figure A5.23. The lower leg (here the right one) is kept in extension at the knee during the entire maneuver. The foot is pointed down.

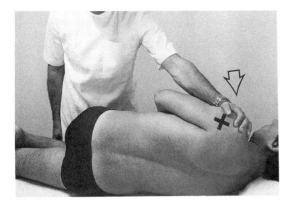
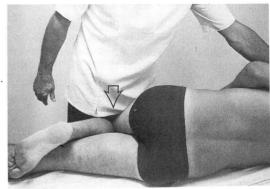
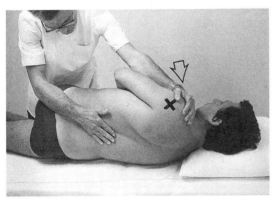
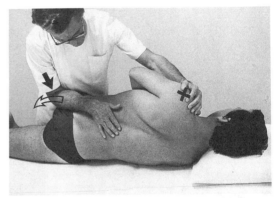

Figure A5.24.   Different phases of the manipulation.

The examiner's left hand is placed on the patient's left shoulder and firmly maintained; this is the "fixed point" (Fig. A5.24, *top left*), and it does not move during the manipulative thrust. The physician then places the right forearm against the patient's upward-facing ischium. The vector of manipulation applies a downward and distractive force to the patient's left hemipelvis, resulting in traction in flexion, with slight left rotation.

During this procedure, the physician stands close to the table. The physician's right knee blocks the patient's left thigh to maintain it firmly as well as to assuage any patient fear of falling off the table.

Taking up the Slack.   Once in position, the physician rotates the patient's body (which must move as a block) anteriorly (Fig. A5.24, *top right*). The ischial pressure is then increased to produce pelvic rotation (from right to left) while the left hand firmly fixates the shoulder (Fig. A5.24, *bottom left*).

Manipulative Thrust.   Once the slack has been taken up, the examiner suddenly increases the pelvic rotation with the right elbow on the ischium. The manipulative thrust is applied downward and to the right (Fig. A5.24, *bottom right*).

N.B.   The anterior rotation of the patient's trunk is well shown in Figure A5.26, as is the blocking of the patient's left thigh by the right knee of the examiner.

The technique shown in Figures A5.25 and A5.26 can be compared with the movement used in archery. The left hand pushes back the left shoulder, while remaining fixed at the time of manipulative thrust. At the same time, the right forearm pulls in the opposite direction, downward on the pelvis (Figs. A5.25 and A5.26 *a* and *b*; Fig. A5.22*b*).

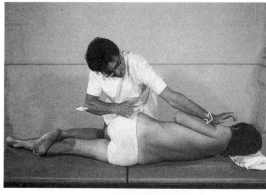

Figures A5.25.

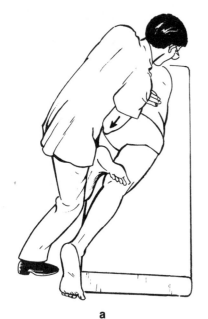

a

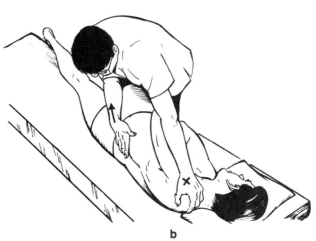

b

Figures A5.26.

Variation of the Manipulation in Flexion (Fig. A5.27):

The patient lies on the right side. Here, the physician does not use the hand to fixate the patient's shoulder, but instead, passes the forearm under the patient's axilla. The left hand now approximates the right one. This technique allows better control of the segment to which the rotation is applied.

By varying the amount of shoulder inclination and thigh flexion and the direction of the manipulative thrust by a few degrees, the physician can execute a precise and effective manipulation, but this maneuver does not allow as forceful an axial traction as the preceding one.

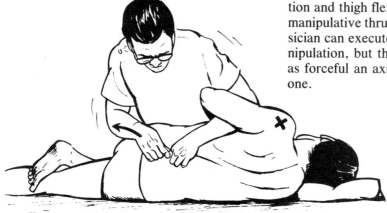

Figure A5.27.

(Basic) Lateral Decubitus Technique in Extension

Positioning. The patient lies on the side (on the right side for left rotation). For extension of the lumbar spine, the left leg is flexed at the knee, and the dorsum of the foot rests against the right popliteal fossa. The plane of the shoulders is perpendicular to the plane of the table. The lower leg is placed on the table in extension to facilitate the spinal extension. The examiner, standing in front of the patient, fixates the patient's shoulder with the left hand and maintains it during the entire maneuver (Fig. A5.28). The examiner's right hand is the active hand. It makes contact with the lateral

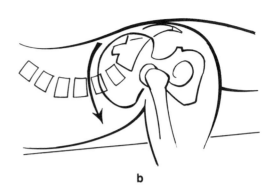

b

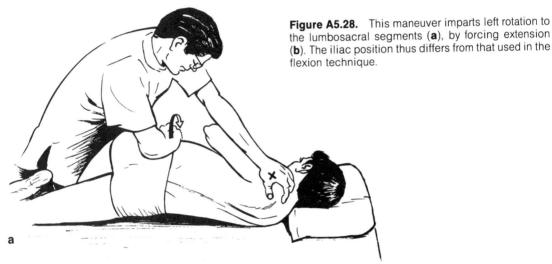

a

Figure A5.28. This maneuver imparts left rotation to the lumbosacral segments (**a**), by forcing extension (**b**). The iliac position thus differs from that used in the flexion technique.

iliac crest. The forearm is perpendicular to the plane of the back.

The iliac hand brings the patient's body into rotation around an axis that passes from head to toes, while the left hand, opposing the global movement, maintains the left shoulder of the patient in the position it had at the start (Figs. A5.28b and A5.29).

Figure A5.29. The contact with the iliac position can also be made with the forearm.

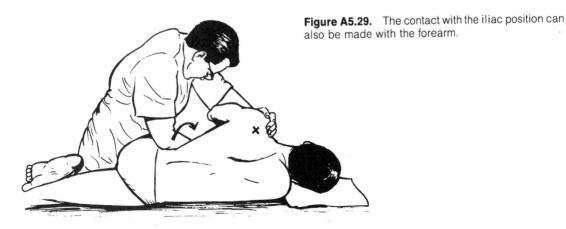

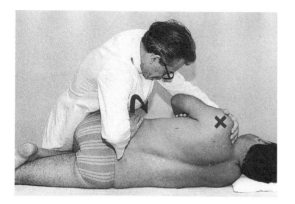

Figure A5.30. **Left.** Positioning. **Right.** Taking up the slack. Manipulative thrust.

The aim of the maneuver is to produce rotation of the lumbosacral spine (in this example, left rotation) and force the extension. The iliac placement thus differs from the one described in flexion (Figs. A5.28–A5.30).

Note the difference between the positions of the examiner in Figure A5.30, *left* and *right*, showing the moment of the forward manipulative thrust and the arm that is perpendicular to the axis of the patient's body.

Taking up the Slack. The physician then progressively rotates the left iliac crest anteriorly, bringing the lumbosacral spine into extension and left rotation (Fig. A5.28*a*).

Manipulative Thrust. The thrust is applied perpendicular to the axis of the spine, inferiorly and anteriorly (Fig. A5.30). The patient's left shoulder is firmly fixated by the examiner's left hand throughout the maneuver.

N.B. During the entire maneuver, the physician's thighs must maintain pressure against the patient's left thigh and knee, so that the patient is not concerned about falling from the table (Fig. A5.31).

Variation

The technique shown in Figure A5.32 is sometimes more comfortable for the examiner. The superior leg of the patient (the right one) is placed between the examiner's thighs. The technique is then the same as that described above.

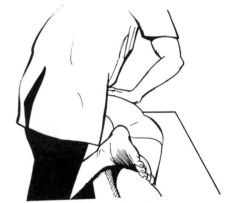

Figure A5.31.

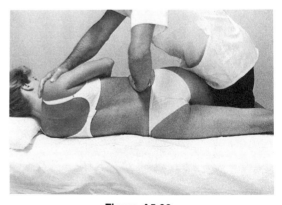

Figure A5.32.

Technique Lateral Decubitus in Neutral Position (without Extension or Flexion)

First Technique (Fig. A5.33, left)

The positions for both patient and physician are the same as in the technique described above. The active hand (the right one) is applied to the left edge of the sacrum. As in the technique in extension, the forearm is perpendicular to the plane of the patient's back. Thus no component of the thrust produces anterior pelvic rotation, as in the extension technique, nor any posterior rotation, as occurs with the flexion technique.

Second Technique (Fig. A5.33)

The patient is supine, with arms teriorly and left leg flexed at the hip From the patient's right side, the ex left hand grasps the patient's wrists fi block trunk movement. The examiner's hand then grasps the patient's left leg, d to the knee, to bring the hip into 90° of flexi The examiner then pulls in the thigh with thrust directed downward.

Figure A5.34 summarizes the various permutations and combinations of the lumbar lateral decubitus technique (described above and shown in Figs. A5.22–A5.33.) Much of what distinguishes these techniques is due to the angle and direction of the manipulative thrust executed.

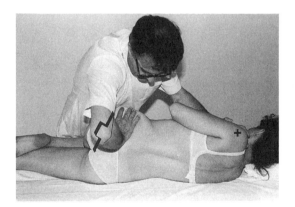
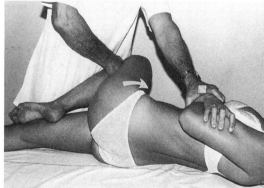

Figure A5.33.

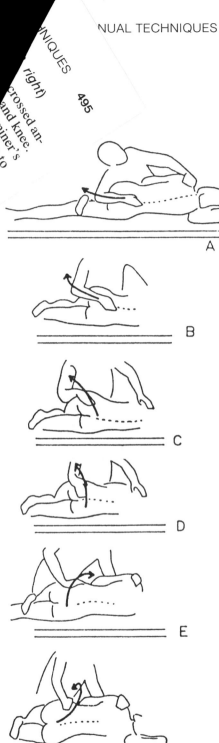

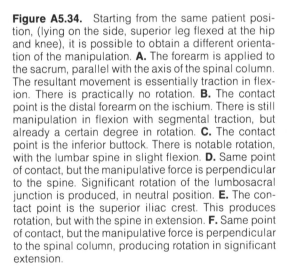

Figure A5.34. Starting from the same patient position, (lying on the side, superior leg flexed at the hip and knee), it is possible to obtain a different orientation of the manipulation. **A.** The forearm is applied to the sacrum, parallel with the axis of the spinal column. The resultant movement is essentially traction in flexion. There is practically no rotation. **B.** The contact point is the distal forearm on the ischium. There is still manipulation in flexion with segmental traction, but already a certain degree in rotation. **C.** The contact point is the inferior buttock. There is notable rotation, with the lumbar spine in slight flexion. **D.** Same point of contact, but the manipulative force is perpendicular to the spine. Significant rotation of the lumbosacral junction is produced, in neutral position. **E.** The contact point is the superior iliac crest. This produces rotation, but with the spine in extension. **F.** Same point of contact, but the manipulative force is perpendicular to the spinal column, producing rotation in significant extension.

(Basic) Astride Technique

This maneuver has already been described for the thoracic spine. It is the technique of choice for rotational manipulation of the thoracolumbar junction and can be utilized in the lower lumbar spine as well. It may also be combined with other coordinates including flexion, extension, rotation, or lateroflexion. It can be used in mobilization or in manipulation, and permits both assisted and resisted manipulative techniques. Moreover, this is an excellent position for examining and testing lumbar motion and detecting subtle degrees of painful limitation.

Manipulation in Pure Rotation

Positioning.   The patient is seated astride the end of the table, back to the examiner. Several arm positions are possible, including hands folded behind the neck (Fig. A5.35, *bottom left*); arms crossed anteriorly (Fig. A5.35, *top right*); and one hand behind the neck, with the other grasping the opposite elbow (Fig. A5.35, *bottom right*).

The hand-on-neck position is generally preferable if significant lateroflexion or rotation is desired, but the position chosen will depend on the size of both patient and examiner (see "(Basic) Epigastric Support Technique" in Appendix 4).

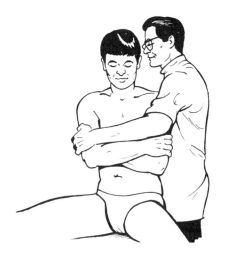

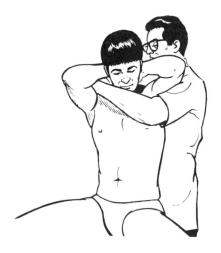
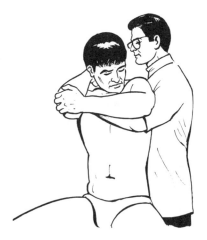

Figure A5.35.   Different patient arm positions.

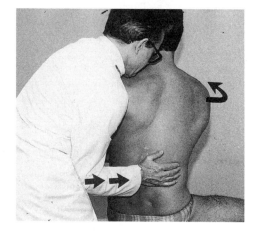

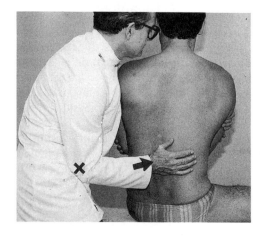

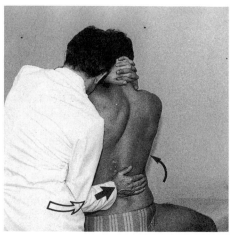

Figure A5.36. The three phases of manipulation. **Top left.** Positioning. **Top right.** Taking up the slack. **Bottom right.** Manipulative thrust. **Top left** and **top right** show the patient in the arms-crossed position, while to the **right**, the hands-on-neck position is shown. The rest of the maneuver follows the usual techniques.

For left rotation, the examiner passes the left forearm in front of the patient's thorax and grasps the right arm near the elbow. The examiner's right thenar eminence is applied to the right transverse process of the vertebra to be manipulated.

The forearm is held horizontally, perpendicular to the patient's trunk. However, if a variable-height table is not available, the examiner's legs are flexed to adjust the position. The right elbow may remain free, but it is best to place it against the anterior iliac crest (Fig. A5.36).

Taking up the Slack. At the start of the maneuver, the physician is slightly to the patient's left. The examiner's left hand brings the trunk into left rotation. Simultaneously, the examiner uses small gliding steps to pivot around the patient, while firmly maintaining the contact on the transverse process and progressively taking up the slack to end range in rotation. At that moment, most of the examiner's weight has been shifted to the right foot.

Manipulative Thrust. With the elbow still in contact with the iliac crest, the manipulative thrust is executed by transmitting pelvic rotation to the right forearm. (Fig. A5.36).

This technique has been described in detail above (see Appendix 4, ''(Basic) Sitting Astride Technique, In Rotation'').

Manipulation in Rotation Combined with Lateroflexion, Flexion, or Extension

This technique allows one to combine rotation with lateroflexion, flexion, or extension.

For example:

- Manipulation in left rotation and left lateroflexion (Fig. A5.37).
- Manipulation in left rotation, flexion, and left lateroflexion (Fig. A5.38). In this variation, the thumb is applied to the patient's spinal segment.
- Manipulation in left rotation, extension, and left lateroflexion (Fig. A5.39).

The manipulation can also be executed with combined contralateral lateroflexion. Certain authors consider this to be a sacroiliac manipulation because the spinal segmental motion is blocked by the lateroflexion. The maneuver acts on the ipsilateral sacroiliac joint (Fig. A7.8).

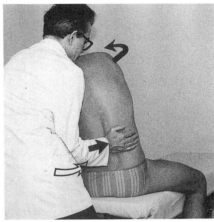

Figure A5.37.

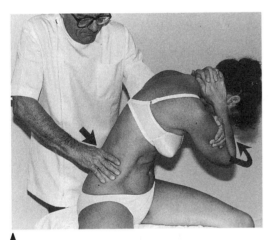

Figure A5.38. Lower lumbar manipulation into left rotation, with the spine in left lateral flexion and forward flexion.

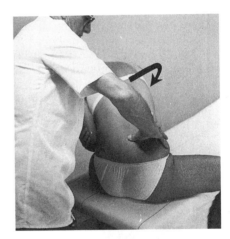

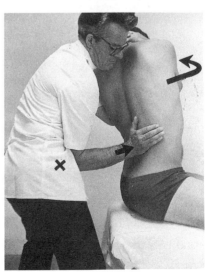

Figure A5.39. Manipulation at L3 into left rotation to the left, with the spine in extension and left lateral flexion.

(Accessory) Double Knee Technique (Fig. A5.40)

Positioning. The patient is seated on a stool, fingers crossed behind the neck. The physician is seated behind on the table, at a slightly higher level than the patient, with the balls of the feet resting on a bar of the stool so that the two knees are in contact with the segment to be manipulated. The heels are lowered as the examiner passes the forearm under the patient's axillae and grasps the wrists (Fig. A5.40).

Taking up the Slack. This is executed in two steps. First, the examiner slightly flexes the arms, pulling the patient back by the shoulders until a firm resistance is felt. Care is taken not to increase pressure on the patient's neck, to avoid altering the flexion applied at the start. The patient's hands must be tightly clasped. Second, the examiner then lifts the heels, which increases the pressure of the knees against the spine. This takes up the slack (Fig. A5.41).

Manipulative Thrust. The examiner briefly pulls both arms slightly upward and back.

This powerful maneuver must be executed gently. As with all manipulation, it must be strictly painless. (Fig. A5.40 shows the starting

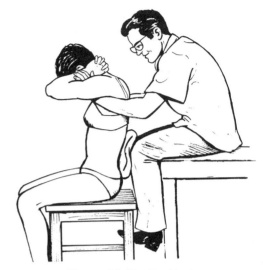

Figure A5.40. Positioning.

position; Fig. A5.41, the intermediary position; and Fig. A5.42, the position at the end. Fig. A5.41. shows taking up the slack (first step); Fig. A5.40, positioning; Fig. A5.42., taking up the slack (second step) and manipulative thrust.)

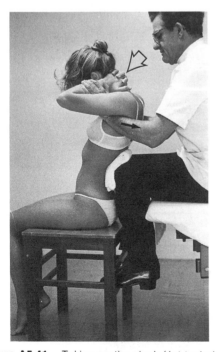

Figure A5.41. Taking up the slack (1st technique).

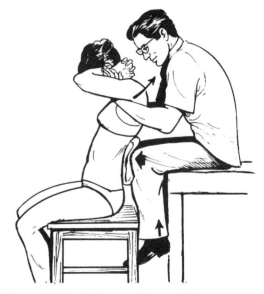

Figure A5.42. Taking up the slack (2nd technique) and manipulative thrust.

(Accessory) Belt Technique

This technique allows one to perform manipulation in pure rotation, rotation with ipsilateral lateroflexion, and rotation with contralateral lateroflexion. It is a powerful and delicate maneuver. The arms act as such powerful levers that the risk of patient injury is significant in the untrained examiner's hands.

In Pure Rotation

Figures A5.43–A5.46 illustrate right rotation. The effect of the maneuver is on the thoracolumbar junction.

Positioning.   The patient is prone and is attached to the table with a large belt over the sacrum.

For a manipulation in right rotation, the physician squats on the patient's right side, facing the shoulders (Fig. A5.43). The patient's right arm is on the physician's right shoulder. The physician's right hand grasps the patient's left shoulder, while the patient's left hand, flat, is placed against the examiner's back (Fig. A5.43). During the positioning, the patient must remain in the center of the table. Therefore, the physician must rise and move forward over the examining table (Fig. A5.43). Finally, the examiner places the left hypothenar eminence over the transverse process of the target vertebra (Fig. A5.44).

Figures A5.43–A5.46 show manipulation in pure rotation on the thoracolumbar junction.

Taking up the Slack.   The physician gradually leans forward, moving the patient with the

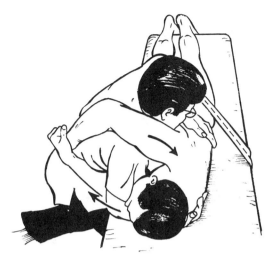

Figure A5.43.

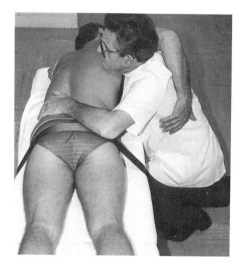

Figure A5.44.   Positioning.

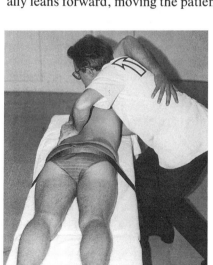

Figure A5.45.   Taking up the slack.

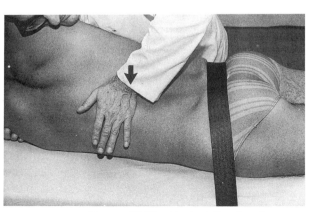

Figure A5.46.   Manipulative thrust.

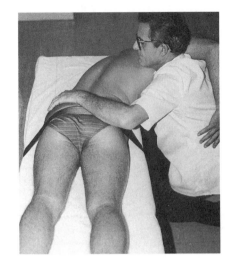

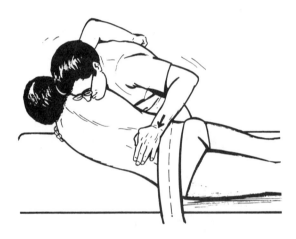

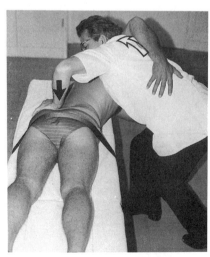

Figure A5.47. Manipulation with lateral flexion performed on the lumbosacral spine.

shoulder, and slowly rises half way up on the knees (Fig. A5.45). This imparts a degree of rotation to the patient's trunk, acting maximally on the thoracolumbar junction.

Manipulative Thrust. A slight push forward of the right shoulder gives the manipulative thrust (Figs. A5.45 and A5.46). This manipulative thrust must be measured. During the entire maneuver, the patient's chest should not move excessively on the table. The lumbar hand assists the movement by applying pressure over the left transverse process of the vertebra to be manipulated (Fig. A5.46). The patient's right shoulder should not, at any time, lose contact with the table. The patient must not be lifted up when the physician rises. During the maneuver, the examiner must maintain the patient on the table and watch that the patient does not rise. The patient is simply turned on the axis. As the physician's shoulder drives forward and slightly downward, the patient's lower shoulder is pulled toward the examiner (Fig. A5.43). The lumbar spine should not be in extension.

In Rotation with Ipsilateral Lateroflexion

A component of ipsilateral lateroflexion allows the manipulation to act on the lumbosacral and lower lumbar segments. Figure A5.47 illustrates right rotation and lateroflexion.

Positioning. The physician pulls in the patient and brings the head and shoulders off the end of the table (Fig. A5.47). The rest of the maneuver is applied as above. Figure A5.47 shows the different actions. The right arm of the examiner must assure that the patient remains "glued" to the table. The patient must not, in any case, be lifted. When the top of the patient's chest comes over the end of the table, the examiner must pull it downward when pressing with the right shoulder.

Taking up the Slack and the Manipulative Thrust. These are executed as in the preceding maneuver.

In Rotation plus Contralateral Lateroflexion

Figure A7.9 is an example of left rotation and right lateroflexion. This maneuver acts on the lower lumbar segments, and the proponents of sacroiliac joint dysfunction also consider it to act on the SI joint. It is described in Appendix 7.

A6. Rib Techniques

The techniques used in the treatment of the costal sprains are often the same as those used for examination. When examining, the aim is to try to evoke tenderness caused by either rib elevation or depression.

The same maneuvers are utilized for treatment, with the addition of a thrust at end range in the pain-free direction.

(ACCESSORY) FIRST TECHNIQUE (FOR THE INFERIOR RIBS)

In Figure A6.1*A*, the 12th rib is painful when depressed and pain free when elevated. Therefore, manipulation is performed in elevation. The patient is seated astride the end of the table with arms crossed overhead. The examiner positions the patient's trunk in left lateroflexion. The patient is instructed to breathe calmly as the examiner grasps the rib to be manipulated with the fingertips of the right hand and maintains it in traction. At the end inspiration, the pressure is suddenly increased with a very slight thrust.

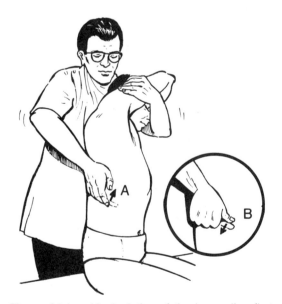

Figure A6.1. Manipulation of the lower ribs: first technique.

In contrast, if the rib is painful with elevation, it must be manipulated in depression (Fig. A6.1*B*). The patient is positioned in left lateroflexion. The examiner's thumb is applied to the superior edge of the rib to be manipulated. At end expiration, the manipulative thrust is applied lightly.

SECOND TECHNIQUE (FOR THE INFERIOR RIBS)

This maneuver is similar to the preceding one. To facilitate lateroflexion of the patient's trunk (in this example, to the left), the examiner's foot (left) is placed on the table so that the knee (left) rests under the patient's axilla (left). The rest of the maneuver is performed as in the preceding technique (Fig. A6.2).

Manipulation for the Last Ribs: Second Technique

The patient is seated astride at the end of the table or on a stool. The physician's knee passes under the patient's axilla contralateral to the side of the rib to be manipulated. This induces trunk lateroflexion, which opens up the region to be treated. The principle is the same as in the preceding technique. Depending on the case, one must either (*a*) slowly elevate the affected rib by grasping its inferior boarder with the fingertips (Fig. A6.2, *left*) or (*b*) slowly depress the affected rib with maintained pressure that is exaggerated at end expiration (Fig. A6.2, *right*)

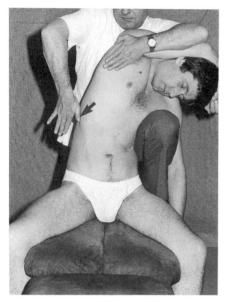 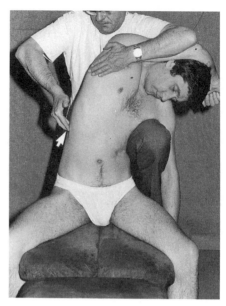

Figure A6.2.   Manipulation of the lower ribs: second technique.

Variation: Patient Standing (Fig. A6.3)

In certain difficult cases, the technique shown in Figure A6.3 is used. The physician has one foot on the manipulation table, the other on the stool. The patient, standing in front, rests the axilla on the physician's knee (here the right one). The left arm is raised vertically with the elbow flexed and the hand placed behind the neck. The physician applies traction to the patient's left elbow and thus increases the right trunk lateroflexion to open up the costal region on which the manipulation will be performed, according to the same principles as outlined in the above two above techniques (*A* and *B*).

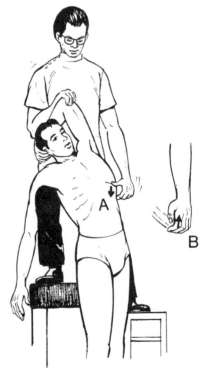

Figure A6.3.

THIRD TECHNIQUE (FOR THE MIDDLE AND INFERIOR RIBS)

The patient is seated astride the end of the table, hands crossed behind the neck or arms crossed on the chest (depending on the patient's morphology). To manipulate a right rib, the examiner grasps the patient's right arm with the left hand and applies the right hand, flat, on the thorax, parallel to the ribs (Figs. A6.4 and A6.5).

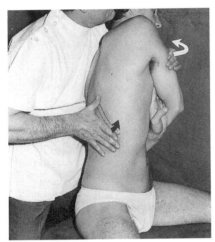

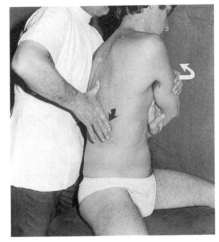

Figure A6.4. Manipulation in elevation. The examiner applies the lateral aspect of the index finger against the inferior border of the rib to be manipulated. The upward pressure is maintained throughout the entire maneuver. With the left arm, the patient's trunk is placed into combined left rotation and left lateroflexion. The right hand assists the movement. At end range, the patient is instructed to breathe slowly and deeply. At end inspiration, a brief and light thrust is given, synchronously, with the left hand (which accentuates the trunk rotation) and the right index finger (which accentuates the pressure upward). This is done while the thumb applies downward pressure against the superior border of the angle of the posterior rib.

Figure A6.5. Manipulation into depression. This maneuver is performed in a similar manner to that used with rib elevation. In this case, the palmar aspect of the index finger is applied to the superior edge of the rib. With this finger, the examiner applies constant downward pressure to the rib while the left arm brings the trunk into rotation and left lateroflexion. The active finger maintains the downward rib pressure. At the same time, the thumb applies upward counterpressure to the inferior edge of the posterior angle of the rib, elevating it. At end expiration, the pressure is gently and precisely increased to perform the manipulation, while a slight thrust is applied with the left hand to increase the rotation of the trunk to the left.

TECHNIQUE FOR THE FIRST RIB

The patient lies on the back, with the arm on the side of the rib to be treated lying along the body. For a left rib, the examiner, on the right side of the patient, places the right hand flat on the table, palmar side up, the thenar eminence resting on the posterior part of the first or second rib at the level of its angle. The other hand rests on the anterior part of the rib, near the sternum. This hand will execute the manipulative thrust, downward or upward, while the thoracic hand applies counterpressure (Fig. A6.6). This maneuver is delicate, requiring close attention when taking up the slack and precision when applying the terminal thrust.

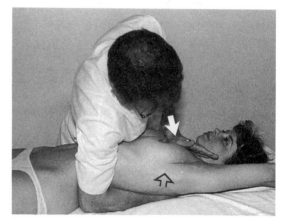

Figure A6.6.

TECHNIQUE FOR AN ANTERIOR COSTAL SPRAIN

The patient is supine. The examiner places the thumb on the superior edge of the rib to be manipulated and assists the downward movement of the rib during expiration. The pressure is maintained and is gently but progressively increased (Fig. A6.7). For this maneuver, it is more comfortable to position the patient's ipsilateral arm as shown in the figure. The maneuver is reversed when rib elevation is indicated (Fig. A6.8), applying the thumb to the rib's inferior edge with both thumbs opposed end to end.

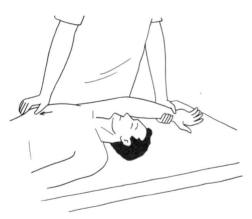

Figure A6.7.

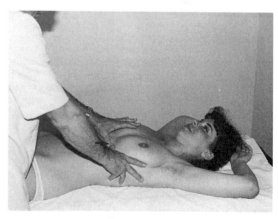

Figure A6.8.

A7 · So-Called Sacroiliac Joint Techniques

GENERALITIES

At the turn of the century, in the English-speaking world, joint sprains were thought to be responsible for most cases of lumbosciatic pain. The first published postmanipulative paraplegia resulted from a manipulation performed under general anesthesia by an orthopedic surgeon to treat an "SI joint sprain" (Goldwaith).

When Barr and Mixter discovered the herniated disk in 1930, it was in a young patient with a refractory acute sciatica attributed to an "SI joint sprain." They thought that the source of the sciatic pain might be a tumor. Mixter operated and discovered a "tumor" compressing the S1 root. This "tumor," thought first to be a chondroma, was a herniated disk. Micromechanical pathology of the SI joint has been forgotten for quite a long time in traditional medicine but still has a place for most manipulators. Important for chiropractors and osteopaths, it varies for the manipulative physicians, depending on the school. After having believed that SI joint microdisplacements were frequent, J. Cyriax thought they were rare, then concluded that they did not exist (1976).

Although the slight but real joint mobility has been proven, the existence of micromechanical pathology has not yet been validated. On the other hand, the techniques used to "unblock" these joints are perfectly effective in certain lumbar and lumbosacral dysfunctions. The question then is whether these so-called SI joint techniques act on the lumbosacral spine or on the SI joints themselves.

Semiology of SI Joint Disorders in Traditional Medicine

The clinical signs that are diagnostic of SI joint problems (inflammatory or infectious) in traditional medicine are far from specific, but it is interesting to recall them. The principal ones are

- Posterior pain caused by gapping or compressing the iliac wings with the patient supine (Fig. A7.1, *top left* and *top right*) or by compression of the superior iliac crest with the subject side lying, which gives a similar result.
- The tripod sign (Coste et al.): The patient is prone, and the examiner applies pressure on the sacrum with the heel of the hand, which irritates the SI joints and causes pain if they are affected.
- Gaenslen's maneuver: The subject is supine, and the examiner leans on the patient's flexed hip and knee (in this example, the right one), bringing them into hyperflexion. The patient's other leg hangs over the end of the table while the examiner exaggerates this movement by pushing the contralateral thigh downward into extension. This maneuver induces maximal SI joint nutation on one side (Fig. A7.1, *bottom left*) with counternutation on the other.
- This maneuver has the same aim. The patient is positioned in side lying (in this example on the left) and is instructed to bring the downward-facing hip and thigh into full flexion with the arms. The examiner grasps the patient's left (upward-facing) knee and brings the thigh into hyperflexion. After applying the left hand to the right iliac crest, the examiner hyperextends the upward thigh (Fig. A7.1, *bottom right*).

These maneuvers have both poor specificity and poor sensitivity, even in cases of inflammation of the SI joints. On the other hand, they can be painful in some cases of lumbosacral dysfunction.

Semiology Proposed by Supporters of SI Joint Blockage

Certain authors and most of the school of manual medicine believe that SI joint blockages are possible and even frequent. The diagnostic criteria are based on a certain number of signs that vary considerably depending on the school or author.

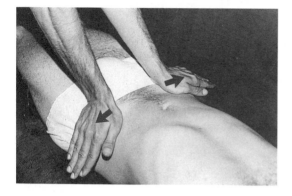
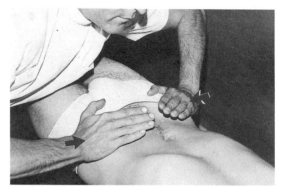
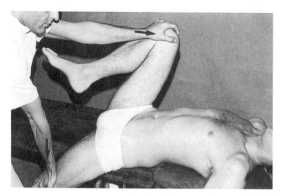
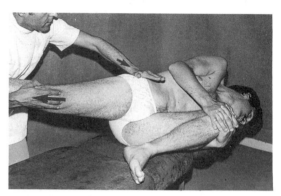

Figure A7.1.   Classical maneuvers for SI joint examination.

They are numerous and include:

- Positions and variations of gaps of different landmarks: posterior superior iliac spines, sacral apex, tubercle of S2, ischium, etc. when the subject bends forward, stands on one leg, or raises the knee to the chest.
- Modifications in tissues of the regions close to the SI joint and the influence of certain maneuvers on these modifications.
- Joint mobility tested by palpation.

We now review these proposed signs.

J. B. Mennell's Signs

Mennell believed that these "blockages" or "SI joint up-slips" were frequent. Among the numerous causes of SI joint sprains, movements such as getting out of the tub or turning back suddenly when one is seated in a chair are the most frequent. He recommended a series of examination maneuvers, for the most part osteopathic techniques, which would rotate the iliac crest either forward or backward to test the blockage or the freedom of movement. Note that it was presumed that these maneuvers selectively mobilized the SI joint and the SI joint only. However, this is not certain.

In case of blockage, the following signs should be found:

- With the patient seated, the posterior superior iliac spine (PSIS) is lower than the one on the opposite side if the iliac wing is blocked in posterior rotation on the sacrum. It comes back to the same level after an adequate manipulation (this sign is described by the osteopaths).
- There is an antalgic attitude in case of "acute SI joint sprain" (antalgic scoliosis concave at the blocked side).
- A false Lasègue's sign can exist. But contrary to what happens with discogenic sciatica, dorsiflexion of the foot does not increase pain if it is an SI joint sprain.
- Lateroflexion is not painful in patients with SI joint sprain (unless it is acute).

• In cases of pure sciatica, it has a nerve root topography. To demonstrate clinically the mobility of the SI joints, Mennell measured the distance between both PSISs of a patient, first sitting, then prone. In the latter position, he noted that the processes are 1.5 cm closer. We tried to find this sign and did not succeed. This measurement technique is quite difficult and subject to significant error. Colachis et al., using pins inserted in the iliac bones, found the opposite of Mennell's results; that is, the processes were slightly closer in the sitting position. But out of 12 cases, the maximum closeness was 1.5 mm, which is not clinically detectable.

Osteopathic Signs

As always in osteopathy, SI joint dysfunction is detected by palpation techniques. According to M. C. Beal, the diagnosis of "anterior sacrum" (i.e., blockage in nutation) or "posterior sacrum" (blockage in counternutation) is made according to classical osteopathic palpation.

Blockage in Nutation

• Local modification of the soft tissues with hypersensitivity to palpation over the superior part of the joint.
• "Strained" gluteal muscles in the part adjacent to the superior pole of the joint.
• "Tension" in the following muscles: adductor magnus (both superior heads), rectus femoris, and sartorius.
• The interval between the median part of the sacrum and the ilium at the level of the superior pole seems increased in relation to the other side and to the normal.
• The anterior superior iliac spine (ASIS) is higher on the blocked side than on the other.
• The PSIS is felt relatively lower on the blocked side (sign noticed by Mennell and Piédallu).
• There is an apparent ipsilateral leg length shortening (false short leg) noticed on examination in supine.
• Finally, palpation reveals loss of mobility in the SI joint that is blocked, at its superior pole.

Blockage in Counternutation

• Local modification of the soft tissues with hypersensitivity to palpation over the inferior part of the joint.
• "Strained" gluteal muscles over the inferior part of the joint.
• "Tension" to palpation of the following muscles: inferior heads of the adductor magnus, pyriformis.
• The interval between the median part of the sacrum and the ilium is decreased in relation to the opposite side and to the normal.
• The ASIS seems relatively lower.
• The PSIS seems relatively higher than the contralateral one.
• Palpation reveals loss of mobility in the SI joint at the level of its inferior pole.

Motion testing is performed as follows: The patient is prone as the examiner passes the hand under the iliac crest on the side opposite. The pelvis is gently rocked, while the examiner places the other hand over the SI joint region to assess the degree of "joint play" that is present or lacking. In addition, the source of the motion restriction is determined to be at either the superior or the inferior pole of the joint.

Signs Based on Alterations in Bony Landmarks

The various bony landmarks change position when the subject moves from sitting to standing, bends the trunk forward, stands on one foot, or raises the knee to 90°. Best-known in France is Piédallu's test. These tests seem to have been especially developed in the chiropractic group. Those most used seem to be the ones perfected by Gillet, Liekens, and Gitelman. The bony location points are the PSIS, the sacral apex, the tubercle of S2, and the ischium (Fig. A7.2).

Piédallu's Test (Fig. A7.3). Pascal Piédallu, speaking about the osteopathic arguments, finds that they are "indisputable, but too subjective."

The tactile changes in the periarticular tension correspond to reality. Probably one day, an appropriately sensitive apparatus will be able to record them. But as long as the researcher will have only his training and his tactile subjectivity to detect them, the personal bias and subjectivity makes a truly objective assessment impossible. The same can be said for the control of the joint mobility

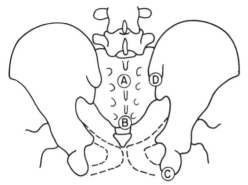

Figure A7.2. Contact points for motion testing performed on the SI joints: *A*, tubercle of S2; *B*, tubercle of S5 (the lowest); *C*, ischium; *D*, posterior superior iliac spine.

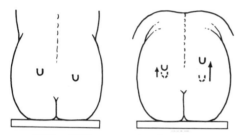

Figure A7.3. PSIS upward migration sign of P. Piédallu.

which, however, in difficult cases, remain the principal criteria.

He proposed a test that evaluated the "upward migration of the posterior superior iliac spine" for blockage in nutation (Fig. A7.3).

- The PSIS is lower on the blocked side of the patient sitting on a hard surface (in standing position also, but that can be due to a real short leg on that side).
- If the patient is asked to bend forward at the waist, sitting or standing, the PSIS goes up during flexion, while the PSIS on the normal side (higher at the start) is pulled to a much lesser extent and is lower than that on the blocked side at the end of the flexion.

This could be explained by the blockage and the contractures making the sacrum interdependent on the iliac on the blocked side, while there is a certain "play" on the free side.

Other Tests

- The standing patient, facing a wall, leans forward against it with arms extended. The examiner places a thumb on each of the PSISs. The subject raises the right knee as high as possible to assess the right SI joint (certain authors think that 90° is ideal). Normally, the PSIS on the side of the raised knee goes down more than that on the stationary side. If there is blockage, it does not descend (Fig. A7.2).
- The patient stands with the legs extended and slightly apart. The examiner places a thumb on each PSIS and grasps the iliac crest with the other fingers. The patient is asked to laterally flex slowly to the right and to the left. Normally, the PSIS remains at the same level.
- The patient stands with legs extended. The thumb is placed on the lowest posterior tubercles of the sacrum, with the index finger on the PSIS. The patient bends forward. Normally, flexion results in divergence of the two fingers by 12 mm. The same maneuver is repeated on the other side. In case of blockage, diversion no longer occurs.
- The patient stands with the legs extended. The examiner places the left thumb on the sacral tubercle of S2 and the right thumb on the PSIS. The patient raises the right leg with knee flexed. If the right SI joint is free, the iliac spine goes down 5 mm in relation to the sacral point location; if the right SI joint is blocked, it does not go down. The test is repeated on the other side. Normally, the sacrum must be felt moving forward and downward, whereas the ilium moves backward and upward. The movement detected would be 6–12 mm. If there is blockage, the sacrum and ilium move together; there is no separation. Note the similarity of these tests to Piédallu's test.

Tests of Sell and Neumann

The German School of Manual Medicine also examines for SI joint dysfunction. Neumann selected the tests that seemed to him to be the most reliable and the most sensitive for revealing SI joint blockage. He describes two pathologic situations in the SI joint:

1. There is loss of the normal play (hypomobility).

2. There is excess of movement in relation to the normal play (hypermobility).

Only the first case is amenable to a manipulative treatment.

The tests of SI joint blockage, according to Neumann, are

• Decrease in joint play.
• Reflex dysfunction in the S1, S2, and S3 regions.

Decrease in Joint Play. This is evaluated by maneuvers called "spring tests." The first test is similar to the osteopathic test discussed above. The patient lies prone and the examiner palpates the SI joint with one hand. The finger used for palpation is placed over the SI joint space, with the fingertip touching the sacrum and the ilium. With the other hand, the examiner grasps the anterior part of the iliac crest and gives rapid vibrating thrusts to the iliac crest. If the vibrations are properly transmitted to the palpating hand, the conclusion is that there is blockage, and if they are poorly transmitted, it means that the articulation is free.

In the second test, the SI joint is also palpated, with the subject and the examiner's hand in the same positions while the other hand does spring pressures on the caudal part of the sacrum. If the SI joint that is tested is free, a small part of the thrust is transmitted to the sacrum. If the articulation is blocked, it is felt completely.

For the third test, the patient is supine. The finger used for palpation is in the same position as for the preceding tests. The hand used for mobilization grasps the leg below the knee, flexes the hip to 90°, and adducts the leg until the slack is taken up in the SI joint. The joint is repetitively mobilized at end range with a gentle repetitive springing movement. The finger palpating the SI joint feels whether it moves or not.

Neumann insists on the difficulty of palpating a joint whose mobility is subtle.

Reflex Signs. The muscles receiving their innervation from S1, S2, and S3—the glutei, hamstrings, calf muscles, and some adductors—are affected and present with taut bands with or without trigger points. Taut muscle bands have been found one fingerbreadth outside the PSIS in the medial part of the gluteus maximus while the rest of the muscle is hypotonic. These cords are a good sign of SI joint blockage according to Sell and Neumann.

These signs decrease if traction is applied to the leg on the locked side, associated with a caudal support on the sacrum. On the other hand, they increase with the opposite maneuver, that is, support on the base of the sacrum with traction to the contralateral lower limb (Sell).

Other Signs.   Neumann also looked for

• A sign similar to Piédallu's sign with the patient standing, then sitting. If it was positive, it might mean there was a blockage of the SI joint; but it could also result from a reflex blockage of superior cervical origin or of L1-L2 (Gutmann).
• The pseudo-Lasègue sign (after Mennell).
• A decrease in the adduction of the thigh on the side of the blocked SI joint.

Palpation of the iliopsoas muscle below ASIS in the inguinal canal is tender. In fact, Neumann declares that the diagnosis of SI joint blockage is made on the convergence of several signs, as they are rarely present together.

Personal Opinion

The diverse signs that are proposed to recognize a SI joint blockage are subtle, as Piédallu and Neumann note. When they are clear, they certainly correspond to a dysfunction. But it is unclear whether the latter arises from blockage of the SI joints.

In almost all cases in which the responsibility of the SI joint seems possible, clinical examination of the spine on the basis of segmental pain (PMID), as we do it, shows the probability of the lumbosacral or thoracolumbar origin of the problem.

The impairment of these segments also explains the tissue changes that are perceptible to palpation (cellulotenoperiosteomyalgic syndrome).

• In the thoracolumbar junction syndrome, the tissue dysfunction involves the subcutaneous tissues overlying the SI joints, with pain and thickening on palpation (pain and perturbations that one would be tempted to assign to the subjacent articulation).
• Irritation of the lower lumbar facets and posterior rami brings perturbations in the retrosacral musculoligamentous tissues.
• The posterior ramus of S1 contributes to the innervation of the SI joint.

The perturbations in texture and sensitivity of the tissues that are found on palpation make it, moreover, difficult to appreciate SI joint mobility by palpation, if it is any way possible. Piédallu's sign seems often, like the other signs, to only indicate a slight antalgic attitude. SI joint sprains can certainly be seen in very particular cases (e.g., the end of pregnancy, a fall on the ischium, or a fracture of the pelvis), but even in these cases, the clinical picture is not very specific. Those who think that SI joint blockages are possible use palpation tests to diagnose them, as they use palpation tests to diagnose segmental vertebral dysfunctions, focusing only on the mobility, not on the provoked pain that we believe is essential to the concept of painful minor intervertebral dysfunction, which we propose to explain pain coming from the spine.

The problem could be summed up as follows. In certain cases, subtle signs of examination lead to the diagnosis of SI joint blockage. The improvement of these signs by maneuvers that are considered to have a specific action on these joints is taken as confirmation of that diagnosis. Unfortunately, no diagnostic sign is specific for SI joint dysfunction, and no manipulation acts only on the SI joint. Thus it seems difficult to describe in the present state, a "syndrome of SI joint blockage" that would be well defined, with clear and objective signs of examination.

N.B. A very interesting study was done by B. Sturesson et al. involving the movement of the SI joint in 25 patients who were considered to have a problem at that level (according to Lewit's criteria, similar to Neumann's). The movements were studied, with radiologic stereophotogrammetric instrumentation, at extreme range and under the influence of loads. The authors noticed that the mobility of the joint is limited, even in young patients. Rotation of 2.5° between the extreme positions and translation of 1 mm was measured (0.1–1.6 mm). There was no difference between a symptomatic and an asymptomatic SI joint.

The authors remark that their measures are far from the 6° of Weisl or of the 9° or 10° estimated by Grieve. If these results are confirmed, it would greatly relieve our doubts about the reality of the blockages of this joint and the possibility of testing its mobility by palpation.

SO-CALLED SI JOINT MANIPULATIVE TECHNIQUES

The techniques that we describe here or that we recall are considered by proponents of SI joint blockage to be maneuvers capable of treating them; they also act strongly on the lumbar spine and even the thoracolumbar region.

Two types of blockages in general are considered, one in nutation, the other in counternutation. The maneuvers thus are aimed at freeing the blocked movement by moving the iliac crest forward in relation to the sacrum, for a blockage in nutation (Fig. A7.4a), or by moving the sacrum forward in relation to the iliac crest, for a blockage in counternutation (Fig. A7.4b). Some authors consider only the global loss of mobility of the SI joint and do not differentiate these two types (Neumann). For others, there are an infinite number of ways in which the SI joint can be blocked and as many tests to differentiate them!

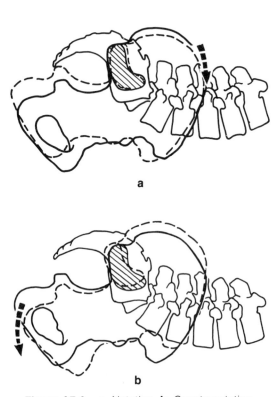

Figure A7.4. **a.** Nutation. **b.** Counternutation.

First Technique

The lateral decubitus maneuver in extension, as described for the lumber spine (Fig. A7.5), is often proposed as a SI joint manipulation destined to correct a blockage in the "anterior sacrum" or a blockage in nutation.

Second Technique

The aim of the second technique is an anterior rotation of the iliac crest (Fig. A7.6). The patient is prone. The examiner stands on the side opposite the target SI joint (in this example, the left one). The left lower limb of the patient is placed in extension, and the examiner then steps over it so that the patient's left leg is held against the examiner's popliteal crease. This pulls the patient's left lower limb into extension and adduction. The examiner then grasps the anterior part of the patient's iliac crest with the left hand and reinforces this action with the right hand.

He then takes up the slack with the left leg,

which increases the adduction while firmly maintaining the counterpressure of the hands on the iliac crest. Once the slack has been taken up, a sudden thrust of the hands, downward and slightly outward on the iliac crest, will result in manipulation.

Third Technique

The maneuver shown in Figure A7.7 is a maneuver in flexion with contact on the right PSIS. The examiner applies a posterior rotation to the ilium capable of treating a blockage in the "posterior sacrum" (blockage in counternutation).

Fourth Technique

This astride technique (Fig. A7.8) with combined right lateroflexion and left rotation is

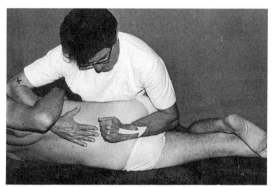

Figure A7.7.

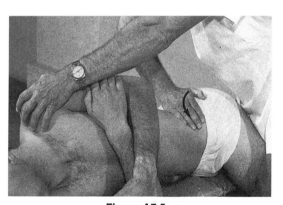

Figure A7.5.

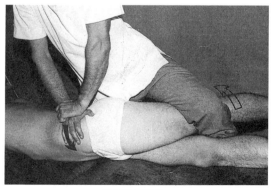

Figure A7.6.

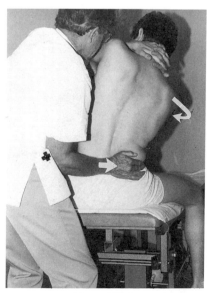

Figure A7.8.

considered to act on the right SI joint whose blockage in "posterior sacrum" would be corrected. The heel of the right hand is applied to the right superior part of the sacrum.

Fifth Technique

Figure A7.9 shows a maneuver in left rotation and right lateroflexion of the lumbosacral spine. The belt is fixed above the PSISs. It is also a manipulation for blockage in "left anterior sacrum" (in nutation). The examiner's right hand presses on the right PSIS.

Sixth Technique

Traction on the Leg

Certain American osteopathic doctors, especially Fryette, consider sudden axial traction of the lower limb to be one of the best techniques of SI joint manipulation. According to him, it must be applied with precision, so that its action is precisely localized on the SI joint.

With One Examiner. The patient is supine. The examiner grasps the patient's leg above the malleoli. The patient is asked to relax and to keep the leg well relaxed. The examiner slowly swings the leg with small and slow movements, and then leans progressively backward, with arms slightly bent. Slowly the leg is pulled toward the examiner, applying axial traction. With the slack taken up, the examiner strong and brief traction.

Two positions of the lower limb are possible:

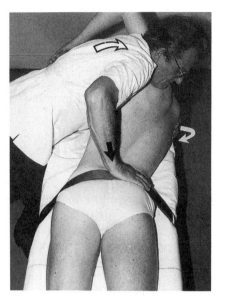

Figure A7.9.

1. The leg is level with, or slightly below, the level of the table. This partially takes up the slack of the anterior muscles (Fig. A7.10).
2. The leg is above the table, taking up the slack of the hamstring muscles (Fig. A7.11). In the first case, it would produce an anterior rotation of the iliac crest, thus unblocking a sacrum blocked in nutation ("anterior sacrum") and in the second case, would act on a sacrum blocked in counternutation ("posterior sacrum").

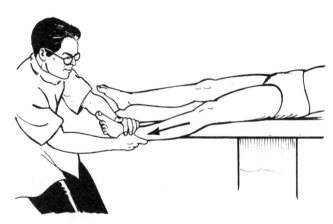

Figure A7.10. Manipulation of SI joint blockage in nutation according to Fryette.

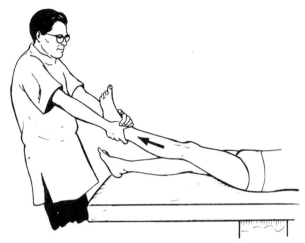

Figure A7.11.   Manipulation of SI joint blockage in counternutation according to Fryette.

This maneuver can be useful in certain lumbar problems not necessarily of SI joint origin. It is delicate in its application, as taking up the slack can be painless while the sudden traction can cause a sharp pain and could seriously aggravate a discogenic problem that it can sometimes relieve.

With Two Examiners.   A similar technique can be done with two examiners (Figs. A7.12 and A7.13).

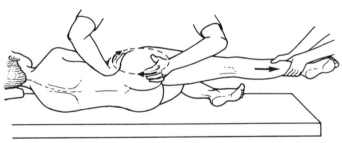

Figure A7.12.   For blockage in nutation: manipulation "anterior rotation of the iliac spine." The patient lies on the side. The first examiner maintains the ilium in rotation anteriorly, and, in so doing, presses on the iliac spine, which is pushed forward toward the is-chium, which is pushed cephalad. At the same time, the second examiner pulls briskly, with the leg slightly elevated and slightly extended (see Fig. A7.10), while the first examiner firmly maintains that pressure.

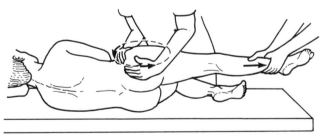

Figure A7.13.   For a blockage in counternutation: manipulation "posterior rotation of the iliac spine." The patient is lying on the side. The first examiner maintains the iliac in rotation posteriorly, placing one hand on the anterior iliac crest and the other at the level of the ischium so that the two hands exert a force that results in a posterior rotation. The second examiner pulls briskly on the leg, which is slightly elevated and in flexion (see Fig. A7.11), while the first examiner maintains the pressure firmly.

BIBLIOGRAPHY

ALAJOUANINE T. et coll. — Le rôle des positions anormales et prolongées de la tête et du cou dans le déterminisme de certains accidents vasculaires du tronc cérébral. *Bull. Mém. Soc. Méd. Hôp. Paris*, 1958, *74*, 1-2, 21-26.

ALAJOUANINE T., PETIT-DUTAILLIS D. — Compression de la queue de cheval par une tumeur du disque intervertébral; opération, guérison; présentation du malade. *Bull. Soc. Nat. Chir.*, 1928, *54*, 1452.

ALAJOUANINE T., PETIT-DUTAILLIS D. — Le nodule fibrocartilagineux de la face postérieure des disques intervertébraux. Etude clinique et thérapeutique d'une variété nouvelle de compression radiculo-médullaire extradurale. *Presse Méd.*, 1930, *38*, 1749.

ALAJOUANINE T., NICK J. — L'algie occipitale d'origine psychique ou syndrome d'Atlas. *Sem. Hôp. Paris*, 1949, *25*, 852-854.

ALI CHERIF A., DELPUECH F., HABIB M., SALAMON G., KHALIL R. — Thrombose vertébrobasilaire après manipulation du rachis cervical. *Ann. Med. Phys.*, 1983, *25*, 459-465.

ALLBROOK D. — Movements of lumbar spinal column, *J. Bone Joint Surg.*, 1957, *39B*, 339.

ANDERSON J.A.D. — Problems of classification of low back pain. *Rheumatol. Rehabil.*, 1977, *16*, 34-36.

ASTEGIANO P.A. — La medicina ortopedica et le terapia manuale. *Medicina Ortopedica*, 1988, *6*, 27-40; et 1989, *1*, 11-21.

AUBRY Y. — *Essai de traitement des algies vasculaires de la face par manipulations vertébrales*. Thèse Méd., Nancy, 1987.

AWAD E.A. — Interstitial myofibrositis. Hypothesis of the mechanism. *Arch. Phys. Med.*, 1973, *54*, 440-453.

AYERS C.E. — Lumbosacral backache. *Boston, M. and S.J.*, 1927, *196*, 9-16.

BADELON B. — Détection par la rachimétrie systématique des facteurs de risque chez l'enfant qui ne souffre pas. *J. Int. Ped.*, 1982, *23*, 3025-3045.

BADELON B., BOULIER A., DUMAS M., FAHE J. — Facteurs constitutionnels ou acquis favorisant le surmenage du segment mobile vertébral lombaire. *In :* Simon L., Rabourdin J.-P., *Lombalgies et médecine de rééducation*. Paris, Masson, 1983.

BAER W.S. — Sacroiliac strain. *Bull Johns Hopkins Hosp.*, 1917, *28*, 159-163.

BAGDLEY C.E. — The articular facet in relation to low back pain and sciatic radiation. *J. Bone Joint Surg.*, 1941, *23*, 2, 481.

BAKLAND O., HANSEN J.H. — The "axial sacroiliac joint". *Anat. Clin.*, 1984, *6*, 29-36.

BARBOR R. — A treatment for chronic low back pain, pp. 661-664. *In : Comptes rendus du 4e Congrès International de Médecine Physique*, Amsterdam, Excerpta Medica, 1966.

BARD M., LAREDO J.D. — Scanner ou radiculographie dans la sciatique. *In :* Sèze S. de et coll. *L'actualité rhumatologique 1986 présentée au praticien*, pp. 181-192. Paris, Expansion Scientifique Française, 1986.

BARCELO P., VILASECA J.M. — Clinica y radiologia de las afecciones degenerativas de las pequenas articulationes vertebrales. *In : Comtemporary Rheumatology*, pp. 218-233. Amsterdam, Elsevier, 1956.

BARJON M.C. — La dystrophie rachidienne de croissance et ses conséquences. *In :* « *Actualités en rééducation fonctionnelle et réadaptation*, 4e série (sous la direction de L. Simon), Paris, Masson, 1979.

BARRE J., LIEOU Y.C. — Syndrome sympathique cervical postérieur. *Paris Med.*, 1925, *15*, 266-269.

BARRIE J.B. — *Etude de l'innervation des plans cutanés de la région lombo-fessière*. Mémoire pour le C.E.S. de R.R.F., Marseille, 1976.

BARTELINK D.L. — The role of abdominal pressure on the lumbar intervertebral discs. *J. Bone Joint Surg.*, 1957, *39A*, 718-725.

BARTSCHI-ROCHAIX W. — Le syndrome de migraine cervicale en pathologie cervicale. *Méd. Hyg.*, 1957, *15*, 606-607.

BEAL M.C. — Motion sense. *J. Am. Osteop. Ass.*, 1953, *53*, 151-153.

BEAL M.C. — The subjective factors of palpatory diagnosis. *The DO*, 1967, *7*, 91-93.

BEAL M.C. — Osteopathic basics. *J. Am. Osteop. Ass.*, 1980, *79*, 456-459.

BEAL M.C. — The sacroiliac problem : review of anatomy, mechanics and diagnosis. *J. Am. Osteop. Ass.*, 1981, *81*, 667-679.

BENASSY J. — Metamerical topography of the cord and its roots. *Paraplegia*, 1970, *8*, 75-79.

BENCE Y., COMMANDRE F., REVELLI G., VIANI J.L., BISSCHOP G. DE, DUMOULIN J. — Données électromyographiques dans les épicondylalgies. Etudes à propos de 122 cas. *Rhumatologie*, 1978, *30*, 91-98.

BENN R.T., WOOD P.H.N. — Pain in the back. An attempt to estimate the size of the problem. *Rheumatol. Rehabil.*, 1975, *14*, 121.

BENOIST M., KAHN M.F. — Le syndrome polyalgique idiopathique diffus : du nouveau sur la polyenthésopathie (fibromyalgie primitive, fibrosite). *In :* Sèze S. de, Ryckewaert A., Kahn M.F., Guérin C., *L'actualité rhumatologique 1987 présentée au praticien*, pp. 78-89. Paris, Expansion Scientifique Française, 1987.

BENOIST M., DEBURGE A., HERIPET G., BUSSON J., RIGOT J., CAUCHOIX J. — Treatment of lumbar disc herniation by chymopapaïn chemonucleolysis. A report of 120 patients. *Spine*, 1982, *7*, 285-290.

BIOT B., DUPRAT A., STAGNARA P. — Les douleurs

commmunes des scolioses de l'adulte. *Ann. Med. Phys.*, 1978, *XXI*, 3, 337-343.

BOCH C.A., DAMERON F.B., DOW M.J., SKOWLUND H.V. — Study on normal range of motion in the neck utilizing a bubble goniometer. *Arch. Med. Phys.*, 1959, *40*, 390.

BOEGLI S., FUTCHY D., MASSE F. — Syndrome du corset plâtré (Cast syndrome). *Med. Hyg.*, 1978, *36*, 2141-2142.

BOGDUK N., DON LONG M. — Percutaneous lumbar medial branch neurotomy. *Spine*, 1980, *5*, 193-200.

BOGDUK N., TYNAN W., WILSON A.S. — The nerve supply to the human lumbar intervertebral discs. *J. Anat.*, 1981, *132*, 39-56.

BOGDUK N., ENGEL R. — The menisci of the lumbar zygoapophyseal joints. *Spine*, 1984, *9*, 454-460.

BOILEAU-GRANT J.C. — *Grant's atlas of anatomy*, 6th ed., Baltimore, William and Wilkins Co, 1972.

BOLDREY E., MAAS L., MILLER E. — The role of atlantoid compression in the etiology of internal carotid thrombosis. *J. Neurosurg.*, 1956, *13*, 127-139.

BONNAIRE E., BUE V. — De la mobilité des articulations pelviennes. *Ann. Gynecol. Obstet.*, 1899, *52*, 296.

BOULANGER Y., LE NOUVEL P., BRISSOT R., LOUVIGNE Y. — Diagnostic et traitement des cervicalgies communes. *Cah. Reed. Readapt.*, 1972, *12*, 265-271.

BOUMAN H.D. — The physiology of muscle spasm as related to low back pain. *So. Med. J.* 1965, *58*, 534-538.

BOURDILLON J.F., DAY E.A. — *Spinal manipulation, 4th ed.* London, William Heinemann Medical Books, 1987.

BOURREAU F., WILLER J.C. — *La douleur.* 1 vol., Paris, Masson, 1979.

BOSWORTH D.M. — The role of the orbicular ligament in the tennis elbow. *J. Bone Joint. Surg.*, 1958, *37A*, 527.

BOSWORTH D.M. — Surgical treatment of tennis elbow. *J. Bone Joint. Surg.*, 1965, *47A*, 1533-1536.

BOYD H.B. — Tennis elbow. *J. Bone Joint. Surg.*, 1973, *55A*, 1183-1187.

BOYEZ M. — *Les sténoses du canal lombaire (229 observations).* Thèse Méd., Paris, (dact.) 1982.

BRADLEY K.C. — The anatomy of backache. *Aust. N.Z. J. Surg.*, 1974, *44*, 227-232.

BRAIN W.R., WILKINSON M. — *Cervical spondylosis.* London, William Heinemann Medical Books Ltd, 1967.

BREGEON CH., VIALLE M., MERCIER PH., GUY G., BARREAU D., CARON-POITREAU C., RENIER J.C. — Etude tomodensitométrique de 75 sciatiques dont 21 récidivantes. *Rev. Rhum. Mal. Osteoartic.*, 1984, *51*, 559-563.

BRIZARD J. — Torticolis de Grisel. *In :* Sèze S. de, *L'actualité rhumatologique 1971 présentée au praticien*, Paris, Expansion Scientifique Française, 1971.

BRODAL A. — *Neurological anatomy.* 1 vol., Oxford, University Press, 1981.

BRODIN H. , NORDGREN B., BEIJE K. — Recording of spine mobility. *Europa Medicophysica*, 1977, *13*, 151-157.

BRUCHNER F.E., GRECO A., LEUNG A.W.L. — Benign thoracic pain syndrome. Role of magnetic resonance imaging in the detection and localization of thoracic disc disease, *J.R. Soc. Med.*, 1989, *82*, 81.

BRUGGER A. — Les syndromes vertébraux radiculaires et pseudo-radiculaires, I et II, 2 vol., *Acta Rheumatologica*, n° 18 et 19, Paris, Documenta Geigy, 1957.

BUCK C.A., DAMERON F.B., DOW M.J., SKOWLUND H.V. —

Study on normal range of motion in the neck utilizing a bubble goniometer. *Arch. Phys. Med.*, 1959, *40*, 390.

BURTON C.V. — Percutaneous radiofrequency facet denervation. *Appl. Neurophysiol.*, 1976-1977, *39*, 80-86.

CAILLENS J.P. — *L'arthrographie de l'épaule.* Paris, Masson, 1974.

CAILLENS J.P., JARROUSSE Y., GUIBAL C. — Quoi de neuf dans l'immobilisation du tronc au cours de la lombalgie ? *In :* Simon L., Rabourdin J.P., *Lombalgies et médecins de rééducation*, pp. 203-207, Paris, Masson, 1983.

CAILLIET R. — *Neck and arm pain.* Philadelphia, F.A. Davis, 1974.

CAILLIET R. — *Les lombalgies* (Trad. M. Mezzana). Paris, Masson, 1977.

CAILLIET R. — *Soft tissue pain and disability.* Philadelphia, F.A. Davis, 1977.

CAILLIET R. — *Les névralgies cervico-brachiales* (Trad. G. Boruchowitdch). Paris, Masson, 1978.

CALIOT P., CABANNE P., BOUSQUET V., MIDY D. — A contribution to the study of the innervation of the sternocleidomastoid muscle. *Anat. Clin.*, 1984, *6*, 21-28.

CAMBIER J. — Complications neurologiques des manipulations cervicales. *Presse Med.*, 1963, *71*, 7, 382-386.

CAPESIUS P., BABIN E. — *Radiculosaccography with water-soluble constrast media.* New York, Berlin, Heidelberg, Springer Verlag, 1978.

CARDIN H. — Intérêt des mobilisations vertébrales dans le traitement des angors vertébro-coronariens. *Ann. Méd. Phys.*, 1960, *3*, 125-133.

CARRERA G.F. — *Lumbar facet arthropathy in computed tomography of the spine.* Victor M., Haughton M.D. Edinburgh, Churchill Livingstone, 1983.

CASTELLINI A.E., GOLDSTEIN L.A., CHAN D.P.K. — Lumbosacral transitional vertebral and their relationship with lumbar extradural defects. *Spine*, 1980, *5*, 489-497.

CHANTRAINE A. — *Médecine physique.* Paris, Masson, 1982.

CHANTRAINE A. — Les tractions vertébrales. *In :* Simon L., Rabourdin J.P., *Lombalgies et médecine de rééducation*, pp. 167-175, Paris, Masson, 1983.

CHANTRAINE A., CHAPARD R., LUDY J.P., BERGUES J., GABAY R. — Tractions vertébrales par un cadre automoteur. *Rhumatologie*, 1976, *28*, 227-230.

CHARNLEY J. — Orthopedic signs in the diagnosis of disc protusion. *Lancet*, 1951, *i*, 186.

CHEVROT A., ROUDIER M., SELLIER N., VALLÉE C., GIRES F., WYBIER M., PALLARDY G. — Arthrographie des articulations lombaires postérieures. Interêt diagnostique et thérapeutique dans les lombalgies et les sciatiques. *Rhumat. Pratique*, 1986, *4*, 1.

CHEVROT A. — Sciatique d'origine articulaire postérieure. *Presse Méd.*, 1988, *17*, 462.

CHOPIN D., MAHON J. — Aspects évolutifs des scolioses à l'âge adulte. *Rev. Chir. Orthop.*, 1980, *67*, suppl. 11.

CHRISMAN O.D., MITTNACHT A., SNOOK G.A. — A study of the results following rotating manipulation in the lumbar intervertebral syndrom. *J. Neurol. Neurosurg. Psychiatry*, 1960, *23*, 321-327.

CHRISTIANSEN C., RIIS B.J., RODBRO P. — Prediction of rapid bone loss in postmenopausal women. *Lancet*, 1987, *ii*, 1105-1108.

CLAUSTRE J. — Les syndromes canalaires du nerf sciatique. In : La sciatique et le nerf sciatique (sous la direction de Simon L.), pp. 270-278. Paris, Masson, 1980.

CLOWARD R.B. — Treatment of ruptured lumbar intervertebral body fusion. J. Neurosurg., 1953, 10, 154.

CLOWARD R.B. — Cervical discography. Ann. Surg., 1959, 150, 1052-1064.

CLOWARD R.B. — The clinical significance of the sinuvertebral nerve of the cervical spine in relation to the cervical disk syndrome. J. Neurol. Neurosurg., Psychiatry, 1960, 23, 321-326.

COBURN D.F. — Vertebral artery involvment in cervical trauma. Clin. Orthop., 1962, 24, 61-63.

CODMAN E.A. — The shoulder. Boston, Thomas Todd, 1934.

COLACHIS S.C., WORDEN R.E., BECHTOL C.O., STROHM B.R. — Movement of the sacroiliac joint in the adult male : a preliminary report. Arch., Phys, Med., Rehabil., 1963, 44, 490-499.

COLLIS D.K., PONSETTI I.V. — Long term follow up of patients with idiopathic scoliosis not treated surgically. J. Bone. Joint Surg., 1969, 51A, 425-445.

COLOMBO I. — Le manipulazioni e le trazioni vertebrali. In : Farnetti P. : Terapia fisica e reabilitazione (2 vol.), pp. 345-360. Milan, A. Wasserman, 1965.

COLOMBO I. — Manuale di medicina ortopedica, Milano, Ghedini ed., 1988.

COMTET J.J., CHAMBAUD D., GENETY J. — La compression de la branche postérieure du nerf radial. Une étiologie méconnue de certaines paralysies et de certaines épicondylalgies. Nouv. Press. Med., 1976, 5, 17, 1111-1114.

COPEMAN W.S.C., ACKERMAN W.L. — Oedema or herniations of fat lobules as a cause of lumbar and gluteal "fibrositis". Arch. Int. Med., 1947, 79, 22.

COURTILON A., NYS A., HEULEU J.N. — Essai contrôlé des rééducations lombaires dans la lombalgie chronique. Ann. Read. Med. Phys., 1987, 30, 1, 1-20.

COUSTEAU J.P. — Médecine du tennis. Paris, Masson, 1982.

CROCK H.V. — Normal and pathological anatomy of the lumbar spinal nerve root canals. J. Bone Joint Surg., 1981, 63, 13, 487-490.

CYRIAX E.F. — On various conditions that may simulate the referred pain of visceral disease and a consideration from the point of view of cause and effect. Practionner, 1919, 102, 314-432.

CYRIAX E.F. — Collected papers on mechano-therapeutics. London, John Bale, 1924, 472 p.

CYRIAX J.H. — The pathology and treatment of tennis elbow. J. Bone Joint Surg., 1936, 28A, 921-940.

CYRIAX J.H. — Lumbago. The mechanism of dural pain. Lancet, 1945, ii, 427-428.

CYRIAX J.H. — Rheumatism and solt tissue injuries. London, Hamish Hamilton, 1960, 400 p.

CYRIAX J.H. — Lumbago mechanism of dural pain. Lancet, 1945, i, 427.

CYRIAX J.H. — Indications for and against manipulation. In : Beiträge zur manuellen Therapie. Stuttgart, Hippocrates Verlag, 1959.

CYRIAX J.H. — Pros and cons of manipulation. Lancet, 1964, i, 571-573.

DANFORTH M.S., WILSON P.D. — The anatomy of the lumbosacral region in relation to sciatic pain. J. Bone Joint Surg., 1925, 7, 109-160.

DEBURGE A. — Sciatique par sténose du canal lombaire. Presse Med., 1984, 13, 16, 973.

DECOULX P., RIEUNAU G. — Les fractures du rachis dorso-lombaire. Rev. Chir. Orthop., 1958, 44, 232-244 et 1959, 45, 237-294.

DECROIX G., WAGHEMACKER R. et coll. — Electronystagmographie et cupulométrie, moyen objectif d'évaluation sémiologique et de contrôle d'efficacité des manipulations vertébrales. Ann. Med. Phys., 1965, 8, 3-15.

DEGRAVE J. — Injection intradiscale d'aprotinine en ambulatoire. Rev. Med. Orthop. 1987, 8, 3-5.

DELCAMBRE B., CATANZARITI L., MEURIN D. — Les cervicalgies dites communes. Paris, Medicorama n° 224, EPRI.

DELMAS A. — Fonction sacro-iliaque et statique du corps. Rev. Rhum., 1950, 17, 475-481.

DENSLOW J.S., KORR I.M., KREMS A.D. — Quantitative studies of chronic facilitation in human motor neurone pools. Am J. Physiol., 1947, 105, 229-238.

DENSLOW J.S. — Pathophysiologic evidence of the osteopathic lesion : The known, unknown, and controversial. J. Am. Osteop. Ass., 1975, 75, 415-421.

DE PALMA A.F. — Degerative changes in the sternoclavicular and acromioclavicular joints in various decades. Springfield, C.C. Thomas, 1957.

DEPASSIO L. — L'exercice illégal des thérapeutiques manuelles. Thèse Méd., Lyon, 1975.

DEPOORTER A.E. — Indications et contre-indications des manipulations vertébrales. In : Comptes rendus du 4e Congrès International de Médecine Physique. pp. 150-155. Amsterdam, Excerpta Medica, 1966.

DERBOLOWSKY U. — Chirotherapie. Ulm Donau, Karl F. Haug Verlag, 1962.

DOLTO B. — Le corps entre les mains. Paris, Hermann, Ed., 1976, 359 p.

DOLTO B. — Pelvis, plaque tournante entre le tronc et les membres. Ann. Med. Phys., 1967, 10, 337-347 et 1968, 11, 406-415.

DOLTO B. — La notion de poutre composite dans le traitement des lombalgies. Ann. Med. Phys., 1973, 16, 77-94.

DÖRR W.M. — Uber die Anatomie der Wirbelgelenke. Arch. Orthop. Unfall-Chir., 1958/1959, 50, 222-234.

DÖRR W.M. — Nochmals zu den Menisci in den Wirbelgelenken. Z. Orthop., 1962, 96, 457-461.

DOUGLAS W.J. — La pratique et les résultats du travail ostéopathique. Rev. Rhum., 1948, 11, 351-354.

DREVET J.G. — Ecole du dos. Rev. Rhum., 1985, 37, 137-140.

DREVET J.G., PHELIP X., KERN G., STOEBNER P., CHIROSSEL J.P. — Echotomographie musculaire. Approche étiologique de certaines lombalgies. Rev. Rhum. Mal. Ostéoartic., 1985, 52, 397-402.

DREVET J.G., AUBERGE TH., LELONG C., CARPENTIER P., PHELIP X. — Pressions intradiscales aux étages L4-L5 et L5-S1 et discectomies percutanées. Rev. Med. Orthop., 1989, 16, 58.

DUC M., DUC M.L., LEICHTMANN G.A. — L'excrétion urinaire

des catécholamines et de l'acide vanylmandélique au cours de la spasmophilie. *Sem. Hôp. Paris*, 1973, *49*, 22, 1603-1610.

Duc M., Duc M.L., Leichtmann G.A. — La spasmophilie maladie fonctionnelle. *Ann. Med. Nancy*, 1982, *21*, 763-769.

Duc M., Coqueron M. — Les céphalées des spasmophiles. *Rev. Med. Orthop.*, 1985, *2*, 13-17.

Dupuis P.R., Ken Yong-Hing, Cassidy J., Kirkaldywillis W.H. — Radiologie diagnosis of degenerative lumbar spinal instability. *Spine*, 1985, *10*, 262-279.

Durey A., Boeda A. — La pubalgie du sportif. *Prat. Méd.*, 1983, *38*, 41-46.

Durey A., Gaudinat R., Troisier O. — Le syndrome des « deux bouts » de la clavicule. *In* : Simon L., Rodineau J., *Epaule et médecine de rééducation*. Paris, Masson, 1984.

Ectors L., Achslogh J., Saintes M.J. — *Les compressions de la moelle cervicale*. Paris, Masson, 1960.

Egund N., Olsson T.H., Schmid H., Selvik G. — Movements in the sacroiliac joints demonstrated with roentgen stereophotogrammetry. *Acta Radiol. (Diagn.) (Stockh.)*, 1977, *19*, 833-846.

Emminger E. — Die Anatomie und Pathologie des blockierten Wirbelgelenkes. *Hippokrates*, 1967, *38*, 253.

Emminger E. — Les articulations interapophysaires et leurs structures méniscoïdes vues sous l'angle de la pathologie. *Ann. Med. Phys.*, 1972, *15*, 219-237.

Engel R., Bogduk N. — The menisci of the lumbar zygapophyseal joints. *J. Anat.*, 1982, *135*, 795-809.

Epstein J.A., Epstein B.S., Rosenthal A.D., Carrus R., Lavine L.S. — Sciatic caused by nerve root intrapment in the lateral recess. *J. Neurosurg.*, 1972, *36* 584-589.

Falconer M.A., McGeorge M., Begg A.G. — Observations on the cause and mechanism of symptom-production in sciatica and lowback pain. *J. Neurol. Neurosurg. Psychiatry*, 1948, *11*, 13.

Farabeuf L.H. — Sur l'anatomie et la physiologie des articulations sacro-iliaques avant et après la symphysectomie. *Ann. Hyg. Obstet.*, 1894, *41*, 407-420.

Farfan H.F., Sullivan J.D. — The relation of facet orientation to intervertebral disc failure. *Can. J. Surg.*, 1967, *10*, 179-185.

Farfan H.F. — *Mechanical disorders of the low back*, Philadelphia, Lea and Febifer, 1977.

Fassio J.P., Bouvier J.P., Ginestie J.F. — Dénervation articulaire postérieure percutanée et chirurgicale. *Rev. Chir. Orthop.*, 1981, Suppl. II, *67*, 131-136.

Fauchet R. — Localisation lombaire de la maladie de Scheuermann. *In* : Simon L., Rabourdin J.P., *Lombalgie et médecine de rééducation*. Paris, Masson, 1983.

Fauchet R. — Les sciatiques de l'enfant. *In* : Simon L. *La sciatique et le nerf sciatique*. Paris, Masson 1980.

Favarel-Garrigues J.C. — Accidents des anesthésiques locaux. *Concours Méd.*, 1980, *102*, 6539-6540.

Fernstrom V. — Discography studies of ruptured lumbar intervertebral diseases. *Acta Chir. Scand.*, 1960, suppl. 258.

Ferry A., Hubert F., Giorgi Ch., Schmitt D., Sommelet J. — Le syndrome du corset plâtré (The cast syndrom). *Am. Med. de Nancy et de l'Est.*, 1981, *XX*, 5.

Fick R. — *Handbuch der Anatomie und Mechanik der*

Gelenke. I. Teil : Anatomie der Gelenke (in Bardeleben's Handbuch der Anatomie des Menschen). Jena, Fisher, 1904.

Fielding J.W. — Cineroentgenography of the normal cervical spine. *J. Bone Joint Surg.*, 1957, *39A*, 1280-1288.

Finneson B.E. — *Low back pain*, 1 vol., Philadelphia, Toronto, J.B. Lippincot Compagny, 1973.

Fischer A.E. — Uber die Epicondylitis und Styloidesneuralgie, ihre Pathogene und zweckmässige Therapie. *Arch. F. Klin. Chir.*, 1923, *125*, 749.

Ford R.F., Clark D. — Thrombosis of the basilar artery with softening in the cerebellum and brain stem due to manipulation of the neck. *Johns Hopkins Hosp. Bull.*, 1956, *98*, 37-42.

Forest A.J., Wolkind S.N. — Masked depression in men with low back pain. *Rheumatol. Rehabil.*, 1974, *13*, 148.

Frachon M. — *Les accidents neurologiques des manipulations cervicales*. Thèse Méd., Lyon, 1981.

Franceshi de Marchi G. — Intervertebral articulations. An anatomo-histological study. *La Clinica Ortopedica*, 1963, *15*, 26-33.

Françon F. — L'épicondylalgie. *In* : Deuxième série de Conférences cliniques de Rhumatologie pratique. Paris, Vigot, 1949.

Françon F., Fabre M. — La coccygodynie. *Rhumatologie*, 1963, *15*, 35.

Freeman M.A.R., Wyke B.D. — The innervation of the knee joint. An anatomical and histological study in the cat. *J. Anat.*, 1967, *101*, 505-532.

Freudenberg G.H. — *Contribution à l'étude du blocage des apophyses articulaires de la charnière lombosacrée*. Thèse Méd., Paris, 1967, 35 p. (dactyl).

Friedenberg Z.B., Edeiken J., Spencer N., Tolentino S.C. — Degenerative changes in cervical spine. *J. Bone Joint Surg.*, 1959, *41A*, 61-70.

Friedenberg Z.B., Miller W.T. — Degenerative disc desease of the cervical spine. *J. Bone Joint Surg.*, 1965, *47A*, 1231.

Friedman A., Desolapool P., Von Storch. — Tension headache. *JAMA*, 1953, *151*, 174-180.

Frykholm R. — Deformities of dural pouches and strictures of dural sheaths in the cervical region producing nerve root compression. *J. Neurosurg.*, 1947, *4*, 403.

Frykholm R. — Cervical nerve root compression resulting from disk degeneration and root sleeve fibrosis. *Acta Chir. Scand.*, 1951, suppl. 160.

Garcia J.L. — *Les dérangements intervertébraux mineurs de siège cervical supérieur. Etude de leur rôle dans certaines céphalées*. Thèse Méd. Reims, 1977.

Garcia J.L. — Rôle du rachis cervical dans la genèse de certaines céphalées chroniques. *Rhumatologie*, 1980, *32*, 4, 115-124.

Garden R.S. — Tennis elbow. *J. Bone Joint Surg.*, 1961, *43B*, 100-106.

Gardner R.C. — Tennis elbow : diagnosis pathology and treatment. *Clin. Orthop.*, 1970, *72*, 248-253.

Genant H.K., Cann C.E., Ettinger B., Gordon G.S. — Quantitative computed tomography of vertebral spongiosa : a sensitive method for detecting early bone loss after oophorectomy. *Ann. Intern. Med.*, 1982, *97*, 699-705.

GHORMLEY R.K. — Low back pain with special reference to the articular facets with presentation of an operative procedure. *JAMA*, 1933, *101*, 1773-1777.

GILES L.G.F., TAYLOR J.R. — Intra-articular synovial protrusions in the lower lumbar apophyseal joints. *Bull. Hosp. Joint Dis. Hosp. Orthop. Inst.*, 1982, *42*. 248-255.

GILES L.G.F., TAYLOR J.R., COCKSON A. — Human zygapophyseal joint synovial folds. *Acta Anat. (Basel)*, 1986, *126*, 110-114.

GILLOT C. — *Eléments d'anatomie*. Paris, Flammarion et Cie ed., 1966.

GILLOT C. — Confrontations entre certaines variétés de lombalgies et les dispositifs anatomiques rachidiens. *Ann. Med. Phys.*, 1972, *15*, 2, 246-256.

GITELMAN R. — Biomechanical disorders of the lumbar spine and pelvis. In : Haldeman S., *Modern developments in principles and practice of chiropractic*. New York, Appleton-Century-Crofts, 1980.

GLOVER J.R. — Back pain and hyperesthesia. *Lancet*, 1960, *i*, 1165-1169.

GLOVER J.R., MORRIS J., KHOSLA T. — Back pain : a randomized clinical trial of rotational manipulation of the trunk. *Clin. Sci.*, 1973, *3*, 1.

GLOVER J.R. — Arthrography of the joints of the lumbar vertebral arches. *Orthop. Clin. North Am.*, 1977, *81*, 37-42.

GODEBOUT J. DE, STER I, HUBERT M.N., BARRAULT J.J. — Diagnostic clinique des paralysies crurales. In : Simon L., *Actualités en rééducation fonctionnelle*. Paris, Masson, 1977.

GOLDLEWSKI S. — Les anomalies congénitales de la jonction cranio-rachidienne. *Ann. Méd. Phys.*, 1966, *9*, 224-250.

GOLDLEWSKI S., DRY J. — *Les anomalies congénitales de la charnière cervico-occipitale*. Paris, Expansion Scientifique Française, 1964, 54 p.

GOES H. DE, SILVA O. — The radiohumeral meniscus and its responsability to tennis elbow. *Arch. Inter-american. Rheumat.*, 1960, *3*, 582.

GOLDIE I. — Epicondylitis lateralis humeri (Epicondylalgia or tennis elbow). A pathogenetical study. *Acta Chir. Scand.*, 1964, (suppl.), 339.

GOLDTHWAIT J.E. — The lumbosacral articulation : an explanation of many cases of lumbago, sciatica and paraplegia. *Boston Med. Surg.*, 1911, *164*, 365.

GONON P. — Etude biomécanique de la colonne dorsolombaire de D10 à S1 (Etudes mécaniques de certaines méthodes d'ostéo-synthèses postérieures). Thèse Méd., Lyon, 1975.

GONON J.P., DIMNET J., CARRET J.P., MAUROY J.C. DE, FISCHER L.P., MORGUES G. DE. — Utilité de l'analyse cinématique de radiographies dynamiques dans le diagnostic de certaines affections de la colonne lombaire. In : Simon L., Rabourdin J.P., *Lombalgies et médecine de rééducation*. Paris, Masson, 1983.

GOOD M.G. — Die primäre Rolle der Muskulatur in der Pathogenese der rheumatischen Krankenheit und die therapeutische Lösung des Rheumaproblems. *Med. Klin.*, 1957, *13*, 450.

GOUAZE A. — *Neuroanatomie clinique*, 3ᵉ ed., Paris, Expansion Scientifique Française, 1988.

GOUGH J.G., KOEPKE G.H. — Electromyographic determination of moteur root levels in erector spinal muscles. *Arch. Phys. Med.*, 1966, *47*, 9.

GOURJON A. — *De certaines modifications tissulaires, peau et muscles dans les sciatiques radiculaires chroniques*. Thèse Méd., Paris, 1974.

GOURJON A., JUVIN P. — Le syndrome cellulo-ténomyalgique de Maigne. *Cinésiologie*, 1975, *58*, 60-64.

GOURJON A., JUVIN P. — Traitement local du syndrome cellulo-téno-myalgique de Maigne. *Cinésiologie*, 1978, *67*, 89-96.

GOUSSARD J.C., HALMAGRAND N., MAIGNE J.Y., MAIGNE R. — Etude de la sensibilité de l'épicondyle chez le cervicalgique chronique. *Ann. Réad. Med. Phys.*, 1987, *30*, 65-68.

Gray's anatomy par Williams P.L., Warwick R., 36th ed., Edinburgh, Churchill-Livingstone, 1980.

GREENMAN PH. E. — *Concepts and mechanism of neuromuscular functions*. Berlin, Heidelberg, New York, Tokyo, Springer Verlag, 1984.

GREGERSEN G.G., LUCAS D.B. — An in vivo study of axial rotation of the human thoraco-lumbar spine. *J. Bone Joint Surg.*, 1967, *49A*, 247.

GRIEVE G.P. — *Common vertebral joint problems*. Edinburgh, London, Melbourne, New York, Churchill-Livingstone, 1981.

GRIEVE G.P. — *Modern manual therapy of the vertebral column*. Edinburgh, London, Melbourne, New York, Churchill-Livingstone, 1986.

GRISEL P. — Enucléation de l'atlas et torticolis nasopharyngien. *Press. Med.*, 1930, *38*, 50.

GROSSIORD A. — Les accidents neurologiques des manipulations. *Ann. Med. Phys.*, 1966, *9*, 283-299.

GROSSIORD A., HELD J.P. — *Médecine de rééducation*. Paris, Flammarion ed., 1981.

GRUBBER S.A., LIPSCOMB H.J., BONNER-GUILFORD W. — The relative value of lumbar roentgenograms, metrizamide, myelography and discography in the assessment of patients with chronic low back syndrome. *Spine*, 1987, *12*, 282-286.

GUILLEMINET M., STAGNARA P. — Rôle de l'entorse vertébrale dans les rachialgies. *Presse Méd.*, 1952, *60*, 1274-1278.

GUNN C.C., MILBRANDT W.E. — Tennis elbow and cervical spine. *Can. Med. Assoc. J.*, 1976, *114*, 803-809.

GUNTZ M. — *Nomenclature anatomique illustrée*. Paris, Masson, 1975.

GUTMANN G. — Die Chirotherapie. *Hippokrates*, 1963, *17*, 685-692.

HACKETT G.S — *Ligament and tendon relaxation treated by prolotherapy*. (III) 1 vol., Springfield, Charles C. Thomas, 1958.

HADLEY L.A. — *Anatomico-roentgenographic studies of the spine*. p. 175. Springfield, Charles C. Thomas, 1976.

HADLEY L.A. — Accessory sacro-iliac articulations. *J. Bone Joint Surg.*, 1952, *43A*, 247-261.

HALDEMAN S. — Clinical basis for discussion of mechanisms of manipulative therapy. In : Korr I., *Neurobiologic mechanisms of manipulative therapy*. New York, Plenum Press, 1978.

HALDEMAN S. — *Modern developments in principles and practice of chiropractic*. New York, Appleton-Century-Crofts, 1980.

HALMAGRAND N., GOURJON A., GROUSSARD J.C., MAIGNE J.Y. — Infiltration épidurale par voie basse : hiatus sacrococcygien. *Rev. Med. Orthop.*, 1987, *7*, 13-17.

HALMAGRAND N., SEROR P., BEDOS H. — Douleur lombo-abdominale d'origine discale L5-S1, traitée par nucléolyse. A propos d'un cas. *Rev. Med. Orthop.*, 1985, *3*, 29-32.

HANSEN K., SCHLIACK H. — *Segmentale Innervation.* Stuttgart, Georg Thieme Verlag, 1962.

HAPPEY E., HORTON A.G., MACRAE T.P., NAYLER A., — Preliminary observations concerning the fine structure of the intervertebral disc. *J. Bone Joint Surg.*, 1964, *46B*, 563-567.

HIJIKATA S. — A method of percutaneous nuclear extraction. *J. Toden Hospital*, 1975, *5*, 39.

HEIKEL H. — Symptômes de la plante du pied. *Acta Orthop. Scand.*, 1965, *36*, 4, 464-470.

HELD J.P. — Les atteintes de l'axe cérébro-spinal au cours des traumatismes cervicaux mineurs. *Ann. Méd. Phys.*, 1965, *8*, 13-23.

HELD J.P. — Pièges et dangers des manipulations cervicales en neurologie. *Ann. Méd. Phys.*, 1966, *9*, 251-260.

HELD P.G., PIERROT-DESEILLIGNY E., RODINEAU J. — Le devenir des sciatiques paralysantes opérées et non opérées. *Ann. Med. Phys.*, 1969, *4*, 394-408.

HERBERT J.J. — Lombalgies. Etude mécanique. Traitements orthopédiques et chirurgicaux. *Rhumatologie*, 1953, *5*, 295-337.

HÉRISSON C., TOUCHON J., BESSET A., BILLIARD M., SIMON L. — Fibrosite et perturbations du sommeil. *Ann. Réad. Med. Phys.*, 1988, *31*, 177-186.

HEULEU J.N., AUGE R. — La massokinésithérapie dans les lombalgies et lombosciatiques. *Encycl. Méd. Chir.*, Instantanés médicaux n° 19.

HIRSCH C.S., PAULSON S., SYLVEN B. SNELLMAN O. — Biophysical and physiological investigations on cartilage and other mesenchymal tissues : characteristics of human nuclei pulposi during aging. *Acta Orthop. Scand.*, 1953, *22*, 175-183.

HIRSCH C., SCHAJOWICZ F. — Studies on structural changes in the lumbar annulus fibrosus. *Acta Orthop. Scand.*, 1952, *22*, 184-230.

HIRSCH C., INGELMARK B.E., MILLER M. — The anatomical basis for low back pain. *Acta Orthop. Scand.*, 1963, *33*, 1-17.

HIRSCHBERG G.C., FROESTSCHER L., NAIEM F. — Iliolumbar ligament syndrome as a common cause of low back pain. *Arch. Phys. Med. Rehab.*, 1979, *60*, 415-419.

HOHMANN G. — Tennisellenbogen. *Verh. Dtsch. Orthop. Ges.*, 1927, *21*, 349--354.

HOLT E.P. — Fallacy of cervical discography. *J. Ann. Med. Ass.*, 1964, *188*, 799.

HOVELACQUE A. — Le nerf sinu-vertébral. *An. Anat. Path. Med.*, *Chir.*, 1925, *2*, 435-443.

HOVELACQUE A. — *Anatomie des nerfs crâniens et rachidiens et du système grand sympathique* (1 vol.), 873 p., Paris, G. Doin ed., 1927.

HUNTER G.A. — Non traumatic displacement of the atlanto-axial joint. *J. Bone Joint Surg.*, 1968, *50B*, 44.

ILLOUZ G., LIMON J. — L'épicondylalgie. Etude de 130 cas. Notes préliminaires sur l'électrodiagnostic. *Ann. Med. Phys.*, 1974, *2*, 17, 214-224.

INGELRANS P., OBERTHUR H. — Les arthrites chroniques sacro-iliaques non tuberculeuses. *Rev. Orthop.*, 1949, *35*, 5.

IMMAN V.T., SAUNDERS J.B. — Referred pain from skeletal structures. *J. Nerv. Ment. Dis.*, 1944, *99*, 660-667.

IMMAN V.T., SAUNDERS J.B. — Anatomico-physiological aspects of injuries to the intervertebral disk. *J. Bone Joint Surg.*, 1947, *29*, 461.

INOUE H. — Three dimensional observation of collagen framework of intervertebral discs in rats, dogs and humans. *Arch. Histol. Jpn*, 1973, *36*, 39-56.

ISCH F. — L'apport de l'électromyographie dans l'étude du fonctionnement des muscles paravertébraux chez l'individu normal et le scoliotique. *Kinésithérapie Scientifique*, 1971, *79*, 7-11.

JACKSON R.P., SIMMONS E.H., STRIPINIS D. — The incidence and severity of back pain in adult idiopathic scoliosis. *Spine*, 1983, *8*, 749-756.

JACKSON H.C., WINKELMANN R.K., BICKEL W.H. — Nerve endings in the human lumbar spinal column and related structures. *J. Bone Joint Surg.*, 1966, *48A*, 1272-1281.

JAN M. — Indications chirurgicales de l'arthrose vertébrale cervicale. *Cah. Méd., Lyonnais*, 1983, *16*, 951-959.

JANEL M. — *Hyperexcitabilité neuromusculaire et céphalées d'origine cervicale. Intérêt des manipulations cervicales.* Thèse Méd. Nancy, 1983.

JAYSON M.I.V. — *The lumbar spine and back pain.* 2nd ed. Turnbridge Wells, Kent, Pitman Medical, 1980.

JESEL M. — Cervicobrachialgies graves d'origine discale. Intérêt du traitement chirurgical. *Ann. Med. Phys.*, 1982, *1*, 111-118.

JESEL M. — Les algies cervicales, cervico-brachiales aiguës d'origine radiculaire ou myélopathique. *In : Cervicalgies non traumatiques en 1989.* Edition Française du *JAMA*, Mai 1989, numéro hors série.

JESEL M. — Technique de stimulo-détection avec détection de la réponse musculaire évoquée par aiguille électrode en dérivation bifilaire. *Lyon Med.*, 1984, *17*, 211-216.

JESEL M., WASSER PH., HIRSCH E., FOUCHER G. — Constatations neurologiques et électrologiques chez 36 patients atteints d'une épicondylalgie chronique. *Ann. Read. Med. Phys.*, 1986, *1*, 29, 47-56.

JOHNSTON H.M. — The cutaneous branches of the posterior primary divisions of the spinal nerves and their distribution in the skin. *J. Anat. Phys.*, 1908, *43*, 80-92.

JUDOVICH B., BATES W. — *Pain syndromes*, 3rd ed. Philadelphia, F.A. Davis and Cie. Pub., 1954.

JUNG A., KEHR P. — *Pathologie de l'artère vertébrale et des racines nerveuses.* Paris, Masson, 1972.

JUNG A., BRUNSCHWIG A. — Recherches histologiques sur l'innervation des corps vertébraux. *Presse Med.*, 1932, *40*, 316.

JUNG A.M. — Du syndrome cervico-céphalique dans les arthroses et traumatismes du rachis cervical. *Cinésiologie*, 1972, *47*, 49-82.

JUNGHANNS H. — Die anatomischen Besonderheiten des 5. Lendenwirbels und der letzten Lendenbandscheibe. *Arch. Orthop. Unfall-Chir.*, 1933, *33*, 2.

JUNGHANNS H. — Pathologie der Wirbelsäule. *In :* Henke-Lubarsch : *Handbuch der speziellen pathologischen Anatomie und Histologie.* Tome IX, vol. 4, pp. 280-284. Berlin, 1939.

JUNGHANNS H. — Erkennung und Behandlung versebragener Krankheiten. *Med. Klin.*, 1958, 208-213 et 252-256.

JUNGHANNS H. — Die insufficientia intervertebralis und ihre Behandlungsmöglichkeiten In : Beitrage zur manuellen Therapie. Stuttgart, Hippokrates Verlag, 1959.

JUNGHANNS H. — Die patho-physiologishen Grundlagen für die manuelle Wirbelsäulentherapie. In : Comptes rendus du 4e Congrès international de Médecine Physique, pp. 141-144. Amsterdam, Excerpta Medica, 1966.

JURMAND S.H. — Les injections péridurales de cortioïdes dans le traitement des lombalgies et des sciatiques d'origine discale. Rev. Rhum., 1973, 40, 471-464.

JUVIN R., DUBOS G., CHIROSSEL P.J., RICHARD J. — Des cervicalgies pièges chez le sujet âgé : les fractures méconnues de l'odontoïde. Rev. Med. Orthop., 1985, 1, 3-7.

KAHN M.F. — Réflexions sur les aspects médico-légaux des lombalgies. Rev. Rhum., 1973, 40, 733-739.

KAPLAN E. — Treatment of tennis elbow by denervation. J. Bone Joint Surg., 1959, 41A, 147-151.

KAPANDJI I.A. — Physiologie articulaire. (3 vol.) Paris, Maloine 1980.

KEEGAN J.J., GARRETT F.D. — The segmental distribution of the cutaneous nerves. Anat. Rec., 1948, 102, 409-437.

KEEGAN J.J. — Dermatome hypoalgesia with posterolateral herniation of lower cervical intervertebral disk. J. Neurosurg., 1947, 4, 115.

KELLER G. — Die Bedeutung der Veränderungen an den kleinen Wirbelgelenken als Ursache des lokalen Ruckenschmerzes. Auswertung der histologischen Befunde. Z. Orthop., 1953, 83, 517-547.

KELLGREN J.H. — On the distribution of pain arising from deep somatic structures with charts of segmental pain areas. Clin. Sci., 1939, 4, 35-46.

KELLGREN J.H. — The anatomical source of back pain. Rheumatol. Rehabil., 1977, 16, 3-12.

KENESI C. — Traitement chirurgical de l'épicondylalgie par désinsertion des épicondyliens, résection de l'apophyse et section du ligament annulaire. Ann. Réad. Med. Phys., 1986, 29, 2, 163.

KERR F.W.L. — A mechanism to account for frontal headache in cases of posterior fossa tumours. J. Neurosurg., 1961, 18, 605-609.

KERR F.W.L. — Evidence for a peripheral etiology of trigeminal neuralgia. J. Neurosurg., 1967, 26, 168-174.

KERR F.W.L. — Central relationship of trigeminal and cervical primary afferents in the spinal cord and medullon. Brain Res., 1972, 43, 561-572.

KERR F.W.L. — Craniofacial neuralgias. Advances in pain research and therapy (Vol. 3). New York, Raven Press, J. Bonica ed., 1979.

KEYES D.C., COMPERE E.L. — The normal and pathological physiology of the nucleus pulposus of the intervertebral disc; anatomical, clinical and experimental study. J. Bone Joint Surg., 1932, 14, 897.

KLEYN A. DE, NIEUWENHUYSE P. — Schwindelänfalb und Nystagmus bei einer bestimmten Stellung des Kopfes. Acta. Oto-Laryng. (Stockh.), 1927, 11, 155.

KOLHER R. — In : Rissanen P.M. Acta Orthop. Scand., 1964, 34, 54-56.

KOPPEL H.P., THOMPSON W.A.L. — Peripheral entrapment neuropathies. Baltimore, William and Wilkins Cie, 1963.

KORR I.M. — Clinical significance of the facilitated state

symposium on the functionnal implications of segmental facilitation. J. Am. Osteopath. Assoc., 1955, 54, 265-282.

KORR I.M. — Neurobiologic mechanisms in manipulative therapy. New York, Plenum Publishing Corp., 1978.

KORR I.M. — Bases physiologiques de l'ostéopathie, (2e ed.). Paris, Maloine, 1982.

KOS J., WOLF J. — Les ménisques intervertébraux et leur rôle possible dans les blocages vertébraux. Ann. Méd. Phys., 1972, 15, 203-218.

KOSTUIK J.P., BENTIVOGLIO J. — The incidence of low back pain in adult scoliosis. Spine, 1981, 6, 268-272.

KOTTKE F.J., MUNDALE M.O. — Range of mobility of the cervical spine. Arch. Phys., Med., 1959, 40, 379.

KRAEMMER J., LATURNUS H. — Lumbar intradiscal instillations with Aprotinine. Spine, 1982, 7, 73-74.

LACAPÈRE J. — Rhumatismes et syndromes radiculaires douloureux. Rev. Rhum., 1933, 20, 1.

LACAPÈRE J. — Névralgie cervico-brachiale. Sem. Hôp. Paris, 1950, 26, 2685-2690.

LACAPÈRE J., GUÉRIN CL. — Algies cervico-brachiales et angor. Monde Méd., 1957, n° 1000, 209.

LACAPÈRE J., MAIGNE R. — Présentation d'un serre-tête pour tractions cervicales. Rev. Rhum., 1957, 24, 299.

LAMY C., FARFAN H.F. — Vertebral body shockabsorber to the spine. J. Bone Joint Surg., 1976, 58B, 1, 141.

LAROCHE G., MEURS-BLATTER L. — Sur quelques erreurs graves par méconnaissance de la cellulite. Presse Méd., 1941, 42-43, 521-523.

LASSALE B., BENOIST M., MORVAN G., MASSARE C., DEBURGE A., CAUCHOIX J. — Sténose du canal lombaire. Etude nosologie et sémiologique. A propos de 163 cas opérés. Rev. Rhum., 1983, 50, 39-45.

LAVEZZARI R. — L'ostéopathie. Paris, Doin, 1949, 188 p.

LAVEZZARI R. — Une observation d'artérite oblitérante. Homéopathie Fr., 1949, 10, 462-464.

LAVEZZARI R. — Ulcération gastrique post-traumatique, guérison par l'ostéopathie. Homéopathie Fr., 1951, 1, 90-93.

LAVIGNOLLE B., SENEGAS J., GUERIN J., BARAT M. — Dégénérescence discale, syndrome des facettes et rhizolyse percutanée. Ann. Med. Phys., 1982, 25, 255-262.

LAVIGNOLLE B., VITAL J.M., SENEGAS J., DESTANDAU J., TOSON B., BOUYX P., MORLIER P., DELORME G., CALABET A. — An approach to the functional anatomy of the sacroiliac joints in vivo. Anat. Clin., 1983, 5, 169-176.

LAZARETH J.P. — Traitement des lombalgies chroniques par thermocoagulation percutanée des articulations postérieures à propos de 55 cas. Thèse Méd., Paris, 1987.

LAZORTHES G. — Le système nerveux périphérique. Paris, Masson ed., 1971.

LAZORTHES G. — Sciatiques paralysantes. Ann. Med. Phys., 1969.

LAZORTHES G., GAUBERT J. — Les innervations des articulations vertébrales interapophysaires. In : Compte rendu de l'association des anatomistes (43e réunion). Lisbonne, 1956, 488-494.

LAZORTHES G., GAUBERT J. — Le syndrome de la branche postérieure des nerfs rachidiens. Presse Med., 1956, 64, 2022.

LAZORTHES G., ESPAGNO J., ARBUS L., LAZORTHES Y., ZADEH O. — Pathogénie, urgence chirurgicale et pronostic des sciatiques paralysantes. *Ann. Med. Phys.*, 1969, *12*, 4, 388-393.

LAZORTHES G. — Les branches postérieures des nerfs rachidiens et le plan articulaire vertébral postérieur. *Ann. Méd. Phys.*, 1972, *15*, 192-203.

LAZORTHES G., ZADEH J. — Constitution et territoire cutané des branches postérieures des nerfs rachidiens. *Rev. Med. Orthop.*, 1987, *10*, 5-9.

LEDOUX M., HALMAGRAND N. — Recherche d'une rééducation adaptée aux syndromes de la charnière dorso-lombaire récidivants. *Rev. Med. Orthop.*, 1986, *6*, 23-27.

LE GO P. — De quelques phénomènes paravertébraux spontanés ou provoqués dans les affections viscérales. Déductions thérapeutiques. Thèse, Paris, 1934.

LE GO P., MAIGNE R., TOUMIT R. — Le traitement des lombalgies et des sciatiques aiguës en médecine physique. *Informations Med. SNCF.*, 1956, *60*, 47.

LE GOAER M. — Intérêt du traitement sclérosant de Hackett dans les hyperlaxités ligamentaires vertébrales et sacro-iliaques post-traumatiques. *Ann. Méd. Phys.*, 1960, *6*, 162-166.

LE GOAER M. — Techniques manipulatives de l'arrière-pied. *Ann. Méd. Phys.*, 1961, *4*.

LELONG C., DREVET J.G., AUBERGE TH., PHELIP X. — Manifestations cliniques et radiologiques des hernies discales antérieures lombaires. *Rev. Med. Orthop.*, 1988, *12*, 51-54.

LEMAIRE V. — Les infiltrations articulaires et péri-articulaires des dérivés cortisoniques. *Concours Med.*, 1982, *104*, 3239-3245.

LERICHE R. — Effet de l'anesthésie à la novocaïne des ligaments et des insertions tendineuses dans certaines maladies articulaires. *Gaz. Hôp. (Paris)*, 1930, *103*, 1294.

LESAGE Y. — Les manipulations des articulations périphériques. *Cinésiologie*, 1984, *23*, 97, 363-430.

LESCURE R. — Etude critique d'un traitement par manipulation dans les algies d'origine rachidienne .Thèse, Paris, 1951.

LESCURE R. — Le pseudo-asthme infantile par insuffisance respiratoire mécanique. Ses caractéristiques et sa rééducation. *Ann. Méd. Phys.*, 1959, *1*, 57.

LEVERNIEUX J. — Les tractions vertébrales. Paris, Expansion Scientifique Française, 1961, 124 p.

LEVERNIEUX J., FOSSIER J. — Les tractions vertébrales sur la cervico-occipitalgie. *Sem. Hôp. Paris*, 1959, *35*, 559-563.

LE VIET D. — Les syndromes canalaires du poignet typiques et atypiques. *Rev. Med. Orthop.*, 1986, *5*, 5-13.

LEWIN T., MOFFET B., VIIDIK A. — The morphology of the lumbar intervertebral joints. *Acta Morphol. Neerlando-Scandinavica*, 1962, *4*, 299-319.

LEWIS T. — *Pain*. New York, Mac Millan, 1942.

LEWIS K. KELLGREN J.H. — Observations relating to referred pain, viscero-motor reflexes and other associated phenomena. *Clin Sci.*, 1939, *4*, 47.

LEWIT K. — Beitrag zur reversiblen Gelenksblockierung. *Zeitschr. Orthop.*, 1968, *105*, 150.

LEWIT K. — *Manuelle Medizin im Rahmen der medizinischen Rehabilitation*. München, Urban und Schwarzenberg, 1977.

LEWIT K. — *Manuelle Therapie*. Leipzig, Johan Ambrosino Barth, 1973.

LEWIT K. — Untersuchungsgang und Diagnose vertebragenen Störungen. *In* : Levit K. *Manuelle Medizin im Rahmen der medizinischen Rehabilitation*. München, pp. 146-154, Wien, Baltimore, Urban und Schwarzenberg, 1977.

LIDDELL E.G.T., PHILIPS C.G. — Pyramidal section in the cat. *Brain*, 1944, *67*, 1-9.

LIEOU Y.C. — Syndrome cervical postérieur et arthrite chronique de la colonne vertébrale cervicale. Etude clinique et radiologique. Thèse Med., Strasbourg, 1928.

LIVINGSTON W.K. — *Pain Mechanisms. A physiologic interpretation of causalgia and its related states*. New York, Mac Millan Co., 1943.

LORA J., LONG D. — So called facet denervation in the management of intractable back pain. *Spine*, 1976, *1*, 121-126.

LOUBOUTIN J.Y., CHALES G., GROSBOIS B., PAWLOTSKY Y. — Les pseudo-lombalgies communes. *Ann. Med. Phys.*, 1980, *2*, 146-149.

LOUIS R. — Lombalgies et crénothérapie. *In* : Simon L. Rabourdin J.-P. *Lombalgies et médecine de rééducation*. Paris, Masson, 1983.

LOUYOT P. — Algies dorsales professionnelles. *Sem. Hôp. Paris*, 1958, *34*, 2670-2679.

LOVETT R.W. — *Lateral curvature of the spine and round shoulders*. Philadelphia, Bilkeston Beard and Cº publ., 1907.

LUSCHNITZ E., RIEDERBERGER I., BAUCHSPIED B. — Das röntgenologische Bild der Osteonecrosis pubica post traumatica. *Fortschr. Roentgen.*, 1967, *1*, 107, 113-118.

LYNTON G.F., GILLES-JAMES R., TAYLOR J.R. — Innervation of lumbar zygapophyseal joint synovial folds. *Acta Orthop. Scand.*, 1987, *58*, 43-46.

MAC NAB I. — *Backache*. Baltimore, The Williams and Wilkins Co., 1979.

MAC NAB I., CUTHBERT H., GODFREY C.M. — The incidence of denervation of sacro-spinales muscles following spinal surgery. *Spine*, 1977, *2*, 4, 294.

MAGNUSSON P.B. — Differential diagnosis of causes of pain in the lower back accompanied by sciatic pain. *Ann. Surg.*, 1944, *119*, 878-891.

MAIGNE J.Y. — Les tendinites de l'angulaire de l'omoplate. *In* : Simon L., Rodineau J. *Epaule et médecine de rééducation*. Paris, Masson, 1984.

MAIGNE J.Y., MAIGNE R., GUÉRIN-SURVILLE H. — Anatomical study of the lateral cutaneous rami of the subcostal and iliohypogastric nerves. *Surg. Radiol. Anat.*, 1986, *8*, 251-256.

MAIGNE J.Y., DOURSOUNIAN L., TOUZARD R.C., MAIGNE R. — Traitement chirurgical du syndrome des perforantes. Résultats sur quatre cas. *Rhumatologie*, 1987, *396*, 177-180.

MAIGNE J.Y., HALMAGRAND N., LAZARETH J.P., MAIGNE R. — Lombalgies et thermocoagulation percutanée. Résultats sur 55 patients. *Rhumatologie*, 1987, *39*, 183-186.

MAIGNE J.Y., BUY J.N., ECOIFFIER J., MAIGNE R. — Etude tomodensitométrique de l'arc postérieur de la charnière thoraco-lombaire. *Rev. Méd. Orthop.*, 1987, *7*, 3-7.

MAIGNE J.Y., BUY J.N., THOMAS M., MAIGNE R. — Rotation de la charnière thoraco-lombaire. Etude tomodensitométrique chez 20 sujets normaux. *Ann. Rééd. Med. Phys.*, 1988, *31*, 239-244.

MAIGNE J.Y., LAZARETH J.P., GUÉRIN-SURVILLE H., MAIGNE R. — The lateral cutaneous branches of the dorsal rami of the thoraco lumbar jusction. An anatomical study on 37 dissections. *Surg. Radiol. Anat.*, 1986, *8*, 251-256.

MAIGNE J.Y., LAZARETH J.P., MAIGNE R. — Etude anatomique de l'innervation cutanée lombo-sacrée. Application à la physiopathologie de certaines lombalgies. *Rev. Rhum.*, 1988, *55*, 107-111.

MAIGNE J.Y. — Etude anatomique du rameau cutané des branches postérieures thoraciques hautes. *Rev. Med. Orthop.*, 1989, *16*, 9-11.

MAIGNE R. — Voir en fin de bibliographie.

MACKENZIE J. — *Symptoms and their interpretation.* London, Shaw and Sons, 1st ed., 1909.

MACKENZIE J. — Some points bearing on the association of sensory disorders and visceral disease. *Brain*, 1983, *16*, 321-354.

MAITLAND G.D. — *Vertebral manipulation*, 4th ed., London Butterworth, 1977.

MALDAGUE B.E., MALGHEM J.J. — Unilateral arch hypertrophy with spinous process tilt. A sign of arch deficiency. *Radiology*, 1976, *121*, 567-574.

MALDAGHE B., MALGHEM J. — Aspects radiologiques dynamiques de la spondylolyse lombaire. *Acta Orthop. Belg.*, 1981, *47*, 4-5, 441-457.

MALMIVAARA A., VIDEMAN I., KUOSMA E., TROUP J.D.G. — Facet joint orientation, facet and costovertebral joint osteoarthrosis, disc degeneration, vertebral body osteophytosis, and Schmorl's nodes in the thoraculumbar junctional region of cadaveric spines. *Spine*, 1987, *12*, 5, 458-463.

MALMIVAARA A., VIDEMAN T., KUOSMA E., TROUP J.D.G. — Pain radiographic, discographic, and direct observation of Schmorl's nodes in the thoracolumbar junctional region of the cadaveric spine. *Spine*, 1987, *12*, 5, 453-457.

MALMIVAARA A. — *Thoracolumbar junctional region*, (1 vol.), Helsinki, Institute of occupational Health, 1987.

MARGUERY O. — Tennis de haut niveau et pubalgies. Une pathologie croissante liée au tennis moderne. *Rev. Med. Orthop.*, 1986, *6*, 29-32.

MAY E., DEBRAY CH., FELD J. — Cellulite en bande et rhumatisme vertébral. *Presse Med.*, 1942, *32*, 437-438.

MENNELL J.M. — *Joint pain.* London, J.A. Churchill Publ., 1964.

MENNELL J.B. — *The Science and Art of joint manipulation* (2 vol.) London, J. and A. Churchill, Ltd., 1952.

MEYER R., KIEFFER D., VAUTRAVERS P., KUNTZ J.L., ASH L. — Paraplégie après infiltrations épidurales cortisoniques. *Rhumatologie*, 1979, *31*, 339.

MICHELSEN J.J., MIXTER W.J. — Pain and disability of shoulder and arm due to herniation of the nucleus pulposus of cervical intervertebral disks. *New. Engl. J. Med.*, 1944, 231.

MIEHLKE K, SCHULZE G., EGER W. — Klinische und experimentelle Untersuchungen zum Fibrosistis Syndrom. *Z. Rheumaforsch.*, 1960, *19*, 310-330.

MILLION R., NILSEN K.M., JAYSON M.N., BAKER B.D. — Evaluation of low back pain and assessment of lumbar corsets with and without back supports. *Ann. Rheum. Dis.*, 1981, *40*, 449-454.

MILLS G P. — The treatment of tennis elbow. *Br. Med. J.*, 1928, *1*, 12-13.

MITCHELL P.E., HENDRY N.G., BILLEWICA W.Z. — Chemical background of intervertebral disc. prolapse. *J. Bone Joint Surg.*, 1961, *43A*, 327.

MIXTER W.J., BARR J.G. — Rupture of the intervertebral disc with involvement of the spinal canal. *New England J. Med.*, 1984, *211-210*.

MOLDOFSKY H. — Sleep and musculoskeletal pain. *Am. J. Med.*, 1986, *81*, (suppl. 3A), 85-90.

MOONEY V., ROBERTSON J. — The facet syndrome. *Clin. Orthop.*, 1976, *115*, 149-156.

MOORE M. Jr. — Radiohumeral synovitis. *Arch. Surg.*, 1952, *64*, 501-505.

MORRIS J.M., LUCAS D.B., BRESLER B. — The role of the trunk in the stability of the spine. *J. Bone Joint Surg.*, 1961.

MORGAN F.P., KING T. — Primary instability of lumbar vertebral as a common cause of low back pain. *J. Bone Joint Surg.*, 1957, *39B*, 6.

MORVAN G., MASSARE C., LEQUESNE M. — *La tomodensitométrie ostéoarticulaire* (1 vol.), 190 p., Paris, Documenta Geigy, 1985.

MURRAY, LESLIE C.F., WRIGHT V. — Carpal tunnel syndrome, humeral epicondylitis and the cervical spine. *Br. Med. J.*, 1976, *I*, 1439-1442.

NACHEMSON A. — Adult scoliosis and back pain. *Spine*, 1979, *4*, 6, 513-517.

NACHENMSON A., LEWIN T., MAROUDAS A., FREEMAN. — In vitro diffusion of dye through the end plates and the annulus fibrosus of human lumbar intervertebral discs. *Acta Orthop. Scand*, 1970, *41*, 589-607.

NADE S., BELL S., WYKE B.D. — The innervation of the lumbar spinal joints and its significance. *J. Bone Joint Surg.*, 1980, *62B*, 255.

NARAKAS A., CRAWFORD G.P. — Les aspects étiopathogéniques, cliniques, anatomopathologiques ainsi que le traitement chirurgical dans l'épicondylite chronique. *Therapeutische Umschau*, 1977, *34*, 2, 70-80.

NARAKAS A. — Traitement chirurgical de l'épicondylalgie. *In : Coude et médecine de rééducation*, pp. 129-141. Paris, Masson, 1979.

NEUMANN H.D. — Diagnosis and treatment of pelvic girdle lesions. *In :* Greenman Ph. *Concepts and mechanismus of neuromuscular functions.* pp. 111-117. Berlin, Heidelberg, New York, Tokyo, Springer Verlag, 1984.

NEUWORTH E. — The vertebral nerve in the posterior cervical syndrome. *New York J. Med.*, 1955, *55*, 1380.

NICK J., ZIEGLER G. — Etude des céphalées cervicales. *Sem. Hôp. Paris*, 1980, *56*, 519-524.

NICK J. — Classification, étiologie et fréquence relative des céphalées. A propos d'une série de 2 350 cas. *Presse Med.*, 1968, *8*, 76, 359-362.

NINGHSIA MEDICAL COLLEGE. — Anatomical observations on lumbar nerve posterior rami. *Chinese Med. J.*, 1978, *4*, 492-496.

NORTON P.L., BROW T. — The immobilizing efficiency of back braces. *J. Bone Joint Surg.*, 1957, *39 A*, 111-134.

NWUGA V.C. — *Manipulation of the spine.* Baltimore, The Williams and Wilkins Co, 1976.

OGDEN J.A. — Subluxation and dislocation of the proximal tiblo-fubular joint. *J. Bone Joint Surg.*, 1974, *56A*, 145-154.

OGER J., BRUMAGNE J., MARGAUX J. — Les accidents des

manipulations vertébrales. *J. Belge Med. Phys. Rhum.*, 1964, *19*, 56-78.

OGSBURY J.S., SIMON R.H., LEHMAN R.W. — Facet denervation in the treatment of low back pain syndrome. *Pain*, 1977, *3*, 257-263.

OLIVIER G., OLIVIER C. — *Mécanique articulaire.* 1 vol., Paris, Vigot édit., 1963.

OSGOOD R.B. — Radiohumeral Bursitis, Epicondylitis, Epicondylalgie. *Arch Surg.*, 1922, *4*, 420.

OROFINO C., SHERMAN M., SCHECHTER D. — Luschka's joint. A degenerative phenomenon. *J. Bone Joint Surg.*, 1960, *42A*, 853-858.

OTTO C.W., WALL C.L. — Total spinal anesthesia : a rare complication of intrathoracic intercostal nerve block. *Ann. Thorac. Surg.*, 1976, *3*, 289-292.

OUDENHOVEN R.C. — Gravitational lumbar traction. *Arch. Phys. Med. Rehabil.*, 1978, *59*, 510-512.

PAAR O., ZWEYMUELLER K., SAVER G. — Traitement chirurgical de l'épicondylite humérale. *Der Chirurg.*, 1978, *49*, 8, 520-22.

PAGE L.E. — *The principles of osteopathy.* Kansas City, Academy of applied osteopathy, 1952.

PAMELA F., BEAUGERIE J., COUTURIER M., DUVAL G., GAUDY J.H. — Syndrome de déafférentation motrice par thrombose du tronc basilaire après manipulation vertébrale. *Presse Med.*, 1983, *12*, 24, 1548.

PARIS S.V., NYBERG R., MOONEY V.T., GONYEA W. — Three level innervation of the lumbar facet joints. *International Society for the study of the lumbar spine.* New Orleans, Louisiana, ISSLS, May 1980.

PATURET G. — *Traité d'anatomie humaine*, (3 vol.), Paris, Masson, 1958.

PAYNE T.L., LEAVITT F., GARRON D.C., KATZ R.S., GOLDEN H.E., GLICKMAN P.B., VANDERPLATE C. — Fibrositis and psychologic disturbance. *Arth. Rheum.*, 1982, *25*, 213-217.

PAYNE E.E., SPILLANE J.D. — The cervical spine an anatomical study of 70 specimen. *Brain*, 1957, *80*, 571.

PEDERSEN H.E., BOUNK C.F.J., GARDNER E. — The anatomy of lumbosacral posterior primary rami and meningeal branches of spinal nerves (Sinu-vertebral nerves). *J. Bone Joint Surg.*, 1956, *38*, 377-391.

PEILLON M. — Traitement des maladies de la charnière lombosacrée. *Ann. Med. Phys.*, 1958, *1*, 1, 18-33.

PEILLON M. — Cinesithérapie de la région cervicale. *Ann. Med. Phys.*, 1959, *2*, 213-222.

PELOUX (DU) J. — Douleurs des scolioses lombaires de l'adulte. *Ann. Readap. Med. Phys.*, 1988, *31*, 53s-66s.

PENNING L. — *Functional pathology of the cervical spine.* Amsterdam, Excerpta Medica Foundation, 1968.

PENNING L., TÖNDURY G. — Entstehung, Bau und Funktion der meniscoïden Strukturen in den Halswirbelgelenken. *Z. Orthop.*, 1963, *98*, 1-14.

PHELIP X. — Le syndrome dit sympathique postérieur de Barré et Lieou. *Prat. Med.*, 1983, *17*, 48-51.

PERL E.R. — Pain, peripheral and spinal factors. *In : The Research status of spinal manipulative therapy monography.* Washington, National Institutes of Health, 1976.

PIEDALLU P. — *L'ostéopathie.* Bordeaux, Biere ed., 1947.

PIEDALLU P. — Problèmes sacro-iliaques. *L'homme sain*, 1952, *2*, 1.

POULETTY J., BESSON J. — Injections intra-articulaires et matériel stérile à usage unique. *Ann. Med. Phys.*, 1973, *16*, 347-355.

PRATT-THOMAS H.R., BERGER K.E. — Cerebellar and spinal injuries after chiropractic manipulation. *JAMA*, 1947, *9*, 133, 600-603.

PRIVAT J.M. et CH., FREREBEAU J., BENEZECH J., GROS C. — Cruralgies symptomatiques d'origine tumorale, traitement chirurgical et rééducation post-opératoire. *In : Actualités en rééducation fonctionnelle et réadaptation.* 2ᵉ série (sous la direction de Simon L.). Paris, Masson, 1977.

PUTTI V. — New conception in the pathogenis of sciatic pain. *Lancet*, 1927, *2*, 53-60.

PUTTI V. — *Lombartrite e sciatica vertebrale.* (1 vol.) Bologna, Cappelli Edit., 1936.

PUTTI V. — Lady Jones' lecture on new concepts in the pathogenesis of sciatic pain. *Lancet*, 1927, *2*, 53-60.

RABISCHONG P., LOUIS R., VIGNAUD J., MASSARE C. — Le disque vertébral. *Anat Clin.*, 1978, *1*, 55-64.

RAMSEY R.H. — The anatomy of the ligamenta flava. *Clin. Orthop.*, 1966, *44*, 129-140.

RANCUREL G., FREYSS G., KIEFFER E. — L'insuffisance vertébrobasilaire de type postural hemodynamique. *Sem. Hôp. Paris*, 1986, *62*, 2741-2754.

RAOU R.J.P. — *Recherches sur la mobilité vertébrale en fonction des types rachidiens.* Thèse, Paris, 1952.

REES W.E.S. — Multiple bilateral subcutaneous rhizolysis of segmental nerves in the treatment of the intervertebral disc syndrome. *Ann. Gen. Pract.*, 1971, *26*, 126-127.

RENIER J.C., AUDRAN M., SERET P., SECHER V. — Contribution à la connaissance de l'évolution naturelle de l'ostéoporose. *Rev. Rhum.*, 1985, *53*, 451-457.

RENOULT C. — *Epicondylalgie, épicondylite, épicondylose ou coude du tennis.* Thèse Med. Paris, 1954, 73 pages dactyl.

RENOULT M. — *La coccygodynie, algie statique.* Thèse, Paris, 1962.

REVEL M., AMOR B. — Rééducation de la musculature lombo-pelvienne dans la lombalgie. *In :* Simon L., Rabourdin J.P., *Lombalgies et médecine de rééducation.* Paris, Masson, 1983.

REVEL M., BUADES C., LE TALLEC R. — *Traitement de la lombalgie commune. Technologie kinésithérapie.* Paris, Lamarre-Poinat, 1981.

REVEL M., AMOR B. — Les orthèses de protection lombaire. *In :* Simon L., Rabourdin J.P., *Lombalgies et médecine de rééducation.* Paris, Masson, 1983.

REYNOLDS D.V. — Surgery in the rat during electrical analgesia induced by focal brain stimulation. *Science*, 1969, *164*, 444-445.

RIEDERER J., RETTIG H. — Beobachtungen eines akuten Basedow nach chiropraktischer Behandung der Halswirbelsäule. *Med. Klin.*, 1955, *50*, 1911-1912.

RIEUNAU G. — Pièges et dangers des manipulations vertébrales en orthopédie. *Ann. Méd. Phys.*, 1966, *9*, 260-272.

RIGGS B.L., MELTON L.J. — Involutional osteoporosis. *N. Engl. J. Med.*, 1986, *314*, 1676-1686.

RINZLER S.H., TRAVELL J. — Therapy directed at somatic component of cardiac pain. *Am. Heart J.*, 1948, *35*, 248.

RISSANEN P.M. — The surgical anatomy and pathology of the supraspinous and interspinous ligaments of the lumbar spine. *Acta Orthop. Scand.*, 1960, suppl. 46.

RISSANEN P.M. — Comparison of pathologic changes in vertebral discs and intervertebral ligaments of the lumbar spine in the light of autopsy. *Acta Orthop. Scand.*, 1964, *34*, 54-56.

RODINEAU J., SAILLANT G. — *Pathologie du membre supérieur du joueur de tennis.* Paris, Masson, 1985.

ROGER B., LAZENNEC J.Y., ROY-CAMILLE R., LAVAL-JEANTET M. — Lombo-sciatalgies post-opératoires et IRM. *Rev. Med. Orthop.*, 1988, *6*, 13.

ROLES N.C., MAUDSLEY R.H. — Radial tunnel syndrome; resistant tennis elbow as nerve entrapment. *J. Bone Joint Surg.*, 1972, *54B*, 499-508.

ROOFE P.G. — Innervation of annulus fibrosus and posterior longitudinal ligaments. *Arch. Neurol. Psychiatry*, 1940, *44*, 100.

ROUSSAT J. — *Responsabilité médicale en matière d'accidents des manipulations du rachis cervical.* Mémoire pour le diplôme d'Etudes médicales relatives à la réparation juridique du dommage corporel, Paris, Université Paris V, 1977.

ROUVIÈRE H. — *Anatomie humaine.* (3 vol.) 11e ed., Paris, Masson et Cie, 1973.

ROY-CAMILLE R., SAILLANT G., RODINEAU J., COULON J.P. — Disques lombaires et spondylolisthésis. *In : Lombalgies et médecine de rééducation*, Paris, Masson, 1983.

RUBIN D. — Cervical radiculitis diagnosis and treatment. *Arch. Phys. Med.*, 1960, *41*, 580-586.

RUNGE F. — Zur Genese und Behandlung des Schreibe-krampfes. *Berliner Klin. Wochen*, 1973, *X*, 245.

RYCKEWAERT A., LEMAIRE V., AMBROSINI C., SEZE S. DE. — Arthrites bactériennes aiguës suppurées après injection intra-articulaire de dérivés cortisoniques. *Rev. Rhum.*, 1973, *40*, 189-193.

SAINT-CLAIR STRANGE F.G. — Debunking the disc. *Proc. Roy. Soc. Med.*, 1966, *40*, 952.

SAMUEL J., KENESI C. — Où en est la chirurgie de l'épicondylite rebelle ? *In : L'actualité rhumatologique 1975 présentée au praticien*, pp. 253-260, Paris, Expansion Scientifique Française, 1975.

SANCHEZ A., JARDIN F., MARGAIRAZ A., GREFFE B. — Rachianesthésies involontaires par la xylocaïne ou du danger des infiltrations rachidiennes. *Nouv. Presse Méd.*, 1977, *6*, 2165.

SATO A. — The somatosympathetic reflexes : their physiological and clinical significance. *In : The research status of spinal manipulative therapy.* NINCDS Monograph No. 15. Washington, DHEW, 1975.

SATO A., SCHMIDT R.F. — Spinal and supraspinal components of the reflex discharges into lumbar and thoracic white rami. *J. Physiol. (London)*, 1971, *212*, 839-850.

SCHMINCKE A., SANTO E. — Zur normalen pathologischen Anatomie der Halswirbelsäule. *Zbl. Allg. Path. Bath. Anat.*, 1932, *55*, 369.

SCHIANO A., SETRICK-NAIM M., DOBBELS E., BARDOT A., SERRATRICE G. — Les anomalies transitionnelles sont-elles un risque de lombalgies ? *In :* Simon L., Rabourdin J.P., *Lombalgie et médecine de rééducation*, pp. 104-107, Paris, Masson, 1983.

SCHMID H.J.A. — Iliosacrale Diagnose und Behandlung, 1978-82, *Manuelle Medizin*, 1985, *23*, 101-108.

SCHMORL G., JUNGHANNS H. — *Clinique et radiologie de la colonne vertébrale normale et pathologique.* Paris, Doin ed., 1956.

SCHNEIDER D.Y. — Current concepts of the Barre syndrome or the posterior cervical sympathetic syndrome. *Clin. Orthop.*, 1962, *24*, 40-48.

SCHWARTZ G.A., GEIGER J.K., SAPNO A.V. — Posterior inferior cerebellar artery syndrome of Wallenberg after chiropractic manipulation. *Arch. Intern. Med.*, 1956, *3*, 352.

SCHWARZ E. — Manuelle Medizin und innere Medizin. *Schweiz Rundsh Med. (Praxis)*, 1974, *63*, 837.

SELLIER N., VALLEE C., CHEVROT A., FRANTZ N., REVEL M., AMOR B., MENKES C.I., PALLARDY G. — La sciatique par kystes synoviaux et diverticules articulaires lombaires à développement intra-rachidien. Etude saccoradiculographique, tomodensitométrique et arthrographique. *Rev. Rhum.*, 1987, *54*, 4, 297.

SENEGAS J., LAVIGNOLLE B. — Syndrome des facettes. *In :* Simon L. Rabourdin J.P. *Lombalgies et médecine de rééducation.* Paris, Masson, 1983.

SERRANO-VELLA R. — *La discographie. Confrontations anatomo-radiologiques et cliniques dans l'étude du disque intervertébral lombaire.* Thèse Med. Marseille, 1972.

SERRATRICE G. — Les acroparesthésies du membre supérieur. *Marseille Med.*, 1977, *137*, 9-28.

SERRE H., SIMON L., BARJON M.C., CLAUSTRE J. — Le canal carpien en pratique rhumatologique. *Rev. Méd.*, 1964, *24*, 127-132.

SERRE H. — Les cruralgies. *In : Rapport de la 3e Conférence internationale des maladies rhumatismales.* Aix-les-Bains, 1956, pp. 381-397.

SÈZE S. DE. — *Algies vertébrales d'origine statique.* Paris, Expansion Scientifique Française, 3e éd., 1951.

SÈZE S. DE. — La sciatique dite banale, essentielle ou rhumatismale et le disque lombo-sacré. *Rev. Rhum.*, 1939, *6*, 986-1036.

SÈZE S. DE. — Huit entretiens sur le rôle du disque intervertébral. Le rôle du disque dans les lombalgies chroniques. *Rev. Rhum.*, 1951, *18*, 500-506.

SÈZE S. DE, DJIAN A., ABDELMOULA M. — Etude radiologique de la dynamique cervicale dans le plan sagittal; une contribution radio-physiologique à l'étude pathogénique des arthroses cervicales. *Rev. Rhum.*, 1951, *18*, 111.

SÈZE S. DE — Les attitudes antalgiques dans la sciatique disco-radiculaire commune. *Sem. Hôp. Paris*, 1955, *39*, 2291-2312.

SÈZE S. DE, CAROIT M., MAITRE M. — Le syndrome douloureux vertébral tropho-statique de la post-ménopause. *Sem. Hôp. Paris*, 1961, *37*, 3505-3524.

SHEALY C.N. — Percutaneous radiofrequency denervation of spinal facets treatment for chronic back pain and sciatica. *J. Neurosurg.*, 1975, *43*, 448.

SHEEHAN S. — Syndromes of basilar and carotid artery insufficiency diagnosis and medical therapy. *Southern Med. J.*, 1961, *54*, 465-470.

SHERRINGTON C.S. — *The integrative action of the nervous system.* New-Haven Yale Univ. Press., 1906, 1947

SIMON L. — Pièges et dangers des manipulations cervicales en rhumatologie. *Ann. Méd. Phys.*, 1966, *9*, 272-283.

SIMON L., BLOTMAN F., CLAUSTRE J. — *Abrégé de rhumatologie*, 4e éd., Paris, Masson, 1984.

SIMON L. — *Actualités en rééducation fonctionnelle et réadaptation*. Une série annuelle : 1 (1976) à 14 (1989).

SIMON L. — *La sciatique et le nerf sciatique*. Paris, Masson, 1980.

SIMON L. — *Lombalgie et médecine de rééducation*. Paris, Masson, 1983.

SIMON L. — *Rachis cervical et médecine de rééducation*, Paris, Masson, 1985.

SINCLAIR D.C., FEINDEL W.H., WEDDELL G., FALCONER M. — *J. Bone Joint Surg.*, 1948, *30B*.

SIRBRANDIJ S. — Instability of the proximal tibio-fibular joint. *Acta Orthop. Scand.*, 1978, *49*, 621-626.

SIRBRANDIJ S. — Instability of the proximal tibio-fibular joint. *Acta Orthop. Scand.*, 1978, *49*, 621-626.

SMYTH M.J., WRIGHT V. — Sciatica and the intervertebral disc. *J. Bone Joint Surg.*, 1958, *40A*, 1041.

SMYTHE H.A. — Fibrositis as a disorder of pain modulation. *Clin. Rheum. Dis.*, 1979, *5*, 823-968.

SMYTHE H.A. — Referred pain and tender point. *Am. J. Med.*, 1986, *81* (suppl. 3A), 90-92.

SOUTHWORTH J., BERSACK S. — Anomalies of the lumbosacral vertebra in 550 individuals without symptoms referable to the low back pain. *AJR*, 1950, *64*, 624-634.

STEINDLER A. — Low back pain an anatomic and clinical study. *J. Iowa M. Soc.*, 1925, *15*, 473.

STILL A.T. — *Philosophy of osteopathy*. Kirksville, A.T. Still, 1899.

STEWART T.D. — The age incidence of neural arch defects in alaskan natives, considered from the stand point of etiology. *J. Bone Joint Surg.*, 1953, *35A*, 937-950.

STILWELL Jr D.L. — The nerve supply of the vertebral column and its associated structures in the monkey. *Anat. Rec.*, 1958, *125*, 2, 139.

STODDARD A. — *Manual of osteopathic technics.*, London, Hutschinson Med. Publications, 1959.

STOOKEY B. — Compression of the spinal cord and nerve roots, by herniation of the nucleus pulposus, in the cervical regions. *Arch. Surg.*, 1940, *40*, 417.

STOVELL P.B., BEINFIELD M.S. — Treatment of resistant lateral epicondylitis of the elbow by lengthening of the Extensor Carpi Brevis tendon. *Surg. Gynecol. Obstet.*, 1979, *149*, 4, 526-528.

STURESSON B., SELVIK G., UDEN A. — Movements of the sacroiliac joints. A roentgen stereophotogrammetric analysis. *Spine*, 1989, *14*, 157-161.

STUCK R.M. — Discographie cervicale. *Am. J. Roentgenol.*, 1961, *86*, 975-982.

SUH C.H. — The fundamentals of computer-aided X-ray analysis of the spine. *J. Biomech.* 1974, *7*, 161-169.

SUREAU Cl. — Notions nouvelles sur l'anatomie et la physiologie de l'articulation sacro-iliaque. *Presse Med.*, 1959, *67*, 947-948.

TAILLARD W. — *Les spondylolisthésis*. Paris, Masson, 1957, 180 p.

TAILLARD W.F. — Etiology of spondylolisthesis. *Clin. Orthop.*, 1976, *117*, 30-39.

TAPTAS J.N. — *Maux de tête et névralgies, douleurs cranio-faciales*. Paris, Masson, 1953.

TATLOW W.F.T., BAMMER H.G. — Syndrome of vertebral artery compression. *Neurology*, 1957, *7*, 331.

TAVERNIER L. — L'épicondylite tenace guérie par énervation sensitive régionale. *Rev. Orthop.*, 1946, *32*, 61-62.

TAYLOR J.R., TWOMEY T. — Age changes in lumbar zygapophyseal joints observations on structure and function. *Spine*, 1986, *11*, 739-745.

TEIRICH LEUBE H. — Berufsbeschwerden und « Beschäftigungsneurosen » bei Musikem. *Arztl. Prax.*, 1960, *12*, 879.

TELLIER M. — Traitement du syndrome tropho-statique de la post-ménopause par la rééducation fonctionnelle. *Ann. Méd. Phys.*, 1959, *2*, 7-11.

TERRIER J.C. — *Manipulation, Massage*. Stuttgart, Hippokrates Verlag, 1958.

TERRIER J.C. — Les bases de la thérapeutique manipulative de la colonne vertébrale. *Méd. Hyg.*, 1959, *17*, 390-391.

TERRIER J.C. — Massage manipulatif de la région lombaire. *Kinésithérapie Scientifique*, 1983, *215*, 11-16.

TESTUT L., LATARJET A. — *Traité d'anatomie humaine* (5 vol.). Paris, Doin, 1948.

TEYSSANDIER M.J. — Effet des contraintes et du cisaillement sur les joints intervertébraux dorsolombaires. *Cinésiologie*, 1978, *67*, 72-78.

TEYSSANDIER M.J., BRIFFOD P., ZIEGLER G. — Intérêt de la diélectrolyse de kétoprofène en rhumatologie et en petite traumatologie. *Sciences Médicales*, 1977, *8*, 157-162.

TEYSSANDIER M.J. — Pénétration des tissus biologiques par les rayonnements. *Rev. Med. Orthop.*, 1987, *8*, 27-31.

THEOBALO G.W. — Role of cerebral cortex in apperception of pain *Lancet* 1949 *2* 41-94.

THIEBAUT F., ISCH F., ISCH-TREUSSARD C. — Etude électromyographique de l'équilibre de suspension. *C.R. des séances de la société de Biologie*, 1952, *146*, 1385-1387.

THIERRY-MIEG J. — Technique des manipulations vertébrales utilisées dans le traitement des cruralgies discales. Indications, contre-indications et accidents. *Sem. Hôp. Paris*, 1967, *43*, 401-405.

TISSINGTON W.F., TATLOW B., BROWN ST. JOHN. — Radiographic studies of the vertebral arteries in cadavers, influence of position and traction on the head. *Radiology*, 1963, *81*, 80-88.

TOMLINSON K.M. — Purpura following manipulation of the spine. *Br. Med. J.*, 1955, no. 4224, 1260.

TÖNDURY G. — Uber den ramus meningiecus nervi spinalis. *Praxis*, 1937, *26*, 3.

TÖNDURY G. — Le développement de la colonne vertébrale. *Rev. Chir. Orthop.*, 1953, *39*, 553-569.

TÖNDURY G. — *Angewandte und topographische Anatomie*. Stuttgart, Georg Thieme Verlag, 1970.

TÖNDURY G. — Beitrag zur Kenntniss der kleinen Wirbelgelenke. *Z. Anat. Entw. Gesch.*, 1940, *110*, 568-575.

TÖNDURY G. — *Entwicklungsgeschichte und Fehlbildungen der Wirbelsaule*. Stuttgart, Hippokrates Verlag, 1958.

TÖNDURY G. — Anatomie fonctionnelle des petites articulations du rachis. *Ann. Méd. Phys.*, 1972, *15*, 173-191.

TOOLE J.F., TUCKER S.H. — Influence of head position

upon cerebral circulation. Studies on blood flow in cadavers. *Arch. Neurol. (Chicago)*, 1960, *2*, 616-623.

TORTEL J.L. — Le psoas douloureux. Une extension du syndrome de la charnière dorso-lombaire de Maigne. *Rev. Med. Orthop.*, 1987, *7*, 19-20.

TOUCHON J., BILLIARD M., BESSET A., SIMON L., HÉRISSON C. — Fibrositis syndrome : polysomnographic and psychological aspect. *In : VIIth European Congress on sleep Research*, Zeged, Hongrie, 1986.

TRAVELL J. — Basis for the multiple uses of local block of somatic trigger area (procaine infiltration and ethyl chloride spray). *Mississippi Valley Med. J.*, 1949, *71*, 13.

TRAVELL J., TRAVELL W. — Therapy of low back and of referred pain in the lower extremity by manipulation and procaine infiltration. *Arch. Phys. Med.*, 1946, *27*, 537-547.

TRAVELL J. — Referred pain from skeletal muscle. *New York State J. Med.*, 1955, Febr. *1*, 331-340.

TRAVELL J., RINZLER S., HERMAN M. — Pain and disability of the shoulder and arm. *JAMA*, 1942, *120*, 417-422.

TRAVELL J., SIMONS D. — Myofacial pain and dysfontion. The trigger point manual. Baltimore, William and Wilkins, 1983.

TROISIER O. — *Sémiologie et traitement des algies discales et ligamentaires du rachis*, (1 vol.), Paris, Masson ed., 1973.

TROISIER O. — Douleurs rachidiennes d'origine ligamentaire. *In : Proceeding du 4e Congrès international de Médecine physique*, 1964. Excerpta Medica n° 76, p. 119.

TROISIER O., GOUNOT-HALBOUT M.C., DUREY A. — La pathologie de la position extrême. *Ann. Med. Phys.*, 1969, *12*, 27-44.

TROISIER O. — La discographie dans les lumbagos à répétition et dans la lombalgie chronique. *In :* Simon L., Rabourdin J.P., *Lombalgies et médecine de rééducation*. Paris, Masson, 1983.

TROISIER O., GOZLAN E., DUREY A., RODINEAU J., GOUNOT-HALBOUT M.C., PELLERAY B. — Traitement des lombosciatiques par injection intradiscale d'enzymes protéolytiques. 80 observations. *Nouv. Press. Med.*, 1980, *9*, 227-230.

TROISIER O., KISSEL-REGNIER C. — Le traitement des tendinites épicondyliennes par la ténotomie souscutanée. *Ann. Réad. Med. Phys.*, 1986, *29*, 1, 85-90.

TSOUDEROS Y., HELD J.P. — Endorphines et douleur. *Concours Med.*, 1982, *104*, 12, 1869.

UNSWORTH A., DOWSON D., WRIGHT V. — Cracking joints. *Ann. Rheum., Dis.*, 1971, *30*, 348.

UPTON A.R.M., COMAS A.J. — The double crush hypothesis in nerve entrapment syndromes. *Lancet*, 1973, *2*, 359-362.

VAN STEENBRUGGHE G., PANTHIER G., MAIGNE J.Y., MAIGNE R. — Etude contrôlée des ondes courtes magnétiques pulsées dans le traitement de la pathologie douloureuse commune. A propos de 141 cas. *Ann. Réad. Med. Phys.*, 1988, *31*, 227-232.

VAUTRAVERS PH. — Traitement physique des lombalgies. *J. Med. Pratique*, 1988, *16*, 14-17.

VERBIEST H. — A radicular syndrome from developmental narrowing of the lumbar vertebral canal. *J. Bone Joint Surg.*, 1954, *26B*, 230-238.

VITTE E., FREYSS G., RANCUREL G. — Insuffisance vertébrobasilaire hémodynamique posturale données récentes. *Encycl. Méd. Chir.*, Instantanés médicaux, 1984, *55*, 38.

VRIES H.A. DE, CAILLIET R. — Vagotonis effect of inversion therapy upon resting neuromuscular tension. *Am. J. Phys. Med.*, 1985, *64*, 3, 119-129.

WAGHEMACKER R. — A propos des manipulations. *Echo Méd. Nord*, févr. 1952.

WAGHEMACKER R. — Les bases physiologiques des manipulations vertébrales. Réunion Internationale de Médecine physique et de Réhabilitation. 7-6-61, Turin. *Minerva Fisioterapica*, 1962, *7* (suppl. n° 4, pp. 21-24).

WAGHEMACKER R. — Contrôle de l'efficacité des manipulations vertébrales dans le syndrome de l'artère vertébrale par l'électronystagmographie et la cupulométrie. *Ann. Méd. Phys.*, 1965, *8*, 3-15.

WAGHEMACKER R. — Applications nouvelles de la cinésithérapie grâce aux progrès de la cinésiologie. *Ann. Méd. Phys.*, 1965, *8*, 51-67.

WAGHEMACKER R., CÉCILE J.P., BUISE A. — Dissociation du syndrome péri-arthrite de l'épaule grâce aux renseignements fournis par l'arthrographie : les conséquences au point de vue rééducation. *Ann. Méd. Phys.*, 1963, *6*, 1-21.

WAGHEMACKER R., LASSELIN et BERTIN J. — Douleurs vertébrales, syndromes radiculaires associés et médecine psycho-somatique. *Rev. Rhum.*, 1955, *9*, 693.

WAGHEMACKER R., MAIGNE R. — La récupération fonctionnelle du rachis lombaire. *Réadaptation*, 10, 1959.

WAGHEMACKER R. — Une preuve objective de l'efficacité des manipulations vertébrales : syndrome cervical et électronystagmographie. *Cinésiologie*, 1972, *44*, 1.

WALLACE D.J. — Fibromyalgia : unusual historical aspects and new pathogenic insights. *M. Sinai J. Med.*, 1984, *51*, 2, 124-130.

WEISL H. — The articular surfaces of the sacro-iliac joint and their relation to the movements of the sacrum. *Acta Anat.*, 1955, *23*, 80-91.

WEISL H. — The ligaments of the sacro-iliac joint examined with particular reference to the function. *Acta Anat.*, 1954, *20*, 201-213.

WERNE S. — The cranio vertebral joints. *Acta Orthop. Scand.*, 1957, *28*, 165.

WETTERWALD F. — Rôle thérapeutique du mouvement. *In : Manuel pratique de kinésithérapie*. Paris, Alcan, 1912.

WIBERG G. — Back pain in relation to the nerve supply of the intervertebral disc. *Acta Orthop. Scand.*, 1949, *19*, 211.

WIESEL W., TSOURMAS N., FEFFER H.L., CITRIN C.M., PATRONAS N. — Study of computer assisted tomography. The incidence of positive CAT Scans in an asymptomatic group of patients. *Spine*, 1984, *6*, 549-551.

WILDER D.G., POPE M.H., FRYMOYER J.N. — Functional topography of the sacroiliac joint. *Spine*, 1980, *5*, 575-579.

WILHELM A., GIESELER H. — Die Behandlung der Epicondylitis humero-radialis durch Denervation. *Der Chirurg.*, 1962, *33*, 3, 118-121.

WINCKLER G. — *Manuel d'anatomie topographique et fonctionnelle*. Paris, Masson, 1964.

WOLF J. — Chondrosynovial membrane serving as joint cavity lining with a sliding and barrier function. *Folia Morphol. Prague*, 1969, *17*, 291-208.

WOLFE F. — Development of criteria for the diagnosis of fibrositis. *Am. J. Med.*, 1986, *81* (suppl. 3A), 99-104.

WOLFF H.D. — *Neurophysiologische Aspekte der manuellen Medizin.* Berlin, Heidelberg, New York, Tokyo, Springer Verlag, 1983.

WOLFF H.D. — The theory of joint play : distance and coherence. *In :* Greenman Ph.E., *Concepts and mechanism of neuromuscular punctions.* Berlin, Heidelberg, New York, Tokyo, Springer Verlag, 1984.

WOLFF H.G., WOLF S. — *Pain.* Oxford, Blackwell Scientific Publications, 1958, 108 p.

WOLFF H.G. — *Headache and other head pain.* 2nd Ed. Oxford, New York, University Press, 1963.

WOLINETZ E. — Sur six cas de thrombose du tronc basilaire. *Sem. Hôp. Paris,* 1963, *27,* 1305-1308.

WYKE B. — The neurology of low back pain. *In :* Jayson M.I.V., *Lumbar Spine and Back Pain,* London, Pitman Press, 1980.

WYKE B. — Receptor systems in lumbosacral tissues in relation to the production of low back pain. *In :* White A.A., Gordon S.L., *AAOS Symposium on Ideopathic Low Back Pain,* St Louis, C.V. Mosby, 1982.

WYKE B.D. — The neurology of joints. *Ann. Roy. Coll. Surg., Engl.,* 1967, *41,* 25-50.

WYKE B.D. — The neurology of joints : a review of general principles. *Clin. Rheumatic Dis.,* 1981, *7,* 223-239.

WYKE B.D. — The neurological basis of thoracic spinal pain. *Rheumatology Phys. Med.,* 1970, *10,* 350.

WYKE B.D., POLAVEK P. — Articular neurology. The present position. *J. Bone Joint Surg.,* 1975, *57B,* 401.

YUNUS M., MASI A.T., CAIABRO J.J., MILLER K.A., FEIGERBAUM J. — Primary fibromyalgia : clinical study of 50 patients with matched normal controls. *Sem. Arth. Rheuma.,* 1981, *11,* 151-171.

YUNUS M., MASI A.T. — Juvenile primary fibromyalgia syndrome. *Arth Rheum.,* 1985, *28,* 138-145.

YUNUS M., KALYAN-RAMAN U.P., KALYAN-RAMAN K., MASI A.T. — Pathologic changes in muscle in primary fibromyalgic syndrome. *Am. J. Med.,* 1986, *81,* (suppl. 3A), 38-42.

ZIEGLER G., TEYSSANDIER M.J., EULLER K. — Lombalgies et radiculalgies lombaires communes *Cahiers Sandoz,* décembre 1975, *30.*

ZIEGLER G., BOSQUE-OLIVA A., EULLER L. — La sciatique commune après 40 ans. *In :* Simon L. *La sciatique et le nerf sciatique.* Paris, Masson, 1980.

ZIEGLER G., EULLER-ZIEGLER L., GRISOT C., BRIFFOD P. — Les injections intra- et péri-articulaires de corticoïdes en 1983. *Concours Med.,* 1983, *9,* 5, 227-231.

ZIMMERMAN A. — Le traitement non chirurgical des pubalgies. *In :* Premières Journées colmariennes de Chirurgie du genou et de Traumatologie sportive, 12 et 13 mars 1982 (polycopié).

ZUCKSCHWERDT L., EMMINGER E., BIDERMANN F., ZETTEL H. — *Wirbelgelenk und Bandscheibe.* Stuttgart, Hippokrates Verlag, 1955.

THE AUTHOR'S PRINCIPAL BIBLIOGRAPHIC REFERENCES

Textbooks

MAIGNE R. — *Les manipulations vertébrales,* 1ʳᵉ éd. 1960, 3ᵉ éd. 1964. Paris, Expansion Scientifique Française, 1960, 1964.

MAIGNE R. — *Douleurs d'origine vertébrale et traitements par manipulations.* 1ʳᵉ éd. 1967, 3ᵉ éd. 1978. Paris, Expansion Scientifique Française, 1967, 1978.

MAIGNE R. — *Orthopedic medicine* (trad. W.T. Liberson), Springfield (Ill.), Ch. Thomas, 1972, 1976, 1979.

MAIGNE R. — *Die manuelle Wirbelsaülentherapie,* (trad. I. Junghanns). Stuttgart, Hippokrates Verlag, 1961.

MAIGNE R. — *Wirbelsaülenbedingte Schmerzen und ihre Behandlungen durch Manipulationen,* (trad. I. Junghanns). Stuttgart, Hippokrates Verlag, 1979.

MAIGNE R. — *Manipulaciones columna vertebral y extremidades* (trad. C. Caballe Lancry), Madrid, Norma ed., 1979.

MAIGNE R. — Manipulations of the spine. Manipulations and mobilisation of the limbs. *In :* Basmadjian J.V., *Manipulation, traction and massage,* Baltimore, London, William and Wilkins Pub., 1980, 1985.

MAIGNE R. — *La terapia manuale in patologia vertebrale e articolare* (trad. P.A. Astegiano), Torino, Libreria Cortina ed., 1979.

Painful Minor Intervertebral Dysfunction

MAIGNE R. — Sémiologie des dérangements intervertébraux mineurs. *Ann. Med. Phys.,* 1972, *15,* 275-293 (Lire la page 281 après la page 276 et avant la page 278).

MAIGNE R. — Die klinischen Zeichen der geringlugigen intervertebralen Störung. *Manuelle Medizin,* 1974, *5,* 115-118.

Segmental Vertebral Syndrome

MAIGNE R. — Le massage dans les sciatiques. *Communication au Congrès National de Médecine physique, Nice, 1961.*

MAIGNE R. — La douleur musculaire dans la sciatique radiculaire commune. *Ann. Méd. Phys.,* 1969, *12,* 45-54.

MAIGNE R. — Cordons musculaires douloureux dans certaines sciatiques et cruralgies rebelles. *Cinésiologie,* 1970, *37,* 231.

MAIGNE R. — Les infiltrats cellulitiques conséquences d'algies radiculaires et causes de douleurs rebelles. *Vie Méd.,* 1971, *52,* 2043-2046.

MAIGNE R. — Articulations interapophysaires et pathologie douloureuse commune du rachis. *Ann. Méd. Phys.,* 1972, *15,* 262-275.

MAIGNE R. — Sémiologie des dérangements interverté-braux mineurs. *Ann. Med. Phys.*, 1972, *15*, 277-289.

MAIGNE R. — Dérangements intervertébraux mineurs et syndrome cellulo-téno-myalgique. Conceptions nouvelles des mécaniques des douleurs vertébrales communes. *Rev. Méditer. Sci. Méd.*, 1978, *5*, 337-348.

Zygapophyseal Joints and Posterior Primary Rami

MAIGNE R. — A propos du mécanisme de la douleur dans les dorsalgies dites des « couturières ». Le point inter-scapulo-vertébral. *Rev. Rhum.*, 1967, *34*, 636-641.

MAIGNE R. — Articulations interapophysaires et patho-logie douloureuse commune du rachis. *Ann. Méd. Phys.*, 1972, *15*, 262-275.

MAIGNE R. — Diagnostic et mécanisme d'un « dérange-ment intervertébral mineur ». *Cinésiologie*, 1973, *47*, 1-24.

MAIGNE R. — Origine dorso-lombaire de certaines lombalgies basses. Rôle des articulations interapophy-saires et des branches postérieures des nerfs rachi-diens. *Rev. Rhum.*, 1974, *41*, 12, 781-789.

MAIGNE R. — Responsabilité du rachis cervical dans les céphalées communes. *Cinésiologie*, 1972, *73*, 73-84.

MAIGNE R. en coll. avec MAIGNE J.Y., LAZARETH J.P. — Etude de l'innervation cutanée lombo-sacrée. Application à la physiopathologie de certaines lombalgies. *Rev. Rhum.*, 1988, *55*, 2, 107-111.

Interscapular Pain of Cervical Origin

MAIGNE R. — Dorsalgies, séquelles des traumatismes cervicaux mineurs. *Communication au 3e Congrès de Thérapie manuelle, Nice, 1962.*

MAIGNE R. — La dorsalgie bénigne interscapulaire. Son origine cervicale fréquente. *Rhumatologie*, 1964, *14*, 457.

MAIGNE R. — Sur l'origine cervicale de certaines dorsal-gies bénignes et rebelles de l'adulte. *Rev. Rhum.*, 1964, *31*, 497-503.

MAIGNE R. — A propos du mécanisme de la douleur dans les dorsalgies. Le point interscapulo-vertébral. *Rev. Rhum.*, 1967, *34*, 636-641.

MAIGNE R. — La dorsalgie interscapulaire. Manifestation de la souffrance du rachis cervical inférieur. « Le point cervical du dos ». *Sem. Hôp., Paris*, 1977, *53*, 18-19, 1067-1072.

MAIGNE R. — Dorsalgie commune et dérangement inter-vertébral mineur cervical. *Rhumatologie*, 1977, *29*, 23-34.

Low Back Pain of Thoracolumbar Origin

MAIGNE R. — Articulations interapophysaires et patho-logie douloureuse du rachis. *Ann. Méd. Phys.*, 1972, *15*, 262.

MAIGNE R. — Origine dorso-lombaire de certaines lombalgies basses. Rôle des articulations interapophy-saires et des branches postérieures des nerfs rachi-diens. *Rev. Rhum.*, 1974, *41*, 12, 781-789.

MAIGNE R. — Une origine méconnue et fréquente de lombalgies basses : les articulations interapophysaires de la charnière dorso-lombaire. Rôle des « Posterior rami » des nerfs rachidiens D11, D12, L1. *Union Med. Canada.*, 1975, *104*, 1676-1684.

MAIGNE R., LE CORRE F., JUDET H. — Lombalgies basses rebelles d'origine dorsolombaire. Traitement chirurgical par excision des capsules articulaires postérieures. *Nouv. Press. Méd.*, 1978, *7*, 7, 565-568.

MAIGNE R. — Les lombalgies après chirurgie discale. Leur origine dorsolombaire fréquente (Etude de 52 cas). *Rhumatologie*, 1978, *30*, 329-335.

MAIGNE R., LE CORRE F., JUDET H. — Premiers résultats d'un traitement chirurgical de la lombalgie basse rebelle, d'origine dorso-lombaire. *Rev. Rhum.*, 1979, *46*, 177-183.

MAIGNE R. — Low back pain of thoracolumbar origin. *Arch. Phys. Med. Rehabil.*, 1980, *61*, 389-395.

MAIGNE R. — Lombalgies et branches postérieures des nerfs rachidiens de la charnière dorso-lombaire. *Ann. Med. Phys.*, 1980, *23*, 150-168.

MAIGNE R. — Chirurgie et électrocoagulation dans les lombalgies d'origine haute. *In :* Simon L., Rabourdin J.P., *Lombalgies et médecine de rééducation.* Paris, Masson, 1983.

MAIGNE R. — Lombalgies et branches postérieures des nerfs rachidiens. *Med. Hyg.*, 1984, *42*, 3281-3288.

The Thoracolumbar Junction Syndrome

MAIGNE R. — Un syndrome nuevo y frequente : el sindrome D12-L1 (Lumbalgias bajas, dolores seudovis-cerales, falsos dolores de la cadera). *Rehabilitacion*, 1977, *11*, 197- 210.

MAIGNE R. — Le syndrome de la charnière dorso-lombaire. Lombalgies basses, douleurs pseudo-viscérales, pseudo-douleurs de hanche, pseudo-tendinite des adducteurs. *Sem. Hôp. Paris*, 1981, *57*, 11-12, 545-554.

MAIGNE R. — Douleurs pseudo-viscérales d'origine dorso-lombaires. *In :* Simon L., *Actualité en rééducation fonctionnelle et réadaptation.* Paris, Masson, 1979.

MAIGNE R. — Pubalgies, pseudo-tendinite des adduc-teurs et charnière dorso-lombaire. *Ann. Med. Phys.*, 1981, *24*, 313-319.

Shoulder Pain and the Cervical Spine

MAIGNE R. — Pseudo-tendinites d'épaule et rachis cer-vical. *Ann. Med. Phys.*, 1975, *18*, 196-203.

MAIGNE R. — Douleurs d'épaule et rachis cervical. *In :* Simon L., *Epaule et médecine de rééducation,* pp. 98-100. Paris, Masson, 1984.

Headache of Cervical Origin

MAIGNE R. — La céphalée sus-orbitaire. Sa fréquente origine cervicale. Son traitement. *Ann. Med. Phys.*, 1968, *11*, 241-246.

MAIGNE R. — Un signe évocateur et inattendu de céphalée cervicale : « La douleur au pincé-roulé du sourcil ». *Ann. Med. Phys.*, 1976, *19*, 416-434.

MAIGNE R. — Signes cliniques des céphalées cervicales. Leur traitement. *Med. Hyg.*, 1981, *39*, 1174-1185.

MAIGNE R., MAIGNE J.Y. — Sémiologie des céphalées cervicales ou diagnostic clinique des céphalées cer-vicales. *In :* Simon L., *Actualités en rééducation fonction-nelle et réadaptation,* pp. 123-130. Paris, Masson, 1982.

Epicondylar Pain

MAIGNE R. — Le traitement des épicondylites. *Rhumatologie*, 1957, *9*, 293-295.

MAIGNE R. — Epicondylalgies, rachis cervical et articulation huméro-radiale. À propos de 150 cas. *Ann. Med. Phys.*, 1960, *3*, 299-311.

MAIGNE R. — Cotation et diagnostic d'une épicondylalgie. *Cinésiologie*, 1975, *56*, 113-114.

MAIGNE R. — Evaluation et orientation thérapeutique des épicondylalgies. *In :* Simon L., *Coude et médecine de rééducation*, pp. 123-128. Paris, Masson, 1979.

MAIGNE R. — Les manipulations dans le traitement des épicondylites. Le facteur cervical. Le facteur articulaire. *Ann. Réadapt. Med. Phys.*, 1986, *29*, 57-64.

Pubalgia

MAIGNE R. — Pubalgies, pseudo-tendinite des adducteurs et charnière dorso-lombaire. *Ann. Med. Phys.*, 1981, *24*, 313-319.

MAIGNE R. — La pubalgie peut être une douleur ténopériostée d'origine rachidienne. *Cinésiologie*, 1982, *21*, 213-220.

MAIGNE R. — Pubisschmerzen und Tendiniden der Adduktoren vertebralen Ursprung. *Manuelle Medizin*, 1986, *24*, 109-113.

Perforating Branch Syndrome of T12 and L1

(Voir aussi Syndrome de la jonction dorso-lombaire).

MAIGNE R., MAIGNE J.Y. — Syndrome des branches perforantes latérales des nerfs sous-costal et abdomino-génital (D12 et L1) : une cause méconnue de douleurs de hanche d'origine vertébrale ou locale. *Ann. Réadapt. Med. Phys.*, 1986, *29*, 29-37.

MAIGNE R., MAIGNE J.Y. — Syndrome des branches perforantes latérales des nerfs sous-costal et ilio-hypogastrique. *Rev. Rhum.*, 1986, *53*, 307-301.

Miscellaneous

MAIGNE R. — Les entorses costales. *Rhumatologie*, 1957, *1*, 35-41.

MAIGNE R. — Douleurs de sein d'origine vertébrale ou pariétale. *Senologia*, 1980, *5*, 287-292.

MAIGNE R. — Pathologie mécanique de l'articulation tibiopéronière supérieure. *In :* Simon L., *Actualités en rééducation fonctionnelle et réadaptation*, pp. 112-118. Paris, Masson, 1981.

MAIGNE R. — Douleurs et pseudo-blocages du genou d'origine vertébrale. *Ann. Med. Phys.*, 1981, *3*, 320-325.

MAIGNE R. — Das Syndrom der Ubergangszonen der Wirbelsäule. (Syndrome des zones transitionnelles). *Manuelle Medizin*, 1984, *22*, 122-124.

MAIGNE R., MAIGNE J.Y. — Le syndrome du ligament ilio-lombaire. Mythe ou réalité ? *Ann. Reed. Med. Phys.*, 1987, *30*, 439-446.

Manipulation

MAIGNE R. — Manipulations vertébrales et manipulateurs. *Sem. Hôp. Paris*, 1953, *29*, 1944-1949.

MAIGNE R. — Les manipulations vertébrales : indications, contre-indications, techniques et résultats. *J. Méd. Paris*, 1955, *11*, 405-418.

MAIGNE R. — *Les manipulations vertébrales.* Paris, Expansion Scientifique Française, 1960.

MAIGNE R. — L'application rationnelle des manipulations vertébrales. *In : Proc. of the IVth International Congress of Physical Medicine. Paris, 1964*, pp. 145-149. Amsterdam, Excerpta Medica, 1966.

MAIGNE R. — The concept of painlessness and opposite motion in spinal manipulations. *Am. J. Phys. Med.*, 1965, *44*, 55-69.

MAIGNE R. — Le choix des manipulations dans le traitement des sciatiques. *Rev. Rhum.*, 1965, *32*, 366-372.

MAIGNE R. — Une doctrine pour les traitements par manipulations : la règle de la non-douleur et du mouvement contraire. *Ann. Méd. Phys.*, 1965, *8*, 37-47.

MAIGNE R. — Fundamentos fisiopatologicos de la manipulacion vertebral. *Rehabilitacion*, 1976, *10*, 427-442.

MAIGNE R. — Manipulations vertébrales et thromboses vertébro-basilaires. *Angéiologie*, 1969, *21*, 287-288.

(Voir aussi J.Y. MAIGNE pour articles faits en collaboration).

Achevé d'imprimer
sur les presses de l'Imprimerie Soulisse et Cassegrain
79000 NIORT
en octobre 1989

N° d'imprimeur : 2727

INDEX

Page numbers in *italics* denote figures; those followed by "t" denote tables.